Vijaya D Joshi's

Manual of
Practical
Physiology

A Comprehensive Guide for Practical and *Viva Voce* Examinations

As per the latest NMC Guidelines | Competency Based Medical Education (CBME)
Curriculum under Graduate Medical Education Regulation

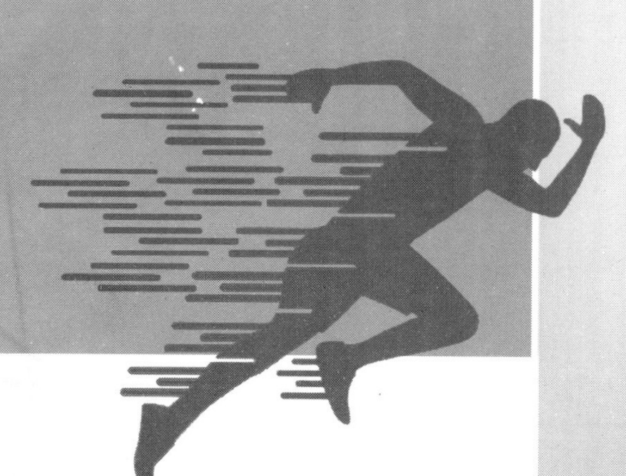

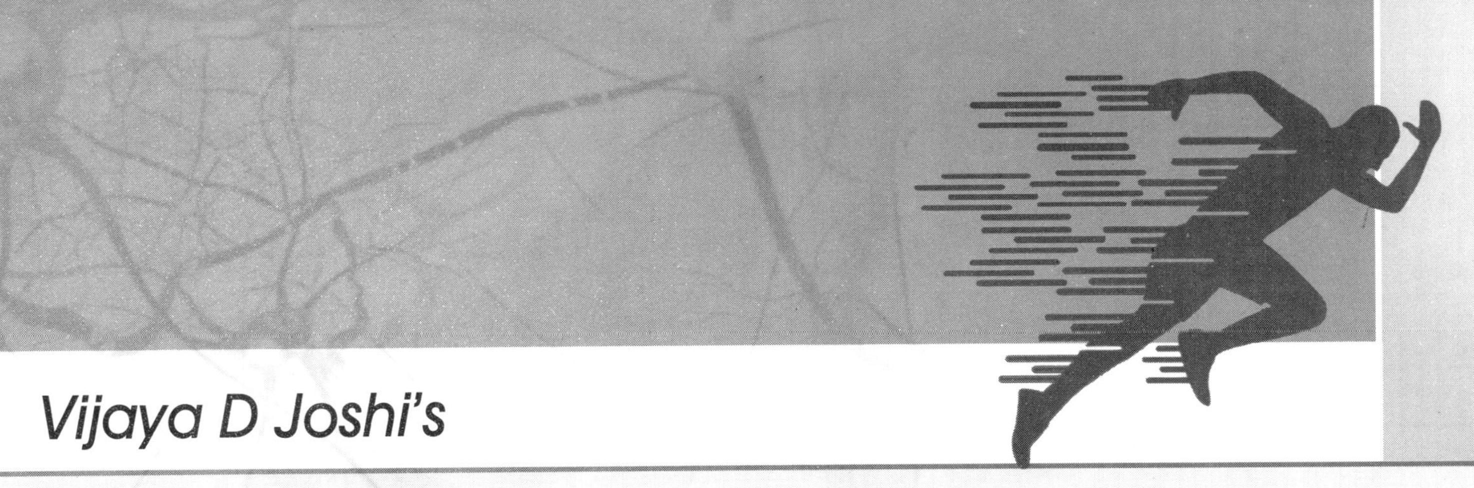

Vijaya D Joshi's

Manual of Practical Physiology

A Comprehensive Guide for Practical and *Viva Voce* Examinations

As per the latest NMC Guidelines | Competency Based Medical Education (CBME) Curriculum under Graduate Medical Education Regulation

Sadhana Joshi Mendhurwar

MD (Physiology)
Professor and Head
Department of Physiology
Dr DY Patil School of Medicine
Nerul, Navi Mumbai, Maharashtra, India

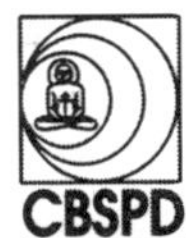

CBSPD

CBS Publishers & Distributors Pvt Ltd

New Delhi • Bengaluru • Chennai • Kochi • Kolkata • Lucknow • Mumbai
Hyderabad • Jharkhand • Nagpur • Patna • Pune • Uttarakhand

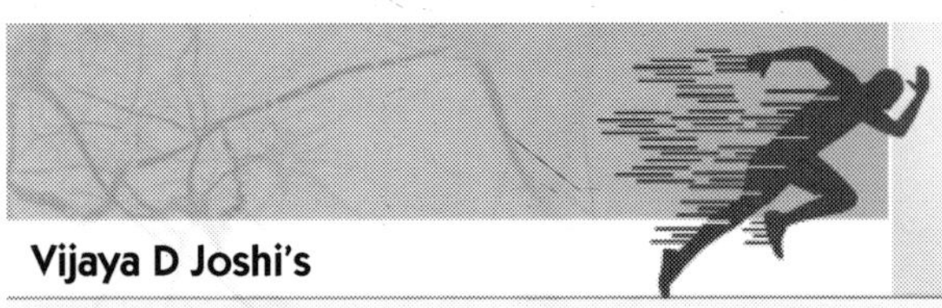

Vijaya D Joshi's

Manual of Practical Physiology

A Comprehensive Guide for Practical and
Viva Voce **Examinations**

ISBN: 978-81-979890-4-9

Copyright © Authors and Publisher

First Edition: 2025
Reprint: **2026**

Published by Satish Kumar Jain and produced by Varun Jain for

CBS Publishers & Distributors Pvt Ltd

4819/XI Prahlad Street, 24 Ansari Road, Daryaganj, New Delhi 110 002, India
Ph: 011-23266838, 23289259

Website: www.cbspd.com
e-mail: delhi@cbspd.com

Corporate Office: 204 FIE, Industrial Area, Patparganj, Delhi 110 092, India
Ph: 011-4934 4934   Fax: 011-4934 4935   e-mail: publishing@cbspd.com; publicity@cbspd.com

Branches

- **Bengaluru:** Seema House 2975, 17th Cross, KR Road, Banasankari 2nd Stage, Bengaluru 560 070, Karnataka, India
  Ph: +91-80-26771678/79   Fax: +91-80-26771680   e-mail: bangalore@cbspd.com
- **Chennai:** 18/8B, Subbarayan Street, Shenoy Nagar, Chennai 600 030, Tamil Nadu, India
  Ph: +91-44-42032115, 26681266   e-mail: chennai@cbspd.com
- **Kochi:** 42/1325, 1326, Power House Road, Opp KSEB, Power House, Ernakulum Kochi 682 018, Kerala, India
  Ph: +91-484-4059061-65,67   Fax: +91-484-4059065   e-mail: kochi@cbspd.com
- **Kolkata:** 147, Hind Ceramics Compound, 1st Floor, Nilgunj Road, Belghoria, Kolkata 700 056, West Bengal, India
  Ph: +91-33-25633055/56   e-mail: kolkata@cbspd.com
- **Lucknow:** Basement, Khushnuma Complex, 7 Meerabai Marg (behind Jawahar Bhawan), Lucknow 226 001, UP, India
  Ph: +910522-4000032   e-mail: tiwari.lucknow@cbspd.com
- **Mumbai:** PWD Shed, Gala no 25/26, Ramchandra Bhatt Marg, Next to JJ Hospital Gate no. 2,
  Opp. Union Bank of India, Noorbaug, Mumbai 400 009, Maharashtra, India
  Ph: +91-22-66661880/89   e-mail: mumbai@cbspd.com

Representatives

- **Gujarat**   • **Hyderabad**   • **Jharkhand**   • **Nagpur**   • **Patna**   • **Pune**   • **Uttarakhand**

For trade terms please contact customercare@cbspd.com
For general enquiries please contact info@cbspd.com

Printed at: Mudrak, Noida, UP, India

to

---

the eternal loving memory of my mother
Late Dr (Mrs) Vijaya D Joshi,
a highly dedicated doctor and academician,
who continues to be a fountain of inspiration to me.
My friend, philosopher and guide – her altruism continues
to lighthouse my path of duty as a medical doctor and teacher

Preface

I have great pleasure in introducing the book *Vijaya D Joshi's Manual of Practical Physiology: A Comprehensive Guide for Practical and Viva Voce Examinations* (As per latest CBME Curriculum) for undergraduate students of physiology.

The revised Competency-Based Medical Education (CBME) curriculum necessitates students to acquire various skills independently as first-year medical undergraduate students in their practical exams. The guiding philosophy is to provide early clinical exposure to students, thereby laying a solid foundation for a life-long journey of embracing integrated medical knowledge and skills.

This book is divided into five major sections—Haematology, Clinical Physiology, Human Experimental Physiology, Charts, Calculations, and Endocrine Disorders, and Amphibian Experimental Physiology. Each chapter covers not only the practical details but also lists various common *viva voce* questions typically asked during that practical. The book also covers all aspects of competency-based practical and clinical examinations, that help students to prepare for practical examinations. Any comments and suggestions from the readers will be highly appreciated.

I am very much thankful to Dr Vijay D Patil (Chancellor, DY Patil Deemed University, Nerul, Navi Mumbai) and Dr Shivani V Patil (Pro-Chancellor, DY Patil Deemed University, Nerul, Navi Mumbai) for their constant support and encouragement to work on the book. My special thanks to our respected Dean Dr Rajiv Rao, DY Patil School of Medicine for his continuous motivation and support. I would like to express my gratitude to all my teachers, colleagues, and students. Special thanks to my postgraduate student, Dr Shubhi Tamrakar for her assistance.

I would like to acknowledge all those who have been involved in the preparation of this book, especially Mr SK Jain (Chairman and Managing Director), Mr Varun Jain (Director), Mr YN Arjuna (Senior Vice President—Publishing, Editorial and Publicity) and his team Mrs Ritu Chawla (GM—production), Arun Sharma (DTP Operator), Dr Yashi Bajpai, Dr Ashu Singh and Binay Kumar (Editors) for the book in its present form.

Sadhana Joshi Mendhurwar

Contents

SECTION 5: Experimental Physiology

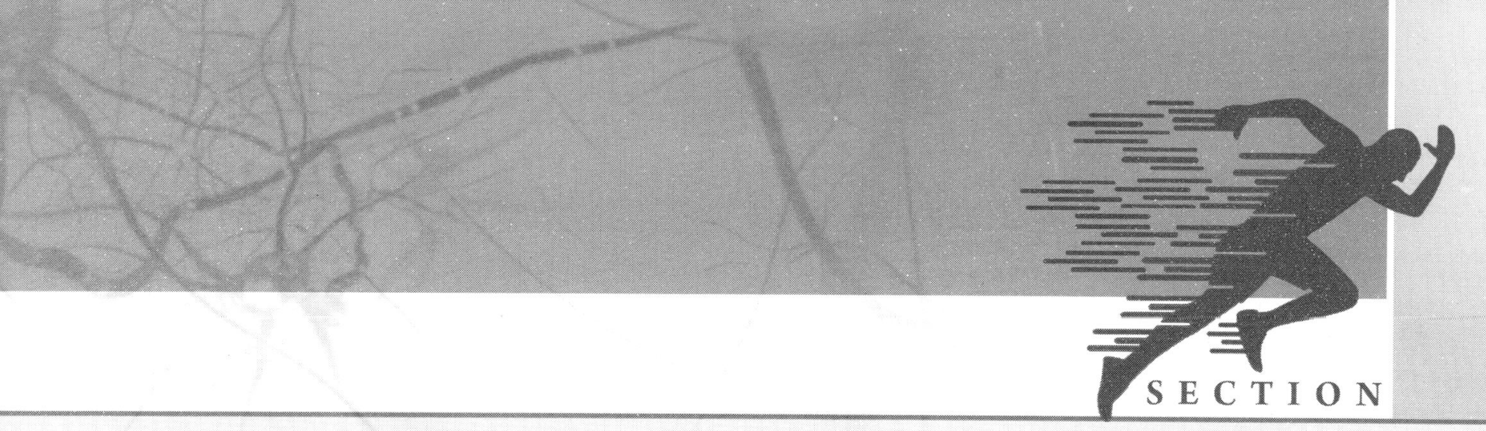

Haematology

Chapter Outline

- Introduction to Haematology
- Study of Compound Microscope
- Methods of Collection of Blood
- Haemoglobinometry
- Determination of Total WBC Count
- Determination of Total RBC Count
- Determination of Differential WBC Count
- Determination of Bleeding Time and Clotting Time
- Determination of ESR
- Determination of Blood Indices
- Determination of Packed Cell Volume (Haematocrit)
- Determination of Blood Groups
- Determination of Osmotic Fragility and Specific Gravity of Blood
- Determination of Reticulocyte Count
- Determination of Platelet Count

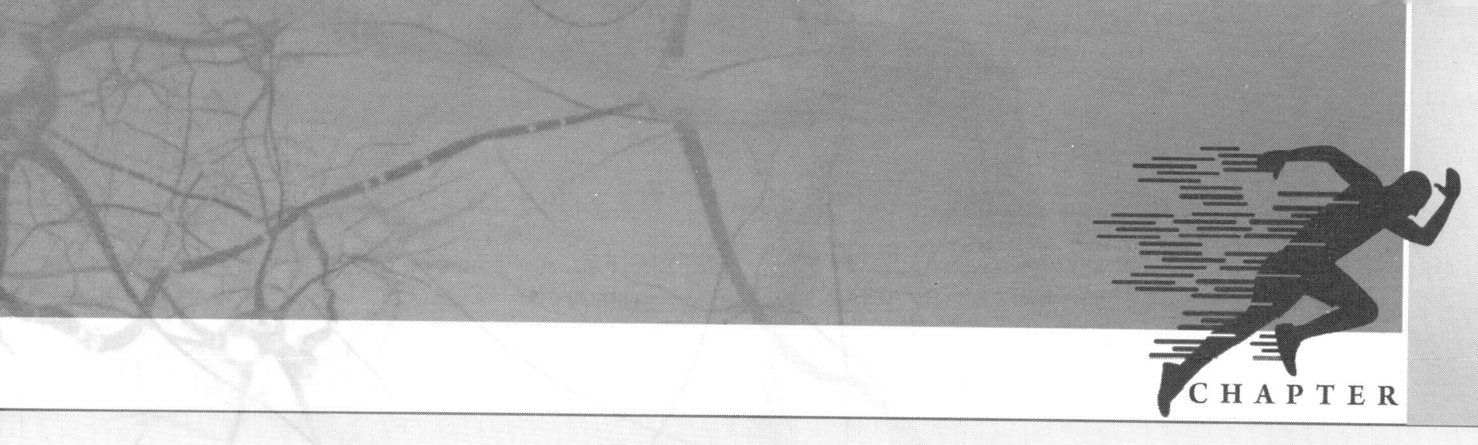

Introduction to Haematology

Learning Objectives
After completion of this practical, the students shall be able to:
- Define haematology
- Name routine haematological tests
- Enumerate functions and components of blood

■ INTRODUCTION

- Hematology is the science that deals with the study of blood.
- In a 70 kg normal adult person, blood volume is about 5–5.5 litres. There are several haematological investigations, that are routinely performed in laboratories. All haematology tests do require adequate skill; however, recently most of the investigations have been done by automated machines. Blood samples for all these haematological tests are obtained by taking a prick (capillary blood) or by puncturing the vein (venous blood). Arterial blood samples are required for some specific blood investigations.

■ COMPONENTS OF BLOOD

Blood has two types of major components—(1) cells, and (2) plasma.

Cellular Component

- Cellular component contain red blood cells, white blood cells, and platelets (thrombocytes).

- Red blood cells (RBCs) constitute the highest number, they are present in millions (4–5.5 million/mm^3 of blood). RBCs help in the transport of gases. White blood cells (WBCs) are in the range of thousands (4,000–11,000/mm^3 of blood). WBCs assist the defence function of the body.
- Platelets are in 1 to 3 lakhs/mm^3 of blood. Platelets help in the arrest of bleeding (hemostasis).

Plasma Component

- The fluid component of blood is plasma. Plasma contains fibrinogen and clotting factors.
- Plasma carries various substances like nutrients, hormones, waste products, etc.

■ SERUM

When fibrinogen is removed from plasma (during the process of coagulation), what remains is serum. Various investigations do require serum for tests (e.g. serum protein, serum glucose, serum triglycerides, etc.).

■ BLOOD SAMPLES

- Blood samples for various haematological tests can be obtained by capillary puncture (collection of blood from capillaries) and venepuncture (collection of blood from veins).
- For some investigations, one requires arterial blood, e.g. arterial blood gas (ABG) analysis.

■ ROUTINE HAEMATOLOGICAL TESTS INCLUDE

- Estimation of haemoglobin (Hb)
- Total RBC count
- Total WBC count
- Differential WBC count
- Erythrocyte sedimentation rate (ESR)
- Packed cell volume (PCV)
- Platelet count
- Blood group
- Bleeding time and clotting time
- Osmotic fragility of blood
- Specific gravity of blood.

Study of Compound Microscope

■ INTRODUCTION

The microscope was invented by Leeuwenhoek. A microscope is known to magnify the image of an object. We should know about the basic construction of a microscope.

Various types of microscopes are available; a compound microscope is frequently used in medical laboratories. In physiology, it is mainly used to study different cell counts and morphology of different cells.

■ COMPOUND MONOCULAR MICROSCOPE

It has the following parts **(Fig. 2.1)**

Base

It supports a microscope on the working table. The base of the microscope has a horseshoe-shaped foot, which gives stability to the microscope. To the foot of the microscope, the limb is attached which bears an optical system.

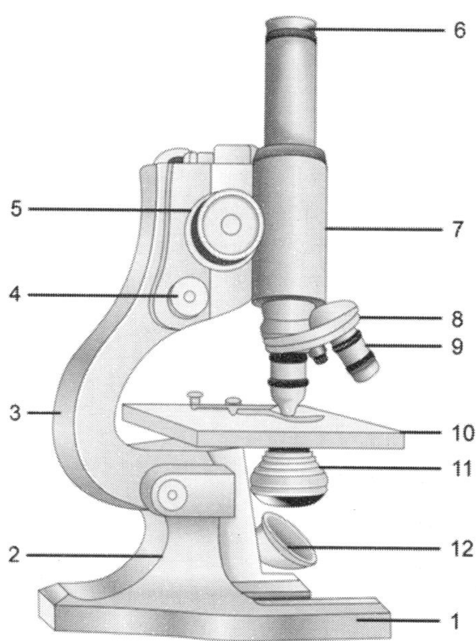

Fig. 2.1: Parts of the compound microscope (1: Base; 2: Pillars; 3: Handle; 4: Fine adjustment screw; 5: Coarse adjustment screw; 6: Eyepiece; 7: Body tube; 8: Fixed and revolving nose piece; 9: Objectives; 10: Stage; 11: Condenser; 12: Mirror)

Body Tube

It is a vertical tube, which can be raised or lowered when required.

Coarse and Fine Adjustment Screws

- Body tubes can be raised or lowered by these screws. With a coarse adjustment screw, the body tube is raised or lowered quickly. With a fine adjustment screw, the body tube is raised or lowered slowly. These adjustments help to focus the object properly.

- Coarse and fine screws are mounted on top of the handle. One pair of each is present on either side. Even if one screw is rotated, the member on the opposite side automatically rotates simultaneously. Usually, the left hand is used for moving coarse or fine adjustment screws.

Fixed Stage

It is a square platform with an aperture in the center on which the slide is placed. Light passes through the aperture and then through the slide. It is attached to the limb below the objective lens.

Mechanical Stage

- It is fixed stage and is calibrated. It has two screws— one for moving slides horizontally and the other for moving slides forward and backwards.
- Stage is fitted with condenser and iris diaphragm.
- The condenser has two lenses mounted into a short cylinder. The condenser can be raised or lowered with the screw. The iris diaphragm is placed below the condenser and controls the amount of light entering the microscope.

Mirror

A mirror is fitted below the condenser to reflect light from the source into the condenser. Mirror has two surfaces: Plain (flat surface) and concave. The mirror can be rotated in all directions. A plane mirror is used in daylight and a concave mirror when the source of light is from one point, like a bulb.

Nose Piece

It is attached to the lower end of the body tube. It has objective lenses of different powers. By revolving the nose piece, any lens can be placed over the slide to be observed.

Objective Lenses

There are three objective lenses with different magnifying powers as given below:

1. **Objective labeled "10x"** magnifies the image 10 times. It is called as low power.
   Magnification with low power would be 100 times (10 × 10).
2. **Objective labeled "40x or 45x"** magnifies the image 40–45 times. It is called as high power. Magnification using high power would be 400 times (40 × 10).
3. **Objective labeled "90x or 100x"** magnifies the image 90–100 times. It is called an oil immersion lens. Magnification with oil immersion lens would be 900–1000 times.

Eyepiece

- The eyepiece is placed at the top of the body tube.
- Usually, two or more eyepieces with different powers are supplied. An eyepiece may have a movable pointer such an eyepiece is called a demonstration eyepiece.
- **Formation of image**: Lenses initiate the magnifying process. A real, inverted, and enlarged image is formed in the upper part of the tube. A field lens is present near the lower plane of the eyepiece, which collects diverging rays of the primary image. These are further magnified by an eye lens from the eyepiece.

■ USE OF MICROSCOPE

The slide to be examined is put on the fixed stage. Objects can be seen under low and high power.

Low Power Adjustment

- Low power objective is placed in position.
- A concave mirror is used.
- Condenser occupies a lower position.
- The diaphragm is adjusted to prevent glare and light is adjusted.
- Body tube is lowered with the help of coarse adjustment so that the low-power objective is about 1 centimeter from the slide.
- Slide is then seen through the eyepiece of the microscope.
- Focusing is done gradually first with coarse adjustment and then finally with fine adjustment. Care is taken not to break the slide.
- The whole slide is scanned and then part of the slide to be seen is selected. The objective is turned to high power.

High Power Adjustment

- High power objective is placed in position. A plain mirror is used.
- Condenser is taken up.
- High power objective is brought near the slide by using coarse adjustment.
- By looking through the eyepiece, light is adjusted.
- Focusing is done gradually first with coarse and finally with fine adjustment to get the best possible view.
- Objective should never be lowered by using coarse adjustment when one is looking through the eyepiece.
- Iris diaphragm is adjusted to cut the thin peripheral rim of rays.

Oil Immersion Adjustment

- Oil immersion lens is placed in position. The plain mirror is used. The condenser is taken high up.

- A drop of cedarwood oil is put on the slide (refractive index of cedarwood oil is same as that of glass).
- Using coarse adjustment oil immersion objective is brought down till it just touches the oil drop.
- Looking through the eyepiece final focusing is done with fine adjustments to get the best possible view.
- Focusing should be done gradually and carefully to prevent the breaking of the slide or damaging of the lens.
- After completing the examination, the objective is raised and the slide is taken out.

■ PRECAUTIONS

- When not in use, the microscope should be kept covered.
- The microscope must be kept clean and free from dust.
- Oil on the objective should be first removed with a dry, soft cloth and then cleaned with a small quantity of xylene/acetone.
- The lenses should be cleaned with a small quantity of isopropyl alcohol (90%).
- Low- and high-power objectives and eyepieces are cleaned with soft linen or polishing cloth. Glass should never be touched with a finger.
- Lowering of the optical tube should not be done when one is looking through the eyepiece.
- If the microscope has to be moved, it should be held upright using a handle and hand below the foot.

■ OTHER TYPES OF MICROSCOPES

- **Binocular microscope**: It is used to prevent strain on the eyes, especially when one has to use the microscope for a long time.
- **Dissecting microscope**: Binocular microscope used for microdissection.
- **Electron microscope**: It has a very high resolving power as compared to ordinary light microscopes.
- **Phase-contrast microscope**: It is useful in the examination of living, unstained material, as well as fixed specimens. It is valuable as a research tool.
- **Polarizing microscope**: It is used to detect certain birefringent substances in the tissue, such as suture material, barium, etc. Any ordinary microscope with polarized filters can be used for this purpose.
- **Dark-field microscope**: It is especially useful for studying very minute organisms.
- **Fluorescence microscope**: When ultraviolet light strikes a fluorescent substance the visible light is emitted. Any conventional microscope can be converted into a fluorescence microscope by introducing a light source, rich in ultraviolet radiations by adding a dark-field condenser and a suitable filter system.

- **Differential-contrast microscope**: This microscope helps in the formation of pseudo-three-dimensional images.

■ COMMON STATIONS – SPOTS IN PRACTICAL EXAMINATION (2/3 MARKS)

- Focus given slide under high power/low power/oil immersion.
- How is the objective of the microscope cleaned?
- Enlist any four adjustments required to be done to adjust the microscope under high power.
- Enlist any four adjustments required to be done to adjust the microscope under low power.
- Enlist any four adjustments required to be done to adjust the microscope under oil immersion.
- Enlist different types of microscopes you know.

■ OBJECTIVE STRUCTURED PRACTICAL EXAMINATION (OSPE)

Procedure station 1: Make microscopic adjustments for focusing under low power.

S. No.	Assessment criteria	Marks assigned	Marks given
1.	Bring the condenser to the lowest position		
2.	Change to concave mirror and slightly open iris diaphragm		
3.	Place the slide on the stage		
4.	Bring a lower objective in position and make coarse adjustments to focus the image		
5.	Use fine adjustment for final focusing of image		
6.	Report and viva on haematology experiment		
7.	Total		

Procedure station 2: Make microscopic adjustments for focusing under high power

S. No.	Assessment criteria	Marks assigned	Marks given
1.	Make use of a plain mirror		
2.	Slightly raise the condenser and partially opens the iris diaphragm		
3.	Place slide on the stage		
4.	First focus under low power		
5.	Bring high-power objective in position and make coarse adjustments to focus the image		
6.	Make fine adjustments for final focusing		
7.	Report and viva on haematology experiment		
8.	Total		

Procedure station 3: Make microscopic adjustments for focusing under an oil immersion lens.

S. No.	Assessment criteria	Marks assigned	Marks given
1.	Change to plane mirror		
2.	Bring the condenser to highest position and open the iris diaphragm completely		
3.	Place slide on the stage and put a drop of oil on the center of the smear		
4.	Bring oil immersion objective into position		
5.	Bring the center of the slide under the view, so that the objective touches the oil		
6.	Make coarse and then fine adjustments to focus the image		
7.	Report and viva on haematology experiment		
8.	Total		

■ KEY POINTS TO REMEMBER

- A compound monocular microscope is used commonly for all haematology practicals.
- 10X is the power of the lens when one focus under low power and 45X when focus under high power.
- Cedarwood oil is used when you focus under oil immersion as it has a refractive index the same as a mirror. Always, any object first has to be examined under low power and then high power.

Methods of Collection of Blood

■ INTRODUCTION

- Blood is collected for various investigations, e.g. haematological, biochemical, serological, and culture.
- For different haematological examinations, collection of blood from the vein is preferred.
- When a small quantity of blood is required, capillary blood is used, e.g. estimation of haemoglobin, red blood cell (RBC) count, white blood cell (WBC) count, blood groups, bleeding, and clotting time.
- The composition of venous blood is almost the same as that of capillary blood.
- For some investigations, arterial blood is preferred. Aseptic precautions are very important while collecting blood.

■ VENOUS BLOOD (Venipuncture)

Sites for Collection

Antecubital fossa (median cubital vein), dorsum of hand in adults, and femoral vein in children **(Fig. 3.1)**.

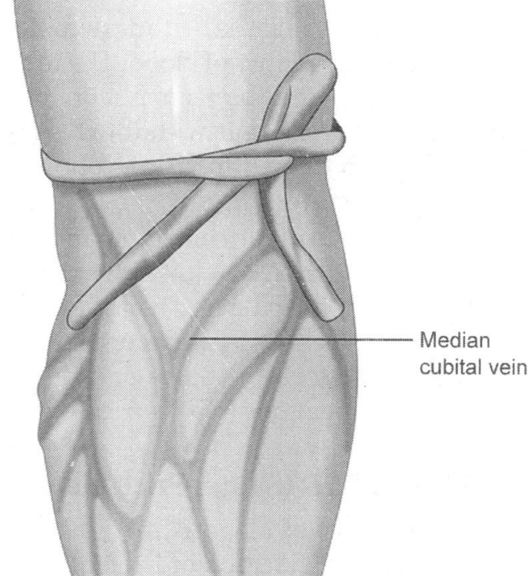

Fig. 3.1: Application of tourniquet for collection of blood by venipuncture.

Precautions

- Before collecting blood, the operator should wash hands and preferably wear disposable plastic or thin rubber gloves.
- Skin over the vein should be cleaned properly. Cleaning of the skin prevents entry of bacteria into the body through the puncture.
- Blood should be withdrawn slowly and delivered gently in the container and mixed properly with an anticoagulant.
- Syringe and needle should be disposed of properly.

Procedure

- Patient is asked to sit on a chair.
- The antecubital vein of the left arm (or right arm) is usually chosen for collecting the blood. Alternatively, veins of the back of the hand or leg can be chosen.
- A tourniquet is placed around the arm. The patient is asked to open and close the fist repeatedly to cause engorgement of the vein.
- After washing hands with soap, the operator should wear disposable plastic, thin rubber gloves. Operators must take care while handling syringes and needles to avoid injury.
- Disposable and dry plastic syringe is used. A disposable needle (sharp and dry) of 18 or 19 G is used. A syringe with a needle is held in the right hand in such a way that the nozzle is in opposition to the patient's skin.
- Skin is cleaned with 70% alcohol and is punctured 0.5 cm below the point where the vein is to be punctured and along the same line of the vein (it prevents counterpunching of the vein).
- Then needle is pushed along the line of the vein to puncture it. When the vein is punctured, blood appears in the syringe.
- The piston of the syringe is withdrawn slowly to collect the required quantity of blood. The tourniquet is removed and the index finger is put on the butt of the needle, and the syringe is withdrawn. A piece of sterile cotton swab dipped in 70% alcohol is firmly pressed at the puncture.
- Blood is transferred to a bulb containing anticoagulant and is thoroughly mixed with anticoagulant by holding the bulb in the palms of hands and rotating it. The bulb is closed either by a cork or a cotton swab. Blood collected is stored in bulbs and bulbs differ according to investigations to be carried out.

■ CAPILLARY BLOOD (Finger Prick Method)

When a small quantity of blood is required, capillary blood is used, e.g. for estimation of haemoglobin, RBC count, WBC count, differential count, blood groups, bleeding, and clotting time **(Fig. 3.2)**.

Sites for Collection

- The ball of the finger, usually the ring finger of the left hand is used
- Ear lobe
- Heel or big toe in infant

Precautions

- Before collecting blood, the operator should wash hands and preferably wear disposable plastic or thin rubber gloves.

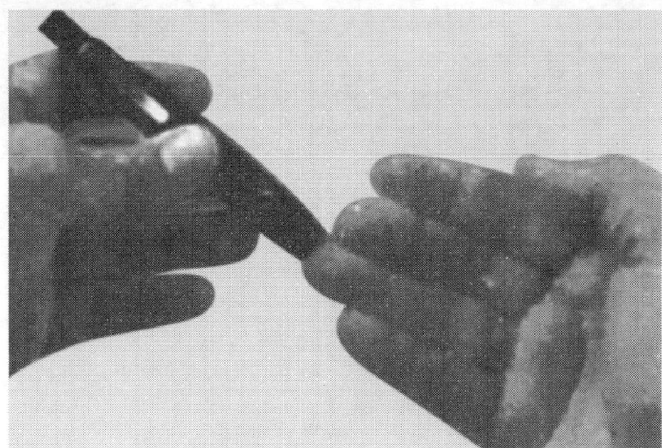

Fig. 3.2: Method of collection of capillary blood

- The pricking needle should be a flat needle with cutting edges having sharp points. It should not be blunt or rusted.
- All apparatus is kept ready before the prick.
- Aseptic precautions should be observed before pricking.
- After a required quantity of blood is collected, a sterile cotton swab should be put and pressed at the site of the prick till the bleeding stops.

Procedure

- The area to be punctured is cleaned with spirit or alcohol. It is allowed to dry.
- Sterile lancets or sterilized disposable needles are used.
- Apparatus (e.g., pipette, slides, etc.) should be kept ready before the prick as blood has to be used immediately after it is withdrawn.
- Bold prick (3–5 mm depth) is given to cause free flow of blood easily so that the finger need not be pressed.
- Fingers should not be squeezed for collecting blood (as it takes tissue fluid out, which dilutes the blood).
- The first drop of blood is wiped with the cotton (as it is diluted with tissue fluid), and then blood is collected.

■ ANTICOAGULANTS

Anticoagulants prevent blood clotting. They are added to a blood sample (mainly blood collected by venipuncture) and sent to laboratories **(Table 3.1)**.

S. No.	Name of bulb	Content	Use
	TABLE 3.1: Anticoagulants		
1.	Wintrobe bulb	NH4 oxalate, K oxalate	Haematological investigations
2.	Fluoride bulb	K oxalate, Na fluoride	Blood sugar
3.	Chemistry bulb	K oxalate (0.2 mg)	Blood urea
4.	Citrate bulb	3.8% Na citrate	For ESR
5.	Plain bulb	—	Serological investigation
6.	Paraffin bulb	Double oxalate and 1 ml liquid paraffin	Blood gases

Commonly Used Anticoagulants

Ammonium Potassium Oxalate

A stock of solution of ammonium oxalate 1.2 g, potassium oxalate 0.8 g, and distilled water up to 100 ml is prepared. About 0.5 ml of this solution is placed in a suitable container and dried at 37°C in a water bath. This much amount of oxalate is sufficient for 5 ml of blood (a bulb prepared in such a way is called Wintrobe's bulb).

Mode of Action

Oxalate precipitates calcium, which is required for clotting.

Uses

It is used only *in vitro*. It is used for the estimation of complete blood count (CBC), erythrocyte sedimentation rate (ESR), and packed cell volume (PCV).

Ethylenediaminetetraacetic Acid

Sodium and potassium salts of ethylenediaminetetraacetic acid (EDTA) are used as anticoagulants for routine haematological work. Excess of EDTA (>2 mg/ml) causes shrinkage of RBCs and degenerative changes in cells.

Mode of Action

Chelates calcium from the blood and acts as an anticoagulant.

Uses

All routine haematological investigations except coagulation studies.

Sodium Citrate

It is the choice of anticoagulant for coagulation studies. It is prepared by dissolving 32 g of trisodium citrate in one liter of distilled water. 3.8% of Na citrate is isotonic with blood but causes its dilution. It is used for the determination of ESR (Westergren's method). The ratio of citrate is 1:4 (One part of citrate is used for 4 parts of blood).

Mode of Action

Chelation of calcium in blood.

Uses

- In a blood bank for storing blood
- Various coagulation studies
- Estimation of ESR by Westergren's method.

Heparin

- It is an effective anticoagulant
- It does not alter the size of RBCs

- It is the best anticoagulant, as it is a natural constituent of blood
- It can be used *in vivo* as well as *in vitro*.

Mode of Action

Prevents action of thrombin and also promotes deactivation of thrombin. By these actions, it prevents the formation of fibrin from fibrinogen.

Uses

- Blood gas analysis and pH assays
- Osmotic fragility test.

Dicoumarol Derivatives

Mode of Action

It competes with vitamin K and therefore a synthesis of clotting factors (Vitamin K-dependent clotting factors) is hampered.

Uses

It can be used only *in vivo*.

Sodium Fluoride

It is usually mixed with oxalate (as fluoride itself is not a very strong anticoagulant). Used for preparing blood specimens for plasma glucose estimation.

Mode of Action

Fluoride inhibits glycolytic enzymes and thus prevents the loss of glucose.

■ COMMON STATIONS – SPOTS IN PRACTICAL EXAMINATION (2/3 MARKS)

Q.1. **Any of the anticoagulants can be kept.** Write uses of the same and the mechanism of their action as an anticoagulant.

Q.2. **Figure of fingerpick/venipuncture.** Identify, and enumerate the precautions, and procedures to do the same.

Q.3. **Name anticoagulant that can be used only** *in vivo*. What is the physiological basis of them used only *in vivo*? (refer to above).

■ KEY POINTS TO REMEMBER

- Blood can be collected from capillaries, arteries and veins for different haematological investigations.
- Various anticoagulants are allowed to mix with blood in order to prevent coagulation of blood, once blood is taken out from a patient.
- It is very important to follow all aseptic precautions while collecting blood.
- Following the correct procedure while collecting blood ensures minimum technical errors.

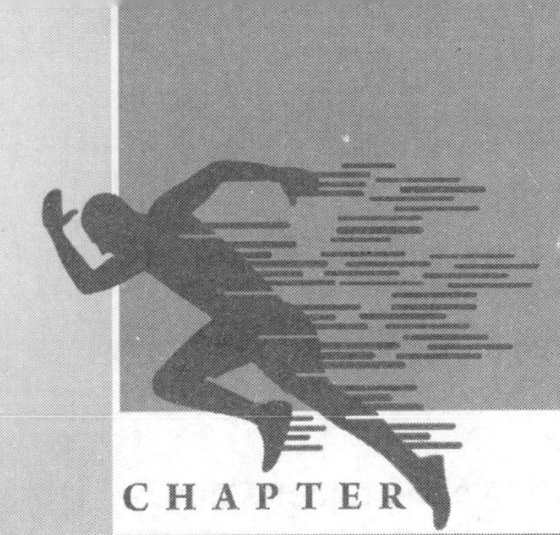

Haemoglobinometry

Learning Objectives

After completion of this practical, the students shall be able to:

- Estimate Hb by Sahli's method
- Prick finger with all aseptic precautions
- List the advantages and disadvantages of Sahli's method
- State principle used for Sahli's method
- Name other methods of estimation of haemoglobin (Hb)
- Give normal values of Hb, its functions and its physiological variations
- List common conditions of increase and decrease in Hb concentration
- Define anaemia
- Give common causes of anaemia and classification of anaemia.

Aim

To estimate Hb by Sahli's method.

Apparatus

- Sahli's haemometer, pricking needle or lancet, dropper, spirit or alcohol N/10 hydrogen chloride (HCl), and distilled water.

Sahli's haemometer contains:

- Haemoglobin pipette (with 20 mm^3 mark)
- Haemometer tube (graduated with % and 100 g/dl)
- Glass rod or stirrer
- Coloured standards

Principle

Haemoglobin is converted into a compound called acid hematin by mixing with N/10 HCl. The brown-coloured compound is matched with the standard provided in Sahli's haemometer.

Procedure

- The haemometer tube is first filled with N/10 HCl by using a dropper up to mark 20.
- For estimating haemoglobin, capillary blood is collected by a finger prick with all aseptic precautions.
- When the proper size of drop is formed, the tip of the pipette is applied to it, and blood is filled exactly up to 20 mm^3 (**Fig. 4.1**). If air bubbles are collected procedure is repeated.
- Blood sticking to the tip of the pipette is wiped off.
- Blood from the Hb pipette is immediately transferred into the haemoglobin tube, in which N/10 HCl is put (**Fig. 4.2**). Contents are mixed well with a stirrer.
- After waiting for 10 minutes (time required for conversion of Hb to acid hematin brown-coloured compound), acid hematin is formed.
- Drop-by-drop water is added to it every time mixing properly with a stirrer. Against the daylight, it is matches with the coloured standards.

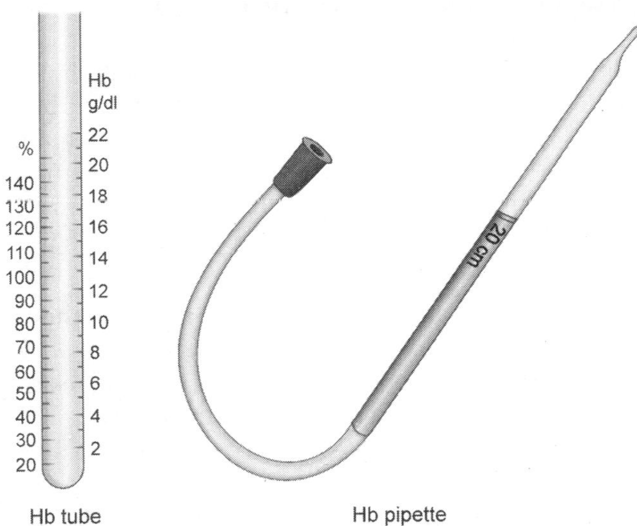

Fig. 4.1: Haemoglobin (Hb) tube and Hb pipette

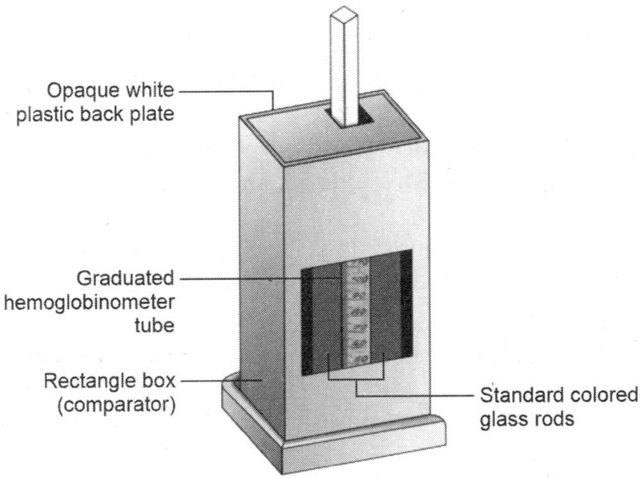

Fig. 4.2: Haemoglobinometer

- Once, it matches with coloured standards, lower meniscus reading is taken as Hb (100 g/dl or %).
- The result is expressed as either % or 100 g/dl.
- According to Sahli's method, 14.5/100 g/dl is considered to be 100%.

Normal Values of Haemoglobin

- **In males**: 14–18/100 g/dl of blood
- **In females**: 12–15/100 g/dl of blood

Advantages of Sahli's Method

- The method is very simple
- Method is less time-consuming

Disadvantages of Sahli's Method

- There is about 8–10% error in the estimation of haemoglobin.
- This method only measures the amount of haemoglobin present in reduced and oxygenated form. Haemoglobin in other different forms (carboxyhaemoglobin, methaemoglobin, etc.) cannot be estimated by this method.
- The brown colour of acid hematin does not remain stable. It begins to fade after some time. Therefore, the method is less accurate. The coloured glass standard of the haemometer also fades with time.

Precautions

- Proper aseptic precautions are a must.
- Once you clean the finger with spirit, allow it to dry on its own (do not blow).
- Squeezing of the finger is avoided.
- Hb tube to be filled exactly to 20 mark.
- Haemoglobin pipette to be filled exactly 20 mm^3.
- Care is taken that blood mixes properly with N/10 HCl.
- For complete conversion of Hb to acid hematin, a 10-minute waiting period is required.
- Matching is done properly against standards provided against the daylight.

Common Experimental Errors

- N/10 HCl not taken accurately.
- Blood taken more or less in Hb tube.
- Squeezing finger after prick, while collecting blood.
- Not mixing blood properly with N/10 HCl.

■ IMPORTANT QUESTIONS AND ANSWERS

Q.1. How much is normal Hb?
- **In males**: 14–18/100 g/dl of blood
- **In females**: 12–15/100 g/dl of blood

Q.2. What is the principle of Sahli's method?

Principle: N/10 HCl mixes with Hb to form acid hematin (brown-coloured compound), which is matched with coloured standards.

Q.3. What are the other methods of haemoglobin estimation?

Other methods of haemoglobin estimation are:
- **Cyanmethaemoglobin method (haemoglobin cyanide)**
  - In this method blood is diluted in a solution containing sodium bicarbonate, potassium cyanide, and potassium ferricyanide (Drabkin's reagent).
  - All forms of haemoglobin (except sulfhaemoglobin) are converted to cyanmethaemoglobin (takes about 10 minutes), and therefore an accurate estimation of haemoglobin is obtained. This is one of the commonly practised methods for Hb estimation.
- **Haldane's method**
  - Haemoglobin is converted to carboxyhaemoglobin by passing carbon monoxide gas through blood. Its colour is matched with standard.

- **Tallquist method**
  - A drop of blood is put on a piece of filter paper. The colour of this drop is matched with the standard.
  - This method is fast and so used for mass screening (but less accurate).
- **Alkaline hematin method**
  - This method gives a true estimate of total haemoglobin as all haemoglobin compounds (including meth- and sulfhaemoglobin) are converted to alkaline hematin.
- **Estimation of the iron content of blood**
  - Iron is separated from blood by the action of sulfuric acid and is estimated. 1g of haemoglobin contains 3.35 mg iron.
  - According to iron content, haemoglobin concentration can be calculated. It is an accurate method.
- **Oxyhaemoglobin method**
  - Haemoglobin is fully oxygenated by treating it with ammonium hydroxide or sodium carbonate. This is the quickest method for general use.
- **Direct reading haemoglobinometers**
  - These instruments have a built-in filter and a scale calibrated for direct reading of haemoglobin in g/100 ml or g/litre.
- **Spectrophotometry**
  - This is a very accurate method. In this, blood is diluted (1–200 or 1–250) with cyanide ferricyanide solution and absorbance is measured at 540 nm and haemoglobin is calculated.
- **Determination of specific gravity of blood by copper sulfate method**
  - This is a quick method of approximate estimation of haemoglobin on a mass scale, e.g. during blood donation, camps, etc.
- **Automated haemoglobinometry**
  - Many automated techniques are there to estimate Hb. Automatic dilutors and pipettes are used.
- **Non-automated haemoglobinometry**
  - Disposable, self-measuring dilution micropipettes are available in the market. The pipette gets filled with blood (by capillary action) and then blood is mixed with reagent (provided) and then a reading is obtained on the spectrophotometer.

Q.4. What happens, if N/10 HCl is taken more in quantity?

- When haemoglobin content is normal, if N/10 HCl taken is more, it does not make any difference.
- But, if a person has severe anaemia then it will give an error in the result as by taking more N/10 HCl you are diluting the blood more.

Q.5. What happens, if N/10 HCl is taken in a lesser quantity (<20% mark)?

- In Sahli's method of estimation of haemoglobin, for conversion of entire haemoglobin present in the blood to acid hematin dilute HCl up to 20% mark is required.
- If a lesser amount of HCl is taken, enough amount of HCl is not available to convert Hb into acid hematin.
- The Hb value can come less than the actual Hb value in that person.

Q.6. What are the disadvantages of Sahli's method?

- There can be 8–10% of error in the estimation of Hb.
- All forms of Hb cannot be measured. It estimates only oxyhaemoglobin and reduced haemoglobin.
- Acid hematin colour developed is not stable and it fades with time.
- The coloured standard provided also fades with time.

Q.7. What is the O_2-carrying capacity of blood?

- One gram of Hb combines with 1.34 ml of O_2. Thus, if one knows the Hb values of the person, O_2-carrying capacity can be calculated.

Q.8. Why Hb is more in males? Why Hb count is low in females?

- **In males**, the testosterone hormone stimulates RBC production (erythropoiesis), therefore Hb count is high.
- **In females**, Hb count is low: Due to loss of blood during menstruation and estrogen inhibits erythropoiesis.

Q.9. Why Hb is more in newborns?

- Haemoglobin concentration in a newborn baby is high. It may be as high as 20 g/100 ml of blood. Newborns have more number of active sites of red bone marrow.

Q.10. What are the functions of haemoglobin?

The functions of haemoglobin are:

- It transports oxygen (oxygen gets attached to the iron part of the heme molecule).
- It transports carbon dioxide. CO_2 is attached to the amino group of the protein part of haemoglobin (globin), forming the carbamino compound. It is therefore possible for haemoglobin molecules to carry O_2 and CO_2 simultaneously.
- Haemoglobin is a major protein in the blood. It acts as a buffer and thus prevents drastic changes in the pH of the blood.
- Haemoglobin also acts as a buffer for maintaining the concentration of PO_2 constant in the interstitial fluid (40 mm Hg). This is possible because of the sigmoid shape of the O_2 dissociation curve.

Q.11. What is anaemia?

- Anaemia is defined as the decreased oxygen-carrying capacity of blood due to a decrease in the Hb level of blood below the lower limit of normality for that particular age and sex.

Q.12. Give etiological and morphological classification of anaemia.

Etiological classification:

- **Blood loss anaemia** caused due to acute or chronic blood loss– acute blood loss as in accident, chronic blood loss as in piles.
- **Anaemia caused due to impaired red cell formation.** Impaired red cell formation is due to the following causes:
  - Inadequate supply of nutrients essential for erythropoiesis (iron deficiency, folic acid deficiency, vitamin B12 deficiency, etc.)
  - Depression of erythropoietic activity of bone marrow (aplastic anaemia and leukaemia).
- **Anaemia due to excessive destruction of red blood cells.** This includes all hemolytic anaemia (extracorpuscular and intracorpuscular defects).

Morphological classification :

- **Hypochromic microcytic anaemia:** RBCs are microcytic and hypochromic, thus MCV, MCH and MCHC values are less than normal. This morphology is typical of iron deficiency anaemia.
- **Macrocytic normochromic/hypochromic anaemia:** RBCs are large in size. Thus, MCV is more, and MCHC may be normal or low. This type of RBC picture is typical with vitamin B12 or folic acid deficiency (megaloblastic anaemia).
- **Normocytic normochromic anaemia:** All blood indices MCV, MCH and MCHC are normal. Such a picture is typically seen when there is chronic blood loss, renal failure (due to deficient erythropoietin secretion) or bone marrow failure.

Q.13. Which blood indices can be calculated with haemoglobin values?

From haemoglobin values, the following indices are calculated:

- Mean corpuscular haemoglobin (MCH) (27–32 pg).
- Mean corpuscular haemoglobin concentration (MCHC) (32–38%).
- Colour index (CI). Its normal value is 0.8–1.2
- All blood indices help in diagnosing the type of anaemia.

Q.14. What are the common causes of iron deficiency anaemia?

Common causes of iron deficiency are:

- Excessive blood loss during menstruation
- Increased demands- infancy, childhood, and pregnancy
- Pathological blood loss due to peptic ulcer, haemorrhoids, ulcerative colitis, etc.
- Deficient diet
- In infants, diminished iron stores at birth
- Daily requirement of iron in males is 0.5–1 mg. In females of reproductive age, it is 1–2 mg

- Diet normally should contain 10–20 mg of iron of which 10% or less is absorbed.

Q.15. What are the common causes of the increase or decrease in Hb count?

Conditions that decrease Hb concentration

- **Physiological:**
  - Hb less in females as compared to males
  - Pregnancy (Haemodilution)
- **Pathological:**
  - Different types of anaemia
  - Excess antidiuretic hormone secretion (hemodilution)
- **Experimental errors:**
  - Finger is squeezed while collecting blood
  - Blood taken less than 20 cumm mark

Conditions that increase Hb concentration

- **Physiological:**
  - High altitude (hypoxia)
  - Newborns
  - Excess sweating
- **Pathological:**
  - Severe diarrhoea and vomiting
  - Congenital heart diseases
  - Emphysema of the lungs
  - Polycythemia vera
- **Experimental errors:**
  - Blood taken more than 20 mm^3 mark
  - Fading of colour plate

Q.16. Describe the cyanmethaemoglobin (Haemoglobin cyanide) method.

- Blood is diluted in a solution containing potassium cyanide and potassium ferricyanide. The absorbance of the solution is measured in a spectrophotometer at a wavelength of 540 nm or in a photoelectric calorimeter with a yellow-green filter.
- Diluent (cyanide-ferricyanide) is prepared as follows– 200 mg of potassium ferricyanide, 50 mg of potassium cyanide, 140 mg of potassium dihydrogen sulphate and 1 ml of non-ionic detergent. Then water is added to make a solution to 1 litre.
- This dilution when added to blood, haemoglobin cyanide is formed. About 20 microliter of blood is added to 4 ml of diluent in a tube, is inverted many times and then allowed to stand for five minutes (so that the reaction is complete). Then absorbance of a solution is compared with the standard (in a photoelectric calorimeter).
- Advantages of this method (refer to Q3).

Q.17. How much is the daily requirement of iron, vitamin B12 and folic acid?

- The daily requirement of iron in males is 0.5 to 1 mg and that in females (of reproductive age) is 1 to 2 mg.

A normal diet contains 10 to 20 mg of iron, out of which 10% is absorbed.

- Vit. B12 daily required by adults is 2 to 4 µg and that of folic acid is 200 µg. The body store of vitamin B12 is about 2 to 5 mg and folic acid is 5 to 20 mg. Deficiency of vitamin B12 and folic acid may not appear early due to their storage, even if they are not taken in the diet for long.

Q.18. What are the common causes of deficiency of folic acid?

- It includes decreased intake, nutritional deficiency/impaired absorption (e.g. coeliac disease, tropical sprue, etc.) or increased demands (e.g. pregnancy, haemolytic anaemia, etc.).
- Due to a deficiency of maturation factors RBCs remain large in size (megaloblastic anaemia).

Q.19. Enumerate different varieties of normal Hb.

- **HbA1**: The most common types of adult Hb (its globin contains two alpha and two beta chains
- **HbA2**: This type of adult Hb contains two alpha and two delta chains.
- **Fetal Hb (HbF)**: It contains two alpha and two gamma chains, HbF gradually disappears after one year of age.
- **HbA 3**: Altered form of Hb found in old RBCs.
- **Embryonic Hb**: It is made up of two alpha and two epsilon chains in the first three months of intrauterine life.
- **HbA 1c**: Some amount of normal Hb is glycosylated. It can be more than 3 to 5% of normal % of Hb. If it exceeds, it is considered prediabetic or diabetic stage (depending on the level of HbA1c).

Q.20. Give information on haemoglobin.

It is a conjugated protein present in RBCs. It is made up of heme and globin iron part of the haem is recycled while protoporphyrin forms bilirubin (converted to bile salts and bile pigments). Globin component is broken into amino acids and recycled again for Hb synthesis.

■ OBJECTIVE STRUCTURED PRACTICAL EXAMINATION (OSPE)

Procedure station: Take a known quantity of blood in a Hb pipette and dilute it with acid haematin with the help of the apparatus provided.

S. No.	Assessment criteria	Marks assigned	Marks given
1.	Check Hb pipette, its patency and Sahli's haematometer given		
2.	Check all apparatus for cleanliness and patency		
3.	Take N/10 HCl to the given mark		

Contd...

Contd...

S. No.	Assessment criteria	Marks assigned	Marks given
4.	With all aseptic precautions (check above for details) take capillary blood up to designated mark on the pipette		
5.	Blow out the blood in Hb tube in which N/10 HCl is taken		
6.	Report and viva haematology experiment		
7.	Total		

Procedure station: Find out the Hb of your own blood with the help of Sahli's haemoglobinometer.

S. No.	Assessment criteria	Marks assigned	Marks given
1.	Check Hb pipette, its patency and Sahli's haematometer given		
2.	Check all apparatus for cleanliness and patency		
3.	Take N/10 HCl to the given mark		
4.	With all aseptic precautions (check above for details) take capillary blood up to the designated mark in the pipette		
5.	Blow out the blood in Hb tube in which N/10 HCl is taken		
6.	Mix blood properly with acid hematin, waits for 10 minutes		
7.	Drop by drop add water in the Hb tube and each time mix the content well		
8.	Match the colour of acid hematin in Hb tube with standards against the daylight		
9.	Report and viva on haematology experiment		
10.	Total		

■ COMMON STATIONS – SPOTS IN PRACTICAL EXAMINATION (2/3 MARKS)

Q.1. Diagram/instrument of Sahli's haematometer: Identify and answer any one or two questions (check above).

Q.2. Diagram/instrument of Hb tube, Hb pipette: Identify and answer any one or two questions (check above).

Q.3. Picture of pallor: What is the clinical sign? What is it due to? Write morphological classification of anaemia.

Q.4. If in a 20-year-old male Hb is 14.5 g%–find out the O_2 carrying capacity of his blood (clue- 1 g of Hb combines with 1.34 ml of O_2).

■ CASE-BASED SCENARIO/PROBLEM-BASED

Case 1: A 25-year-old lady comes with c/o fatigue, palpitations, and H/o heavy bleeding during menstruation. O/E pallor ++ MCV-60, MCH-17 picograms, PCV 28.

- What is the reason for pallor in this lady?
- What will be the physiological basis of treatment?
- What can be the morphology of RBCs?
- Why PCV is less? (clue-iron deficiency anaemia, microcytic, microchromic, thus less MCV and MCH) less PCV as well.

Case 2: A 58-year-old man comes with c/o weakness and more loss of blood due to piles. He has been on and off bleeding due to piles for the last 8 to 10 years.

- What chronic blood loss will cause?
- What will be the morphological picture of the RBCs in him? (clue- normocytic normochromic with chronic small amount of blood loss).

Case 3: A paediatrician comes for a visit to check the newborn (born one day before). He checks the newborn thoroughly. Newborn's Hb was found to be 20 g%.

- What is the normal range of Hb in a newborn?
- Why is Hb more in newborns as compared to adults? Give its physiological basis.

Case 4: A 25-year-old male comes with c/o pallor and fatigue. He also complains of problems with respect to focus (concentration) and short-term memory. He also c/o intermittent tingling and numbness in his hands and feet. His Hb is 10.9 g, MCV(123 cubic microns), MCH 37.6 picograms and MCHC 33.5 picograms. Serum antibodies for the intrinsic factor test is negative.

Blood smear: Anisocytosis++, Poikilocytosis++, large RBCs

- What condition probably the patient is suffering from?
- What is megaloblastic anaemia
- Why serum intrinsic factor test was done?
- What will be the physiological basis of treatment (clue vit B12 injections)

Case 5: 7-year-old boy c/o fatigue, body ache and dark-coloured stools for last two days. On examination– pulse 90 beats/min other vitals normal, Hb 7g%, retic (reticulocyte) count 4%, no bilirubin present in urine, total bilirubin 6 mg/dl and high indirect bilirubin.

- What could be your probable diagnosis? (Haemolytic jaundice).

- Write steps in bilirubin metabolism. (Haem–biliverdin-unconjugated bilirubin-gets converted in the liver into conjugated bilirubin- bilirubin glucuronides excreted in bile- in the intestine it is converted to stercobilin, remaining 20% converted as urobilin and excreted in urine)
- What is indirect bilirubin?
- What is the physiological basis of raised reticulocyte count? (clue- stimulation of erythropoiesis process).

Haemolytic jaundice: Excess production of bilirubin glucuronide, increasing quantity of stercobilin formation (dark-coloured stools with excess faecal stercobilinogen) and no bilirubin in urine.

Case 6: A 45-year-old female comes with c/o fever and pain in her abdomen for 4 days. She also has c/o dark-coloured urine and pale stool.

On examination– icterus ++ Hb 11.7 g%, serum bilirubin 5 mg/dl, direct bilirubin levels higher than indirect bilirubin levels.

- What is the probable diagnosis? (obstructive jaundice)
- Physiological basis of signs and symptoms.

Obstructive jaundice: Occurs due to obstruction to bile secretion in the intestine. Thus no faecal stercobilin formed leading to pale-coloured stool and conjugated bilirubin is excreted in urine (dark-coloured urine).

■ KEY POINTS TO REMEMBER

- *Normal Hb values in males:* 14–18 g/dl and in females: 12–15 g/dl of blood.
- *Sahli's principle:* When blood is mixed with HCl, acid hematin (coloured compound) is formed and its colour is matched with standards.
- Important functions of Hb include carrying O_2 from lungs to tissues, CO_2 from tissues to lungs, and Hb acts as a buffer.
- Hb values are more in males, and infants, and are less in females.
- The most commonly practised method for Hb estimation is cyanmethaemoglobin and the most accurate method is an estimation of the iron content of the blood.
- We can diagnose different types of anaemia with the help of blood indices. Iron deficiency anaemia is most common in our country. Common symptoms of anaemia are pallor, fatigue, and muscle weakness.

Determination of Total WBC Count

Learning Objectives

After completion of this practical, the student shall be able to:
- Identify and differentiate between red blood cell (RBC) and white blood cell (WBC) pipettes
- Focus Neubauer's chamber under low power for WBC counting
- Prick the finger with all aseptic precautions
- Dilute the blood in a pipette for WBC count and list precautions for diluting blood
- Charge the Neubauer's chamber and list the precautions for charging the chamber
- Calculate the area and volume for the WBC count. Give the normal value of the WBC count
- Give the composition and function of each constituent of Turk's fluid
- List common causes of leukocytosis and leukopenia
- Give structure and function of leukocytes
- Describe the steps of leukopoiesis.

Aim

To count white blood cells in a given sample of blood.

Apparatus

Microscope, lancet or needle, WBC diluting fluid, WBC pipette **(Fig. 5.1)**, Neubauer's chamber.

White Blood Cell Diluting Fluid (Turk's Fluid) Composition

- 1% glacial acetic acid (for hemolyzing RBCs)

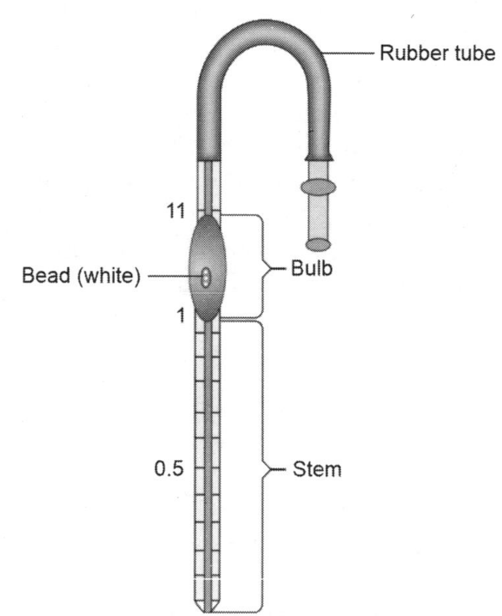

Fig. 5.1: White blood cell (WBC) pipette

- Gentian violet (to stain nuclei of WBCs)
- Distilled water (to make a solution 100 ml, which also helps in the hemolysis of RBCs).

Principle

- For counting WBCs blood is diluted with diluting fluid, which removes red cells by hemolysis and stains nuclei of WBCs by gentian violet.
- It is part of a routine haematological investigation to assess the nature and severity of infection along with differential WBC count.

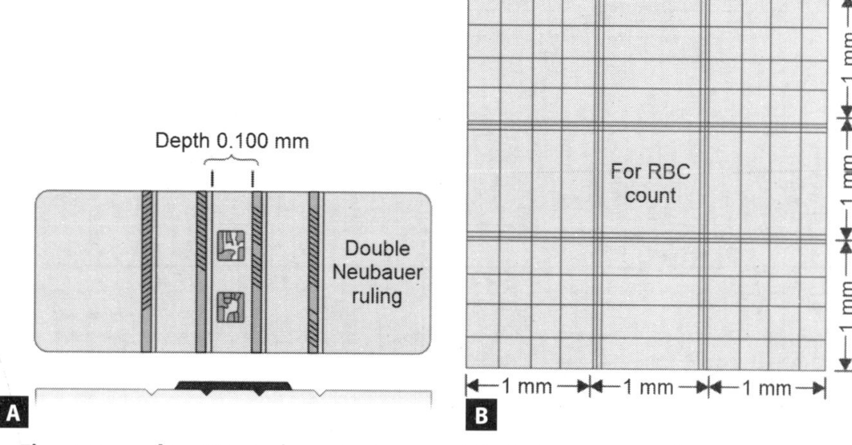

Figs. 5.2A and B: (A) Neubauer's chamber; (B) WBC squares for four corner square

Neubauer's Chamber (Fig. 5.2A)

- It is a single solid heavy glass slide. It has a transverse bar at its centre. The surface of this bar is 0.1 mm below that of the rest of the slide.
- It is separated from the remainder of the slide by two transverse grooves, one on each side running parallel to it.
- The base is divided at its centre by a groove, which allows the setting up of two preparations. The surface of the bar is ruled by two sets of small squares.
- Each ruling is a square of 3 mm × 3 mm. This square is further divided into nine equal squares each having area of 1 mm^2 (1 mm × 1 mm).
- Out of these nine squares, four corner squares are used for WBC count. The area of each corner square is 1 mm^2.
- The space between the coverslip and the upper surface of the bar is 0.1 mm. Thus, when the coverslip is put depth is 0.1 mm. Therefore, the volume of fluid in each square would be equal to 0.1 mm^3.
- Each square is further divided into 16 equal squares by single lining **(Fig. 5.2B)**.
- The central square is for counting of RBCs.

Procedure

- Clean and dry pipette, coverslip, and Neubauer's chamber are taken.
- Patency of the WBC pipette is checked.
- Neubauer's chamber is focused on WBC squares under low power. The coverslip is put.
- Without disturbing adjustment of the microscope, Neubauer's chamber is kept along with a coverslip on the table.
- With usual aseptic precautions finger is pricked for the proper size of blood drop to form.
- Blood is collected up to 0.5 mark in the WBC pipette (if air bubbles are collected, the procedure is repeated). The tip of the pipette is wiped.

- Immediately, WBC diluting fluid is sucked up to 11 marks in the WBC pipette.
- Pipette is taken horizontally in palms and gently rotated.
- Neubauer's chamber along with the coverslip is kept ready on the table.
- The stem part of the pipette is discarded (as it contains only diluting fluid).
- Neubauer's chamber is charged.

Charging of the Chamber

- First two or three drops (from the stem portion of the pipette containing only diluting fluid) are discarded.
- Then the chamber with coverslip put on it is charged as follows. The pipette is held at an angle of 45° to the surface of the chamber.
- A small drop is allowed to form at the tip of the pipette.
- Its point is applied to the narrow slit between the coverslip and the chamber.
- Fluid runs under the coverslip by capillary action. Bubble formation is avoided.
- If drop of fluid put is large and fluid overflows then the chamber and coverslip are washed, dried, and the chamber is recharged.
- Neubauer's chamber is focused under low power **(Fig. 5.3)**.
- White blood cells are identified as clear, nucleated, and refractile bodies.
- Drawing WBC squares in notebook and number of WBCs in each square is noted.
- Rule of counting is obeyed in order to prevent recounting of cells.
- Final result is calculated.
- WBC count is written as WBC count per mm^3 of blood.

Precautions

- Pipette, Neubauer's chamber, and coverslip should be dry and clean.
- Check the patency of the WBC pipette.

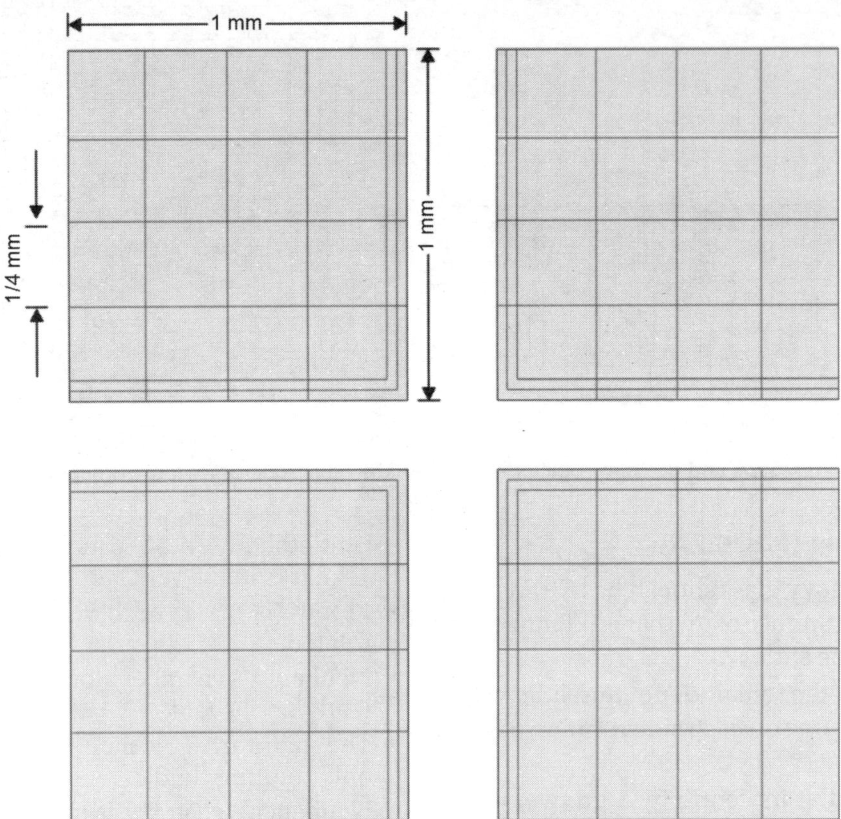

Fig. 5.3: Neubauer's chamber squares for counting white blood cells (WBCs)

- Do not squeeze your finger.
- Blood should be collected exactly up to the 0.5 mark. Wipe off the tip of the pipette.
- Diluting fluid to be collected exactly up to 11 marks.
- Avoid overcharging or undercharging of Neubauer's chamber.
- Avoid counting cells twice.

Technical Errors

- Blood taken in the pipette more or less than 0.5 mark.
- Diluting fluid taken more or less than 11 marks.
- Use of defective pipettes.
- Overcharging or undercharging of Neubauer's chamber.
- Improper counting of cells.
- Mistake in calculations.
- Mistaking dirt or clumped red cell for leukocytes.

■ CALCULATIONS

Neubauer's Chamber

- For counting WBC count, Neubauer's chamber is to be focused under low power. Neubauer's chamber is divided in nine equal squares (3 mm × 3 mm). Out of nine squares, four corner squares are used for WBC counting. So, each square has area of 1 mm². When coverslip is put depth is 1/10, so, volume of each square is 0.1 mm³.
- As we are counting in four squares volume is 0.4 mm³.

Dilution Factor

- Blood is taken up to 0.5 mark and diluting fluid up to 11 mark. After that, few drops (up to 1 mark) are discarded as the stem of the pipette contains only diluting fluid.
- Therefore, 0.5 parts of blood get diluted in 10 parts of diluting fluid. Thus dilution factor becomes 1:20.

WBCs are counted in four corner square each having volume of 0.1 mm³ of fluid.

The total volume in which WBCs are counted is 0.4 mm³.

Total number of WBCs counted in four squares is—say "N"

0.4 mm³ contains "N" cells.

Therefore, mm³ contain N × 10/4------cells.

The dilution factor is 1:20

Therefore, total WBC count = N × 10/4 × 20

= N × 50

■ IMPORTANT QUESTIONS AND ANSWERS

Q.1. How do you identify the WBC pipette? How dilution becomes 1:20?

The WBC pipette has:

- 0.5, 1, and 11 mark.

- The size of the bulb is smaller (as compared to the RBC pipette).
- White bead in the bulb.
- *Dilution:* 0.5 parts of blood get diluted in 10 parts of diluting fluid, dilution factor becomes 1:20.

Q.2. How much is the normal WBC count? In which condition RBC pipette is used for WBC counting?
- Normal WBC count is 4,000–11,000/mm^3 of blood.
- In leukaemia (abnormal proliferation of WBC), as the count is high you have to dilute the blood more; therefore, in such conditions, we use RBC pipette for WBC counting.

Q.3. What is the physiological significance of doing the WBC count?
Leukocytes constitute a mobile defence of the body. The total WBC count is done to assess the subject's ability to defend his/her body against microbial invasion.

Q.4. What are leukocytes?
- WBCs (leukocytes) are part of the body's defence system that provides protection against infection. Development of leucocytes is called as leucopoiesis.
- In embryo WBCs develop from mesoderm at birth, granulocytes are developed by bone marrow. Lymphocytes and monocytes develop from stem cells in bone marrow (myeloid stem cells forming granulocytes and monocytes, lymphoid stem cells forming lymphocytes)
- Circulating WBCs number is controlled in the normal range and works for the body in defence of any foreign particle, bacteria or virus.

Q.5. What is leukocytosis?
WBC count of more than 11,000/mm^3 is termed as leukocytosis.

Q.6. What are the physiological conditions causing leukocytosis?
Physiological conditions causing leukocytosis are:
- Newborn, infants (up to 1 year) (15000–20000/cu mm of blood)
- After exercise
- After meals (raised BMR post meals that increase marginal pooling of cells in circulation)
- Mental stress
- Exposure to increased temperature
- Parturition (due to tissue injury, haemorrhage and exertion)
- Pregnancy (at full-term)

Q.7. Why WBC count increases after exercise?
During exercise, there is disruption of the margination of leukocytes along the vascular endothelium. Therefore, leukocytes are released from the margination pool into general circulation.

Q.8. What are the pathological causes of leukocytosis?
Pathological causes of leukocytosis are:
- Acute bacterial infection (with pyogenic bacteria), e.g. boils, abscess, pneumonia, etc.
- Chronic bacterial infections (tuberculosis)
- Tissue injury (infections, burns, and post-surgery)
- Haemorrhage
- Inflammatory disorders

Q.9. What is leukopenia? Can it be physiological?
Leukopenia is decreased in WBC count below 4,000 mm^3 of blood. Very rarely, it can be physiological (sometimes in severe cold).

Q.10. What are the pathological causes of leukopenia?
Pathological causes of leukopenia are:
- Infections: Typhoid fever and paratyphoid fever
- Repeated exposure to X-ray or radium
- Aplasia of bone marrow
- Aplastic anaemia
- Cytotoxic therapy
- Malnutrition

Q.11. What is leukaemia? Enumerate its types.
- It is a cancerous condition where there is abnormal proliferation of WBCs and infiltration of tissues by leukemic cells.
- They can be myeloid (involving neutrophils) or lymphatic (involving lymphocytes) and can be acute and chronic.
- Immature forms of WBC (myeloblasts) may start appearing in blood when bone marrow activity increases in leukaemia.

Types of leukaemia	Characteristic features
Acute lymphoblastic leukaemia	Most common in children (present with anaemia, moderate increase in leucocytes and increased number of lymphoblasts)
Acute myeloblastic leukaemia	Most common in adolescents and middle age (15 to 40 year age group) high WBC count, and increase in number of myeloblasts
Chronic myeloid leukaemia	Most common in the 4th/5th decade of life. Slow onset, WBC count in lack. More number of metamyelocytes seen
Chronic lymphoblastic leukaemia	Most common after the age of 50, slow onset, marked lymphadenopathy and raised lymphocytes

Q.12. How leukocytes are classified?
Depending on the presence or absence of WBCs are classified as granulocytes and agranulocytes granules.

Granulocytes	Agranulocytes
• Neutrophils • Eosinophils • Basophils	• Lymphocytes • Monocytes

Q.13. Describe the functions of WBCs.

Monocytes and Neutrophils

- *Phagocytosis:* They destroy invading organisms, viruses, and other injurious agents mainly by phagocytosis.
- Neutrophils can destroy 5–20 bacteria before they become inactivated; whereas monocytes can destroy 100 bacteria before they become inactivated. After phagocytosis bacteria are destroyed, with the help of various lysosomal enzymes and bactericidal agents.

Eosinophils

They are produced in large numbers in parasitic infections. They attach themselves by way of special surface molecules to the parasites and release substances that kill parasites.

Basophils

They are similar to large mast cells located immediately outside many of the capillaries. Function of basophils are release of heparin, histamine, and bradykinin in inflamed tissue. Basophils also play an important role in allergic reactions.

Lymphocytes

B lymphocytes are responsible for the humoral type of immunity (by production of antibodies) and T lymphocytes produce cellular immunity.

Q.14. Describe stages of granulopoiesis.

- Pluripotent haemopoietic stem cells → CFU-S (Colony Forming Unit- Spleen) → CFU-GM (Colony Forming Unit → Myeloblast → Promyelocyte → Myelocyte → Neutrophil myelocyte → Neutrophil metamyelocyte → Neutrophil (same way eosinophil and basophil are formed).
- Cell division is limited to myeloblasts, promyeloblasts and myelocytes. In later stages, only cell differentiation happens (no cell division).
- In the metamyelocyte stage nucleus appears and granules become prominent.

Q.15. Describe stages of formation of monocytes and lymphocytes.

- Pluripotent haemopoietic stem cell (PHSC) CFU-S → CFU- GM → Monoblast → Promonoblast → Monocyte
- Pluripotent haemopoietic stem cell (PHSC) → Lymphoid stem cell (LSC) → Lymphoblast → Large lymphocyte → Small lymphocyte.
- Foci of lymphocytes in bone marrow and thymus are engaged in rapid proliferation which is not specifically related to antigenic stimulation. Lymphocytes migrate from these sites to other locations in the body.
- In lymph nodes and spleen as well there is active proliferation of lymphocytes, especially in response to antigenic stimulation.

▌OBJECTIVE STRUCTURED PRACTICAL EXAMINATION (OSPE)

Procedure station 1: To dilute blood for total WBC count.

S. No.	Assessment criteria	Marks assigned	Marks given
1.	Identifie WBC pipette. Check for its patency and cleanliness		
2.	Keep an adequate amount of WBC diluting fluid ready		
3.	Take all aseptic precautions		
4.	Suck blood exactly in the pipette up to 0.5 mark. Wipe the tip of the pipette		
5.	Suck diluting fluid up to the 11 mark. Avoiding entry of air bubbles		
6.	Hold the pipette horizontally in your palms and roll it, so that blood mixes properly with diluting fluid		
7.	Keep it on the table		
8.	Report and viva on haematology experiment		
9.	Total		

Procedure station 2: To charge Neubauer's chamber for total WBC count.

S. No.	Assessment criteria	Marks assigned	Marks given
1.	Take clean and dry coverslip and Neubauer's chamber		
2.	Focus Neubauer's chamber under low power and look for WBC squares		
3.	Without disturbing adjustment of the microscope, keep Neubauer's chamber with a coverslip, on the table		
4.	Discard first two drops from the pipette containing diluting fluid		
5.	Charge Neubauer's chamber properly (as explained above)		
6.	Report and viva on haematology experiment		
7.	Total		

Procedure station 3: To determine the total WBC count of your own blood.

Procedure: Explained above.

S. No.	Assessment criteria	Marks assigned	Marks given
1.	Take clean and dry coverslip and Neubauer's chamber		
2.	Focus Neubauer's chamber under low power and looks for WBC squares		
3.	Without disturbing adjustment of the microscope, keep Neubauer's chamber with a coverslip, on the table		
4.	Discard first two drops from the pipette containing diluting fluid		
5.	Charge Neubauer's chamber properly (as explained above)		
6.	By focusing under low power counts WBCs in four squares (as explained above)		
7.	Derive the formula for WBC counting and finds and writes the result (as explained above)		
8.	Report and viva on haematology experiment		
9.	Total		

■ COMMON STATIONS – SPOTS IN PRACTICAL EXAMINATION (2/3 MARKS)

Q.1. Diagram/instrument of Neubauer's chamber, Turk's fluid, WBC pipette: To identify and answer any one or two questions (check above).

Q.2. Dilution factor in total WBC count is 1:20 justify.

Q.3. Enumerate 2 technical errors and 2 counting errors while counting WBC count.

■ CASE-BASED SCENARIO/ PROBLEM-BASED

Case 1: A 35-year-old man c/o high fever, cough for 2 days. His blood report shows Hb-13 g%, WBC count – 15000, and neutrophil count raised. Pulse – 105/min, Resp rate – 15/ min, BP – 120/70 mm Hg.

- What must be the reason for the increase in his WBC count?
- Enumerate two conditions that increase WBC count physiologically.
- How do neutrophils fight back infections?

Case 2: A 12-year-old girl c/o fever on and off for the last 2 to 3 months. Her blood report shows Hb– 12 g%, WBC count – 1.5 lakh/cu mm of blood.

- What can be the possible reasons for the increase in her WBC count?
- What further investigation can you suggest? (clue-differential count, bone marrow biopsy) (refer to Q11).

■ KEY POINTS TO REMEMBER

- Normal WBC count is 4,000–11,000 per mm^3 of blood.
- Dilution factor in WBC count is 1:20 and Turk's fluid is used as diluting fluid.
- The stem part of the pipette has to be discarded before charging Neubauer's chamber.
- An increase in WBC count is called leukocytosis and a decrease is called leukopenia.
- Abnormal proliferation of WBC is leukaemia.
- WBC acts as a defence system of our body where neutrophils and monocytes work by phagocytosis.
- T lymphocytes are responsible for cell-mediated immune response and B lymphocytes are responsible for antibody-mediated immune response.

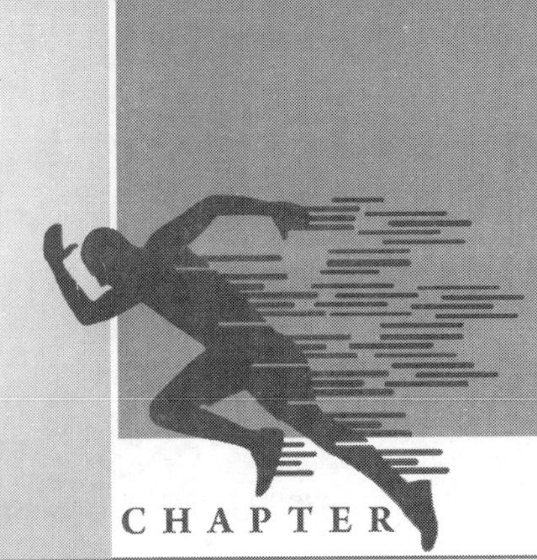

Determination of Total RBC Count

Competency:
PY 2.11: Estimate RBC count of blood.

Learning Objectives
After performing this practical, students shall be able to:
- Identify red blood cell (RBC) pipette
- Focus Neubauer's chamber under high power and identify RBC squares
- List the precautions taken while pricking the finger
- Suck the blood exactly up to 0.5 mark
- Give the composition and function of each constituent of RBC diluting fluid
- Charge the Neubauer's chamber and list all the precautions while diluting the blood
- Give normal dilution factor for RBC count and normal value of RBC count in males and females
- Give physiological and pathological variations in RBC count
- Define anaemia and polycythemia and enlist functions of RBCs
- Enumerate stages of erythropoiesis
- List precautions and errors while doing an RBC count
- Calculate the area and volume for RBC squares and count and enter the number of cells in respective squares
- Express results in millions/cu mm of blood

Aim
To estimate the total red blood cell count of blood.

Principle
Blood is diluted by diluting fluid and then the RBC count is calculated by multiplying the count by the dilution factor.

Apparatus
Microscope, Neubauer's counting chamber, RBC pipette, spirit, and lancet or pricking needle, cotton swab, RBC diluting fluid **(Fig. 6.1)**.

Composition of RBC Diluting Fluid
- Sodium chloride 0.5 g (for isotonicity)
- Sodium sulfate 2.5 g (anticoagulant)
- Mercuric chloride 0.25 g (preservative)
- Distilled water 100 ml.

Procedure
- Dry and clean Neubauer's chamber and coverslip are taken.

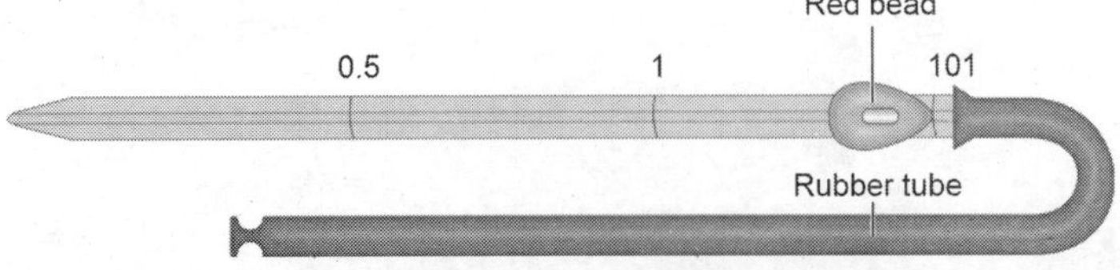

Fig. 6.1: Red blood cell (RBC) pipette

- Patency of the RBC pipette is checked.
- With usual aseptic precautions, the finger is pricked.
- Blood is collected in RBC pipette exactly up to the 0.5 mark.
- If air bubbles come, the procedure is repeated.
- Blood sticking to the tip of the pipette is wiped with the help of cotton.
- RBC diluting fluid is sucked up to 101 mark of RBC pipette.
- The pipette is held horizontally in palms and gently rotated, so that blood mixes properly with diluting fluid (mixing occurs in the bulb part of the pipette).
- Coverslip is put on a ruled area of Neubauer's chamber.
- RBC squares of Neubauer's chamber are focused under low power.
- Without disturbing the adjustment of the microscope, Neubauer's chamber is kept along with the coverslip on the table.
- Discard a few drops from the pipette (as stem of the pipette contains only diluting fluid).
- Charge the Neubauer's chamber as explained [in white blood cell (WBC) count practical].
- Charged Neubauer's chamber (along with coverslip) is put under the microscope (low power already focused).
- For counting RBCs, Neubauer's chamber is focused on high power.
- Counting of RBCs is done under high power in four corners and one central square.

Rule for Counting

- Any cell, which is lying in the upper or left border of that square, is counted in that particular square. This prevents counting of the same cell twice.
- Your observations are entered in corresponding squares drawn in the notebook.
- RBC count is expressed in millions per cubic millimeter of blood.

■ CALCULATIONS

Neubauer's Chamber

- The central square is used for RBC count. It is lined by triple lines. It is further subdivided into 25 equal squares by triple ruling. RBCs are counted in five such squares **(Figs. 6.2 and 6.3)**.
- Usually, four corner squares and one central square are chosen for counting. Each of these 25 squares is further divided into 16 equal squares by a single ruling. The area of the smallest square therefore is:
  $= 1/5 \times 1/5 \times 1/4 \times 1/4 = 1/400 \text{ mm}^2$, and

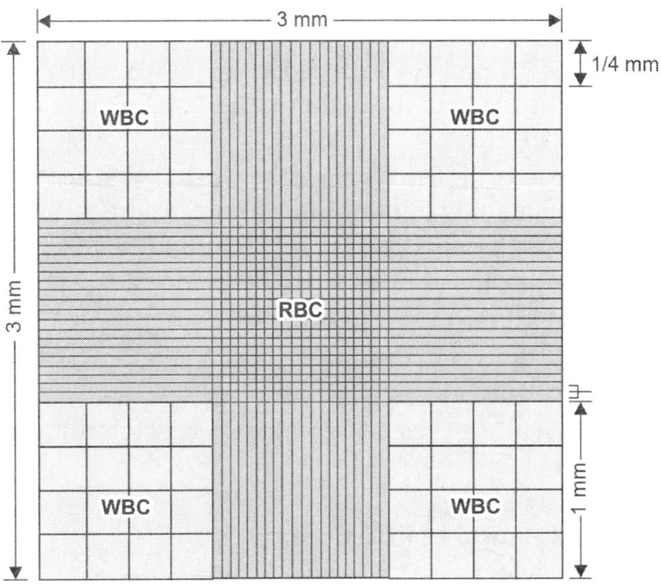

Fig. 6.2: Neubauer's chamber: Central square for red blood cell (RBC) count; (WBC: White blood cell)

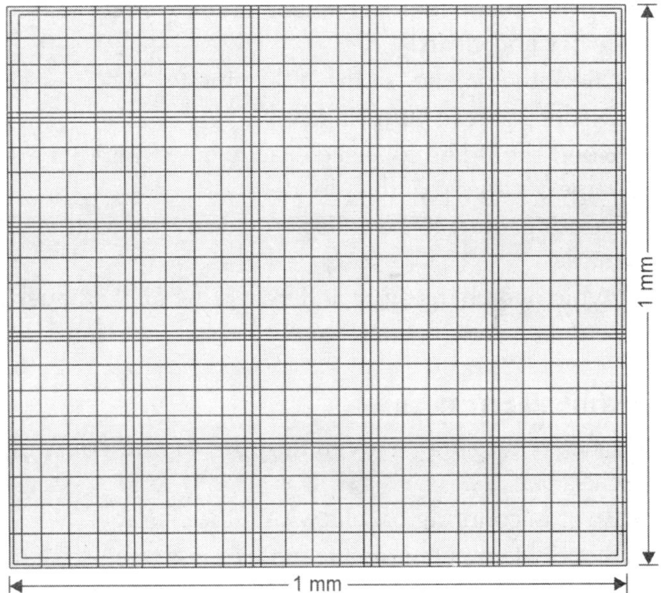

Fig. 6.3: Central square red blood cell (RBC) counting (high power)

The volume of each small square is:
$= 1/400 \times 1/10 = 1/4000 \text{ mm}^3$

RBCs are counted in 80 such small squares (5 larger squares each containing 16 small squares and 5 RBC squares under high power).

Therefore, the total volume in which RBCs are counted is:
$1/4000 \times 80 = 1/50 \text{ mm}^3$

If "N" is the total number of RBCs in five squares, to convert it to a number of cells present in a volume of 1 mm^3, N is multiplied by 50.

Dilution Factor

- In RBC count, we take blood up to 0.5 mark and diluting fluid up to 101 mark. Diluting fluid we take up to 101 mark.
- One part of the fluid (stem of the pipette) we discard as it contains only diluting fluid. Thus 0.5 parts of blood get diluted in 101 parts of diluting fluid.
  Therefore, the dilution factor becomes 1:200.
  Thus,
  Total RBC count/mm^3 = N × 50 × 200
  = N × 10,000
  The count is expressed in millions per cubic millimeter of blood.

Normal Range of RBC Count

- In adult males: 5–6.5 million/mm^3 of blood
- In adult females: 4–5.5 million/mm^3 of blood

Precautions

- Pipette, Neubauer's chamber, and coverslip should be dry and clean
- Check the patency of the WBC pipette
- Do not squeeze your finger
- Blood should be collected exactly up to the 0.5 mark. Wipe off the tip of the pipette.
- Diluting fluid to be collected exactly up to the 101 mark
- Avoid overcharging or undercharging of Neubauer's chamber. Avoid counting cells twice.

Technical Errors

- Undercharging or overcharging of the counting chamber
- Error in counting of cells within the chamber
- Blood taken in the pipette more or less than 0.5 mark
- Diluting fluid taken more or less than 101 mark
- Use of defective pipettes
- Overcharging or undercharging of Neubauer's chamber
- Improper counting of cells
- Mistake in calculations

■ IMPORTANT QUESTIONS AND ANSWERS

Q.1. How much is the normal RBC count?
- In adult males: 5–6.5 million/mm^3 of blood.
- In adult females: 4–5.5 million/mm^3 of blood.

Q.2. How do you identify the RBC pipette?
The RBC pipette has:
- Markings 0.5, 1, and 101

- Larger bulb size
- Red bead in bulb part of the pipette

Q.3. What are other uses of RBC pipette?
Besides for RBC count, the RBC pipette can be used for:
- Sperm count
- Leukemia (abnormal proliferation of WBCs)
- Platelet count

Q.4. Why dilution factor for RBC is more than that for WBC?
- As RBCs are in millions (WBCs are in thousands) they have to be diluted more than WBCs
- In RBC count: The dilution factor is 1:200
- In WBC count: The dilution factor is 1:20

Q.5. What happens, if you take blood more or less than 0.5 mark?
- If blood is taken in the pipette less than 0.5 mark, there will be an error in the result. As less blood is taken count will be less than the actual RBC count in that person.
- If blood is taken in the RBC pipette more than the 0.5 mark, there will be an error, as more blood is taken count will be more than the actual (in both cases it is considered that diluting fluid is taken up to 101 mark).

Q.6. What happens, if diluting fluid is taken more or less than 101 marks?
If diluting fluid is taken more or less, the dilution of blood will differ and the count will be wrong.

Q.7. What are the functions of the red bead present in the RBC pipette?
- It helps in mixing contents of the bulb (i.e. blood and diluting fluid).
- The red bead helps the RBC pipette to be differentiated from the WBC pipette (which has a white bead).

Q.8. What happens to WBCs while one is doing RBC count?
WBCs are not lysed and can be seen when one is doing RBC count but their number is much less as compared to RBCs and they are not stained. Therefore, they do not interfere while the RBC count is being done.

Q.9. What are the units of marking on the pipette?
RBC pipette has markings as 0.5, 1, and 101. These markings do not have any units. They are arbitrary markings, like those of a WBC pipette.

Q.10. What are the functions of RBCs?
- *Oxygen (O$_2$) transport:* RBCs are a major vehicle for oxygen transport in blood.
- *Viscosity of blood:* RBCs are responsible for one-third of the viscosity of blood.

Q.11. Describe the shape and size of red blood cells.
- The mean diameter of RBC is 7.2–7.4 μ.
- The shape of RBC is described as biconcave disc.
- The normal lifespan of RBC is 120 days.

Q.12. What is the site of the formation of RBCs?
- In early embryonic life, nucleated red cells are produced in the yolk sac.
- During the middle trimester of gestation, RBCs are mainly formed in liver and spleen.
- During the last month of gestation, red cells are exclusively formed in bone marrow.
- Up to the age of 5 years, red cells are formed by bone marrow essentially of all the bones.
- After the age of 20 years, the marrow of membranous bones and proximal ends of long bones form RBCs.

Q.13. How is erythropoiesis controlled?
- Erythropoiesis is the process of formation of red blood cells.
- The main function of RBCs is to supply oxygen to the tissues. Whenever there is a decrease in the number of RBCs, hypoxia (inadequate supply of O_2 to tissues) is produced. Hypoxia stimulates the production of erythropoietin in the kidneys, which in turn stimulates erythropoiesis **(Flowchart 6.1)**.

Q.14. What are the factors required for erythropoiesis?
Factors required for erythropoiesis are:
- **First-class proteins**: First-class proteins in adequate amounts. Severe amino acid deficiency due to protein deprivation results in depression of erythropoiesis.
- **Iron:** It forms the part of heme molecule and is therefore essential.
- **Copper**: It is required for the incorporation of iron into protoporphyrin during the final stage of synthesis of heme. Copper is also believed to facilitate iron turnover in the body.
- **Vitamin B12** (cyanocobalamin) and folic acid: They play an important role in the biosynthesis of nucleotide precursors of nucleic acids. There is a need for an active synthesis of nucleic acids because of rapid proliferation of erythrocyte precursors.

- **Ascorbic acid** (vitamin C): Vitamin C facilitates turnover of iron in the body.
- **Pyridoxine** (vitamin B6): Pyridoxal 6 phosphate is a coenzyme required in the synthesis of aminolevulinic acid, which is the first step in the biosynthesis of porphyrin rings.
- **Trace metals**: Cobalt and zinc.
- **Hormones:** Thyroxine, cortisol, and androgens in adequate amounts.
- Basal secretion of erythropoietin from kidneys is the physiological stimulus for erythropoiesis.

Q.15. What are the common clinical features of anaemia?
Clinical features of anaemia are:
- **Fatigue and weakness**: Tiredness, easy fatigability, and generalized muscular weakness are common and early symptoms.
- **Pallor:** This is the most important sign. It may be seen in the skin, nail beds, mucous membranes, and conjunctiva.
- Dyspnea on exertion (difficulty in breathing)
- Palpitation (feeling your own heartbeat)
- Koilonychia (check the general examination Chapter in clinical physiology)
- Glossitis, angular stomatitis, etc.

Q.16. What are physiological and pathological variations in RBC count?

Physiological variations	
RBC count more in	*RBC count less in*
• Newborns • Males as compared to females • High altitude • High temperature • Exercise • Stress	• Old age • Pregnancy • Females as compared to males

Pathological variations	
RBC count more in	*RBC count less in*
• Polycythemia vera • Conditions causing chronic hypoxia • Severe diarrhoea and vomiting (hemoconcentration)	• All types of anaemia • Excess fluid therapy–hemodilution

Q.17. Why is the RBC count higher in infants?
RBC count is higher in infants because red bone marrow is present in all the bones and therefore RBC production is more.

Q.18. Why RBC count is higher in males?
In males, testosterone secreted by testes stimulates RBC production.

Flowchart 6.1: Feedback mechanism of erythropoiesis

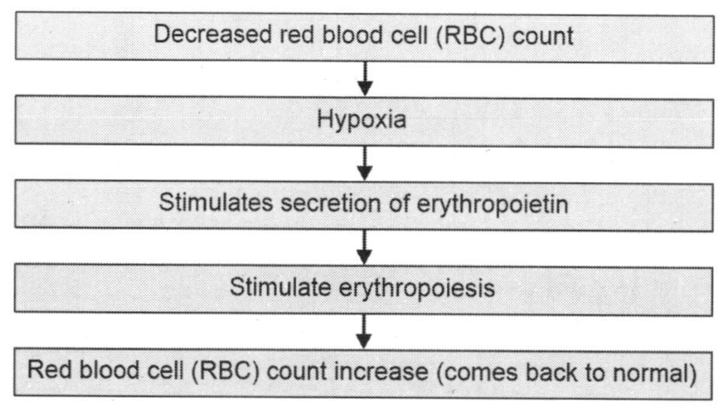

Q.19. Why RBC count is lower in females?

In females, there is menstrual loss of blood after puberty and estrogen probably suppresses erythropoiesis leading to a lesser "RBC" count as compared to males of equivalent age.

Q.20. Why does the RBC count increase with exercise?

Exercise causes a redistribution of RBCs in circulation. Marginal pooling of cells enters the circulation.

Q.21. Why is the RBC count low in pregnancy?

- In pregnancy, there is an increase in plasma volume disproportionately to red cell mass. Thus, there is hemodilution leading to a decrease in RBC count.
- Plasma volume may increase right from the early weeks of pregnancy to a maximum at 24 weeks of pregnancy. Thus, there is hemodilution leading to a decrease in RBC count. In pregnancy average increase in plasma volume is about 43% and the average increase in red cell mass is 25%.

Q.22. How do you diagnose the type of anaemia?

Type of anaemia can be diagnosed by calculating various blood indices.

Q.23. Why RBC count is low in old age and renal disease?

- **Renal diseases**: Erythropoietin is mainly produced in kidneys. This directly affects erythropoiesis and thus production of RBCs. Besides, the excretory function of the kidney is affected, and toxic substances that accumulate may depress RBC production.
- **Old age:** As age advances red marrow is converted to yellow which results in less production of RBCs.

OBJECTIVE STRUCTURED PRACTICAL EXAMINATION (OSPE)

Procedure station 1: To dilute blood for total RBC count.

S. No.	Assessment criteria	Marks assigned	Marks given
1.	Identify RBC pipette. Check for its patency and cleanliness		
2.	Keep adequate amount of RBC diluting fluid ready		
3.	Take all aseptic precautions		
4.	Suck blood exactly in the pipette up to 0.5 mark. Wipes the tip of the pipette		
5.	Suck diluting fluid up to the 101 mark. Avoiding entry of air bubbles		
6.	Hold the pipette horizontally in your palms and roll it, so that blood mixes properly with diluting fluid		
7.	Keep it on the table		
8.	Report and viva on haematology experiment		
9.	Total		

Procedure station 2: To charge the Neubauer's chamber for total RBC count.

S. No.	Assessment criteria	Marks assigned	Marks given
1.	Identify RBC pipette. Check for its patency and cleanliness		
2.	Keep adequate amount of RBC diluting fluid ready		
3.	Take all aseptic precautions		
4.	Suck blood exactly in the pipette up to 0.5 mark. Wipe the tip of the pipette		
5.	Suck diluting fluid up to the 101 mark. Avoiding entry of air bubbles		
6.	Hold the pipette horizontally in palms and roll it, so that blood mixes properly with diluting fluid		
7.	Charge Neubauer's chamber (as described above)		
8.	Report and viva on haematology experiment		
9.	Total		

Procedure station 3: To estimate the RBC count of your own blood.

S. No.	Assessment criteria	Marks assigned	Marks given
1.	Identify RBC pipette. Check for its patency and cleanliness		
2.	Keep an adequate amount of RBC diluting fluid ready		
3.	Take all aseptic precautions		
4.	Suck blood exactly in the pipette up to 0.5 mark. Wipe the tip of the pipette		
5.	Suck diluting fluid up to the 101 mark. Avoiding entry of air bubbles		
6.	Hold the pipette horizontally in your palms and roll it, so that blood mixes properly with diluting fluid		
7.	Charge Neubauer's chamber (as described above)		
8.	By focusing under high power count RBCs in four squares (as explained above)		
9.	Derive the formula for RBC counting and find and writes the result (as explained above)		
10.	Report and viva on haematology experiment		
11.	Total		

▌ COMMON STATIONS – SPOTS IN PRACTICAL EXAMINATION (2/3 MARKS)

Q.1. Diagram/instrument of Neubauer's chamber, RBC fluid, RBC pipette: Identify. Answer any one or two questions (check above).

Q.2. Dilution factor for RBC count is 1:200 justify.

Q.3. Enumerate 2 technical errors and 2 counting errors while counting RBC count.

▌ CASE-BASED SCENARIO/PROBLEM-BASED

Case 1: A newborn blood sample is collected from a pediatric ward, RBC count was 8 million/cu mm of blood

- Give physiological basis for high RBC count (clue-more active sites of red bone marrow)

Case 2: A 23-year-old girl comes with c/o fatigue. On investigation, her RBC count is 2.5 million/cu mm of blood and her Hb is 7.5 g%

- What is the probable cause of the findings? (clue-anaemia), please check above.
- What do you expect her PCV value? and why? (less, as there is anaemia), please check the Chapter 11 on hematocrit.
- Which haematological investigation do you suggest that will help diagnose the type of anaemia?
- Also, check the cases given in the Chapter 4 on Hb estimation.

▌ KEY POINTS TO REMEMBER

- RBC count is higher in males than in females.
- RBCs are seen under high power. RBC dilution factor is 1:200.
- Erythropoiesis is the process of formation of RBCs from pluripotent hematopoietic stem cells to mature RBCs. It takes 7–9 days for the same.
- Various factors required for erythropoiesis are erythropoietin, first-class proteins, vitamin B12, iron, folic acid, trace metals, etc.

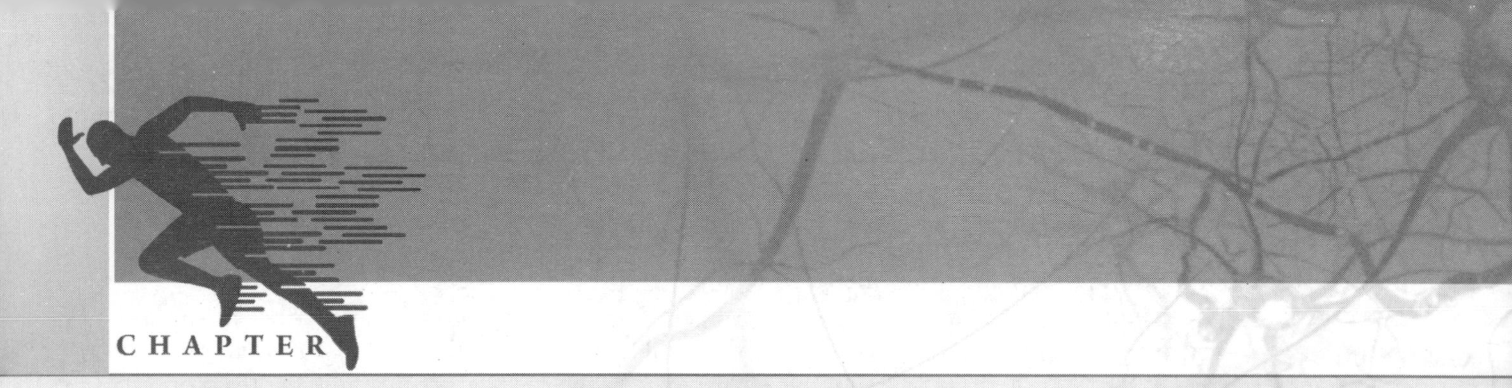

Determination of Differential WBC Count

Competency:

2.11: Estimate differential WBC count.

Learning Objectives

After completing this practical, the student shall be able to:
- List precautions, taken while pricking the finger
- Make a blood smear by wedge method
- Identify red cells, differential leukocytes, and platelets from the smear
- Fix and stain smear
- List criteria of ideal smear
- List and identify morphological features of all the white blood cells (WBCs)
- Give structure and function of various leukocytes
- List common causes of increase and decrease in leukocytes
- Enumerate constituents and functions of each constituent of Leishman's stain
- Give the clinical significance of differential count
- List precautions and errors in differential WBC count practical

Aim

To count different white blood cells.

Apparatus

Microscope, Leishman's stain, lancet or needle, slides, and distilled water.

Principle

A drop of blood is spread to form a thin blood film. It is dried and fixed with methyl alcohol and is stained with a suitable stain for differentiating different types of WBCs. Each type of WBC is identified and counted.

Leishman's Stain

It contains acidic and basic dyes.
- *Eosin:* It is an acidic dye and mainly stains granules of eosinophil.
- *Methylene blue:* It is a basic dye. It mainly stains cytoplasm, nuclei of WBC, and granules of basophils.
- Acetone-free methyl alcohol is fixative (it fixes cells to the slide).

▪ BLOOD SMEAR

Steps in Preparation of Blood Smear

One should know how to prepare a blood smear before learning the procedure of differential count.

Blood smear is prepared in two steps:
1. Making the blood smear.
2. Fixing and staining the blood smear **(Fig. 7.1)**.

Procedure

- Four to five clean and grease-free glass slides are taken.

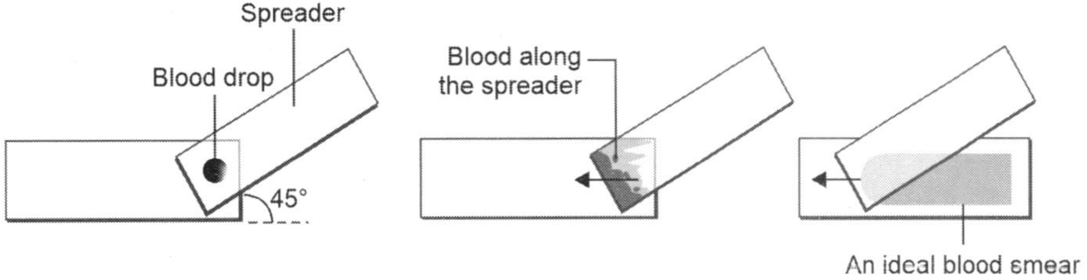

Fig. 7.1: Preparation of blood smear

- Three to four glass slides are put on the table.
- With usual aseptic precautions, the finger is pricked.

Preparation of Blood Smear

- Small drop of blood is put on each slide.
- Other slide (spreader) is put in front of the blood drop at an angle of 45° with the slide on which blood drop is put.
- The spreader slide is moved backwards so that a drop of blood spreads along the edge of the spreader.
- For maintaining the angle of 45°, the spreader is moved along the length of the slide slowly and smoothly.
- Using the same procedures, three to four blood smears are made.
- Blood smears are allowed to dry.

Staining of the Smear

- 10–12 drops of Leishman's stain are put on each slide just to cover the whole of the blood smear.
- It is kept for 2 minutes (time required for fixation of smear). In about 2 minutes, methanol helps to fix the stain.
- Then about 20 drops of distilled water are put along the whole length of the smear.
- Distilled water and stain are mixed by gentle blowing.
- After 5–7 minutes, slides are washed under tap water to remove excess stains.
- Slides are kept upright for drying.
- Smears are first visualized under low power and then high power.
- Best smear is chosen for counting.
- Count is done under high power or oil immersion lens.

Method of Counting

- Counting is started from the left upper corner and then the slide is moved horizontally to the right **(Fig. 7.2)**.
- Counting is done in a zig-zag manner as shown in the diagram.
- Hundred squares are drawn on paper and each cell is identified and is written in the square **(Fig. 7.3)**.
  N: Neutrophil

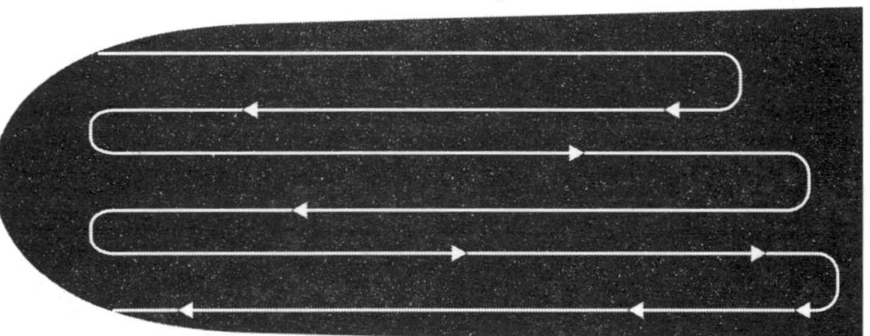

Fig. 7.2: Method for counting of white blood cells (WBCs)

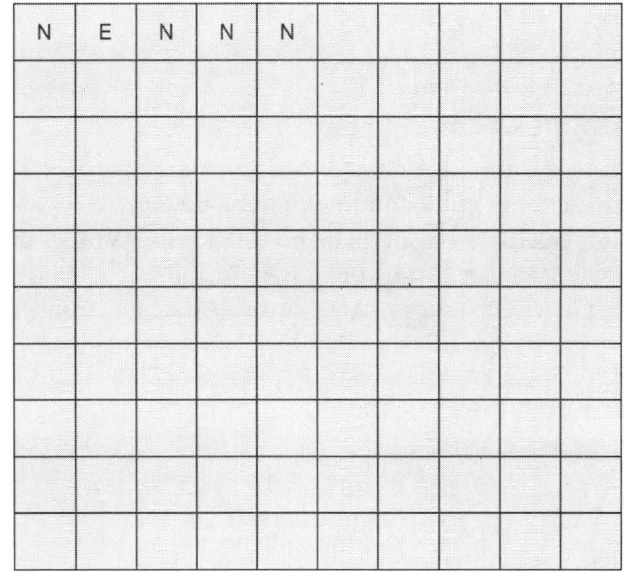

Fig. 7.3: Differential white blood cell (WBC) count

E: Eosinophil
B: Basophil
M: Monocyte
L: Lymphocyte

- The WBCs are identified according to their size, nucleus, and presence, or absence of granules **(Fig. 7.4)**.

Normal Differential Count

- Neutrophils: 50–70%
- Eosinophils: 1–4%

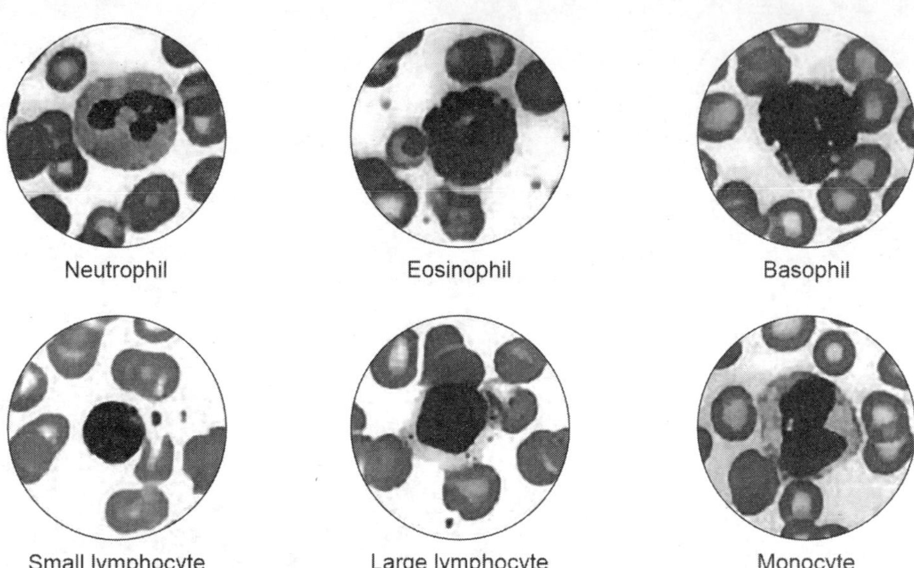

Fig. 7.4: Different types of white blood cells
(For colour version, See plate 1)

- Basophils: 0–1%
- Lymphocytes: 20–30%
- Monocytes: 2–5%

Absolute Count

- It is the total number of a particular type of WBC present per cubic millimetre of blood.
- It is calculated from total and differential WBC count as follows, e.g. suppose eosinophils are 4% and total WBC count is 10,000/mm^3. Absolute count for eosinophils = $10,000 \times 4/100 = 400/\text{mm}^3$

Normal Values for Absolute Count of Differential WBCs

- *Neutrophils:* 2,000–7,000/mm^3
- *Eosinophils:* 10–400/mm^3
- *Basophils:* 0–100/mm^3
- *Monocytes:* 500–800/mm^3

Precautions

- Slides should be clean and grease-free.
- All aseptic precautions should be taken before the prick.
- Glass spreader should have a smooth edge. The spreader slide should be moved steadily with a single quick and smooth movement.
- Smear should be made immediately once a drop of blood is put on the slide. The smear must be completely dry.
- A proper amount of Leishman's stain is put in for fixation of the smear.

- Quality of smear is assessed with naked eyes and microscopically.
- Counting and identification of cells should be done in a zig-zag manner, to avoid errors in counting.

Technical Errors

- Improper way of preparing smear.
- Over or under-staining of smear with Leishman's stain.
- Identifying cells wrongly.

■ IMPORTANT QUESTIONS AND ANSWERS

Q.1. How much is normal differential count?
- Neutrophils: 50–70%
- Eosinophils: 1–4%
- Basophils: 0–1%
- Lymphocytes: 20–30%
- Monocytes: 2–5%

Q.2. How do you differentiate WBCs morphologically?
Refer to **Table 7.1**.

Q.3. What are the criteria for an ideal blood smear?
Criteria for ideal blood smear:
- Good smear should cover ½ to ¾ of the length of the slide.
- It should be tongue-shaped.
- It should be well stained (not overstained not under stained).
- It should not be too thick. Ideally, the smear should be one cell thick with no overlapping of cells.
- There should be no gaps in a smear.

TABLE 7.1: Types of leukocytes (Morphological characteristics)

Granulocytes

Name	Diameter	Nucleus	Cytoplasmic granules
Neutrophil	10–14 µ	Multi-lobed	Violet pink fine granules
Eosinophil	10–14 µ	Bi-lobed (spectacle shaped)	Coarse red granules
Basophil	10–14 µ	The nucleus is not seen clearly and it is overlaid with granules	Coarse blue granules

Agranulocytes

Name	Diameter	Nucleus	Cytoplasmic granules
Monocyte	12–18 µ	Kidney shaped	Large quantity of blue cytoplasm. No granules
Small lymphocyte	7–10 µ	Large round nucleus	Thin rim of cytoplasm surrounding the nucleus. No granules
Large lymphocyte	10–14 µ	Round nucleus	The amount of cytoplasm is greater than that in small lymphocyte. No granules

- Under the microscope, the background of cells should be clear. Leukocytes should show the proper colour of the nucleus, cytoplasm, and granules (under low power RBCs appear as dots). Different types of leukocytes are shown in **Table 7.1**.

Q.4. Why alcohol present in Leishman's stain is acetone-free?

Acetone is a lipid solvent and therefore it dissolves the membrane of WBCs, so acetone-free alcohol is taken.

Q.5. Can any other stain be used to make a blood smear?

Besides Leishman's stain, Wright's stain is also used commonly to make the blood smear. A mixture of methylene azure and methylene blue and eosin can be used (Giemsa's stain) to make a blood smear.

Q.6. Enumerate common staining defects.

- Overstaining of blood smear can cause RBCs to appear deep blue and WBCs to appear dark blue and differentiation of WBCs becomes impossible.
- If the stain is under-stained, nuclei of WBCs may appear lighter than cytoplasm. This can also happen if the blood smear is overwashed.
- If Leishman's stain is old, it can cause precipitation of stain granules on the blood smear.

Q.7. What are the uses of blood smear?

Uses of blood smear:

- Differential WBC count
- Study of red cell morphology
- Study of the morphology of platelets
- Sex differentiation—by Barr body identification

Blood smear: Peripheral blood smear besides, for DLC, also helps to identify the morphology of RBCs and platelets. Blood smears can be preserved which becomes important when we want to asses clinical progress of a patient to treatment/disease.

Q.8. Why is Leishman's stain diluted after 2 minutes and not earlier?

Leishman's stain contains alcohol, which fixes the smear so that it is not washed out by water when the stain is diluted. Therefore, the stain is kept on the smear for 2 minutes for fixation of smear.

Q.9. Which is the largest WBC in the peripheral blood smear?

Monocyte is the largest cell in the peripheral blood.

Q.10. How do you differentiate between neutrophils and eosinophils?

Neutrophils and eosinophils are differentiated on the following criteria:

- **Nucleus**: The nucleus of a neutrophil is usually multilobed. In eosinophils, the nucleus appears spectacle-shaped.
- **Granules**: In neutrophils granules are fine and they take violet pink color. In eosinophils, granules are coarse and they take red colour.

Q.11. How do you differentiate between small and large lymphocytes?

Small and large lymphocytes are differentiated on the following criteria:

- **Size:** The diameter of large lymphocytes is 10–14 µ; whereas the diameter of small lymphocytes is 7–10 µ (almost the same as that of RBC).
- **Nucleus and cytoplasm**: The nucleus is rounded in both but it almost fills the small lymphocyte, so that only a thin rim of blue-coloured cytoplasm appears around it. In large lymphocytes, the amount of cytoplasm is more.

Q.12. How do you differentiate between large lymphocytes and monocytes?

- The size of a large lymphocyte is 10–14 µ in diameter, whereas a monocyte has a diameter of about 15–18 µ.
- In large lymphocytes, the nucleus is rounded; whereas in monocytes, the nucleus is kidney-shaped.
- The amount of cytoplasm is more in monocytes.

Q.13. What is the clinical importance of doing differential count?

- Differential count is vital for the diagnosis of several blood-related diseases. Differential count is done to find out the increase or decrease in different types of WBCs, e.g. in allergic conditions, especially eosinophil count increases.
- Lymphocytosis occurs in chronic bacterial infections.
- Leukopenia occurs with severe bone marrow depression.

Q.14. Why are WBCs observed under an oil immersion lens?

Differential count is done under an oil immersion lens, so that the resolution is good and one is, therefore, able to differentiate types of WBCs better.

Q.15. Describe the functions of different leukocytes.

Neutrophils:

- Act as phagocyte.
- In the process of phagocytosis, many chemicals are released, which are bactericidal.
- First line of defence against bacterial infections.

Eosinophils:

- Involved in allergic reactions.
- Eosinophil granules contain chemicals that neutralize allergens and are larvicidal and parasiticidal.

Basophils:

Releases heparin, histamine, bradykinin, serotonin, and the number of lysosomal enzymes.

Monocytes:

- They are actively phagocytic.
- They remain in circulation for few hours and migrate in tissues to form tissue macrophages. They are second line of defense.
- They protect the body against fungi, bacteria, viruses, and parasites.
- They secrete a number of cytokines, which mediate various immunological responses.

Lymphocytes:

- Mediate immunological responses of the body.
- T lymphocytes mediate cellular immunity.
- B lymphocytes mediate humoral immunity by producing antibodies.

Q.16. What is neutrophilia? When does it occur?

An increase in neutrophil count is known as neutrophilia. Neutrophilia is observed in various physiological and pathological conditions **(Table 7.2)**.

Q.17. What is neutropenia? When does it occur?

A decrease in neutrophil count is known as neutropenia.

It occurs in the following conditions:

Physiological conditions: Physiological neutropenia is very rare.

TABLE 7.2: Various physiological and pathological conditions causing neutrophilia

Physiological conditions	Pathological conditions
Muscular exercise	Acute pyogenic infections, e.g. tonsilitis
Emotional stress	Haemorrhage
After meals	Steroid therapy
Pregnancy	Rheumatic fever
Parturition	Gout
Newborn	Leukaemia

Pathological conditions:

- Typhoid and paratyphoid fever
- Parasitic infections like malaria and kala-azar
- Viral infections like measles, influenza, and viral hepatitis
- Hematopoietic disorder—aplastic anaemia, irradiation by X-ray, radium, etc.
- Hypersplenism
- Drugs, which depress the bone marrow

Q.18. What is lymphocytosis? When does it occur?

Lymphocytosis is an increase in a number of lymphocytes.

It occurs in:

Physiological conditions: Infancy and childhood

Pathological conditions:

- Chronic infections, e.g. tuberculosis and secondary syphilis
- Acute infections, e.g. whooping cough
- Viral infections, e.g. Epstein–Barr virus and cytomegalovirus
- Chronic lymphocytic leukemia

Q.19. What is lymphopenia? When does it occur?

Lymphopenia: It is a decrease in lymphocyte count

It occurs in the following conditions:

- Adrenocorticotropic hormone (ACTH) injection
- Steroid therapy
- Immunosuppressive therapy

Q.20. What is eosinophilia? When does it occur?

An increase in eosinophil count is termed as eosinophilia

It occurs in the following conditions:

- Allergic conditions, e.g. bronchial asthma and hay fever
- Tropical eosinophilia
- Parasitic infections, e.g. filariasis and hookworm
- Skin diseases, e.g. psoriasis and pemphigus
- Collagen diseases

Q.21. What is eosinopenia? When does it occur?

Eosinopenia: It is a decrease in eosinophil count

It occurs in the following conditions:

Physiological conditions:

- Stress
- Injection of ACTH or adrenaline

Pathological conditions:

- Acute pyogenic infections
- Aplastic anaemia
- Steroid therapy

Q.22. What is monocytosis?

An increase in monocyte count is monocytosis. It is seen in the following conditions:

- Certain protozoal infections like malaria and kala-azar
- Infectious mononucleosis
- Collagen diseases
- Subacute bacterial endocarditis

Q.23. What is monocytopenia?

A decrease in monocyte count is monocytopenia. It occurs rarely. It is seen in:

- Bone marrow failure
- Aplastic anaemia
- Septicemia

Q.24. What is basophilia?

Increase in basophil count is basophilia. It is seen in:

- Chronic myeloid leukemia
- Polycythemia

Q.25. What is basophilopenia?

Decrease in basophil count is basophilopenia. It occurs rarely. It is seen in septicemia and aplastic anaemia.

Q.26. What is Arneth count?

- Neutrophil count that is based on a number of lobes in it is called Arneth count. It indicates functional activity of bone marrow. More number of neutrophils are thus bilobed or trilobed.

  The normal count is as follows:

  Stage I (Nucleus with one lobe)– 5 to 10%

  Stage II (Bilobed nucleus)– 20 to 30%

  Stage III (Trilobed Nucleus)– 40 to 50%

  Stage IV (Nucleus with four lobes)– 10 to 15%

  Stage V (Nucleus with five lobes)– 3 to 5%
- There can be a shift to the left which means that there are a greater number of neutrophils with the single-lobed nucleus. This means that there are a greater number of young cells in circulation indicating an increased rate of formation of neutrophils.
- Shift to right occurs when there are a greater number of neutrophils with 4 to 5 lobed nuclei. This means that there are a greater number of old cells in circulation indicating decreased rate of formation of neutrophils. On a similar basis, there is another index known as Smiling's index.

Q.27. What is peroxidase reaction?

Peroxidase reaction: It detects the presence of oxidizing enzymes in the cells that help in differentiating immature cells of myeloid series (peroxidase positive) from lymphoid series (peroxidase negative). Oxidase granules are found in granulocytes, myelocytes and myeloblasts and are absent in young myeloblasts and cells of lymphoid series.

▌ OBJECTIVE STRUCTURED PRACTICAL EXAMINATION (OSPE)

Procedure station 1: To prepare a blood smear from a given sample of blood.

S. No.	Assessment criteria	Marks assigned	Marks given
1.	Select four slides and spreader		
2.	Clean and dry the slides		
3.	Mix the given blood properly and put a drop of blood at one end of the slide		
4.	Place the spreader in front of a drop of blood at an angle of 30–45° and draw the spreader back until it touches the drop of blood (as explained above)		
5.	Let the drop spread along the edge of a spreader		
6.	Move the spreader smoothly and slowly to another end of the slide to make an ideal smear		
7.	Let the smear dry in air and keep it on the table		
8.	Report and viva on haematology experiment		
9.	Total		

Procedure station 2: To examine a stained blood smear provided to you and focus on any leukocyte.

S. No.	Assessment criteria	Marks assigned	Marks given
1.	Select ideal blood smear (criteria please check above)		
2.	Check for uniform distribution and staining of cells focus the smear under high power (condenser in top position and iris, diaphragm fully opened)		
3.	Focus under high power and does fine adjustments, if required		
4.	Focus and identifies different leukocytes (which every leucocyte is asked to focus)		
5.	Report and viva on haematology experiment		
6.	Total		

Procedure station 3: To examine a stained blood smear provided to you and focus on any leukocyte (if asked to focus under oil immersion, all assessment criteria same as given for Q2 but focusing should be done under oil immersion).

Focusing under oil immersion:

- Place a drop of oil on the chosen site of the ideal blood smear.
- Change to oil immersion objective.
- All other microscopic adjustments are the same as given above.

Procedure station 4: To do differential count of your own blood.

S. No.	Assessment criteria	Marks assigned	Marks given
1.	Select four slides and spreader		
2.	Clean and dries the slides		
3.	With all aseptic precautions prick the finger (as explained above) and put a drop of blood at one end of slide		
4.	Place the spreader in front of a drop of blood at an angle of 30–45° and draw the spreader back until it touches a drop of blood (as explained above)		
5.	Let the drop spread along the edge of a spreader		
6.	Move the spreader smoothly and slowly to another end of the slide to make an ideal smear		
7.	Put the stain and water drops (as described above on the smear)		
8.	Let the smear dry in air and keep it on the table		
9.	Start identifying different leucocytes (as described above) and write it down to count a total of 100 cells		
10.	Report and viva on haematology experiment		
11.	Total		

◼ COMMON STATIONS – SPOTS IN PRACTICAL EXAMINATION (2/3 MARKS)

Q.1. Diagram/bottle of Leishman's stain: Identify and give use of each of its constituents and answer any one or two questions (check above).

Q.2. Enumerate criteria for ideal smear: Identify any cell mounted under microscope.

Q.3. Give functions or conditions that increase or decrease cell count.

Q.4. Enumerate any conditions (physiological/pathological) that can increase or decrease specific leucocytes (please check above).

Q.5. Write the significance of doing differential WBC count.

◼ CASE-BASED SCENARIO/PROBLEM-BASED

Case 1: A 16-year-old boy comes with a c/o high-grade fever for 2 to 3 days. Body ache and loss of appetite. O/E all vitals are normal. Blood report shows Hb 13 g%, WBC count– 3500/cu mm of blood platelet counts normal. DLC shows raised neutrophils. Tests for malaria, dengue and typhoid are negative. Rest systemic examination normal.

Based on your physiological knowledge answer the questions:

- What can be the reason for the low WBC count? Give a physiological basis (clue–viral/bacterial infections, WBCs are fighting back infection giving rise to low counts).
- What are the functions of neutrophils?

Case 2: 55-year-old woman c/o weight loss, and fatigue since the last three months. Also c/o loss of appetite. On examination, BP was 130/88 mm Hg and pulse was 78 beats/min afebrile. She shows blood report that she has done 2 days back—Hb–10.8 g% WBC count: 990000 per cubic mm of blood (N–60%, Lymphocytes–4%, Monocytes–1%, basophils–10%). Peripheral smear shows normocytic normochromic RBCs and an excess number of neutrophils and myeloblast.

- What is a probable condition the lady is suffering from? (leukaemia–please refer to Chapter 5; Q11)
- Give the normal value of the WBC count.
- What is cause of the appearance of myeloblast? (refer Chapter 5, Q11)
- Do you suggest any other investigation (clue–bone marrow biopsy).

◼ KEY POINTS TO REMEMBER

- Differential count helps us to understand, which particular WBC has increased or decreased.
- Normally, neutrophils: 50–70%; eosinophils: 1–4%; basophils: 0–1%; lymphocytes: 20–30%; and monocytes: 2–5%.
- Increase in any cell count is written with a suffix as cytosis and decrease in any cell count as penia.
- Differential WBC count is seen under high power and or oil immersion lens.

Determination of Bleeding Time and Clotting Time

Competency:

PY 2.11: Estimate bleeding time and clotting time.

> ### *Learning Objectives*
> At the end of this practical, student shall be able to:
> - Describe the importance of doing bleeding time (BT) and clotting time (CT)
> - Determine BT by Duke's method and CT by capillary tube method
> - Define BT and CT and give their normal values
> - List conditions, which alter BT and CT
> - List precautions taken while doing BT and CT
> - Enumerate steps in coagulation
> - Give normal platelet count and list causes of thrombocytopenia
> - Define purpura and hemophilia.

Aim

Bleeding time and clotting time are determined to assess the integrity of the hemostatic mechanism.

Apparatus

Lancet or needle, capillary tubes, filter paper, and stopwatch.

Bleeding Time (Duke's Method)

Procedure

- The stopwatch is set at zero.
- With all the usual aseptic precautions, finger is pricked (a bold prick of about 5 mm depth is given).
- Blood should flow freely without squeezing the finger.
- Stopwatch is started immediately.
- Drop of blood is blotted on filter paper every 30 second.
- Drop becomes progressively smaller.
- Stopwatch is stopped as soon as bleeding ceases.
- Number of blood drops on filter paper are counted and multiplied by 30 seconds.
- This gives you your bleeding time in seconds (to be converted in minutes) as shown in **Fig. 8.1**.

Precautions

- Take all usual aseptic precautions.
- Use the stopwatch properly—starting exactly when the prick is given till bleeding ceases.
- Give at least 5 mm deep prick.
- Do not squeeze the finger.

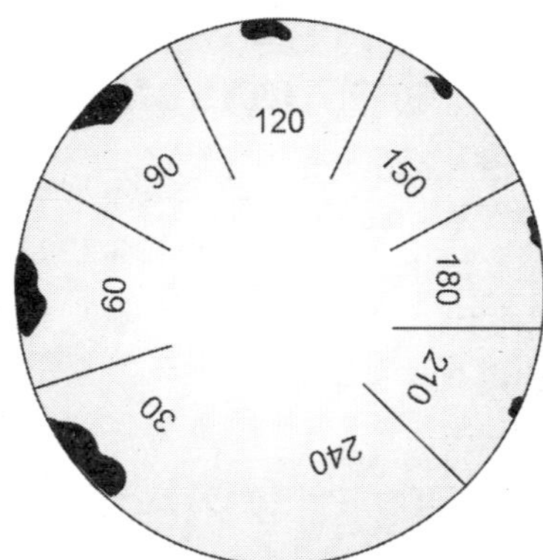

Fig. 8.1: Estimation of bleeding time (Duke's method)

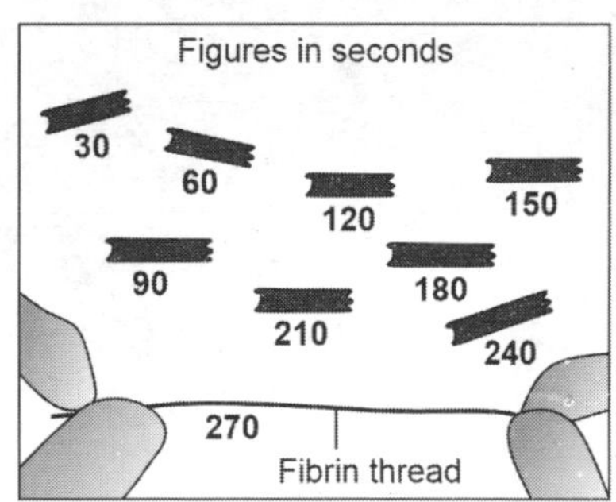

Fig. 8.2: Estimation of clotting time (capillary tube method)

- Do not allow filter paper to press on the bleeding spot.
- Measure bleeding time accurately.

Clotting Time – Capillary Tube Method (Wright's Method)

Procedure

- With all the usual aseptic precautions finger is pricked (3–5 mm depth).
- Stopwatch is started immediately.
- First drop of blood is wiped off.
- Blood is allowed to flow in the capillary tube by keeping one end of the tube into the blood drop. The other end of the capillary tube is kept at the lower level.
- Blood gets collected in the capillary tube by capillary action.
- Every 30 seconds, a small piece of capillary is broken. It is repeated till a fibrin thread appears between two cut ends.
- The time interval between prick and appearance of fibrin thread is clotting time as shown in **Fig. 8.2**.
- Normal value of clotting time is 6 to 8 minutes.

Precautions

All aseptic precautions should be taken.
- A bold prick of 3–5 mm is given.
- Squeezing of finger is not done.
- The stopwatch should be properly started at the time of prick.
- Clotting time is calculated.

■ IMPORTANT QUESTIONS AND ANSWERS

Q.1. What is hemostasis?
Hemostasis: It is the process of stoppage of bleeding. Three major steps are:
1. Vasoconstriction
2. Platelet plug formation
3. Clot formation

Q.2. Bleeding time depends on what?
- Bleeding time depends on the effectiveness of vasoconstriction and platelet plug formation.

Bleeding time depends on:
- Platelet numbers and their functional state
- Functional status of blood vessels
- Extent of the breadth of the wound.

Q.3. What is bleeding time? How much is the normal bleeding time?
It is the time interval between skin puncture and arrest of bleeding. Normal bleeding time is 1–5 minutes (Duke's method).

Q.4. What are the different methods for determining bleeding time?
Bleeding time is determined by:
- **Duke's method (explained above):** Duke's method is a commonly used method for estimation of bleeding time.
- **Ivy's method:** A sphygmomanometer is tied to the forearm of the patient and pressure is raised to 40 mm Hg. Same time approximately 5 cm below the cubital fossa two separate punctures are made. With the help of two separate blotting papers, bleeding time is calculated. When bleeding stops, release the pressure from the sphygmomanometer. Paper on which bleeding time is longer is considered as accurate (normal BT with this method– 5 to 11 minutes). This method is more reliable than Duke's method.

Q.5. What is idiopathic thrombocytopenic purpura (ITP)?
- Purpura is a group of diseases, which occur due to thrombocytopenia (decrease in platelet count). Due to a deficient number of platelets, petechial haemorrhages (small vessels rupture) or purpuric lesions are seen on the skin.
- Acute ITP usually is a self-limiting disorder and may not require any therapy.

Q.6. What is thrombocytopenia?
Thrombocytes mean platelets. Thrombocytopenia is a decrease in platelet count.

Q.7. How much is normal platelet count?
Normal platelet count is $100,000–300,000/mm^3$ of blood.

Q.8. What is the effect of bleeding time and clotting time on purpura?
In purpura as platelet count is decreased, bleeding time is prolonged. As there is nothing wrong with the clotting mechanism, clotting time remains normal.

Q.9. Enumerate conditions causing prolonged bleeding time.
- Thrombocytopenia, i.e. platelet count $<50,000/mm^3$ of blood.
- Disorders of platelet, e.g. thrombasthenia.
- Von Willebrand's disease.
- Any bleeding disorder can be acquired (common) or inherited.

Q.10. What are the different tests used to determine clotting time?

Two methods for determining clotting time are—(1) Capillary tube method, and (2) Lee and White method.

Q.11. Clotting time depends on what?

- Clotting time depends on the effectiveness of the clotting mechanism.
- Presence/absence of any of the clotting factors.

Q.12. What is clotting time? How much is normal clotting time?

Clotting time is defined as the time interval between you prick your finger and clot formation (fibrin thread formation). Normal clotting time is 3–8 minutes.

Q.13. Why bleeding time is less than clotting time?

- *Bleeding time:* It is a time interval between skin puncture and arrest of bleeding. Bleeding is arrested quickly by vascular spasm and platelet plug formation.
- *Clotting time:* It is the interval between skin puncture and formation of a clot. Formation of clot occurs by multiple (enzyme cascade) reactions and therefore it takes a longer time.

Q.14. What are the stages of clot formation?

Stages of clot formation are:

- Activation of Stuart factor
- Formation of thrombin from prothrombin
- Formation of fibrinogen to fibrin

Q.15. What is Lee and White's method of clotting time?

Lee and White method:

- In this method, venous blood is collected.
- One milliliter of blood is transferred in glass tube of 8 mm diameter. The tube is placed in a water bath at 37°C. After every 30 seconds, the tube is tilted to see whether blood is clotted or not.

Q.16. What are the physiological variations in clotting time?

Physiologically clotting time is reduced in:

- Menstruation
- Before and during parturition

Q.17. What are the pathological variations in clotting time?

Clotting time is prolonged in:

- Haemophilia
- Genetic absence or deficiency of any clotting factor
- Liver diseases (can cause excessive bleeding in tissues)
- Vitamin K deficiency
- Anticoagulant therapy
- Disseminated intravascular coagulation.

Q.18. What is prothrombin time (PT)? What is its clinical significance?

- This test measures the clotting time of plasma in the presence of an optimal concentration of tissue extract (thromboplastin) and indicates the overall efficiency of the extrinsic clotting system.
- Normal prothrombin time is 10–12 seconds.
- *Clinical significance:* This test is commonly used to monitor oral anticoagulant therapy. Prolonged PT suggests the possibility of deficiency of factors II, V, VII and X.

Q.19. What is haemophilia?

- Haemophilia occurs due to a deficiency of factor VIII. It is X-linked recessive bleeding disorder. In haemophilia, only clotting time is prolonged (due to a deficiency of clotting factor VIII or IX).
- As platelet function is normal, bleeding time remains normal.
- *Haemophilia A:* It is classical haemophilia and the most common hereditary coagulation disorder (deficiency of factor VIII). Sex-linked disorder and is transmitted by females (they are carriers). There can be h/o repeated bleeding from joints, nose and even minor injuries.
- *Haemophilia B:* It is due to a deficiency of factor IX.
- *Treatment:* It includes clotting factors or blood transfusion.

Q.20. What is Christmas disease?

Christmas disease occurs due to a deficiency of factor IX. It is also called as haemophilia B.

Q.21. What is coagulation?

- It is a chemical irreversible process occurring due to the activation of all the clotting factors of blood.
- Clot is formed by formation of fibrin threads in which blood cells are trapped.

Q.22. What is agglutination?

It is a chemical irreversible process occurring due to reaction between agglutinogen and agglutinin. It causes clumping of red blood cells (RBCs). Later on, RBCs are hemolyzed.

Q.23. Name various tests to assess bleeding disorder.

- Bleeding time (as explained above)
- Clotting time (as explained above)
- Platelet count (as explained above and in the Chapter on platelet count)
- Prothrombin time (as explained above)
- **Clot retraction time:** Total clot retraction takes about 18 to 24 hrs. Clot retraction depends on platelet function. Clot lysis happens by 72 hrs normally.
- **Prothrombin consumption time:** It shows the amount of prothrombin present in serum after clot formation. Usually, more than 90% of prothrombin is converted to thrombin in the coagulation process. Thus more than 5% of prothrombin in serum indicates platelet deficiency.

- **Partial thromboplastin time:** The normal value is 60 to 80 seconds. It is prolonged with a deficiency of more than one clotting factor XII, XI, X, IX, V, II.

Q.24. What are the indications of doing BT and CT?

- Before any major/minor surgery
- Before putting the patient on blood thinners (anti-coagulant therapy)
- Family history of bleeding disorders
- Before biopsy (mainly from bone marrow)

Q.25. What is thrombosis? What is embolism?

- **Thrombosis:** It is the formation of blood clots in an unbroken blood vessel (atherosclerotic plaque formation may trigger it). Common arteries prone to atherosclerosis are –coronary arteries, carotid arteries, and cerebral arteries.
- **Embolism:** A thrombus may break open in small fragments called embolus (pleural-emboli) and can block even a tiny blood vessel of vital organs (e.g. brain, lungs). Besides blood clot, air or fat embolism can occur (common after fracture of bones).

Q.26. Enumerate common anticoagulants, their mechanism of action and their uses.

Name of anti-coagulant	Mechanism of action	Uses
Ammonium potassium oxalate	Precipitates calcium oxalate from plasma and decrease ionic calcium level and retards clotting process	Can be used only *in vitro* Used for estimation of CBC, ESR, PCV
Sodium citrate	Citrate combines with calcium in the blood to form unionized calcium, lack of ionic calcium prevents coagulation (chelation effect)	In blood bank for storing blood coagulation studies ESR (Westergren's method)
Heparin (natural constituent of blood)	Prevents formation of thrombin Prevents formation of fibrin Helps in deactivation of thrombin Increases amount of thrombin adsorbed by fibrin	Can be used *in vivo* and *in vitro* Osmotic fragility test, Blood gas analysis, pH assays
EDTA (ethylenedia-minetetra-acetic acid)	Chelation of calcium ions in blood	All routine haematological investigations except coagulation studies
Dicumarol derivatives	It competes with vitamin K and thus the synthesis of vitamin K-dependent clotting factors	It can be used only *in vivo*

Q.27. Enumerate conditions in which coagulation time is prolonged.

- **Deficiency of factor II (prothrombin), VII, IX and X:** This is observed with vitamin K deficiency, and liver diseases like cirrhosis, and hepatitis.
- **Deficiency of smaller components of factor VIII:** This is observed in classical haemophilia (haemophilia A).
- **Factor IX deficiency:** This is observed in Christmas disease.

Q.28. What is disseminated intravascular coagulation?

- This condition is seen following infection, mismatched blood transfusion, etc. where at many places in the body coagulation is activated which will decrease platelet count and also prolong prothrombin time with simultaneous stimulation of fibrinolysis.
- This can result in life-threatening haemorrhage.

Q.29. What are the indications of anticoagulant therapy?

Indications:

- Treatment of venous thrombosis
- Acute myocardial infarction
- Unstable angina
- Post-surgery

It includes low molecule weight heparin and warfarin. Usually, this is followed by fibrinolytic therapy with drugs like streptokinase, urokinase, and tissue plasminogen activator (TPA).

Contraindications of fibrinolytic therapy: Active internal bleeding, recent cerebrovascular accident, etc.

▋ OBJECTIVE STRUCTURED PRACTICAL EXAMINATION (OSPE)

Procedure station 1: To determine the clotting time of your own blood by capillary tube method.

S. No.	Assessment criteria	Marks assigned	Marks given
1.	Check for all aseptic precautions		
2.	Keep stopwatch ready		
3.	Check patency of capillary tube		
4.	Mark the time and after a prick collects blood in the capillary tube (as explained above)		
5.	Break capillary tube every 30 seconds (please check above)		
6.	Check for clotting and fibrin thread appearance		
7.	Report and viva on haematology experiment		
8.	Total		

Procedure station 2: To determine the bleeding time (by Duke's method) of your own blood by capillary tube method.

S. No.	Assessment criteria	Marks assigned	Marks given
1.	Check for all aseptic precautions		
2.	Keep stopwatch ready		
3.	Check the patency of capillary tube		
4.	After making a prick, mark the time and collect blood drops every 30 seconds until the bleeding stops		
5.	Accurately record the bleeding time		
6.	Prepare reports and be ready for the viva on the haematology experiment		
7.	Total time taken		

■ COMMON STATIONS—SPOTS IN PRACTICAL EXAMINATION (2/3 MARKS)

Q.1. Blotting paper, capillary tube: Identify and write its use in which haematological investigation, answer any one or two questions (check above).

Q.2. Clotting time is more than bleeding time. Give physiological basis.

Q.3. Picture with petechial haemorrhage: Identify and give a reason for the same.

Q.4. Heparin, streptokinase, urokinase kept. Enumerate 2 conditions where they are used.

■ CASE-BASED SCENARIO/PROBLEM-BASED

Case 1: A 8-year-old girl comes with h/o bleeding from an injury on the leg while playing a game. Teacher brought her to casualty as the bleeding was not stoppable after more than 10 minutes.

- Why physician ask for a platelet count immediately?
- What is the role of platelets in stopping the bleeding?
- Any other blood tests you would like to suggest?

■ KEY POINTS TO REMEMBER

- Bleeding time is always less than clotting time.
- Normal platelet count is $100,000–300,000/mm^3$ of blood.
- In haemophilia, clotting time is prolonged and bleeding time is normal; while in purpura, bleeding time is prolonged and clotting time is normal.
- **Coagulation:** It is a chemical irreversible process occurring due to activation of all the clotting factors of blood.
- **Agglutination:** It is a chemical irreversible process occurring due to a reaction between agglutinogen and agglutinin.

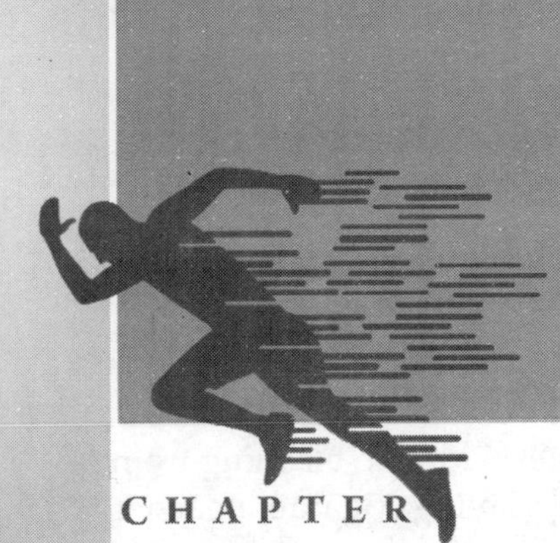

Determination of ESR

Learning Objectives

After completing this practical, the student shall be able to:
- Define what is erythrocyte sedimentation rate (ESR)
- Differentiate between Westergren's tube and Wintrobe's tube
- Give normal values for estimation of ESR and clinical significance
- List common conditions that cause alteration in ESR.

Aim

To determine the rate at which erythrocytes settle down in blood.

Apparatus

Pricking apparatus, Wintrobe's tube, Westergren's pipette with a rack, and blood sample.

Method of Determination

There are two methods for the determination of ESR:
1. Westergren's method
2. Wintrobe's method

Westergren's Method

Anticoagulated blood is taken in the pipette, and left undisturbed in a vertical position. The level of a column

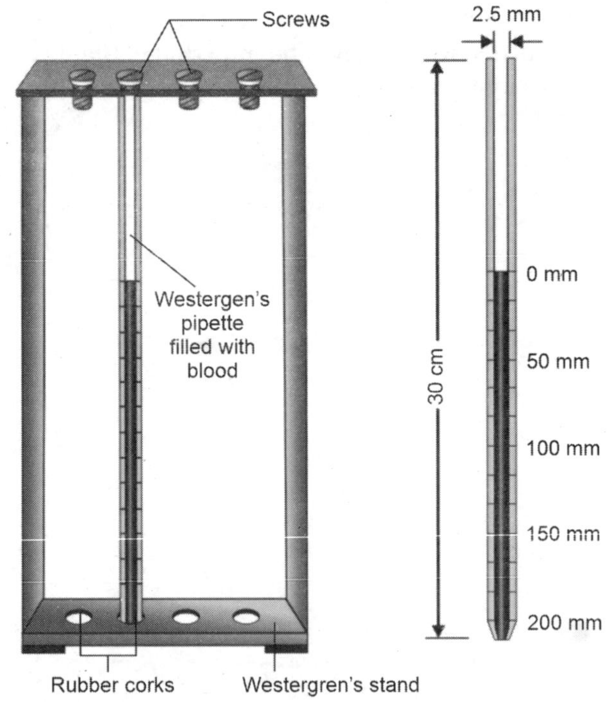

Fig. 9.1: Westergren's pipette with stand

of blood is noted at the beginning and at the end of 1 hour. ESR is noted as mm/at the end of 1 hour **(Fig. 9.1)**.

Westergren's Pipette

- Westergren's tube is open-ended. It is 300 mm in length. It has an internal bore of 2.5 mm.

- It is graduated from 0–200 mm above downwards, only along the lower two-third of length.

Blood Sample

- Sodium citrate (3.8%) is taken as anticoagulant.
- Ratio of blood to anticoagulant is 4:1. Ethylenediaminetetraacetic acid (EDTA) can also be used.

Procedure

- With usual aseptic precautions by method of venepuncture, venous blood is collected.
- Blood is placed in a tube containing 3.8% sodium citrate (4:1 ratio of blood to volume of citrate), and mixed properly. It is kept undisturbed for 1 hour. Observation is recorded at the end of 1 hour.

The normal range of ESR in this method is:

- In males: 3–5 mm at the end of 1 hour
- In females: 4–7 mm at the end of 1 hour

Wintrobe's Method

Ammonium potassium oxalate (ratio of 3:2) is used as an anticoagulant. Fresh EDTA can also be used as an anticoagulant.

Wintrobe's Tube

- Wintrobe's tube is thick-walled cylindrical tube 11 cm (110 mm) in length with internal bore of 3 mm.
- Marking from 0–10 above downwards is used for reading ESR.
- Marking from 0–10 below upwards is for reading hematocrit. It can hold about 1 ml of blood **(Fig. 9.2)**.

Procedure

- With all usual aseptic precautions by venepuncture, venous blood is collected.

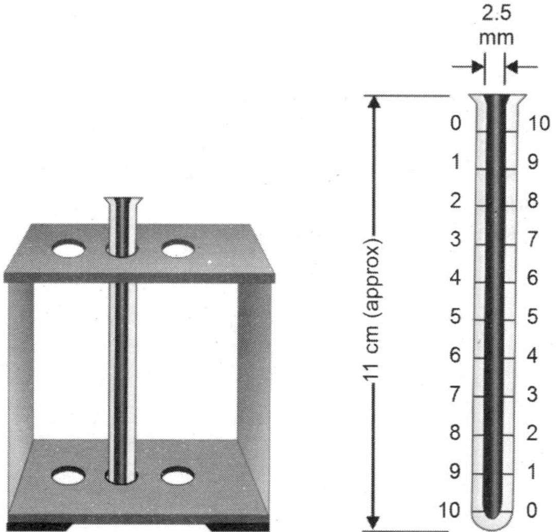

Fig. 9.2: Wintrobe's tube with stand with 0 to 10 above to downwards markings for ESR and 0 to 10 below upwards markings for PCV

- Blood is properly mixed with an anticoagulant. With the help of a Pasteur pipette, Wintrobe's tube is filled up to 0 mark.
- Wintrobe's tube is placed vertically and the time is noted. Observation is recorded at the end of 1 hour.

Normal range of ESR by Wintrobe's method is:

- In males: 0–9 mm at the end of 1 hour
- In females: 0–20 mm at the end of 1 hour

Precautions

- Concentration of anticoagulant should be appropriate.
- Blood should be properly mixed before filling the tubes.
- Blood should be filled exactly till mark zero.
- Tubes should be kept vertical in respective racks.
- Blood column should not contain any air bubbles or blood clots.
- Reading of ESR should be taken after one hour.
- The tube should be dry and clean before filling.
- Test should be carried out within 4 hrs after collecting blood.

■ IMPORTANT QUESTIONS AND ANSWERS

Q.1. What is rouleaux formation?

Rouleaux formation is piling up of red cells, they look like a stack of coins. Sedimentation is faster when the size and number of rouleaux are large (ESR is settling down of RBCs due to rouleaus formation and in PCV settling of cells is accomplished by centrifugation process).

Q.2. What are the advantages and disadvantages of Westergren's and Wintrobe's methods?

Westergren's method	Wintrobe's method
Advantages	**Advantages**
• Column is higher so ESR is measured easily • Test is more sensitive	• PCV can be measured in supernatant plasma used for serological tests • The amount of blood required is less
Disadvantages	**Disadvantages**
• More amount of blood required • PCV cannot be determined • Sodium citrate dilutes RBC (increases ESR)	More chances of air bubbles as the bore of the tube is narrow

Q.3. What are the factors affecting ESR?

Factors affecting/influencing ESR

- **Size of rouleaux:** Lesser the size and a number of rouleaux faster is the sedimentation.
- **Plasma factors:** More the fibrinogen concentration more is the rouleaux formation. (Fibrinogen neutralizes the charges on red cells and makes red cells sticky).

- **Number of red cells**: Polycythemia decreases ESR. Anaemia increases ESR.
- **Viscosity of blood**: The more viscous the blood, the rate of sedimentation decreases and vice-versa.
- **Temperature:** An increase in temperature increases ESR.

Q.4. What is the clinical significance of ESR?

- ESR is not a diagnostic test. It is known to increase in many inflammatory conditions. ESR gives a clue to the physician regarding the progress of the disease and the response of the disease to treatment.
- For prognostic purposes, this test is especially used in tuberculosis and rheumatic fever.

Q.5. What are physiological and pathological variations in ESR?

Physiological variations in ESR	
Increase in ESR:	**Decrease in ESR:**
• Exercise	• High altitude (polycythemia)
• Pregnancy (increased fibrinogen and globulin)	• Infants
• Females	• Males

Pathological variations in ESR	
Increase in ESR:	**Decrease in ESR:**
• Acute infections (pneumonia)	• Polycythemia
• Chronic infections (tuberculosis)	• Decrease fibrinogen level
• Acute noninfective infections (gout)	• Hereditary spherocytosis
• Anaemia	• Sickle cell anaemia
• Collagen diseases	

Q.6. Explain the mechanism of sedimentation of erythrocytes.

Sedimentation can be observed in three stages

- **Preliminary/first stage**: Stage during which time rouleaux formation occurs and aggregates are formed. This happens in the first 10 to 15 minutes.
- **Second stage**: This is the period in which the sinking of the aggregates takes place at a constant speed. This phase occurs for more than half an hour.
- **Third stage**: In this stage, the rate of sedimentation slows as aggregated cells pack at the bottom of the tube. This happens in the last 12–15 minutes (with shorter tube-like Wintrobs's tube, packing may start before an hour has elapsed).

Q.7. How do RBCs remain separate in circulating blood?

In circulatory blood, RBCs are continuously moving. They are known to repel each other due to their negative electrostatic charges (imparted by sialic acid moieties on cell membranes) mutually repel each other. This repulsion force is known as zeta potential.

Q.8. Which anticoagulants are used when ESR is estimated with Westergren's and Wintrobe's method?

- Citrate solution and sodium-potassium oxalate are used as anticoagulants in Westergren's and Wintrobe's methods respectively to prevent clotting of blood.
- Oxalate used, does prevent changes in size and shape of the cell, which is required as we find out PCV after estimating ESR.

■ COMMON STATIONS– SPOTS IN PRACTICAL EXAMINATION (2/3 MARKS)

Q.1. Westergren's tube, Wintrobe's tube, stand: Identify and write its use.

Q.2. Westergren's and Wintrobe's tube: Identify and enumerate the advantages and disadvantages of both.

■ CASE-BASED SCENARIO/PROBLEM-BASED

Case 1: A person suffering from some infection/inflammatory condition, or anaemia with raised ESR values. Comment on the same, and enumerate factors that alter ESR (physiological/pathological).

■ KEY POINTS TO REMEMBER

- ESR is not a diagnostic but a prognostic test.
- ESR indicates the rate at which RBCs settle down, it is high in anaemia and low in polycythemia.
- The normal range of ESR is different in Westergren's and Wintrobe's methods, always ESR in females is always on the higher side (due to fewer RBCs in females).

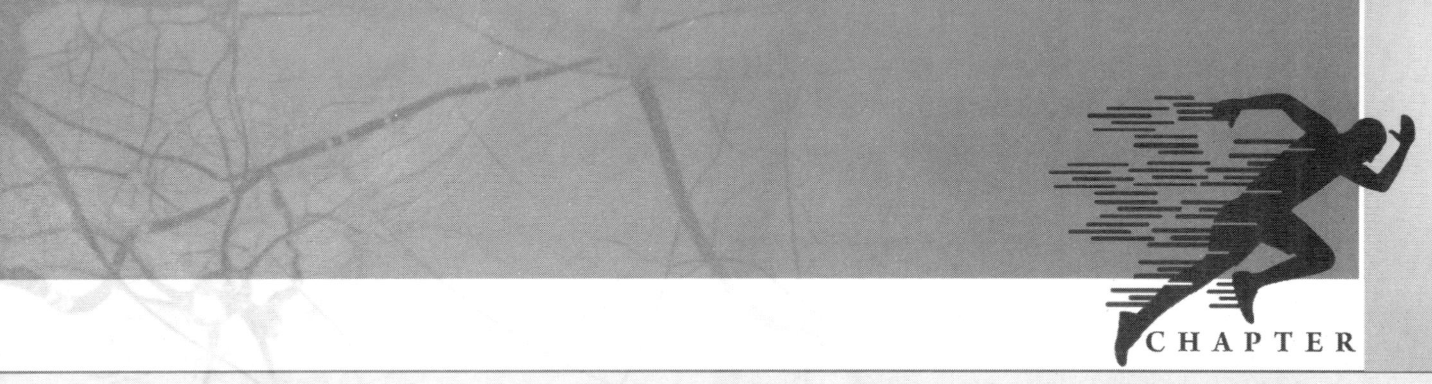

Determination of Blood Indices

Learning Objectives

At the end of this practical, the students shall be able to:
- Enumerate various types of blood indices with normal range and how to obtain them
- Give morphological classification of anaemia
- Enumerate formulas for different blood indices.

Different blood indices are calculated from:
- Hemoglobin (Hb) concentration
- RBC (red blood cell) count
- PCV (packed cell volume)

These indices are helpful in the diagnosis of the type of anaemia.

The following indices are calculated:
- Mean corpuscular volume (MCV)
- Mean corpuscular haemoglobin (MCH)
- Mean corpuscular haemoglobin concentration (MCHC)
- Colour index.

A. Mean Corpuscular Volume

- It is the mean or average volume of each red cell. It is expressed in cubic microns, i.e.

$$MCV = \frac{PCV \times 10}{RBC \text{ counts in million mm}^3}$$

- Normal MCV varies from 82–92 cubic microns.

- **MCV:** It is a very reliable indicator of red cell size. RBCs with normal MCV are called normocytes, those with high MCV are called macrocytes and those with low MCV is called microcytes. Accordingly, anaemia is labelled as macrocytic, microcytic, and normocytic.
- **Macrocytosis:** It is observed in deficiency of vitamin B12 and deficiency of folic acid.
- **Microcytosis:** It is observed in iron deficiency.

Derivation of MCV

If PCV is 45%, i.e. in 1 cu mm of blood PCV = 0.45cu mm
Then, the number of cells in the same volume of blood (1cu mm) = 5 million
Therefore,

$$MCV = \frac{0.45 \text{ mm}^3}{5 \text{ million}}$$

$$= \frac{0.45 \times 1 \text{ mm} \times 1 \text{ mm} \times 1 \text{ mm}}{5000,000}$$

Substituting it:
MCV = 0.45 × 1000 × 1000 × 1000/ 5000000
= 0.45 × 1000/5
= 45 × 10/5
= 90 cubic microns

B. Mean Corpuscular Haemoglobin (Normal range 27 to 32 picograms)

- It indicates the amount of Hb (by weight in picograms) present in each cell.

$$MCHC \text{ (g/dL)} = haemoglobin/haematocrit$$

- Average MCH varies from 27 picograms to 32 pico-grams. When MCH is normal, it is described as normochromic. An increase in MCH is described as hyperchromic and a decrease in MCH is described as hypochromic.

- Accordingly, anaemia can be labelled as normochromic, hyperchromic, or hypochromic.

Derivation of MCH

If Hb = 15 g/100 ml, the RBC count is 5 million/cu mm of blood
Hb is expressed as g/100 ml of blood. It should be converted to picograms
1 g = 10^{12} picograms
Hb = 15×10^{12} picograms/100 ml
RBC count is expressed in cu mm. It should be converted to count per 100 ml because Hb concentration is expressed per 100 ml
Thus, RBC count = 5 million/cu mm of blood
In 1 cu mm = 5000000 × 1000
In 100 cu cm = 5000000 × 1000 × 100
Thus MCV = Hb in picograms per 100 ml/number of RBCs per 100 ml
$$= 15 \times 10^{12}/5000000 \times 1000 \times 100$$
$$= 15 \times 10/5$$
$$= 30 \text{ picograms}$$

C. Mean Corpuscular Haemoglobin Concentration (Normal range: 32–38%)

- It indicates the degree of saturation of RBC with Hb.
- Instead of expressing Hb per cell (as in MCH), it is expressed per volume of the cell.
- Haemoglobin concentration is expressed in terms of percent saturation.
- There is some limit beyond which red cells cannot contain Hb. Therefore, under no conditions, the value of MCHC can be increased.
- The normal range of MCHC is 32–38%. It can never be more than 38%.
- It can be less when there is hypochromic anaemia (usually due to iron deficiency).

$$MCHC = \frac{Hb \text{ (in g/l)}}{RBC \text{ (in millions/µl)}}$$

Derivation of MCHC

Hb is expressed in grams/100 ml (15 g per 100 ml)
Therefore, PCV also should be expressed in ml per 100 ml
Therefore, PCV= 45 ml/100 ml
Therefore
MCHC = Hb in g/100 ml/ PCV in 100 ml × 100
$$= 15/45 \times 100$$
$$= 33.3\%$$

D. Colour Index

- Colour index (CI) is the ratio of the concentration of Hb to red blood cells when both are expressed in the same units, i.e. percentage of normal 14.5 g of Hb/100 ml is considered as 100%.

- The RBC count of 5 million per cubic millimetre is considered as 100%.

$$CI = \frac{14.5 \text{ g Hb/100 ml}}{5 \text{ million RBC in mm}^3}$$

= 100% Hb / 100% RBC count
= 1

- Normal colour index ratio is one. It varies from 0.8 to 1.2.
- Colour index indicates the average amount of Hb per cell (as MCH). But when both Hb concentration and RBC count are simultaneously decreased, the colour index remains within the normal range. Therefore, the colour index is not significant clinically.

■ IMPORTANT QUESTIONS AND ANSWERS

Q.1. What is the importance of calculating various blood indices?
MCV, MCH, and MCHC are helpful in the classification and diagnosis of anaemia. These indices are widely used in clinical haematology.

Q.2. How do you classify anaemia morphologically?
- Anaemia are classified according to size, shape, and % of Hb in RBC.
- MCV is mean corpuscular volume. When, it is in the normal range it is called normocyte. When MCV is less it is called microcyte and more MCV is called macrocytic. Microcytosis is observed with iron deficiency anaemia and macrocytosis in megaloblastic anaemia (vitamin B12 deficiency).
- MCHC is the mean corpuscular haemoglobin concentration. When, it is in the normal range cell is normochromic. When MCHC is less it is called hypochromic.

Depending on the morphology of RBCs we can have different types of anaemia.
- Iron deficiency anaemia is microcytic and hypochromic and vitamin B12 deficiency anaemia is macrocytic normochromic.
- Normocytic normochromic anaemia can be seen with renal diseases, acute blood loss, etc. For other types of classification of anaemia, refer to Chapter 6.

Q.3. Why MCHC cannot go beyond 38%?
MCHC is an average concentration of Hb in the RBC volume. Thus, it cannot extend beyond a certain limit.

▌ COMMON STATIONS – SPOTS IN PRACTICAL EXAMINATION (2/3 MARKS)

- Hb, PCV, and RBC count can be given and asked to find out MCV, MCH, and MCHC. Answer any one or two questions from the above.

Plate 1

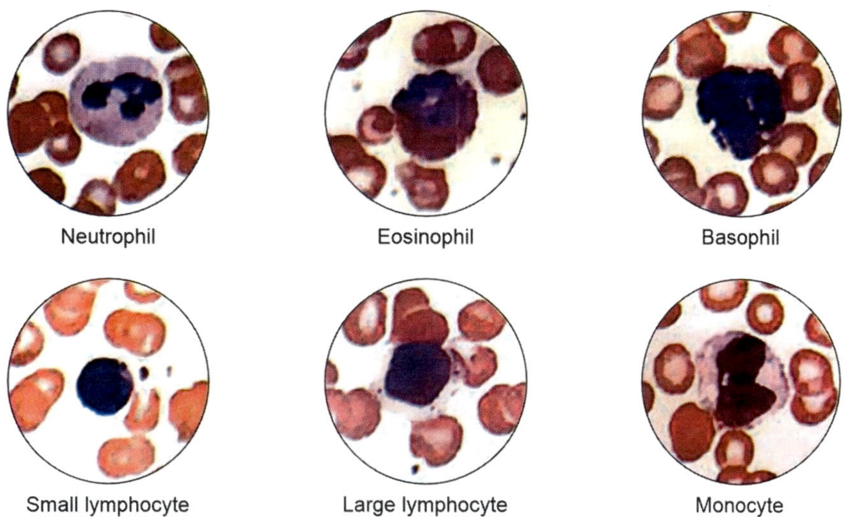

Neutrophil
Eosinophil
Basophil
Small lymphocyte
Large lymphocyte
Monocyte

Fig. 7.4: Different types of white blood cells

Plasma (55%)
Cells (45%)
Buffy coat
(white blood cells, platelets)
Red blood cells

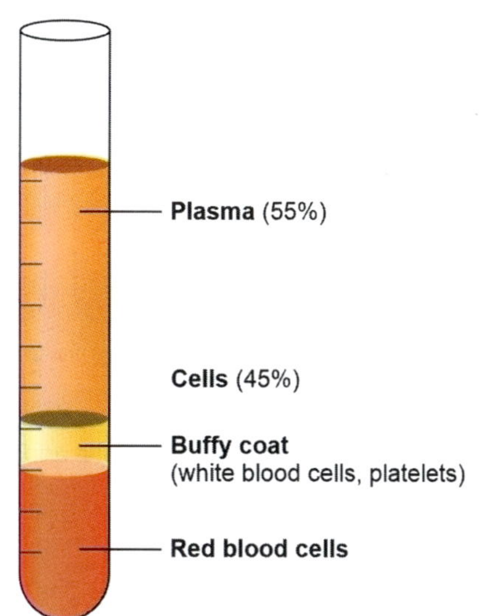

Fig. 11.1: Formation of layers after centrifugation

Plate 2

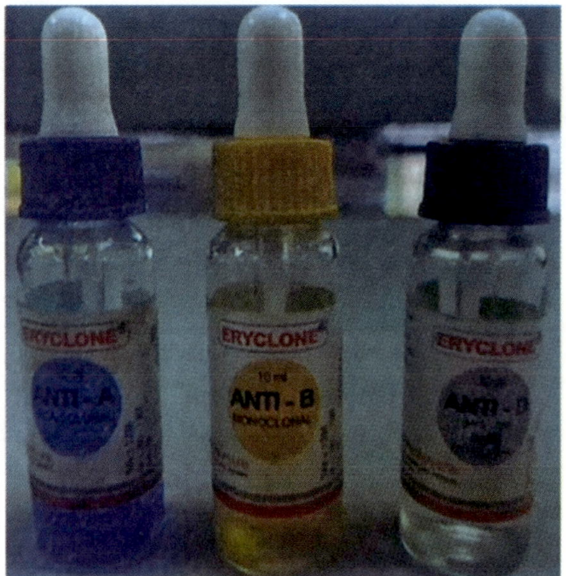

Fig. 12.1: Blood group antisera

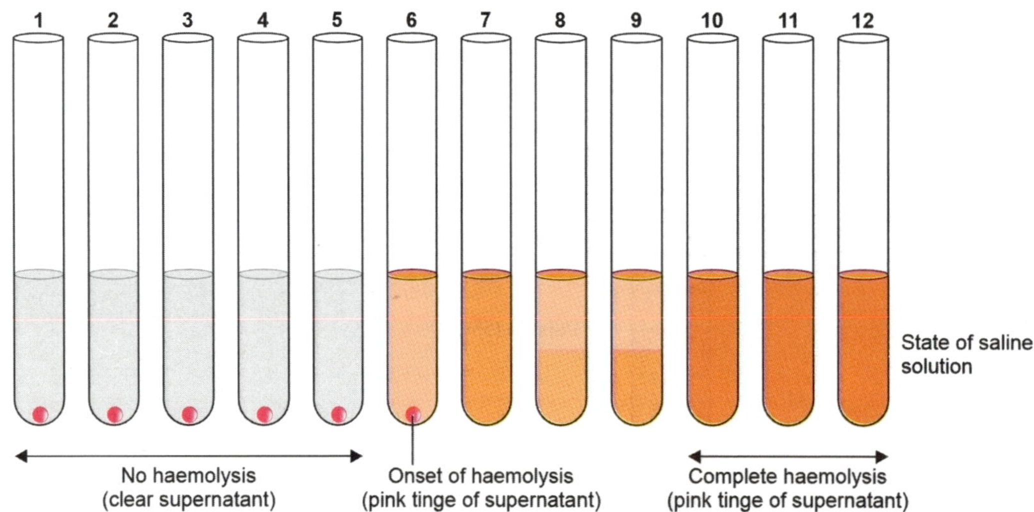

Fig. 13.1: Osmotic fragility– haemolysis starts in the sixth tube and is completed in the 10th tube

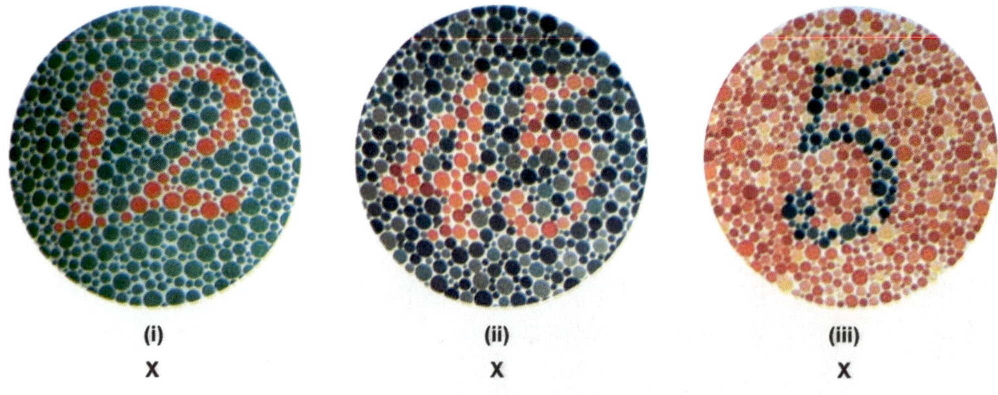

Fig. 50.1: Ishihara's chart

- Tick the correct option for the following statements:
  - **A. Normocytic normochromic anaemia** (e.g. acute blood loss, renal disease)
    MCV – Normal/raised/decreased
    MCHC – Normal/raised/decreased
  - **B. Microcytic hypochromic anaemia** (e.g. iron deficiency anaemia)
    MCV – Normal/raised/decreased
    MCHC – Normal/raised/decreased
  - **C. Macrocytic normochromic anaemia** (e.g. vitamin B12 and folic acid deficiency, i.e. megaloblastic anaemia)
    MCV – Normal/raised/decreased
    MCHC– Normal/raised/decreased

■ KEY POINTS TO REMEMBER

- MCV, MCH, and MCHC are blood indices. With the help of blood indices, one can diagnose the type of anaemia.
- Morphological classification of anaemia is done according to size, shape of RBC, and amount of Hb content of RBC.
- Iron-deficiency anaemia gives rise to microcytic hypochromic anaemia.
- Vitamin B12 deficiency causes macrocytic hypochromic anaemia.

11

Determination of Packed Cell Volume (Haematocrit)

Competency:
PY2.12: Describe the haematocrit test. Note the findings and interpret the results.

Learning Objectives

After completion of this practical, you will be able to:
- Identify the Wintrobe's tube
- Give normal values of packed cell volume (PCV) in men and women
- List conditions that alter PCV
- List precautions and errors in the determination of PCV
- Give physiological basis of alteration in PCV in different conditions.

Packed Cell Volume

- Packed cell volume (PCV) is the volume of red cells expressed as a percentage of the total volume of blood.
- It is called haematocrit. Haematocrit is a reliable indicator of the red cell population. PCV can be measured by the macrohaematocrit method and micro-haematocrit method. Wintrobe's method described in the chapter is the macrohaematocrit method.

Principle

Red blood cells are heavier (specific gravity 1,090) than plasma (specific gravity 1,030). Blood to which anticoagulant is added is placed in a tube and centrifuged. Cells settle down due to centrifugal force. Reading of PCV is expressed as a percentage of volume of whole blood.

Apparatus

Wintrobe's tube (described in Chapter 9 on ESR), centrifuging machine, Pasteur pipette, blood sample [usually ethylenediaminetetraacetic acid (EDTA) or oxalate is used as anticoagulant].

Procedure

- Carefully mix the bulb containing the blood specimen.
- Fill A Pasteur pipette with blood to a 10 cm mark (if the level crosses the mark, remove excess blood with the help of a dropper).
- Place the pipette at the bottom of the Wintrobe's tube and withdraw the pipette as blood gets filled in the tube (prevents air bubbles).
- Centrifuge for 30 minutes at 3,000 rpm **(Fig. 11.1)** and then observe the tubes.

Observation

- In the tube, the uppermost layer is straw-coloured plasma.
- At the bottom, red cells are packed. Their upper limit is noted.
- On the top of red cells is a thin layer of WBCs and above it is a buffy layer of platelets.
- If the uppermost limit of packed red cells is noted as 4.5, then

$$PCV = 4.5 \times 10 = 45\%$$

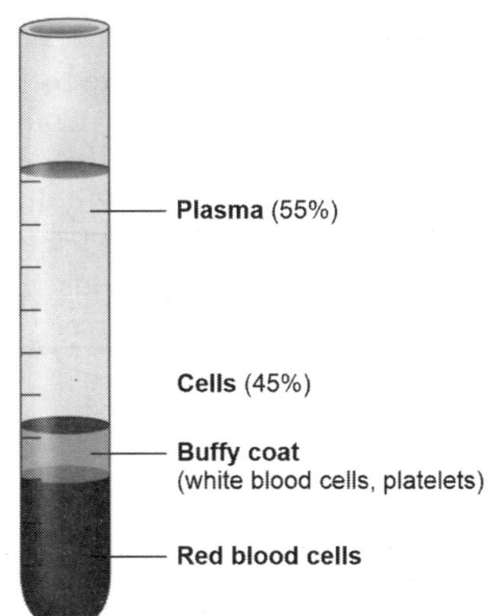

Fig. 11.1: Formation of layers after centrifugation
(For colour version, See plate 1)

Precautions

- Mix the blood thoroughly.
- Anticoagulants should not affect the size and shape of red cells.
- If air bubbles appear, repeat the procedure.
- Take reading exactly at the end of one hour (excluding buffy coat).

Normal Value of PCV

- In males: 38–54%
- In females: 30–47%

■ IMPORTANT QUESTIONS AND ANSWERS

Q.1. What is the clinical significance of PCV?

- It is a reasonable index of red cell population or haemoglobin content.
- Haematocrit (PCV) is useful in the determination of blood indices, which helps in the diagnosis of the type of anaemia.
- Haematocrit is an important determinant of the viscosity of blood.
- It helps to determine the state of hydration of the body.

Q.2. Name of different layers seen in Wintrobe's tube from above downwards.

From above downwards, different layers after plasma are a layer of platelets, a layer of WBCs, and a layer of RBCs.

Q.3. What are the methods for determining PCV?

- **Macrohaematocrit method:** Wintrobe's tubes
- **Microhaematocrit method:** Capillary haematocrit tubes
- **Advanced laboratories:** Automated techniques.

Q.4. What are physiological variations in PCV?

Physiological variations	
Increase in PCV:	**Decrease in PCV:**
• High altitude • Newborns and infants	• Pregnancy (hemodilution) • Less in females than males • More water intake

Q.5. What are pathological variations in PCV?

Pathological variations	
Increase in PCV:	**Decrease in PCV:**
• Hypoxia to the tissues (e.g. emphysema, congenital heart diseases, etc.) • Polycythemia vera • Severe dehydration • Burns • Dehydration	• Different types of anaemia • Conditions causing hemo-dilution • Emphysema of the lungs • Congenital heart disease (any condition that causes inadequate supply of O_2 to tissues)

Q.6. What is true haematocrit/true cell volume?

Even if red cells are fully packed, about 2% of plasma is trapped between the cells. Therefore,

True haematocrit = 0.97–0.99 × observed haematocrit.

Q.7. What is body haematocrit?

Body haematocrit is = 0.87 × observed haematocrit (this correction is required as red cell mass is unequally distributed throughout the body).

Q.8. What information do you get from supernatant plasma?

- Supernatant plasma should be yellowish in colour, which indicates that RBCs are not hemolyzed.
- If it is reddish in colour, it indicates hemolysis (destruction of RBCs).
- Yellow colour of supernatant plasma indicates jaundice; while turbid colour is seen in lipoedema.

Q.9. Why is the haematocrit value of venous blood, normally 3% more than that of arterial blood?

Venous blood is carried from tissues to lungs. Due to chloride shift, the volume of each red cell increases therefore venous haematocrit is more than arterial blood haematocrit.

Q.10. Enumerate factors affecting the speed of packing of cells.

Factors affecting the speed of packing of red cells are:

- Viscosity of suspending fluid
- Density and size of cells
- Centrifugal force

Q.11. What is microhaematocrit?

It is a method to find out PCV with the help of a small quantity of blood collected in a microcapillary tube, which is centrifuged at a higher speed.

COMMON STATIONS–SPOTS IN PRACTICAL EXAMINATION (2/3 MARKS)

- *Wintrobe's tube, centrifuge machine:* Diagram/instrument. Identify and write its uses. Answer any one or two questions from the above.
- *Westergren's tube (PCV):* Identify and label all different layers.
- Hb–10 g%, PCV= 40%. Find out MCV. What happens to MCV with megaloblastic anaemia?
- Hb– 8 g%, PCV= 32%, RBC count 4 million/cumm of blood. Find out MCHC.
  (Check case studies in the Chapter on Hb estimation, and RBC count)

KEY POINTS TO REMEMBER

- Packed cell volume is the volume of red cells expressed as a percentage of the total volume of blood.
- PCV values have been found more in newborns and people staying at high altitudes. Physiologically in males, PCV is more as compared to females.
- Speed of packing of red cells depends upon the size and density of cells, centrifugal force, and viscosity of suspending fluid.

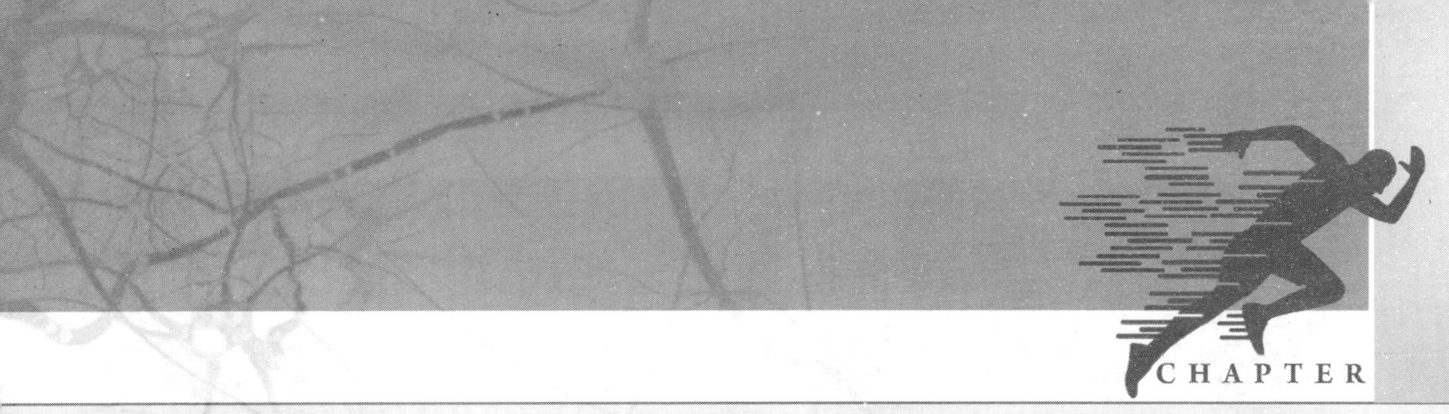

Determination of Blood Groups

Competency:

PY 2.11: Estimate blood groups.

Learning Objectives

After completion of this practical, the students shall be able to:

- Name different blood group systems
- Give the physiological significance of ABO and Rhesus (Rh) system
- Determine the blood group from a given sample of blood
- List the precautions and errors during the determination of blood group
- State Landsteiner's law
- Give importance to the cross-matching of blood and the concept of major and minor cross-matching
- List common hazards of blood transfusion
- Give common indications of blood transfusion.

Aim

To determine the blood group (ABO and Rh).

Apparatus

Glass slides, dropper, porcelain tiles with 12 depressions, normal saline, anti-A serum, anti-B serum, spirit, anti-D serum, and 1% sodium citrate prepared in normal saline.

Different Blood Groups

Depending on the type of agglutinogen present, there are four types of blood groups.

- A group—containing "A" agglutinogen and anti-B agglutinins.
- B group—containing "B" agglutinogen and anti-A agglutinins.
- AB group—containing both "A" and "B" agglutinogens and no agglutinins.
- O group—not containing either "A" or "B" agglutinogens and both agglutinins are present.

Principle

Agglutination reaction happens between antigens present/absent on the RBC membrane and antibodies present/absent in the serum. Depending on the agglutination, blood groups are determined.

Procedure

- Three to four drops of sodium citrate solution are put in one of the depressions on the porcelain tile. It is labelled "D".
- With usual aseptic precautions, the finger is pricked and two drops of blood are mixed with sodium citrate solution placed in the depression "D".
- Thus, red blood cell suspension is obtained.
- Two drops of anti A and Anti B serum **(Fig. 12.1)**, and normal saline are put in three different depressions and they are labelled A, B, and C. Note-separate pipettes are used for anti-A and anti-B to avoid contamination of sera.

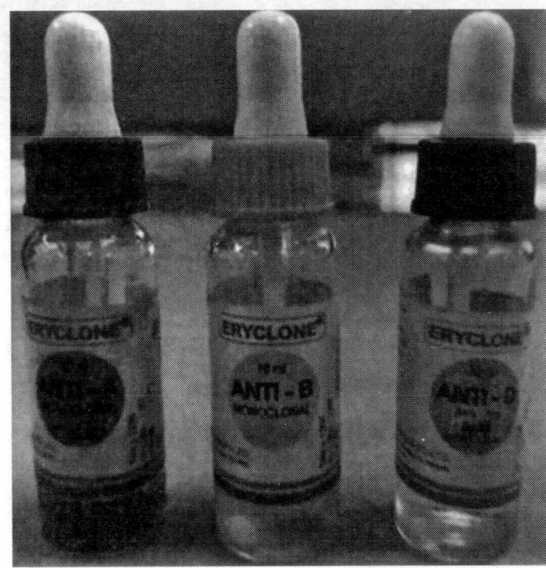

Fig. 12.1: Blood group antisera *(For colour version, See plate 2).*

TABLE 12.1: Determination of blood group		
Anti-A	*Anti-B*	*Blood group*
+	-	A group
-	+	B group
+	+	AB group
-	-	O group

- Two drops of cell suspension (from D) are put in each of these depressions (A, B, and C). It is mixed by blowing.
- After 15 minutes, A, B, and C depressions are observed for the presence or absence of agglutination.
- C depression acts as a control (for comparing between agglutination and no agglutination). In depression, C agglutination does not occur. If by any chance agglutination occurs in this control (C), the whole procedure is to be repeated.
- Blood group is determined depending on the presence of a particular antigen and corresponding agglutinogen on RBC.
- Agglutination is confirmed by taking a drop from each depression on the slide and observing the slide under the microscope.
- By using anti-D serum, the Rh group of the person is determined.
  (*Note:* Agglutination means clumping of RBCs, which happens due to a reaction between agglutinogen and agglutinin. Coagulation occurs due to the activation of clotting factors).

Precautions

- All aseptic precautions are taken.
- Slides and porcelain tile should be dry and clean.
- Labeling on the tile with A, B, and C depressions should be proper.
- Confirm findings under microscope.

■ IMPORTANT QUESTIONS AND ANSWERS

Q.1. What are different blood group systems?
More than 30 blood group systems are known. The important ones are—ABO, Rh, MN, S, P, E, Kell, Duffy, Kidd, etc.

Q.2. What is the basis of the classification of blood groups?
- Human RBCs on their surface (cell membrane) contain a series of glycoproteins and glycolipids, which constitute blood group antigens.
- On the basis of the presence of these antigens, blood group systems are classified **(Table 12.1)**.
- Development of these antigens is genetically controlled.

Q.3. What is the cross-matching of blood?
- Blood is collected from the donor and the recipient. Plasma and red cells are separated in each.
- Then donor's cells are mixed with the recipient's plasma (major cross-matching).
- Recipient's cells are matched with the donor's plasma (minor cross-matching).

Q.4. Why is the matching of the donor's cells with the recipient's plasma called major cross-matching?
There is a high agglutinin concentration in the recipient's plasma. Due to the high concentration of agglutinins reaction can easily take place (between the donor's cells and the recipient's plasma) and therefore matching of the donor's cells with the recipient's plasma is called major cross-matching.

Q.5. Why is matching between the donor's plasma and the recipient's cells called minor cross-matching?
- Reaction of the donor's plasma and recipient's cells is not very important, and usually does not occur on giving a mismatched transfusion; therefore, it is called minor cross-matching.
- Donor's plasma when enters the recipient's circulation, gets diluted with the recipient's blood. Therefore, antibody titer is not high enough to cause agglutinogen.

Q.6. State Landsteiner's law.
- This law states that if an agglutinogen is present on the red cell membrane, the corresponding agglutinin must be absent in plasma and vice-versa.
- This law is applicable to the ABO group system and only the first half of the law is applicable to the Rh group system.

Q.7. What is the importance of the MN system?

The MN system is usually required for paternity tests. MN groups are also useful in genetic and anthropological studies.

Q.8. What is the importance of blood groups?

Importance of blood groups:

- To study human genetics.
- Problems of identity and parentage.
- Study of anthropogeny.
- Association and proneness to disease, e.g. group-A people suffer more from gastric carcinoma, etc.
- Rh group is important for marriage counselling.
- To ensure compatible blood transfusion.

Q.9. What is a blood transfusion?

- Blood transfusion is defined as a collection of whole blood from the donor, and its infusion into the venous blood of the recipient.
- Transfusion can be of whole blood or it can be as packed red cells, white cells, platelets, or fresh frozen plasma.
- Blood transfusion carries a definite risk and therefore should be given only, if other simpler, and safer therapy has proved ineffective.

Q.10. What are the indications for blood transfusion?

Common indications for blood transfusion are:

- Pre- and postoperative
- Acute blood loss
- Chronic anaemia
- Bone marrow failure
- Purpura
- Clotting factor deficiencies
- Thalassemia

Q.11. What are the complications of blood transfusion?

Complications of blood transfusion are:

- Air embolism due to faulty technique of transfusion. Citrate toxicity (tetany) due to the rapid rate of transfusion.
- Febrile reactions—fever and rigour.
- Allergic reactions—itching, urticaria and anaphylactic reaction.
- Circulatory overload—heart failure.
- Hemolytic reactions—jaundice and hemoglobinuria.
- Transmission of diseases—hepatitis, malaria, AIDS, and syphilis.
- Transfusion hemosiderosis.
- Post-transfusion purpura.

Q.12. What is a mismatched blood transfusion?

When incompatible blood is transfused, it is called as mismatched transfusion.

Q.13. What are the hazards of mismatched blood transfusion?

Hazards of mismatched transfusion are as follows:

With mismatched blood transfusion mainly donor's cells agglutinate in the recipient's circulation leading to an immediate severe hemolytic reaction occurs. It is characterized by the following phases:

- **Phase of hemolytic shock:** Severity depends on the rate of intravascular red cell destruction. Common symptoms are fever, breathlessness, vomiting, etc.
- **Post-shock phase:** Because of red cell destruction, there is free haemoglobin in the blood which increases bilirubin leading to jaundice, and haemoglobinuria.
- **Oliguric phase:** With hemolytic reaction, kidneys are damaged due to the development of acute tubular necrosis and renal failure.

Q.14. What is the clinical importance of the Rh group?

- In the Rh group system, natural antibodies against Rh are not present.
- Therefore, by any chance, Rh –ve person receives Rh +ve blood for the first time; the Rh antigen causes sensitization (large numbers of agglutinins are formed against the Rh antigen).
- If a person is given Rh +ve blood next time, he gets a severe reaction.

Q.15. What is erythroblastosis fetalis?

- If Rh (–ve) women bears Rh +ve fetus for the first time, sensitization occurs.
- At the time of delivery, fetal RBCs enter the maternal circulation. Mother gets sensitized and agglutinins against Rh antigens are formed.
- If next time a woman bears Rh +ve fetus again, agglutinins pass through the placenta causing agglutination of fetal RBCs leading to erythroblastosis fetalis.
- Erythroblastosis fetalis can be prevented by desensitizing pregnant Rh –ve mother (having Rh +ve fetus).

Q.16. What precautions should be taken during blood transfusion?

Precautions taken during blood transfusion are:

- Proper aseptic precautions must be taken during transfusion.
- Transfusion should be done only if it is absolutely indicated.
- Donor's and recipient's blood groups should be checked and cross-matched.
- Before starting the transfusion, the label on the blood bottle should be checked for the name and the blood group.
- Transfusion should be given at a slow rate (not more than 20 drops per minute) with blood temperature the same as room temp.

Q.17. What precautions are taken while selecting the donor?

The following precautions are taken for selecting the donor:

- Donor should be healthy.

- Donors should be not suffer from diseases like syphilis, malaria, AIDS, etc. which are spread through blood.
- Donor's haemoglobin and PCV should be within normal range.

Q.18. How is blood stored?

- Blood is collected with complete aseptic precautions. It is stored in a sterile container.
- To each 480 ml of blood 120 ml of ACD mixture is added. Blood stored at 4°C can be used for about 21 days.
- Long-term storage of blood can cause lysis of RBCs and WBCs. Various platelet coagulation factors (factor V and VIII) are destroyed.
- Acid citrate dextrose (ACD) mixture contains—acid citric (monohydrous)—0.48 g, trisodium citrate—1.32 g, dextrose—1.47 g, and distal water to make 100 ml.

Q.19. Why is glucose added to the ACD mixture?

- RBCs in collected blood, tend to swell and hemolyze unless Na^+, K^+ pump remains active to maintain the size of RBCs.
- To remain active Na^+, K^+ pump requires energy which is obtained from glucose.

Q.20. Enumerate various blood fractions used for transfusion.

Blood fractions	Common indications
Packed red cells	Chronic anaemia
Platelet concentrate	Thrombocytopenia
Plasma (human albumin)	Burns
Cryoprecipitate, fibrinogen	Factor VIII deficiency
Fresh frozen plasma	Coagulation disorders

Q.21. What are secretors and non-secretors?

- Some people who secrete blood group antigens in saliva (in all body fluids except CSF) are called secretors.
- People who do not secrete blood group antigens in saliva are called non-secretors.

Q.22. Enumerate differences between coagulation and agglutination.

Coagulation and agglutination: Both are chemical and irreversible processes.

Coagulation	Aglutination
Presence of fibrin threads with RBCs trapped	There is a clumping of RBCs
Occurs due to activation of the coagulation process	Occurs due to a reaction between agglutinogen and agglutinin

Q.23. What is Bombay's blood group?

Bombay blood group: Phenotypes of the blood group lack H antigen on the RBC membrane (have anti-H in serum). Thus there is no antigen A or B in red cells, but plasma does contain anti-A, anti-B and anti-H antibodies.

▌ OBJECTIVE STRUCTURED PRACTICAL EXAMINATION (OSPE)

Aim

To determine the blood group of your own blood/given sample.

Procedure

The procedure for determination of the blood group is given above.

S. No.	Assessment criteria	Marks assigned	Marks given
1.	Arrange all apparatus as required to do the experiment		
2.	With all aseptic precautions, prick the finger and mix it with sodium citrate and add it to each depression of the tile		
3.	Confirm that anti-A, anti-B, and control are taken properly.		
4.	Do all procedures as explained above to find out the blood group of own/ given sample		
5.	Blow contents properly and mix them well		
6.	Confirm agglutination under a microscope		
7.	Report and viva on haematology experiment		
8.	Total		

Please note: For finding out Rh group +ve/-ve anti-D is mixed in the blood sample. Agglutination indicates it is RH +ve. No agglutination Rh –ve.

▌ COMMON STATIONS – SPOTS IN PRACTICAL EXAMINATION (2/3 MARKS)

- **Anti-A, anti-B or anti-D sera bottles** can be shown: Identify any one or two questions from the above.
- **Na citrate bottle:** Write the mechanism of action as an anti-coagulant (clue–chelation of calcium ions retards the process of clotting).

▌ CASE-BASED SCENARIO/PROBLEM-BASED (2/3 MARKS)

Case 1: A 40-year-old lady was advised blood transfusion. As the transfusion started, she developed chills and got a fever.

- What probably the lady is having?
- Enumerate precautions before blood transfusion.
- Enumerate hazards of mismatched blood transfusion

■ KEY POINTS TO REMEMBER

- There are different ways of classifying blood groups. Landsteiner's law states, that if agglutinogen is present on the surface of RBC corresponding agglutinin is absent in plasma and vice-versa.

- **Major cross-matching:** When the donor's cells are mixed with the recipient's plasma and minor cross-matching is when the recipient's cells are mixed with the donor's plasma.

- Erythroblastosis fetalis can be prevented by giving anti Rh antibodies.

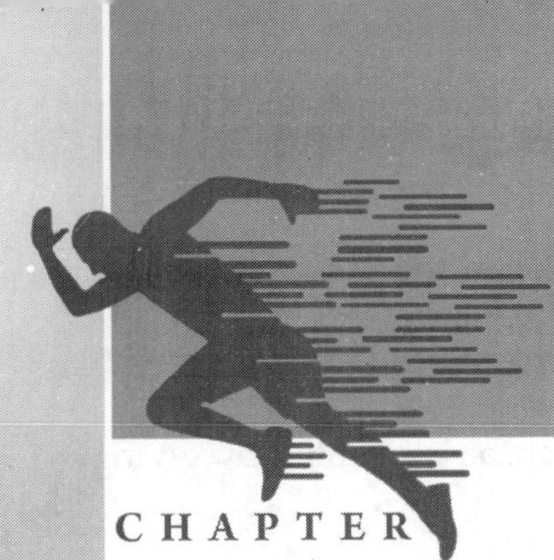

13

Determination of Osmotic Fragility and Specific Gravity of Blood

Competency:

PY2.12: Describe the test for osmotic fragility and specific gravity of blood. Note the findings and interpret the results.

Learning Objectives

At the end of the practical, the students shall be able to:

- Define osmotic fragility of blood
- Understand the clinical significance of osmotic fragility
- Enumerate variations in osmotic fragility
- Describe the significance of this practical in clinical physiology
- Give the principle of determination of blood
- List factors affecting the specific gravity of blood
- List physiological and pathological variations in specific gravity.

A. OSMOTIC FRAGILITY OF BLOOD

■ INTRODUCTION

The osmotic fragility of red cells is defined as the ease with which red blood cells (RBCs) are ruptured (haemolyzed) when exposed to hypotonic solutions. It does assess the integrity of the membrane of red cells. Osmotic fragility helps in the diagnosis of anaemia where physical properties of RBCs are altered.

Apparatus

Test tubes, test tube rack, 1% sodium chloride (NaCl) solution, dropper, and distilled water.

Principle

- Normal red cells remain suspended in isotonic solutions (0.9% saline) without rupturing for many hours.
- When they are suspended in a hypotonic solution, they absorb fluid, swell, and get ruptured.

Procedure

- Arrange test tubes in a rack and label them as 1 to 12.
- In the first test tube, 25 drops of 0.9% NaCl are put (isotonic)
- In the 12th test tube, 25 drops of distilled water are put (nil tonicity)
- Prepare solutions of different hypotonicity by mixing the required number of drops of 1% NaCl and distilled water in test tubes serially from 1 to 12 (one dropper is used to put saline solution and another dropper for distilled water).
- In test tubes from 1–12, solutions of different tonicity are prepared as given in **Table 13.1**.
- One drop of given blood is added to each test tube.

TABLE 13.1: Preparation of solutions of different tonicity

Test tube number	1	2	3	4	5	6	7	8	9	10	11	12
Drops of distilled water	3	9	10	11	12	13	14	15	16	17	18	25
1% saline drops	22	16	15	14	13	12	11	10	9	8	7	0
% saline solution	0.88	0.64	0.60	0.56	0.52	0.48	0.44	0.40	0.36	0.32	0.28	0

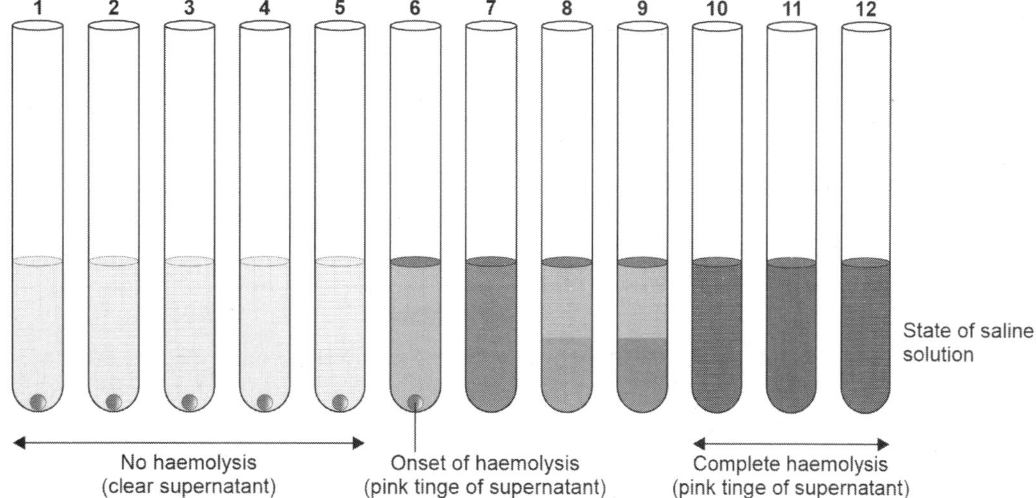

Fig. 13.1: Osmotic fragility–haemolysis starts in the sixth tube and is completed in the 10th tube *(For colour version, See plate 2)*

- Each tube is inverted gently so that blood mixes with saline and again it is kept in a rack.
- These test tubes are kept undisturbed for about an hour.
- Without disturbing tubes, observe the tubes for a percentage of haemolysis **(Fig. 13.1)**.

Observations

- In tube number 1, there is no haemolysis where RBCs settle down and supernatant fluid is clear above.
- In test tube number 12 where complete haemolysis has occurred appears uniformly red. In test tubes, where there is partial haemolysis, RBCs do get settled down but supernatant saline is pink (haemolyzed RBCs).
- Haemolysis begins at 0.46–0.38% NaCl solutions and gets completed at 0.32–0.3% of NaCl solutions.
- RBCs are biconcave in shape and thus have a greater surface area compared to their volume. Any change in the normal volume-to-surface area ratio of RBCs alters the ability of RBCs to accommodate water. Therefore, alteration in the shape of RBCs can make them more fragile.
- When the rate of haemolysis of RBCs is increased, osmotic fragility increases (decreased resistance to rupture) and when the rate of haemolysis of RBCs is decreased osmotic fragility is reduced.

Precautions

- Counting of drops should be very accurate as given above.
- A separate dropper has to be used for pouring distilled water and saline.
- A minimum of half an hour is required for complete haemolysis to occur.

■ IMPORTANT QUESTIONS AND ANSWERS

Q.1. What is the clinical significance of the determination of osmotic fragility of blood?

Osmotic fragility tells us about the shape of RBCs. This test is used as a screening test for the diagnosis of haemolytic anaemia (e.g. sickle cell anaemia, hereditary spherocytosis).

Q.2. What are variations in osmotic fragility?

The fragility of RBCs increases in:

- Hereditary spherocytosis
- Deficiency of glucose-6-phosphate dehydrogenase (G6PD) enzyme
- Venous blood
- Stored blood

Fragility of RBCs decreases in:

- Thalassemia
- Iron deficiency anaemia
- Sickle cell anaemia
- Post splenectomy

Q.3. RBC membrane is selectively permeable. Justify.

RBC membrane is permeable to water, crystalloids, and anions, however, it is not permeable to colloids, cations, plasma proteins and haemoglobin.

Q.4. How does RBC resist haemolysis when put in a hypotonic solution?

- RBCs have a peculiar biconcave shape and thus have a greater surface area as compared to the volume of fluid retained in them.
- Volume/surface area ratio determines the amount of water a cell can accommodate before lysis
- Normal RBC can increase in volume by about 70% before the surface membrane is stretched. Once this limit is reached, lysis occurs.
- Therefore, even if 0.5% NaCl solution is hypotonic there is no haemolysis of RBCs.

Q.5. What is haemolysis?
- Any condition in which the shape of RBCs causes increased volume/surface area ratio, decreases the ability of RBCs to accommodate water before stretching (as explained above).
- This makes RBCs more fragile, and their ability to resist haemolysis in hypotonic solution decreases.
- Various haemolytic agents include—hypotonic saline, distilled water, alternate freezing, and thawing, fat solvents like alcohol, chloroform, etc.
- Vigorous shaking of the test tube filled with blood, leads to mechanical damage to RBCs and their rupture.

Q.6. When can haemolysis take place in the body?
- Haemolysis can take place due to internal or external factors.
- Internal factors include, structural abnormalities of RBCs and external factors include mismatched blood transfusion, bacterial toxins, drug reactions, etc.

■ COMMON STATIONS– SPOTS IN PRACTICAL EXAMINATION (2/3 MARKS)

- 1 to 12 test tubes and rack kept with different tonicity of solutions. Identify experiment. Give its clinical significance. Answer any one or two questions from above (please check).
- RBCs– spherocytes, sickle cell (picture), write what will affect the osmotic fragility test.

■ KEY POINTS TO REMEMBER

- Determining osmotic fragility is a common screening tool for the diagnosis of haemolytic anaemia.
- Test also helps in the diagnosis of spherocytic and non-spherocytic hereditary anaemia.

B. SPECIFIC GRAVITY OF BLOOD

■ INTRODUCTION

- Specific gravity of blood is the ratio of the weight of blood to the weight of equal volume of water at 4°C.
- Normal specific gravity of blood varies from 1,055 to 1,062.
- The specific gravity of RBCs is greater than the plasma.

- Specific gravity depends upon haematocrit, plasma proteins, and water content of the blood. Under normal conditions, it is a good indicator of the haemoglobin (Hb) content of the blood.

Apparatus

Test tubes, dropper, distilled water, and stock solution of copper sulphate with 1.100 of specific gravity.

Principle

- Solutions of different specific gravities are prepared by a proper mixture of solution of copper sulphate and distilled water (ranging from 1.050 to 1.068).
- Specific gravity of blood and each solution is compared by putting a drop of blood in each tube.

Procedure

- Copper sulphate solution of different specific gravities (1.050–1.068) is prepared by mixing distilled water with a stock solution of copper sulphate in different test tubes as shown in **Table 13.2**. Label tubes as 1, 2, 3, and so on.
- Mix the solution in each tube properly. Then oxalated blood whose specific gravity is to be determined is taken in a dropper.
- Pour a drop of blood into each tube with the help of a pipette (from a height of 1 cm above the solution).
- Observe the behaviour of blood drops in each tube.
- Blood drop will sink, if it is heavier and will float if it is lighter.
- This happens when the specific gravity of blood is the same as that of solution.
- Blood drop floats in solution in copper sulphate solution due to the covering of the copper proteinate layer (that is stable only for 15–20 seconds).
- After that, it becomes heavier and sinks in the water.

Precautions

- The ratio of copper sulphate and water must be accurate while preparing the solution.
- Reading has to be taken in 10 to 12 seconds.

TABLE 13.2: Preparation of copper sulphate solution of different specific gravity

Test tube number	1	2	3	4	5	6	7	8	9	10
Copper sulphate solution	4.9	5.1	5.3	5.5	5.7	5.9	6.1	6.3	6.5	6.7
Distilled water	5.1	4.9	4.7	4.5	4.3	4.1	3.9	3.7	3.5	3.3
The specific gravity of the solution	1.050	1.052	1.054	1.056	1.058	1.060	1.062	1.064	1.066	1.068

■ IMPORTANT QUESTIONS AND ANSWERS

Q.1. Why $CuSO_4$ is used in this experiment?

Because $CuSO_4$ is cheap, it is noninflammable and not hygroscopic in nature, so it is used for this experiment.

Q.2. What are the physiological and pathological variations in the specific gravity of blood?

Physiological variations

Increase in specific gravity:	Decrease in specific gravity:
• Newborns	• Pregnancy
• High altitudes	• Excess water intake
• Excess sweating	

Pathological variations

Increase in specific gravity	Decrease in specific gravity:
• Diarrhoea	Any condition where there is
• Dehydration	increased water content of blood
• Vomiting	(e.g. nephrotic syndrome)

Q.3. What is the clinical significance of the determination of the specific gravity of blood?

- If water, salt, and plasma protein concentrations are normal, then the specific gravity indicates total cell volume.
- Thus, this test is used as a screening test for anaemia in blood donors (in World War II, this method helped to assess if blood transfusions are required or not).

Q.4. Enumerate factors affecting the specific gravity of blood.

Factors affecting specific gravity of blood

- Number of RBCs in blood
- Plasma protein concentration
- Haemoglobin content of blood
- Water content of blood

■ COMMON STATIONS – SPOTS IN PRACTICAL EXAMINATION (2/3 MARKS)

- Different test tubes filled with $CuSO_4$ and a drop of blood, identify the experiment and write its clinical use. Answer any one or two questions from the above (please check).
- Enlist various conditions that can alter the specific gravity of blood.

■ KEY POINTS TO REMEMBER

- Specific gravity of blood is the ratio of the weight of blood to the weight of equal volume of water at 4°C.
- Normal specific gravity of blood varies from 1,055 to 1,062.
- It is used as a screening test for anaemia before an emergency blood transfusion.
- Specific gravity of blood depends on the number of RBCs, plasma proteins in the blood and also the Hb content and water content of the blood.

Determination of Reticulocyte Count

Competency:

PY 2.13: Describe steps of reticulocyte count.

Learning Objectives

After completion of this practical, the student shall be able to:

- Describe the significance of doing this count
- Understand the concept of reticulocyte response
- Understand the causes of reticulocytosis and reticulocytopenia
- Describe reticulocyte staining.

Aim

To determine the reticulocyte count of the given blood.

Apparatus

Microscope, needle/lancet, oxalated blood/EDTA blood/fresh blood, reticulocyte stain.

Introduction

- Reticulocytes are precursors of RBCs. Normally, 1% of RBCs are present as reticulocytes. Reticulocytes are stained by supravital staining. After staining blue coloured thread-like network is seen in them and therefore they are called as reticulocytes.
- The number of reticulocytes in the blood indicates erythropoiesis. More demand for red cells stimulates erythropoiesis and that in turn increases the number of reticulocytes also in the peripheral blood. Reticulocytes remain in circulation for about 24 hrs before they become mature RBCs.

Preparation of the Dye

New methylene blue—1 g of new methylene blue is dissolved in 100 ml of iso-osmotic phosphate buffer, pH 7.4 (i.e. 24.3 g/L of NaH_2PO_4 and 21.3 g/L of NaH_2PO_4 for iso-osmotic buffer.

Procedure

- 2 to 3 drops of blood are mixed with 2 to 3 drops of vital stain (reticulocyte staining fluid) in a test tube.
- Mix it gently and keep the test tube in an incubator at 37°C for about 15 minutes.
- Make 3 to 5 moderately thick smears, dry them and then add a drop of blood on the coverslip and inver and press it on the stain.
- Examine under oil immersion lens and then reticulocytes and RBCs in each field are counted.
- A minimum of 1000 red cells are counted (minimum of 10 fields).
- Reticulocytes are large-sized (more than normal RBC) with reticulofilamentous material in cytoplasm stained deep blue.

An automated method to count reticulocytes: Cells are stained with fluorochrome dye (that stains RNA). Cells fluoresce when exposed to ultraviolet light and then counted.

Calculations

If the number of reticulocytes/100 fields = 100

Total number of RBCs in 10 fields   = 300

Therefore,
Total number of RBCs in 100 fields = 3000
Then, % of reticulocytes = 100/3000 × 100
= 3.3%

Normal Range

- In adults: 0.2 to 2%
- In infants: 2 to 6%

Precautions

- They are the same as those taken during differential WBC count (concerning preparation of blood smear).
- Staining time should not be less than 10 minutes.
- Before making blood smears, proper mixing of blood with stain should be carried out.

Automated method: Cells are stained with fluorochrome (which mainly stains RNA) and cells are counted by fluorescence technique. With the automated method, counting is easy and more accurate compared to the manual method.

■ IMPORTANT QUESTIONS AND ANSWERS

Q.1. What is the clinical significance of reticulocyte count?

Clinical significance:

- Reticulocytes are precursors of RBCs. Normally, they are 0.2 to 2% of circulating blood.
- It reflects the erythropoietic activity in the body.
- Reticulocyte count is done to understand if hematinic drugs (given as a part of treatment for anaemia) stimulated erythropoiesis or not.

Q.2. What are the physiological and pathological conditions that increase reticulocyte count? (Reticulocytosis)

Reticulocytosis	
Physiological variations	*Pathological variations*
• Infants • High altitude	• In response to the treatment of anaemia • Chronic haemolytic anaemia • After severe haemorrhage • Excess production of erythropoietin from the kidney

Q.3. What are physiological and pathological conditions that decrease reticulocyte count? (reticulocytopenia)

Physiological conditions causing reticulocytopenia are rare. Pathological conditions for reticulocytopenia are:

- Post splenectomy
- Bone marrow failure
- Aplastic anaemia

Q.4. What is vital and supravital staining?

- *Vital staining:* As the name suggests, it is the staining of live tissues using some dyes or injections.
- *Supravital staining:* It is the staining of living tissues before fixing them (killing them). RNA content of reticulocytes can be detected by exposing living cells to supravital staining.

Q.5. What is reticulocyte response?

- *Reticulocyte response:* It is an increase in the count number of reticulocytes in circulating blood.
- It indicates about the erythropoiesis activity of red bone marrow.
- It can also be assessed to check if the diagnosis of anaemia was correct and the measures taken to correct it (hematinic drugs) are in the right direction or not.
- Increase count of number of reticulocyte counts starting after about a week or so after starting with hematinic drugs (for treating iron deficiency anaemia). The same response is obtained (reticulocyte response) when vitamin B12 is given as a part of treatment for pernicious anaemia.

Standard lab values for RBC

Tests	Normal range	Significance of test
Total RBC count	*Males:* 5–6.5 million/mm^3 of blood *Females:* 4–5.5 million/mm^3 of blood	Number of red cells in the blood
Reticulocytes	0.2 to 2% of total RBC count	Rate of red cell production
Haemoglobin	*Males:* 14–18/100 g/dl of blood *Females:* 12–15/100 g/dl of blood	Hb content of the blood
PCV	*In males:* 38–54% *In females:* 30–47%	Volume of cells in 100 ml of blood
MCV	82 to 92 cubic microns	Size of RBC
MCH	27 to 32 picograms	Concentration of Hb in RBC
MCHC	32 to 38%	Red cell mass

■ COMMON STATIONS: SPOTS IN PRACTICAL EXAMINATION (2/3 MARKS)

Q.1. Identify reticulocytes under a microscope. Write its normal range.

Q.2. What is the significance of doing reticulocyte count? Answer any one or two questions from above.

Q.3. A 22-year-old anaemic person with Hb–10 g% was put on haematinic drugs for 10 days. He was advised to do reticulocyte count by a doctor.

- What is the reason to check for reticulocyte count?
- Do you expect any change in reticulocyte count, Why?

■ KEY POINTS TO REMEMBER

- Reticulocytes are precursors of RBCs and their normal level is 0.2 to 2% of the total RBC count.
- Cells can be stained with supravital staining and counted or by automated techniques.
- Reticulocyte response is important to watch after treatment with hematinic drugs.

Determination of Platelet Count

Competency:

PY2.13: Describe the steps for estimation of platelet count.

Learning Objectives

After completion of this practical, the students shall be able to:

- Name various methods for performing platelet count
- Enumerate and discuss the functions of platelets
- Enumerate procedure for platelet count by ammonium oxalate method
- State normal range of platelet count.

▪ PLATELETS

Platelets play an important role in hemostasis. They are non-nucleated, round or oval-shaped cells. Their size varies from 2 to 4 microns. The inner denser part is chromomere and the outer lighter portion is hyalomere. Hylomere contains microtubules, actin, myosin fibres and thrombosthenin. The remaining cell organelles are present in the chromomere.

Aim

To determine platelet count.

Apparatus

Lancet, Neubauer's chamber, RBC pipette, cotton, spirit, platelet diluting fluid (1% ammonium oxalate).

Procedure

- Focus central square of Neubauer's chamber with a coverslip under high power.
- Without disturbing the adjustment of the microscope, keep Neubauer's chamber on the table.
- With all aseptic precautions, prick the finger and suck capillary blood up to 0.5 mark. Suck diluting fluid after that up to 101 mark.
- Mix it well by holding the pipette in between the palms of the hands.
- Discard the first 2 to 3 drops (as it contains only diluting fluid) and charge Neubauer's chamber.
- Keep charged Neubauer's chamber in moist petridish for 20 to 30 minutes (that will allow platelets to settle down).
- Start counting platelets as done for RBC count, i.e. in 4 corners and one central square (follow the rule of 'L' as counting during RBC count).
- Platelets appear as refractile, bluish tiny particles.

Calculations

Platelets are counted in five squares (as in RBC count) Therefore,

Volume of fluid = $1 \times 1 \times 0.1 = 0.1$ mm^3

If 'N' is the number of platelets counted in 25 RBC squares = 0.1 mm^3 of diluted blood.

Number of platelets per mm^3 will be = N $\times$ dilution factor (200)/0.1.

$$= N \times 10 \times 200$$
$$= N \times 2000$$

Normal range of platelet count: 1.5 to 4.5 lakh/cumm of blood (normal ratio of platelets to RBCs is 1:20).

Precautions

- Thoroughly clean the glassware
- Dilute the blood rapidly and shake it properly (as there is the tendency of platelets to form clumps)
- Wait for 15 minutes for the settling of cells after charging the chamber.
- Remaining precautions (please check Chapter total WBC count and total RBC count).

Automated method: The S Plus coulter counter is used for automated platelet counting.

■ IMPORTANT QUESTIONS AND ANSWERS

Q.1. What are the functions of platelets?
Functions of platelets:

- Platelets help in endothelial support.
- Platelets help in hemostasis as:
  - Platelet plug formation
  - Release of vasoconstrictor substances from platelets
  - Release of platelet factors required for coagulation
  - Due to the presence of actomyosin-like protein in platelets, they are responsible for clot retraction
- Platelets help in the phagocytosis of various substances like carbon particles, immune complexes, viruses, etc.
- Platelets store, synthesize and transport serotonin. They also store and transport heparin.

Q.2. Define thrombocytosis and thrombocytopenia.

- **Thrombocytosis:** It is an increase in platelet count above normal.
- **Thrombocytopenia:** It is a decrease in platelet count below normal.

Q.3. Enumerate physiological and pathological conditions causing thrombocytosis.

Thrombocytosis	
Physiological conditions	*Pathological conditions*
• Exercise • Parturition	• Post-surgery/trauma • Infections • Allergic reactions • Chronic myeloid leukemia

Q.4. Enumerate physiological and pathological conditions causing thrombocytopenia.

- Physiological conditions leading to thrombocytopenia are rare.
- Pathological conditions causing thrombocytopenia are:
  - Idiopathic thrombocytopenic purpura
  - Leukemias
  - Aplastic anaemia
  - Hypersplenism (splenomegaly)
  - Bone marrow infiltration (due to secondary carcinoma or multiple myeloma).

Tendency of bleeding is proportional to the degree of thrombocytopenia. It starts with petechiae, ecchymoses, bleeding from the nose, and gums, menorrhagia, and sudden bleeding anywhere in the body.

Q.5. What is thrombocytopenic purpura?
Please refer to the Chapter on bleeding time and clotting time.

Q.6. How does platelet diluting fluid (1% ammonium oxalate) act?

- It does act as an anticoagulant,
- It preserves platelets, and
- It destroys RBCs.

Q.7. How are platelets formed?

- *Site of formation:* Platelets are formed in bone marrow from megakaryocytes (the largest cell of bone marrow) See below Q.11.
- *Lifespan:* Platelets life span is 10 to 12 days. Senile platelets are removed by the reticuloendothelial system.

Q.8. Discuss the role of platelets in hemostasis.
Hemostasis (prevention of blood loss from the vessel) is achieved as follows:

- *Vascular spasm:* Immediately after the cut or injury to the vessel, the damaged vessel undergoes a temporary spasm (wall of vessels contract). Spasms of the vessels occur mainly due to:
  - *Nervous reflex:* It is initiated due to pain or other impulses originating from traumatized blood vessels.
  - *Local myogenic spasm:* It is initiated due to direct damage to the vessel wall.
  - *Release of vasoconstrictor:* Thromboxane A2 is a vasoconstrictor substance that is released from platelets. This helps in vasospasm of many small blood vessels.
- *Formation of platelet plug:* Small vascular holes are sealed by platelet plug rather than by blood clots as they are very small. If there is a large hole in any of the blood vessels (due to injury) then besides the platelet plug, blood clot formation becomes essential to stop/arrest bleeding.
- *Blood clot formation:* Clot begins to develop within 15 to 20 seconds after trauma if trauma is severe. If trauma is not severe, it might take a few minutes (1–2 minutes) to initiate the process of blood clotting. In the next 3 to 6 minutes, it completely seals the vessel wall. Then the clot retracts to cause further closing of

the hole (with the help of contractile proteins present in platelets).

Q.9. Explain in detail the mechanism of platelet plug formation.

Mechanism of platelet plug formation:

- As platelets come in contact with damaged vascular surfaces, they swell and assume irregular forms due to the formation of pseudopods. Contractile proteins in platelets (actin and myosin) contract and release ADP, and thromboxane A2 that is secreted in blood.
- Platelets become sticky and start sticking to collagen fibres. This indicates that platelets are activated now.
- This activation of platelets at the damaged site of the vessel, sets a vicious cycle to cause activation of more and more platelets that start sticking to originally activated platelets, forming platelet plugs.

Q.10. What is the Rees-Ecker method of platelet count?

- This is another method of estimating platelet count. The method is the same as the ammonium oxalate method. However, the diluting fluid used is named Rees-Ecker diluting fluid.
- Contents of Rees-Ecker fluid
  - Na citrate (3.8%): Acts as anticoagulant
  - Brilliant cresyl blue (0.1g): To stain platelets
  - Formalin/formaldehyde (0.2 ml): For fixation of stain and lysis of RBCs
  - Distilled water (100 ml): Solvent

Principle of Rees-Ecker method: Blood is diluted with solution as mentioned above. Anticoagulant presence prevents coagulation.

Q.11. Describe the development of thrombocytes/ platelets.

- Platelets are developed from megakaryocytes from bone marrow. The development of thrombocytes is called thrombopoiesis.
- *Steps of thrombopoiesis:* Pluripotent stem cells committed stem cells → CFU-Megakaryocytes →

Promegakaryocyte → Granular megakaryocyte → Mature megakaryocyte → Platelets.

◼ COMMON STATIONS – SPOTS IN PRACTICAL EXAMINATION (2/3 MARKS)

- **Platelet diluting fluid bottles:** Identify and write where they are used. Answer any one or two questions from the above.
- **Platelets mounted under the microscope:** Identify any one or two questions from the above.
- A 8-year-old girl comes with h/o injury to her left leg while playing. Her teacher put pressure with cotton at the site of the wound and the bleeding was stopped by the time she reached the hospital. What is the mechanism by which bleeding stopped?

◼ CASE-BASED SCENARIO/PROBLEM-BASED

Case 1: XYZ 28-year-old comes to OPD with c/o fever for 4 days, fatigue and body ache. Since, morning he has seen bluish dots on his abdomen.

On examination, all vitals were normal, WBC count– 8500/cumm of blood, RBC count– 4 million/cumm of blood and platelet count is 35000/cumm of blood. The bleeding time is 11 minutes.

- What does the blood picture suggest?
- What is the reason for bluish spots and prolonged bleeding time? (Please refer to the Chapter on bleeding and clotting time).

◼ KEY POINTS TO REMEMBER

- Platelets play an important role in hemostasis.
- Normal platelet count is 1.5 to 4.5 lacks/cumm of blood.
- There are various physiological and pathological conditions that can alter platelet count.

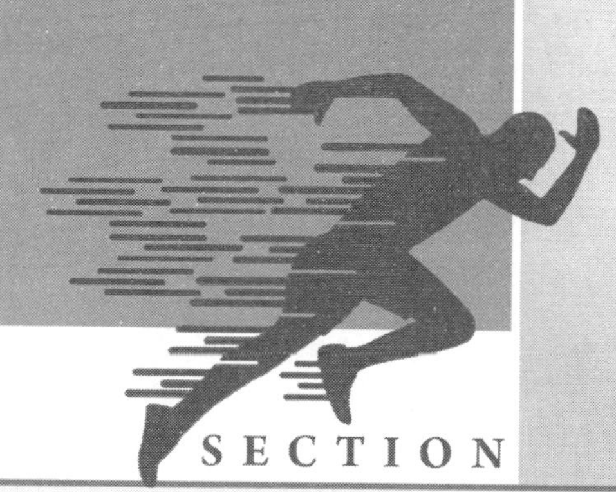

Clinical Physiology

Chapter Outline

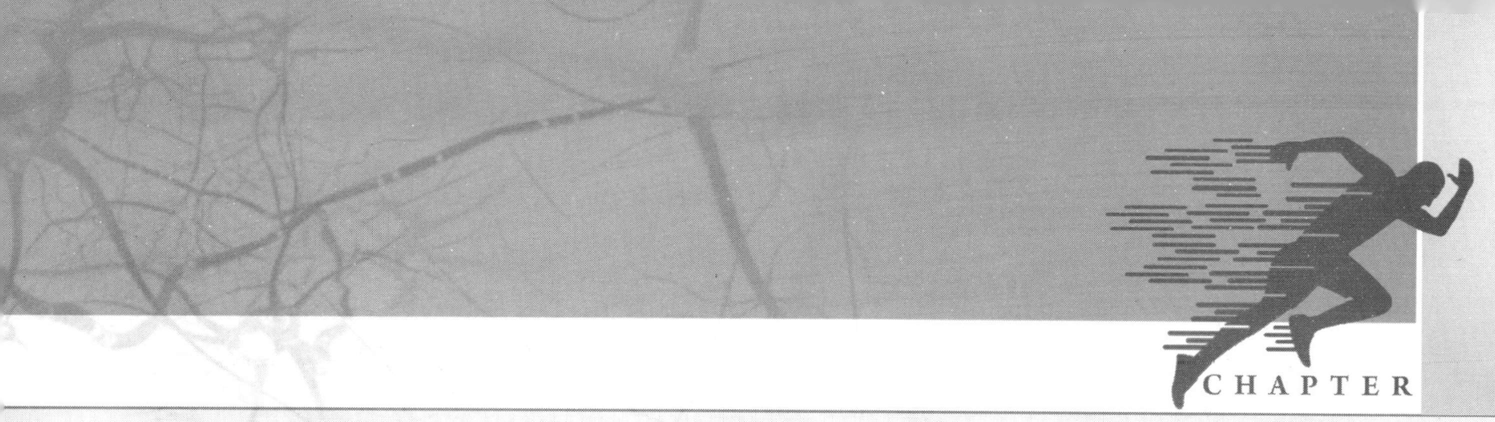

General Examination and History Taking

Competency:

PY 11.13: Obtain history and perform general examination in a volunteer/simulated environment.

Learning Objectives

At the end of this practical, the students shall be able to:
- Enlist the headings under which general examination is carried out
- Take a relevant and detailed history of a patient with efficient communication
- Enlist the parameters that are to be examined in the general examination of the patient
- Evaluate headings under which systemic examination is carried out with the significance of each heading
- Give significance to percussion and enlist the procedure and rules of percussion

◼ CLINICAL EXAMINATION

Clinical examination includes:
- History taking
- General examination
- Systemic examination of the respiratory system (RS), cardiovascular system (CVS), alimentary system, and central nervous system (CNS)

Pre-requisites before Clinical Examination
- Presence of natural light (well-lighted room)
- Standing to the right side of the patient
- Female attendant when the male doctor examines a female patient
- Proper exposure of body parts to be examined.

Objective of History Taking
- The objective of history taking is to understand the reason behind the disturbance in normal function (physiology) and get information about the patient's present illness (origin, progress, and duration) personal habits, family history and past history for diagnosis.
- Patient's complaints are called as symptoms and what the doctor finds on examination are called as signs.
- History taking is an art and skill that one develops over the years and becomes important in order to treat a patient even than a clinical examination.
- Appropriate skill is required to interpret the patient's symptoms and signs that one finds on physical examination.

◼ HISTORY TAKING AND GENERAL EXAMINATION

Step 1

Quick assessment as we look at the patient
- Appearance of patient-relaxed/anxious
- Is he/she depressed/afraid
- Does he/she make good eye contact
- Any difficulty in breathing
- Posture normal or not

Step 2

Basic information of patient
Name, Age, Sex, Occupation, Address, Height, Weight, WC, Waist hip ratio, Marital status.

Step 3

- **Start a conversation with simple questions:** After this information, usually, the conversation should start with a simple question like "What makes you come here today? As far as possible patient should be allowed to narrate in his/her own words but the physician must moderate in between to get complete information.
- **Observing non-verbal communication:** While the patient is narrating in his way what has made him come here, it's very important to observe the body language of the patient, his/her interaction with relatives, if they are there, the logic in which he/she is speaking.
- **Indirect (open-ended) questions:** The doctor does ask usually two types of questions. Indirect questions usually are one that indicates or makes patient to talk (e.g. a physician may say; tell me more about or what you think about or you would like to tell me something else, etc.). These questions are mainly patient-centred.
- **Direct (close-ended) questions**: These are the questions which usually doctor ask and are disease-centred.

Step 4

- **History of present illness:** Origin, duration and progress and treatment taken for the same. Here all chief complain (symptoms) of the patient are noted in chronological order. Character and time duration of a particular symptom may help us understand the defect in normal structure, function as well as the pathological process involved in it, e.g. myocardial infarction or stroke has an acute onset in contrast weight loss, peptic ulcer, and weakness can have a gradual onset.
- From a good history one should understand all the details of any complain. An example of the most common symptom that a patient comes to see a doctor if pain is given below:

Points to be covered for common complaints like pain
Site of pain, character/type of pain, history of referred pain, aggravating factors, severity, time duration, relieving factors.

Step 5

- **Past history:** This includes history of any major illness, operations and specific history of diabetes, hypertension, or epilepsy.

Step 6

- **Family history:** It provides information about infectious or hereditary diseases. In the case of infectious diseases, it becomes important to understand any infectious disease at home/neighbourhood. We also come to know about sanitary conditions and the socio-economic status the patient belongs to.
- Some diseases and allergic conditions run in the family. For some diseases there are genetic trends for a particular disease (in that case h/o first-order relatives become important).

Step 7

- **Personal history:** We record the patient's personal details like appetite, bowel habits, micturition history, sleep history.
- Personal history can vary in different age groups and men and women.

Women	Menstruation history, menarche age, menopause age, obstetric history, history of vaccination for HPV, any treatment for infertility, examination of breast
Children and adolescents	Birth history, detailed immunization history, developmental milestones, learning and behaviour, academic achievements, pubertal development, etc.
Old age	History of chronic disease conditions like diabetes, hypertension, stroke, h/o fall/immobility, impaired senses like vision, hearing, speech, pressure ulcers, and incontinence.

Step 8

Drug history: The patient has to be asked about any particular medicines he/she is taking. One should also ask for taking any herbal or complementary medicines. Enquiring must be made regarding self-medication or taking medicine without prescriptions.

Step 9

Occupational history: Sometimes occupational history becomes important and it may play an important role in the diagnostic process.

Step 10

Alcohol/smoking history/addictions: A detailed history of alcohol, smoking or tobacco use sometimes plays an important role in the diagnostic process and even the progress of disease. If reporting amount of these habits looks excessive then a detailed and specific assessment is required to be done. History of any other addictions should also be enquired.

History/Proforma

Name	Age	Sex	Race
Occupation	Marital status	Residence address	
History of present illness			
Past history			
Family history			
Personal history			
Drug history			
Occupational history			
Alcohol/smoking history			

Conclusion

- One has to understand that after taking history in this way, some situations directly hint to a particular diagnosis and for some cases, your clinical experience and logical analysis of the symptoms of the patient help you to arrive at a diagnosis and treat the patient.
- When you are writing notes it becomes important to keep eye contact with your patient.

■ GENERAL EXAMINATION

After a detailed history taking, we start with a general examination of the patient. In a general survey, we try to understand the patient's physique. If he/she is cachexic, slim or obese (central/general obesity).

The general examination includes:

A: Physique and nutrition of the patient

- Physique and nutrition help many times in providing a clue towards disease. One can note if patient is slim, obese, or cachexic. State of muscle, scalp hair and skin quality can give clue about the nutritional status of a person.
- *Nutrition:* Nutrition of the muscles is to be tested with skin fold thickness and anthropometric measurements like height and weight.

Body mass index (BMI) = Weight (in kg)/height in m² – Asian standards
Normal BMI: 18–23
Overweight: 23.1–28
Obese: 28.1–33
Grossly obese: More than 33

B: Speech

The way in which a person speaks or answers questions or makes eye contact can help to diagnose or understand any of clinical conditions and mental status of the person.

C: Body temperature

- It has to be recorded in mouth, axilla, or rectum. Normal body temperature is about 36 to 37°C, with 0.5 higher temp in the rectum (as compared to mouth temperature).

- Diurnal fluctuations can be seen in temperature with a minimum recorded in the early morning. A close monitoring of patient's temperature with the help of a TPR chart is vital for understanding course of disease.

D: Hands

- Examining hands can be of diagnostic significance for varieties of conditions. Just a simple handshake with the patient can give inputs regarding the neurological or musculoskeletal status of the patient.
- Tremors in hands are common with thyrotoxicosis. Pin-rolling movements are characteristics of Parkinson's disease.

Clubbing of Fingers should be Examined (Figs. 16.1, 16.2)

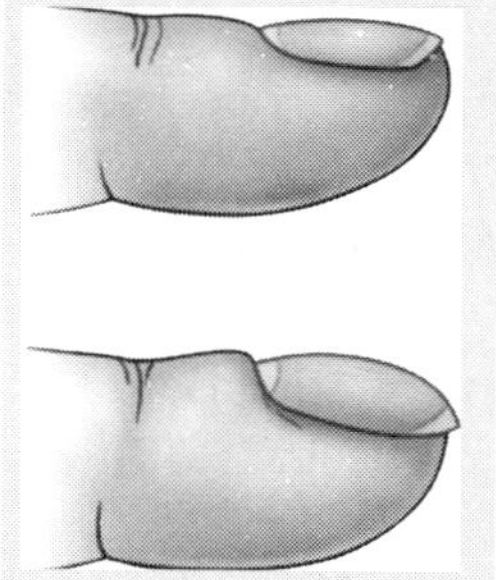

- The normal angle of the fingernail and nail base is 180 degrees. This is called as Lovibond's angle.
- In clubbing tissues at the nail base get thickened leading to a reduction in this angle (**Fig. 16.1**).
- It is seen with a variety of cardiorespiratory disease states.

Fig. 16.1: Clubbing of fingers

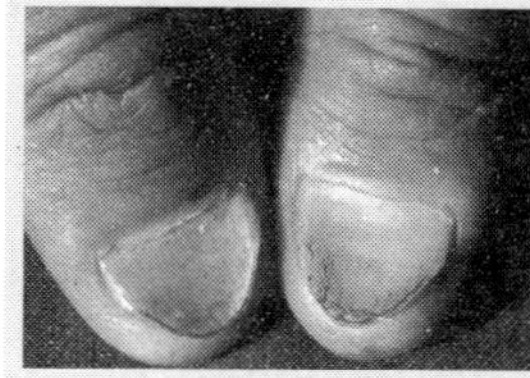

Koilonychia: Nails become soft, and brittle with spoon-shaped concavity. They are characteristically seen with iron deficiency anaemia (**Fig. 16.2**).

Fig. 16.2: Koilonychia (iron deficiency anaemia)

E: Face and neck

- Face can reflect a patient's mood as well as attitude. Besides this, it should be looked for any obvious swelling or eruptions (butterfly irruption – characteristic of SLE (autoimmune disease).
- Look for any obvious parotid swelling or puffiness on the face. Cranial nerve examination (especially facial nerve and III, IV, and VIth cranial nerve, and II and Vth cranial nerve is covered in the cranial nerve examination chapter).
- Neck should be inspected, and palpated for any obvious swelling or pulsations (JVP refer to the examination of the cardiovascular system).
- Neck examined for all groups of lymph nodes (**Fig. 16.3**). Generally small, mobile lymph nodes are found in all normal people. Any enlarged lymph node should be carefully examined to understand any local pathology or malignancy or involvement of the reticuloendothelial system (**Figs. 16.3A and C**).
- Neck circumference can give a clue for diagnosis or risk factors for assessment of obstructive sleep apnea.

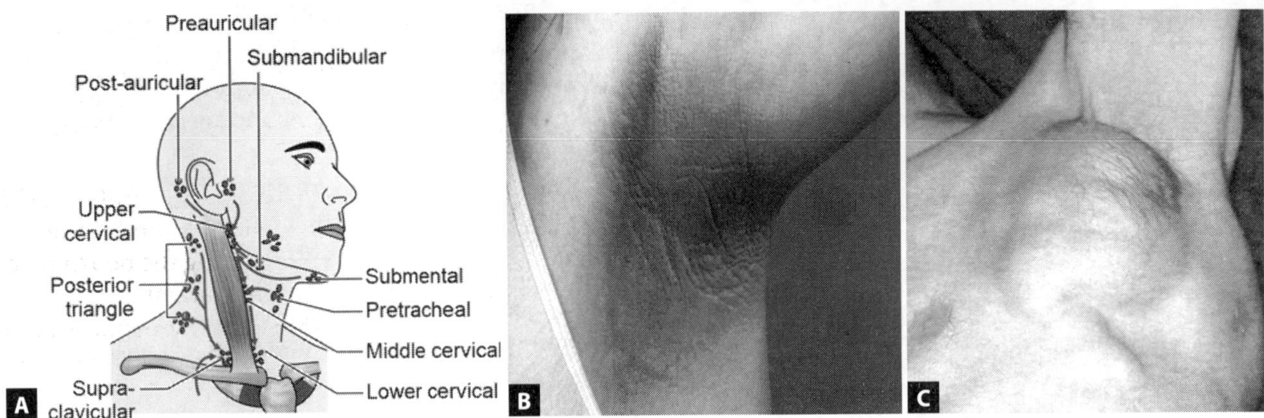

Figs. 16.3A to C: (A) Cervical group of lymph nodes; (B) Acanthosis nigricans; (C) Enlarged axillary lymph node

F: Axilla

- Besides palpating axillary lymph nodes observe for abnormal skin colouring and growth of axillary hair (important in pubertal age as a sign of secondary sexual characteristics).
- **Acanthosis nigricans**: Dark velvety appearance of skin classical with insulin resistance **(Fig. 16.3B)**.

G: Mouth

- Refer to examination of alimentary cavity in chapter 17.
- **Halitosis (bad breath)** is common in people with poor dental hygiene. **Acetone breath** is a sign of diabetic ketoacidosis. The odour of alcohol can be easily recognized.

H: Skin

- One should look for pallor, jaundice (yellowish discolouration of skin, mucous membrane, conjunctiva), and cyanosis whenever examining the skin of the patient.
- Central cyanosis is best observed on lips and conjunctiva. Peripheral cyanosis is observed in the extremities.

I: Breast

- Breast examination is done to understand the size, shape, contour and symmetry of the chest (note any asymmetry or inversion of nipples).
- For any nodule, note down its size, shape, tenderness and consistency.

J: Vital signs

- It includes the pulse, blood pressure and respiration rate of a person. It helps in the diagnosis of the patient for various clinical conditions.
- **Pulse:** Besides radial pulse palpation (for detail *see* Chapter 18- Examination of Pulse) one can palpate for femoral pulse, popliteal pulse, and anterior tibial pulse on the lower extremities.

K: Ear, nose, throat

Ear, nose and throat should be examined in all patients for any discharge, pain, or swelling.

L: Spine, bone, and joints

- Spine and bones should be examined for any obvious abnormal shape or movement. One should also check lateral and forward bending for spine flexibility.
- All possible movements at all joints should be checked for smoothness in movements.

General Examination–Proforma

Personal details		
Name	*Age*	*Address*
Gait-		Speech
Pulse—/min	BP—mm Hg Temp.-	Body constitution- Average/obese/thin
Height weight BMI WC HC WHR		*Skin:* Pallor/cyanosis/any other findings
Eyes: Pallor/jaundice		*Ear, nose, throat:* Any discharge
State of awareness /Level of consciousness		Speech
Mouth: Breath Lips Gums Teeth Tongue		
Neck: Neck circumference Thyroid *Lymph nodes:* Neck Axilla Supratrochlear Groin		
Oedema Spine Bones Joints Genitals		

■ SYSTEMIC EXAMINATION

Each system that is RS, CVS, CNS, or abdomen is to be examined under all the four headings mentioned below.

1. Inspection
2. Palpation
3. Percussion
4. Auscultation

Brief about Systemic Examination

Inspection	*Palpation*
This means observing the patient, which can help you in diagnosis. • It is carried out in good daylight preferably • Body parts to be examined are uncovered • All findings of inspection are confirmed on palpation • Findings on the inspection are noted	• All inspection findings are to be confirmed on palpation • Always stand on the patient's right side and explain what you are going to examine • Examination is done by fingers or flat of the hand • Movement of hand while palpating should be gentle and fingers to be held straight with slight flexion at metacarpophalangeal joints • Findings on palpation are noted

Percussion	*Auscultation*
• It is examined with help of hands and fingers by tapping on different body parts and eliciting different notes • Different notes are recorded on the percussion of different body parts • Normally, three notes are—tympanic note (abdomen), resonant note (lungs), and dull note (on any solid organs like heart, spleen, liver, bone, etc.)	• This means listening with the help of stethoscope • Stethoscope is used to auscultate heart sounds, breath sounds, peristaltic movements and other abnormal sounds like murmurs, pleural rub, etc

Stethoscope

- It consists of two earpieces which are joined by a Y-shaped rubber/metallic tube.
- Other end of the rubber tube contains bell type of chest piece or diaphragm **(Fig. 16.4)**.
- Diaphragm and bell are used to auscultate sounds.

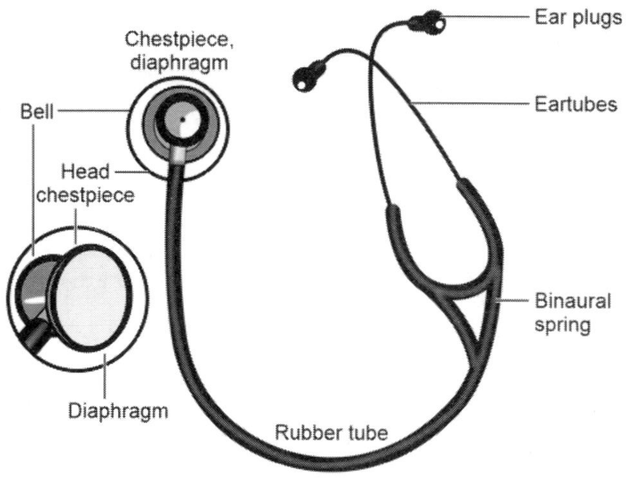

Fig. 16.4: Stethoscope

- Earpiece must fit comfortably in ears. They should be directed forward and medially in direction of ear canals.
- The functioning of diaphragm can be checked by light tapping on it with finger.
- Details of systemic examination with respect to each system are given in the respective chapters ahead.

Important anatomical landmarks for systemic examination	
Midsternal line: Vertical line drawn through centre of the sternum and xiphoid process	**Midclavicular line**: Vertical line from middle of the clavicle (it is parallel to midsternal line)
Mid scapular line: Vertical line on posterior chest wall that extends through apices of scapula	**Anterior axillary line**: Vertical line extending down from the anterior axillary fold
Midaxillary line: Vertical line in between anterior and posterior axillary line	**Posterior axillary line**: Vertical line extending down from posterior axillary fold

■ IMPORTANT QUESTIONS AND ANSWERS

Q.1. What is a general examination?
- General examination is essential part of clinical examination of patient before any systemic examination.
- It involves observation of the patient from head to foot for features of diagnosis. If performed properly it provides adequate clue to diagnosis

Q.2. Under what headings general examination should be carried out?

General examination should be carried out under the following headings:

General appearance of patient: Gait, and decubitus
- **Metal state**: Orientation of patient with respect to time, place, and person.
- **Vital signs**: Temperature, pulse, respiration and BP
- **Built and nutrition**: Height, weight, chest girth, and waist circumference
- **Skin:** For pallor, cyanosis, state of hydration, any obvious skin eruptions, infections, sign of deficiencies, scars, and irruptions
- **Nails:** Cyanosis, and clubbing
- **Head:** Examined for size and shape, girth of head (especially in children)
- **Mouth:** For the smell of breath, and any obvious teeth misalignment
- **Oedema**: Pitting (heart failure, nephrotic syndrome) or non-pitting oedema (Thyroid, filariasis)
- **Lymphadenopathy:** Lymph nodes examined in neck, axilla, supratrochlear and groin.
- **Bone, spine and joints**: For swelling and deformities
- **Ear, nose, and throat**: For any discharge
- **Neck:** For neck veins, lymph node enlargement, and thyroid gland

Q.3. How is general appearance of patient assessed?
- Under general appearance of patient one can assess his/her gait (way he/she is standing, walking) and also one can observe position of patient in the bed. (In cardiac failure patient adapts orthopneic position)
- One can observe patients' eye contact and speech.

Q.4. What is gait of the patient. Enumerate different types of gates.
- It is essential to observe the walking or gait pattern of the patient wherever possible. Many things like patient's comfort while walking, his/her position, dragging of leg, breathless while walking, pain while walking, etc.
- One has to look for turning, arm tilt, pelvic tilt, smooth movements, normal arm swings with walking, etc.

Some common gaits include:
- Unsteady gate (broad base) of cerebellar ataxia
- High stepping gate of sensory ataxia
- Myopathic waddling gate with weak proximal muscles
- Painful gate with some severe pain, and injury.

Q.5. How is mental state assessed in patient?
- By communicating properly with patient, mental status can be assessed very easily, by asking simple questions such as What is today's date? How long you been admitted here? Where do you work? What is your education? Where do you stay, etc.?
- It informs about the patient's orientation in time, place and person. It also informs about his/her level of intelligence.

Q.6. What is the significance of doing anthropometric measurements?
- Patient's height, weight, skin fold thickness is measured. BMI (as mentioned above) is calculated, and is one of the important anthropometric indices of the patient. Besides BMI person's waist circumference, waist-to-hip ratio, waist to height ratio can also be assessed. There are standard set for males, and females for each parameter.
- High BMI is considered as one of the important cardiovascular risk factors for a patient.

Q.7. How mouth/oral cavity is examined?
See Chapter of Examination the alimentary system.

Q.8. What is pallor? Where you should look for pallor?
- Pallor is paleness. It depends on amount and quality of blood in capillaries as well as the quality of the skin.
- Sites to look for – Pallor should be looked at lower palpebral conjunctiva, tongue, soft palate, lips palms nails, etc. **(Fig. 16.5)**.

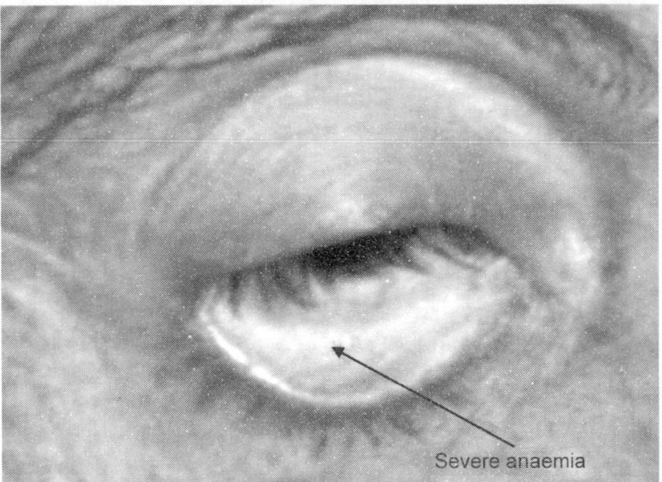

Fig. 16.5: Pallor

Q.9. What is jaundice?
- Jaundice is a yellow discolouration of the skin or mucous membrane. It is seen in the scleral portion, i.e. bulbar conjunctiva.
- It is due to the presence of excess bilirubin (normal bilirubin level 0.2–0.8 mg/100 ml of blood) in body fluids. Jaundice appears when the bilirubin level exceeds 2 mg.

Q.10. Where should be jaundice looked for? What are its types?
- Jaundice should be looked at following sites—Sclera, palms, soles, and skin. When serum bilirubin exceeds the level of 2 mg then it can be observed clinically.
- **Types of jaundice:** Prehepatic (Haemolytic) jaundice, hepatic jaundice and post hepatic (obstructive jaundice). (Check case studies for jaundice in haematology section).

Types of jaundice	Features
Prehepatic (haemolytic)	• Fecal stercobilin and urine urobilinogen is increased • *Van den Bergh test:* Indirect positive
Hepatic	• Fecal stercobilin normal/raised • Urine urobilinogen normal/raised • Biphasic reaction to Van den Bergh test
Post hepatic (obstructive)	• Due to obstruction, bilirubin does not reach the intestine • Fecal and urine urobilinogen absent • *Van den Bergh test:* Direct positive

Q.11. What is cyanosis? Where it is looked for?
Cyanosis is the bluish discolouration of skin and mucous membranes **(Figs. 16.6A and B)**. It is looked at conjunctiva, lips, tongue, nails, skin, etc.

Q.12. What is the physiological basis for cyanosis?
- Cyanosis is produced due to presence of reduced haemoglobin >5 g% in capillary blood.

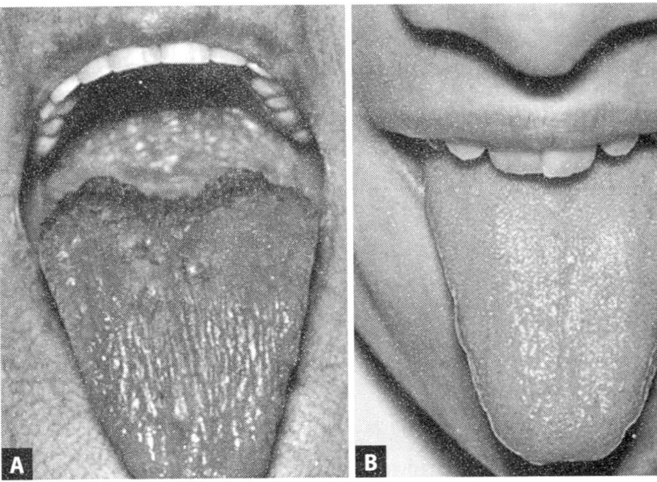

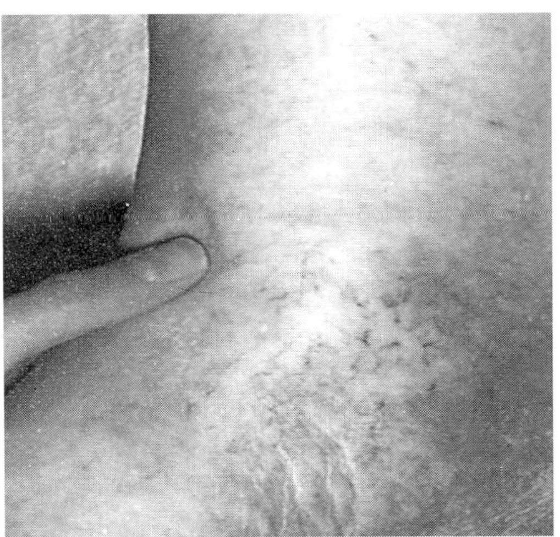

Figs. 16.6A and B: (A) Cyanosis tongue; (B) Normal tongue

Fig. 16.7: Pitting oedema in cardiac failure

- If we consider 15g% of Hb as a standard, then Hb in arterial blood is 95% saturated with oxygen and Hb in mixed venous blood is about 70% saturated with oxygen.
- The amount of reduced Hb in capillary blood is assumed as mean of arterial, and venous content of reduced Hb. Thus, in normal person capillary blood contains 2.5g% of reduced Hb.
- When the concentration of reduced Hb is >5g%, skin and mucous membranes become blue (due to the dark colour of reduced Hb). Patient with severe anaemia may not show cyanosis as the total Hb in him may be <5g%.
- **Cyanosis types**: Peripheral (seen on hands, feet) and central (seen on lips, tongue). Peripheral cyanosis is due to the slow flow of blood through tissues. Central cyanosis is due to inadequate oxygenation of arterial blood or the mixing of arterial blood with venous blood.
- Central cyanosis is seen with congenital heart diseases, patent ductus arteriosus, etc. Peripheral cyanosis is common with heart failure.

Q.13. What is clubbing? State its common causes.

Clubbing: In clubbing of the fingers, the tissues at the base of the nail are thickened and the angle between nail base and adjacent skin of finger is obliterated (Lovibond angle) making nails convex. Degree of clubbing is graded as I to IV.

Physiological basis: The exact cause for the clubbing of fingers is not known. It is observed that there is increased arteriovenous anastomosis in clubbing that causes hypertrophy of the tissues in the nail bed. Sometimes clubbing also has a genetic component.

Common causes:
- Bronchopulmonary diseases:
  - Bronchiectasis

- Bronchogenic carcinoma
- Lung abscess
- Cardiac disease:
  - Congenital heart diseases, e.g. Fallot's tetralogy
  - Subacute bacterial endocarditis
- Chronic abdominal disorders:
  - Ulcerative colitis
  - Crohn's disease

Q.14. What is oedema?

- Swelling of skin and subcutaneous tissue due to accumulation of excess free fluid in interstitial tissue spaces is termed oedema.
- It can be classified as localized or generalized. It can also be classified as pitting and non-pitting **(Fig. 16.7)**.

Q.15. What are the common causes of oedema?
Common causes of oedema:
- Cardiac causes
  - Congestive cardiac failure
- Renal causes
  - Acute glomerulonephritis
  - Nephrotic syndrome
- Hepatic causes
  - Cirrhosis of liver
  - Carcinoma of liver
- Nutritional
  - Anaemia and hypoproteinemia

Q.16. What are the sites where lymph nodes should be palpated?
Enlargement of lymph nodes must be checked in:
- Neck (submental, submandibular, cervical, posterior auricular and occipital groups of lymph nodes) for this doctor has to stand behind the patient and patient's neck slightly flexed.

- Axilla (anterior, posterior, apical, and lateral group of lymph nodes)
- Inguinal group of lymph nodes.

In all the above sites lymph nodes should be palpated for their size, shape, mobility, consistency, and tenderness. Lymphadenopathy is very common with tuberculosis. If lymph nodes are fixed to deep structures, it may indicate a malignant condition.

Q.17. What is the objective of history taking?

- The objective of history taking is to get information about the patient's present illness (origin, progress, and duration), personal habits, past illness, and family history that help in arriving at a diagnosis.
- Ultimately the physician's knowledge, and experience combined with meticulous examination of the patient facilitates the best possible treatment for the patient.

Q.18. What is the importance of examining eyes in general examination?

Eyes should be examined under the following headings:

- **Conjunctiva**–examined for:
  - Pallor
  - Cyanosis
  - Bitot's spots
- **Sclera** – examined for:
  - Jaundice
  - Evidence of haemorrhage (scurvy)
- **State of pupils**
  - Size and shape
  - Reaction to light
- **Cornea** – examined for:
  - Xerophthalmia (dryness)

Q.19. What is the importance of examining the mouth in the general examination?

Mouth should be examined under the following headings:

- **Breath**: Acetone odour-diabetic acidosis
- **Lips**: Pallor, cyanosis
- **Gums**: Bleeding gums-scurvy, gingivitis
- **Tongue**: Pallor, cyanosis, dryness, and ulceration
- **Buccal cavity**: Pallor, ulcerations
- **Tonsil**: Enlargement of tonsils

Q.20. What is the significance of examining skin?

Examination of skin can provide many clues to diagnosis. The skin should be examined under the following headings:

- Pallor
- Cyanosis
- Yellow discolouration/jaundice
- Any allergic eruptions, scaling, etc.
- State of hydration
- Hair loss and texture

Q.21. What are kyphosis, scoliosis and lordosis?

All three conditions are deformities detected in the vertebral column.

- **Kyphosis**: It is the backward bending of the vertebral column. It results in convexity of the spine posteriorly and concavity anteriorly.
- **Scoliosis**: It is the lateral bending of the vertebral column
- **Lordosis**: It is the forward bending of the vertebral column. It results in concavity of the spine posteriorly and convexity anteriorly. Physiological lordosis is seen in pregnancy.

Q.22. What should be the position of the patient and examining doctor?

To carry out the examination doctor should stand on the right side of the patient. The ideal position of the patient is lying down on the table.

Q.23. How do you carry out systemic examination?

Please check above.

Meaning of commonly used terms in clinical practice	
Symptom	Patient's complaints are termed as symptoms, e.g. fever, pain in abdomen, etc.
Sign	The findings of the doctor on examination are termed as signs, e.g. tenderness (pain on touch, pallor, etc.)
Prognosis	It is possible future course/degree of cure of disease
Tenderness	It is pain sensation, a patient feels on touch
Diagnosis	It is the ability to differentiate between different diseases from each other. It is the conclusion drawn by a physician after examining a patient
Differential diagnosis	When the clinical picture does not point out to a definite diagnosis, multiple conclusions are drawn by doctor on examining the patient
Febrile	Having fever

Q.24. What are vital signs?

Vital signs include: Recording of BP, recording of arterial pulse and respiratory rate. Besides this recording of body temperature. Normal body temperature is 98–99 °F (36.6–37.2°C)

(Refer to TPR chart in charts section).

■ OSCE–GENERAL EXAMINATION

Procedure station 1: Check for pallor and give your findings:

S. No.	Assessment criteria	Marks assigned	Marks given
1.	Greet and stand on the right side of the subject		
2.	Take consent and explain the procedure		

Contd...

Contd...

S. No.	Assessment criteria	Marks assigned	Marks given
3.	Ask the subject to sit upright		
4.	Check subject's eyes—lower palpebral conjunctiva, dorsum of the tongue, soft palate, oral mucosa, palms, nails		
5.	Report and viva on clinical examination		
6.	Total		

Procedure station 2: Check for clubbing and report the findings:

S. No.	Assessment criteria	Marks assigned	Marks given
1.	Greet and stands on the right side of the subject		
2.	Take consent and explains the procedure		
3.	Ask subject to sit upright		
4.	Check for subject's tissues of nail bed and checks for the Lovibond angle and checks for convexity of nails		
5.	Report and viva on clinical examination		
6.	Total		

Procedure station 3: Check for icterus and report the findings:

S. No.	Assessment criteria	Marks assigned	Marks given
1.	Greet and stand on the right side of the subject		
2.	Take consent and explains the procedure		
3.	Ask the subject to sit upright		
4.	Check for subject's eyes for yellowish discolouration of sclera, palms and nails as well		
5.	Report and viva on clinical examination		
6.	Total		

Procedure station 4: Check for lymphadenopathy and report the findings

S. No.	Assessment criteria	Marks assigned	Marks given
1.	Greet and stand on the right side of the subject		
2.	Take consent and explains the procedure		
3.	Ask the subject to sit upright and flex his neck		

Contd...

Contd...

S. No.	Assessment criteria	Marks assigned	Marks given
4.	Check for lymph nodes in all areas (mentioned above under the heading of palpation for lymph nodes)		
5.	Report and viva on clinical examination		
6.	Total		

COMMON STATIONS – SPOTS IN PRACTICAL EXAMINATION (2/3 MARKS)

Q.1. Diagrams of pallor, clubbing, icterus, oedema lymphadenopathy, red tongue, cyanosis, kyphosis, scoliosis and lordosis to identify with one or two common clinical conditions causing them.

Q.2. Picture of lymphadenopathy: Identify, and enlist a group of lymph nodes to be palpated. List two conditions causing lymphadenopathy.

Q.3. Percussion figure: Identify, and write rules for eliciting the same.

Q.4. To fill general examination proforma of a normal person.

Q.5. Figure of stethoscope: Identify the figure, label its parts, and give uses.

Q.6. Figure/apparatus: Thermometer, BP apparatus, to identify and write its uses.

Q.7. Enlist prerequisites before clinical examination of a patient.

CASE-BASED SCENARIO/PROBLEM-BASED (2/3 MARKS)

Case 1: In the labour room, after delivery baby did not cry immediately and you observe that in a few minutes baby's tongue and limbs start becoming bluish.

- What probably is the cause of this bluish discolouration?

Case 2: A 35-year-old male has had kyphoscoliosis since birth.

- What is kyphoscoliosis?
- Will this condition affect his lung volumes and capacities and what is its physiological basis?

Case 3: A male 45 years of age comes with fever and throat pain. Examine him for lymphadenopathy.

- What are the groups of lymph nodes one should try to palpate?
- What is the physiological basis of enlarged lymph nodes when there is infection?

Case 4: A 40-year-old male comes with yellowish discolouration of the skin and his serum bilirubin is 3 mg/dl.

- What is the cause of his raised bilirubin levels?
- Examine patient for icterus.

Case 5: A 28-year-lady comes with c/o body aches, fatigue and breathlessness on exertion. On examination, there is pallor present on the tongue and mucous membrane.

- What is pallor? Where it is found.
- What is normal Hb in males and females

■ KEY POINTS TO REMEMBER

- History taking plays an important part in the clinical examination of patients. General examination and systemic examination are important to diagnose and treat patients for various clinical conditions.
- General examination includes an examination of the patient from head to toe.
- Systemic examination is to be carried out under four headings–inspection, palpation, percussion, and auscultation.

Examination of Alimentary System

Competency:

PY 4.10: Demonstrate the correct clinical examination of abdomen in volunteer or simulated environment.

> ### Learning Objectives
>
> After completion of this practical, the students shall be able to:
> - Give headings under which the alimentary system is examined
> - Understand the significance of testing saliva
> - List nine regions of the abdomen
> - Give common conditions causing splenomegaly and hepatomegaly
> - Demonstrate various tests for ascites
> - Demonstrate palpation of the liver, spleen and kidneys and give the findings
> - Demonstrate percussion of the abdomen and give the findings
> - Demonstrate auscultation of the abdomen and give the findings.

■ COMMON SYMPTOMS

Pain in the abdomen, heartburn (acidity), vomiting, diarrhoea, loss of appetite, blood in the stool (malena), change in bowel habits, constipation, anorexia (loss of appetite), sudden weight loss, etc. Many times, symptoms of the alimentary system (GIT) can be non-specific and many times signs of abnormality are noted when the disease reaches an advanced stage. Therefore, a meticulous detailed examination of the alimentary system becomes very important.

■ EXAMINATION OF ALIMENTARY SYSTEM

The oral cavity is the starting point of the alimentary system. Examination of the alimentary system can be divided into:
- Examination of the oral cavity
- Alimentary system examination

Examination of Oral Cavity

- The oral cavity forms the starting point of the open-ended alimentary canal. Thus examination of the alimentary system has to start with examination of the oral cavity first.
- Various diseases can show signs of disease in the oral cavity or mouth. Thus careful assessment of the oral cavity can help clinicians arrive at a diagnosis.
- Besides the examination of the mouth, one has to examine the head and neck along with the oral cavity in a systematic manner.

Headings for Examination of Oral Cavity

- **Breath**: The smell of the breath of a patient can give clues to doctors about various diseases. Various renal conditions, diabetic ketoacidosis, dental infections or dental caries, poor dental hygiene, etc. Can give rise to bad breath.
- **Examination of lips**: Observe lips for pallor, cyanosis or any other discolouration.

- **Examination of gums and teeth**: Observe gums for any discolouration or infection. Inspect teeth for any caries, missing teeth, and implants.
- **Examination of maxilla and mandible**: The maxilla and mandible should be examined for size, shape and contour. Palpate temporomandibular joint with opening and closing of the mouth and auscultate sound with a stethoscope.
- **Examination of buccal cavity**: Inspect the buccal cavity for colour, any swelling scar or lesions.
- **Palpation of lymph nodes**: Preauricular, submental, tonsillar, cervical, and supraclavicular lymph nodes for size, consistency, mobility, and pain if any.
- **Soft and hard palate, pharynx**: The palate is the roof of the mouth and floor of the nasal cavity. Observe the movement of the soft palate with sound and observe the position of the uvula (detail examination of IX and X cranial nerve in CNS Chapter), and look for tonsils (regress in adulthood). This can be done by introducing a tongue depressor in the mouth.
- **Examination of the tongue**: Observe for colour, state of hydration, and normal movements of the tongue (Cranial nerve XII in CNS Chapter), observe root, and body margins upper and lower surface of the tongue. Normally, tongue is pink in colour, with no ulcers, and no paralysis. With anaemia, the tongue might be pale.
- **Examination of taste sensation**: The facial nerve carries taste sensation from the anterior two-thirds of the tongue and the glossopharyngeal nerve carries sensation from the posterior one-third of the tongue [Cranial nerves (VII and IX) in CNS Chapter]. On the dorsal surface of the tongue, there are taste buds. Five basic tastes that can be tested. They are sweet, salty, bitter, sour, and umami.
- **Examination of teeth**: For any caries, missing teeth, and implants, observe for alignment and malocclusion, etc.
- **Palpation of salivary glands**: Palpate for parotid, sublingual, and submandibular glands.

Note: Anatomical deformities or dysfunction of various oral structures like tonsils, hard and soft palate, mandible, tongue, and misalignment of teeth can cause a reduction in upper airway diameter and can make a person prone to various breathing and sleep disorders. Dentists as well as sleep medicine physicians work together to deal with these disorders.

For Examination of the Alimentary System

- Subject should be relaxed in a dorsal recumbent position.
- Abdomen is exposed from xiphisternum to pubis symphysis.

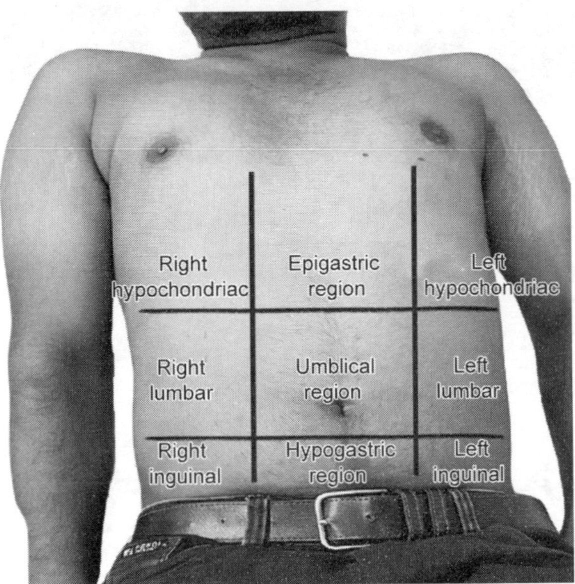

Fig. 17.1: Nine regions of the abdomen (two imaginary vertical and horizontal lines. (1-right hypochondrium, 2-epigastrium, 3-left hypochondrium, 4-right lumbar region, 5-umbilical region, 6-left lumbar region, 7-right iliac fossa, 8-hypogastric region, 9-left iliac fossa, trans-pyloric plane-the midpoint of the line between xiphisternum and (umbilicus [at lower border of L1] Trans-tubercular plane—transverse line joining tubercles that mark the highest point on iliac crest).

Clinically

- Abdomen is divided into nine regions **(Fig. 17.1)**.
- It is divided into nine regions by two vertical planes and two horizontal planes.
- Clinical examination of the alimentary system is carried out by a sequence of examination— inspection, palpation, percussion, and auscultation.

SYSTEMIC EXAMINATION OF THE ALIMENTARY SYSTEM

Inspection

The abdomen should be exposed from the xiphisternum to the pubic symphysis for inspection.

The following points are noted:

- **Size and shape of the abdomen**: Observe the shape, size and contour of the abdomen. Normally abdomen is flat. Look for any sunken and globular abdomen.
- **Abdominal symmetry**: Normally, it is symmetrical. Observe for any obvious bulge on the abdomen.
- **Umbilicus:** Normally, it is retracted and inverted.
- **Movements with respiration**: Normally, abdominal wall rises with inspiration and falls with expiration.
- **State of skin**: Inspect for any scar marks and infection.
- **Veins**: Normally, there are no superficial visible veins on the abdomen. Distended veins on the abdomen are seen with obstruction of the inferior vena cava.

- **Visible pulsations**: Inspect for any visible pulsations on the abdomen. In many thin people, aortic pulsations are seen in the epigastric region.
- **Visible peristalsis**: Except in thin individuals, visible peristalsis is not seen in normal person.
- **Any pigmentation of the abdominal wall**: Linea nigra in midline is observed with pregnancy.
- **Hernial sites**: Observe umbilical, inguinal and femoral regions for any swelling or swelling on coughing
- **Genitalia**: Inspect groins, penis and scrotal sac for any swelling and confirm the position of testes in the normal place.

Palpation

- It is divided into superficial and deep palpation.
- **With superficial palpation**, one should check for tenderness (pain on touch) and consistency of the abdominal wall. Normally abdominal wall is elastic in nature. The doughy feel of the abdomen is observed in tuberculosis of GIT.
- With superficial palpation to rule out hernia, inguinal, umbilical and femoral regions are palpated for the presence of impulse on coughing.
- **Deep palpation** is carried out to palpate the spleen, liver and kidneys.

Palpation of Liver

Method

- The patient should be in a relaxed state. Hips and knees should be flexed (this relaxes abdominal muscles) in a supine state
- Ask the patient to turn his/her head to the opposite side and to take deep breaths.
- Palpation begins in the right iliac fossa and then gradually works towards the right subcostal margin (right hypochondrium). Palpation is done by the flat of the hand placed on the abdomen.
- Hand is pressed inwards and upwards as the patient takes deep inspiration. If the liver is enlarged, it is felt by the radial border of the index finger. Normally, the liver is not palpable (in children sometimes it is palpable). Only when it is enlarged, it becomes palpable.
- Enlarged liver is felt by the radial border of the palpating hand's index finger.
- If the liver is palpable, its degree of enlargement, edge, shape, surface, tenderness (pain on touch) consistency, movement with respiration and pulsations (if any) should be noted **(Fig. 17.2)**.

Common causes of hepatomegaly are:
- Infective hepatitis, malaria, typhoid, amoebic abscess, etc.

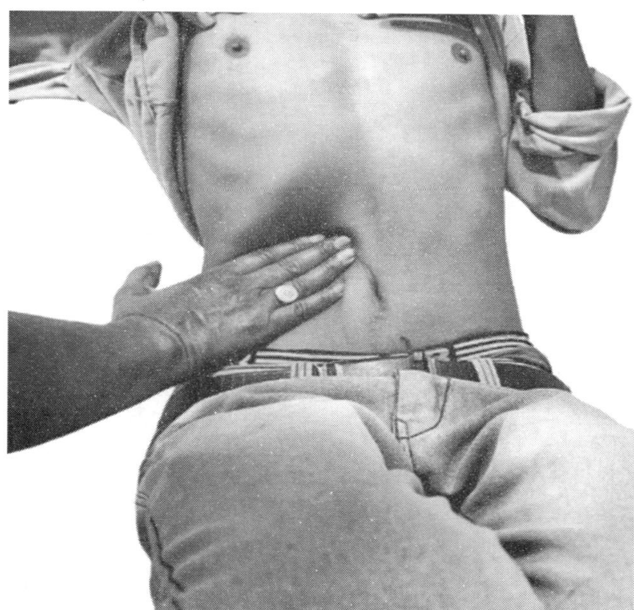

Fig. 17.2: Palpation of liver

Palpation of Spleen

Method

- The patient should be in a relaxed state. Hips and knees should be flexed (this relaxes abdominal muscles) in a supine state.
- Ask the patient to turn his/her head to the opposite side and to take deep breaths.
- Flat of the right hand is placed in the right iliac fossa and the left hand is placed over the lower part of the thoracic cage posterolaterally on the left side. Palpation begins in the right iliac fossa moving upwards and left obliquely towards the left hypochondrium (because the spleen enlarges in this direction). Normally, the spleen is not palpable.
- Spleen can also be palpated with one hand, by keeping flat of the right hand in the right iliac fossa and moving gradually upwards obliquely.
- When the spleen enlarges, it increases twice or thrice its normal size then only it becomes palpable.
- If the spleen is palpable its degree of enlargement, edge, surface, tenderness, and consistency should be noted **(Fig. 17.3)**.

Common causes of splenomegaly are:

Malaria, typhoid, thalassemia, and leukemia, etc.

Palpation of Kidneys

Method—Bimanual Palpation of Kidneys

- The patient should be in a relaxed state. Hips and knees should be flexed (this relaxes abdominal muscles) in a supine state.
- Ask the patient to turn his/her head to the opposite side and to take deep breaths.

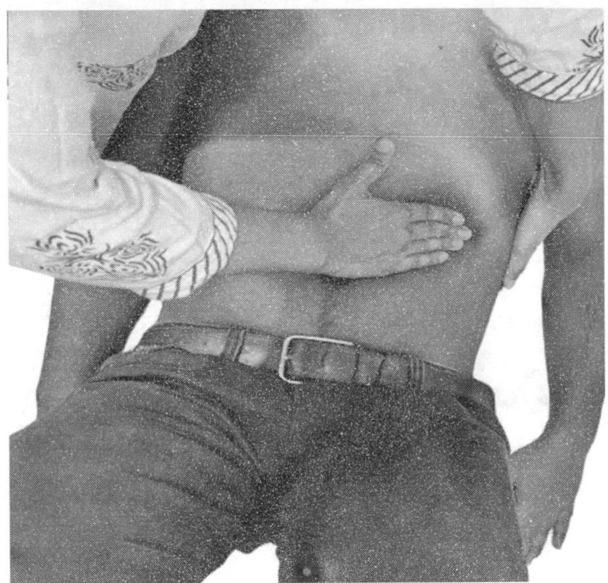

Fig. 17.3: Palpation of spleen

- The left hand of the examiner should be placed behind the costovertebral angle and palpating right hand in the lumbar region.
- With the expiration of the patient, two hands are approximated to feel for a kidney. The procedure is repeated for other kidney palpations. Thus, the right and left kidneys are palpated.
- Normally, they are not palpable. In a thin person, sometimes the right kidney is palpable **(Figs. 17.4A and B)**.

Percussion

- Abdomen is percussed in all nine regions.
- Normally, the tympanic note is elicited on the abdomen.

- On the liver, kidneys, and spleen, the dull note is elicited. Percussion of the abdomen is useful to diagnose ascites (free fluid in the abdomen).
- There are many tests to diagnose ascites clinically. Dullness over major regions of the abdomen is produced due to an enlarged liver, spleen, tumour, ascites, etc. Over 1500 ml of fluid must collect in the peritoneal cavity before its presence can be detected by physical examination.

Common tests to demonstrate ascites are:

Horseshoe-shaped dullness:

- The patient should be in a relaxed state. Hips and knees should be flexed (this relaxes abdominal muscles) in a supine state.
- Ask the patient to turn his/her head to the opposite side and breathe.
- This test can be demonstrated with moderate collection of fluid in the peritoneal cavity with dullness marked in hypogastric regions and flanks giving rise to horseshoe-shaped dullness.
- With moderate collection of fluid and a person lying in the supine position, fluid gets collected in flanks and hypogastric regions. Intestines float upwards in epigastric and umbilical regions (thus this region demonstrates tympanic note) and flanks and hypogastric region demonstrate dull note (due to collection of liquid).
- This can be demonstrated by percussing in various directions away from the umbilicus till a dull note is obtained **(Fig. 17.5)**.

Shifting dullness:

- The patient should be in a relaxed state. Hips and knees should be flexed (this relaxes abdominal muscles) in a supine state.

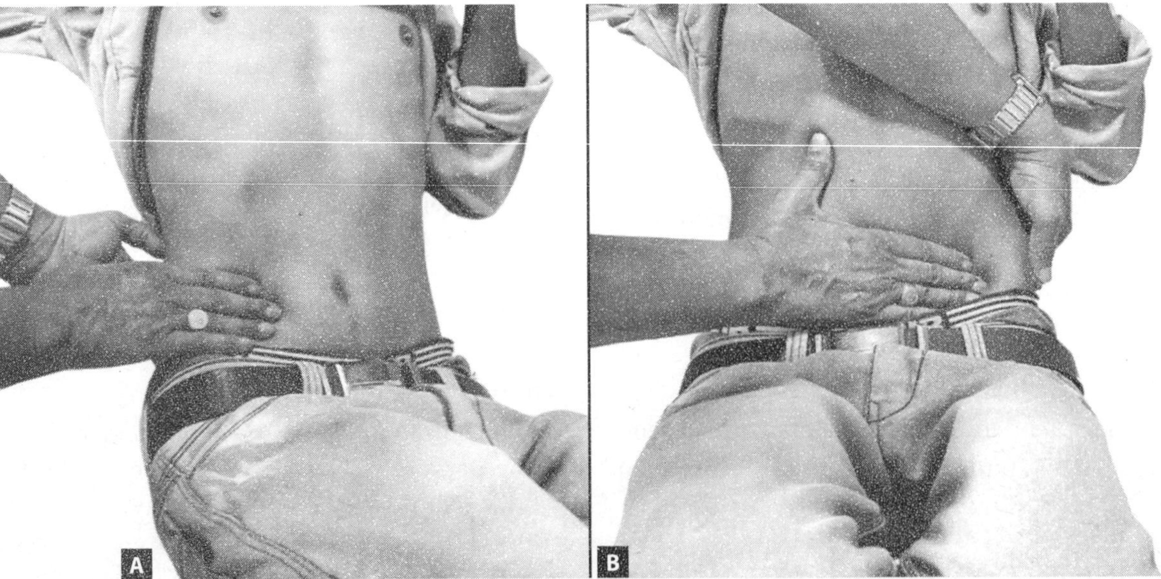

Figs. 17.4A and B: Bimanual palpation of kidneys

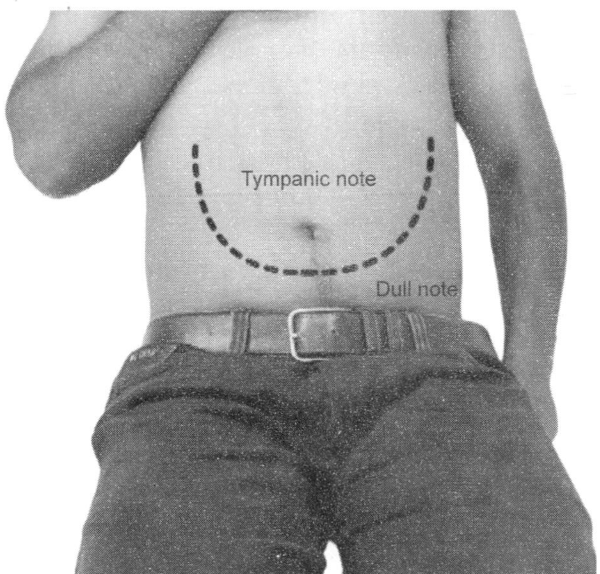

Fig. 17.5: Horseshoe-shaped dullness

- Ask the patient to turn his/her head to the opposite side and breathe.
- Due to the gravity effect when a person is in the supine position, fluid gets collected in flanks and hypogastric regions.
- When you ask the person to turn to one side (say left side), fluid gravitates to the left flank and intestines float up and a tympanic note is observed on the right flank. Simultaneously width of dullness increases in the left flank.
- Thus, dullness shifts. The same test can be repeated by asking a person to sleep right lateral **(Figs. 17.6A and B)**.

Fluid Thrill

- The patient should be in a relaxed state. Hips and knees should be flexed (this relaxes abdominal muscles) in a supine state.
- Ask the patient to turn his/her head to the opposite side and breathe.
- Physician puts hand over one flank and with fingers of other hand gives a tap on another flank. Wave is initiated due to this tap and transmitted to the opposite side.
- To avoid false sensations, we ask the subject/patient to keep his hand vertically and firmly against linea alba **(Fig. 17.7)**.

Auscultation

- In the alimentary system, auscultation is done to listen to bowel sounds (borborygmi).
- Normal bowel sounds are heard as intermittent, low or medium-pitched gurgles in the paraumbilical region.

Observations–Examination of Alimentary System Proforma

Systemic examination of the alimentary system: Any systemic examination is to be done after a complete general examination as shown in Chapter 1 General Examination.

Examination of the oral cavity and throat
Lips   Tongue   Gums   Palate   Tonsils   Pharynx
Inspection of abdomen
Size and shape   Symmetry   Status of umbilicus
Movements with respiration   Visible veins   Skin on abdomen Pigmentation
Visible peristalsis   Hernial sites   Visible pulsations   Genitalia

Contd...

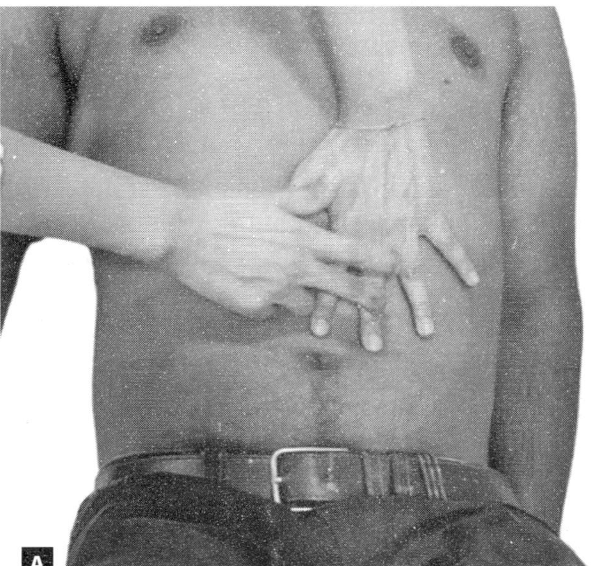

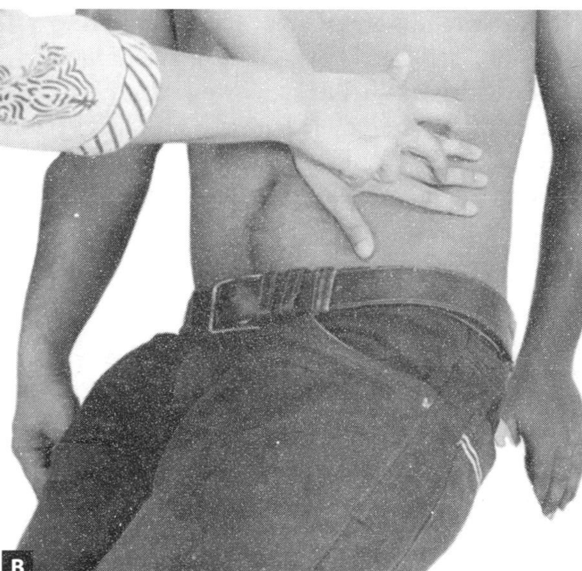

Figs. 17.6A and B: Shifting dullness

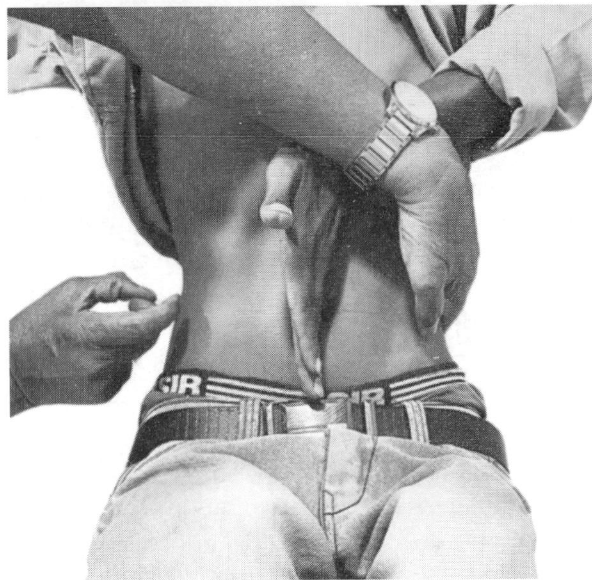

Fig. 17.7: Fluid thrill

Contd...

Palpation
Superficial palpation of the abdomen
Consistency of abdominal wall   Tenderness   Pulsations on abdomen   Hernial sites
Deep palpation of the abdomen
Liver   Spleen   Kidney
Percussion of abdomen
Percussion of the abdomen in nine regions
Horseshoe shaped test   Shifting dullness test   Fluid thrill test
Auscultation of abdomen
Peristaltic sounds

■ IMPORTANT QUESTIONS AND ANSWERS

Q.1. What are the nine regions of the abdomen?
Abdomen is divided into nine regions by two imaginary vertical and horizontal lines (as described above). Nine regions of the abdomen are epigastric, right and left hypochondriac, umbilical, right and left lumbar, hypogastric and right and left iliac fossa (Refer to **Fig. 17.1**).

Q.2. What can be normal variations in size and shape of the abdomen?
- **Flat abdomen:** The rib margins and anterior abdominal wall are more or less at the same level.
- **Globular/round abdomen:** The anterior abdominal wall presents a forward convexity. It may be due to the presence of fetus (pregnancy), flatus (gaseous distension), faeces (chronic constipation), fluid (ascites) and fat (obesity). In all the above conditions, the type of distension is symmetrical. Convexity of the anterior abdominal wall may contribute to loss of abdominal muscle tone.

- **Scaphoid/sunken abdomen:** Abdomen with a forward concavity. It is observed in very thin people, cachexia, prolonged starvation, and dehydration.

Q.3. Enumerate conditions which give rise to abdominal asymmetry.
- Normal abdomen is symmetrical. Lack of symmetry can be noted due to localised bulging.
- It can be observed with enlargement of the liver, spleen, presence of tumour or retraction of the abdominal wall due to any injury of the underlying muscle.

Q.4. Why general examination becomes important before examination of the alimentary system?
- Systemic disease related with respect to the alimentary system can be evident while one is doing general examination of the patient.
- Clubbing of fingers, spider naevi (small telangiectatic superficial blood vessels), yellowish discolouration of skin and mucous membrane (due to raised bilirubin levels) can indicate a liver disease.
- Parotid swelling, erythema on palms can be associated with liver dysfunction and alcohol liver disease.

Q.5. How spleen is palpated? What are common conditions causing splenomegaly?
- Spleen is situated in the left hypochondriac region. Steps to be followed and instructions to be given to the patient for the same are discussed above in detail
- **Common causes of splenomegaly:** Malaria, typhoid, thalassemia.

Q.6. How liver is palpated? What are the common causes of hepatomegaly?
- Liver is situated in the right hypochondriac region. Steps to palpate the liver and instructions given to the patient are discussed above in detail.
- **Common causes of hepatomegaly**—cirrhosis, hepatitis, malaria, typhoid. Normally, liver is situated in right hypochondrium.

Q.7. Is normally visible peristalsis or pulsations observed on inspection of the abdomen?
- In normal person usually there are no visible pulsations (except in thin individuals epigastric pulsations of aorta are visible).
- Visible peristalsis is also not observed in a normal person.

Q.8. Are abdominal veins visible? What is caput medusae?
- Normally on inspection abdominal veins are not visible (except in very thin persons in the subcostal margin).
- **Caput medusae**: It is characteristic presence of distended veins around the umbilicus and is observed

in portal hypertension (it shows anastomosis between systemic and portal veins).

Q.9. What is peritoneum? What is peritoneal fluid?

- Peritoneum is the serous membrane that lines the abdominal cavity and surrounds all abdominal organs.
- Parietal peritoneum lines the abdominal wall and the visceral peritoneum wraps around organs. The space between two is the peritoneal cavity.
- Peritoneal fluid helps to prevent friction of various abdominal organs, normally it is 50 to 75 ml.

In peritonitis, movement of the abdominal wall with respect to respiration is absent or markedly diminished. This is called as **silent abdomen**.

Q.10. What is ascites? Enumerate different tests to elicit ascites.

- Collection of free fluid in the peritoneal cavity is known as ascites.

Tests to elicit ascites are:

- Horseshoe test
- Fluid thrill
- Shifting dullness

Q.11. Which ascites tests will come positive in a normal person?

All three tests (fluid thrill, horseshoe-shaped dullness and shifting dullness) will be negative in a normal person. As ascites is not present in a healthy person. All three tests are hypothetical.

Q.12. What is a puddle's sign?

This sign is elicited to detect the presence of minimal fluid, even 120–150 ml of fluid collection in the abdomen can be detected by this method. First abdomen is percussed in a supine position, in the midline and then patient is asked to sleep in the knee-elbow position and then you elicit dullness near the umbilicus (dependent part).

Q.13. Enumerate common causes of ascites.

Common conditions causing ascites are cirrhosis of liver, congestive cardiac failure, malnutrition, ovarian tumour, nephrosis of kidneys, etc.

Q.14. What is the significance of auscultation of the abdomen?

- Auscultation is a useful way of listening to bowel sounds and deciding whether they are normal, increased (e.g. diarrhoea, hunger) or decreased (intestinal obstruction). Bowel sounds are appreciated with deep expiration and slight application of the bell of stethoscope. Sounds are best heard at the right umbilicus.
- On auscultation of the abdomen, normal peristaltic sounds (borborygmi) are intermittent, low/medium pitched gurgles. The absence of peristalsis (silent abdomen) is common post-operative, intestinal paralysis.

Q.15. How do you palpate the abdomen?

Abdomen is palpated under two headings:

- **Superficial palpation**: It is done to check tenderness, rigidity and consistency of the abdominal wall.
- **Deep palpation**: It is done for palpating the liver, spleen and kidneys (please refer above for details).

Q.16. What is referred pain?

- It is the pain that arises from a visceral organ which is projected or located to a specific site on the body surface that is away from the anatomical location of the organ.

  Example: Pain in appendicitis is felt at the umbilicus, pain arising from myocardium is referred to left arm/shoulder.

Q.17. Besides spleen, liver and kidneys, can any other be palpable in the abdomen?

Other palpable organs in the abdomen:

- **Gallbladder**: Gallbladder has to be palpated in the same way as that of liver. In normal person usually, it is not palpable. If it is enlarged, it may be felt as a firm globular swelling lateral to the edge of the rectus abdominis near the tip of the ninth costal cartilage. It can be due to obstruction of common bile duct, pancreas cancer, gallbladder cancer, etc.
- **Urinary bladder**: Normally, it is not palpable. If there is a retention of urine in the bladder, it can be palpated as a firm swelling above the suprapubic region which may reach till umbilicus.

In females, it has to be differentiated from ovarian cyst, fibroid or gravid uterus (pregnancy)

Aorta and femoral vessels: Normally, aorta is not felt. Sometimes on deep palpation, it may be felt a little above and to the left of the umbilicus. Here fingertips are used for palpation.

Q.18. Enumerate other techniques/investigations to assess alimentary system functions.

Techniques/Investigations include:

- **X-ray:** A plain X-ray abdomen is one of the important investigations while diagnosing acute abdomen. Perforation/obstruction of the abdomen may show free air under the diaphragm on X-ray.
- **Examination of vomitus (if any):** Right from contents of vomitus to smell, amount of mucus, colour, consistency, and presence of blood/bile can give a clue in reaching towards a conclusion in case of alimentary disease.

- **Examination of faeces:** Physical as well as microscopic examination can help to diagnose various clinical conditions.
- **Peritoneal fluid:** Aspiration of peritoneal fluid is done for diagnostic as well as therapeutic purposes.
- **Oesophageal function assessment:** It can be done by barium swallow which can help to detect slow transit or arrest of food bolus in the oesophagus. Various manometric studies do help to find pressure changes with deglutition and localizing functional abnormalities of movements (e.g. achalasia), heartburn, 24 hrs. pH monitoring in the lower oesophagus helps in diagnosis and treatment.
- **Upper gastrointestinal endoscopy:** Direct visualization of different parts of GIT till proximal small bowel is done for diagnostic as well as therapeutic purposes. It can be done with or without sedation and local pharyngeal anaesthesia.
- **Gastric function assessment:** It includes various tests that can assess gastric functions like basal and maximum acid secretion, gastrin levels, tests for *Helicobacter pylori* infection, X-ray, barium swallow studies
- **Liver function tests and pancreatic function tests:** To help assess and diagnose various liver and pancreatic dysfunctions.
- **Small bowel:** Barium swallow and barium follow-through studies can help diagnose various small bowel pathologies like diverticula or neoplasm. Nowadays small bowel enema is an alternative used for barium follow-through studies. Radioisotope studies of the bowel can be done for inflammatory bowel disease.
- **Other tests:** Colonoscopy, proctoscopy, sigmoidoscopy, cholangiography (to assess biliary system), angiography of gastrointestinal arteries ultrasound MRI, CT scan, PET scan includes some of the important investigations used for therapeutic as well as diagnostic purposes for various clinical conditions.

OSCE—ALIMENTARY SYSTEM

Procedure station 1: Inspect abdomen and give your findings.

S. No.	Assessment criteria	Marks assigned	Marks given
1.	Greet and stand on the right side of the subject		
2.	Ask the subject to lie down in a supine position comfortably with knee and hips flexed and explain procedure		
3.	Inspect the abdomen from xiphisternum to pubic symphysis		
4.	Ask the patient to turn his face opposite side and breath		

Contd...

Contd...

S. No.	Assessment criteria	Marks assigned	Marks given
5.	Able to describe size, the shape of the abdomen, abdominal symmetry, state of umbilicus, movement of abdominal wall with respiration		
6.	Able to describe any visible peristalsis, visible pulsations, state of skin, scar marks if present		
7.	Able to check for umbilical, inguinal and femoral sites for hernia (any swelling)		
8.	Report and viva on clinical examination		
9.	Total		

Procedure station 2: Palpate the abdomen superficially and give your findings.

S. No.	Assessment criteria	Marks assigned	Marks given
1.	Greet and stand on the right side of the subject		
2.	Ask the subject to lie down in a supine position with knees and hips flexed and explain the procedure		
3.	Inspect abdomen from xiphisternum to pubic symphysis		
4.	Ask the patient to turn their face opposite side and breath		
5.	Confirm all findings of inspection of the abdomen		
6.	Check and describes the consistency of the abdominal wall and tenderness if present		
7.	Check for umbilical, inguinal and femoral sites for hernia (any swelling)		
8.	Report and viva on clinical examination		
9.	Total		

Procedure station 3: Palpate liver and give your findings.

S. No.	Assessment criteria	Marks assigned	Marks given
1.	Greet and stand on the right side of the subject		
2.	Ask the subject to lie down in supine position comfortably and explains the procedure		
3.	Ask for turning face to opposite side and take deep breath, flexion at knees		
4.	Palpate from right iliac fossa with flat of hand till right subcostal margin		

Contd...

Contd...

S. No.	Assessment criteria	Marks assigned	Marks given
5.	Press hands inwards and upwards with deep inspiration		
6.	Report and viva on clinical examination		
7.	Total		

Procedure station 4: Palpate spleen and give your findings.

S. No.	Assessment criteria	Marks assigned	Marks given
1.	Greet and stand on the right side of the subject		
2.	Ask the subject to lie down in supine position comfortably and explains the procedure		
3.	Ask for turning face to opposite side and take deep breath, flexion at knees		
4.	Palpate from right iliac fossa with flat of right hand and places left hand on the lower part of the thoracic cage on the left side (press left hand downwards and medially)		
5.	Press right hand downwards with each deep inspiration and go obliquely palpating till left subcostal margin (lower part of the thoracic cage)		
6.	Report and viva on clinical examination		
7.	Total		

Procedure station 5: Palpate kidneys and give your findings.

S. No.	Assessment criteria	Marks assigned	Marks given
1.	Greet and stand on the right side of the subject		
2.	Ask the subject to lie down in supine position comfortably and explains the procedure		
3.	Ask for turning face to opposite side and take deep breath, flexion at knees		
4.	Place left hand behind the costo-vertebral angle to maintain forward pressure and right hand up on hypochondrium with fingers pointing towards costal margin		
5.	Try to approximate both hands during expiration for palpating kidney		
6.	Repeat procedure for left kidney palpation (standing on right side of the patient)		
7.	Report and viva on clinical examination		
8.	Total		

Procedure station 6: Percuss abdomen and give your findings.

S. No.	Assessment criteria	Marks assigned	Marks given
1.	Greet and stand on the right side of the subject		
2.	Ask the subject to lie down in supine position comfortably and explains the procedure		
3.	Expose abdomen from xiphisternum to pubic symphysis		
4.	Ask for turning face to opposite side and flexion at knees		
5.	Do percuss all nine quadrants of abdomen		
6.	Report and viva on clinical examination		
7.	Total		

Procedure station 7: Demonstrate horseshoe-shaped dullness test.

S. No.	Assessment criteria	Marks assigned	Marks given
1.	Greet and stands on the right side of the subject		
2.	Ask the subject to lie down in supine position comfortably and explains the procedure		
3.	Expose abdomen from xiphisternum to pubic symphysis		
4.	Ask for turning face to opposite side and, flexion at knees		
5.	Do percuss from the umbilicus away to the periphery to mark horseshoe-shaped dullness		
6.	Report and viva on clinical examination		
7.	Total		

Procedure station 8: Demonstrate fluid thrill test.

S. No.	Assessment criteria	Marks assigned	Marks given
1.	Greet and stand on the right side of the subject		
2.	Ask the subject to lie down in a supine position comfortably and explains the procedure		
3.	Expose abdomen from xiphisternum to pubic symphysis		
4.	Ask for turning face to opposite side with flexion at knees.		
5.	Ask the subject (patient) to keep the edge of his/her hand vertically along linea alba		
6.	Place one hand on the flank and with fingers of the other hand, tap the flank on the opposite side		

Contd...

Contd...

S. No.	Assessment criteria	Marks assigned	Marks given
7.	Report and viva on clinical examination		
8.	Total		

Procedure station 9: Demonstrate shifting dullness test.

S. No.	Assessment criteria	Marks assigned	Marks given
1.	Greet and stand on the right side of the subject		
2.	Ask the subject to lie down in a supine position comfortably and explains the procedure		
3.	Expose abdomen from xiphisternum to pubic symphysis		
4.	Ask for turning face to opposite side with flexion at knees		
5.	Do percuss abdomen (in supine position) from the umbilicus to flank (till dull note is heard)		
6.	Do keep pleximeter at the same place, instructs the subject to turn left lateral (wait for a minute)		
7.	Demonstrate area where there was dull note before, it is tympanic note		
8.	Report and viva on clinical examination		
9.	Total		

Procedure station 10: Auscultate abdomen and give your findings.

S. No.	Assessment criteria	Marks assigned	Marks given
1.	Greet and stands on the right side of the subject		
2.	Ask the subject to lie down in a supine position comfortably and explains the procedure		
3.	Expose abdomen from xiphisternum to pubic symphysis		
4.	Ask for turning face to opposite side and flexion at knees		
5.	Ausculate all areas around the umbilicus		
6.	Report and viva on clinical examination		
7.	Total		

COMMON STATIONS – SPOTS IN PRACTICAL EXAMINATION (2/3 MARKS)

Q.1. Enlist common symptoms patients come with alimentary disease.

Q.2. Figure of physician palpating liver, spleen, kidneys, percussing abdomen for tests of ascites, auscultating abdomen for intestinal sounds: Identify the picture and one or two questions related to it. (as given above)

Q.3. Diagram showing fluid thrill. Identify test. Write the cause for the placement of patient's hand on abdomen in the picture.

Q.4. Diagram of nine quadrants of the abdomen – Identify and label.

Q.5. Diagram showing shifting dullness. Identify test. Write why this test cannot be demonstrated with massive collection of fluid in abdomen.

Q.6. Diagram showing horseshoe-shaped dullness. Identify test. Write areas in which dull note is expected on the abdomen in this patient.

Q.7. Describe normal intestinal sound. What is a silent abdomen?

Q.8. Fill alimentary system proforma for a normal person (please check above for a proforma).

CASE-BASED SCENARIO/PROBLEM-BASED (2/3 MARKS)

Case 1: A 45-year-old male comes for his routine checkup. He is a known alcoholic for the last 15 years. On examination, all vitals are normal. Per abdomen liver is palpable.

- What can be the probable cause of palpable liver?
- Enumerate two conditions that cause hepatomegaly.

Case 2: A 27-year-old male comes with c/o high-grade fever with chills since last two days. On examination patient is febrile 101°C, pulse 110/min, BP 130/80 mm of Hg. Per abdomen spleen is palpable.

- What can be the probable cause of an enlarged spleen?
- Enumerate two conditions that cause splenomegaly.
- What blood investigations you would suggest for such a patient?

Case 3: A 15-year-old school-going girl comes with c/o loose motions since last night. She has c/o body aches and low-grade fever since morning. On examination per abdomen bowel sounds frequency is increased.

- What is the physiological basis of the increased frequency of bowel sounds?
- What are areas where one should auscultate for bowel sounds?

IMPORTANT POINTS TO REMEMBER

- Examination of the oral cavity and saliva forms an important part in the examination of the alimentary system.
- Various tests are available to detect salivary secretion, which are useful in the diagnosis of many oral and systemic diseases.
- Abdomen can be divided into nine regions as right and left hypochondrium, epigastric, right and left lumbar, umbilical, right and left iliac fossa, and hypogastric.
- Common causes of splenomegaly include malaria and typhoid. Common causes of hepatomegaly are cirrhosis, fatty liver, and typhoid.
- Intestinal sounds are auscultated near the umbilical region.

Examination of Arterial Pulse

Competency:
PY 5.12: Record blood pressure and pulse at rest and in different grades of exercise and posture in volunteer or simulated environment.

Learning Objectives

At the end of this practical, students shall be able to:

- Describe the significance of the examination of the pulse
- Define arterial pulse
- List parameters with which the pulse is examined
- Give findings after examining the subject for pulse.
- Enlist common causes of—tachycardia, bradycardia, high- and low-volume pulse
- Give use of three fingers while examining the pulse
- Name different sites to feel for arterial pulse
- List the physiological and pathological variations in pulse rate

■ PULSE

Pulse is defined as a rise in pressure and distension of the vessel wall due to the ejection of blood in the aorta due to ventricular systole. This pressure wave is transmitted along the arterial tree and felt at any peripheral arteries as a pulse.

Pulse is felt at different arteries: Common arteries palpated are radial, external temporal, carotid, brachial, femoral, popliteal, posterior tibial and dorsalis pedis, etc.

Clinical Method of Examination of Pulse (Use of Three Fingers)

The radial artery is palpated with the help of three fingers. The middle finger is used to feel pulse; the index finger is used to vary the pressure on the artery; whereas the distal finger is used to prevent retrograde pulsations from the palmar arch. The following observations are made—rate, rhythm, volume, tension force, character of the pulse wave, condition of the vessel wall and equality **(Fig. 18.1)**.

- **Rate:** Pulse rate is expressed as rate/min. Normal pulse rate is 70–90 beats/min.
- **Rhythm:** Interval between two successive beats if the regular, rhythm is regular. Normally, the rhythm is regular.

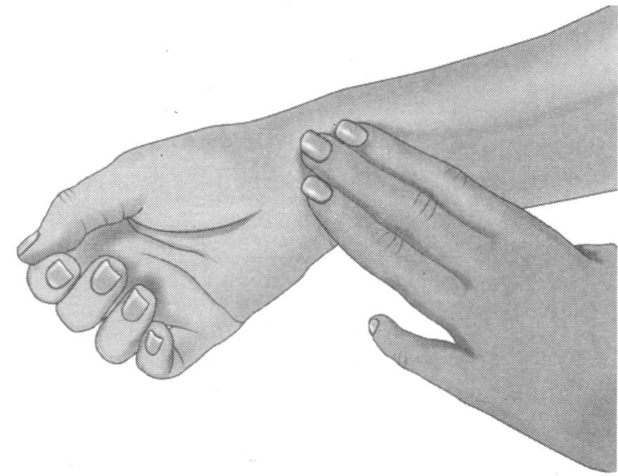

Fig. 18.1: Clinical examination of pulse (radial artery)

- **Volume:** It is the amplitude of movement of the vessel wall during the passage of the pulse wave. It corresponds to pulse pressure (pulse pressure is the difference between systolic and diastolic blood pressure).
- **Tension:** It is pressure applied to the artery, to feel the pulse best. Normally, moderate pressure is necessary to feel the artery. Tension of the pulse gives an idea about diastolic pressure.
- **Force:** It is the pressure required to obliterate the pulse. It roughly corresponds to systolic pressure.
- **Character of the pulse:** Normally, the ascent and descent of the pulse wave are smooth and gradual, but the dicrotic wave is not felt clinically. Different abnormal characteristics of the pulse wave are observed in different clinical conditions.
- **Condition of vessel wall:** Artery is rolled beneath fingers against the underlying bone. Normally, the artery is elastic and is, therefore, not felt. In older person because of atherosclerosis, arteries lose their elasticity and can be felt as a rope-like structure.
- **Comparison on two sides:** For equality.

■ IMPORTANT QUESTIONS AND ANSWERS

Q.1. What is tachycardia?
- A heart rate of more than 100 beats/min is called tachycardia.
- Physiological conditions causing tachycardia: Exercise, anger, emotions, and excitement.
- Common pathological conditions causing tachycardia: Fever, increased body temperature directly stimulates sinoatrial (SA) node, thyrotoxicosis and anaemia.

Q.2. What is bradycardia?
- A heart rate of less than 60 beats/min is called bradycardia.
- Physiological conditions causing bradycardia: Sleep, athletes (increased vagal tone), fear, meditation and pranayama (after practising for many years).
- Common pathological conditions causing bradycardia; myxedema and heart blocks.

Q.3. What does the volume of the pulse suggest?
- Volume of the pulse suggests pulse pressure.
- Pulse pressure is a difference between systolic and diastolic pressure. If normal BP is 120/80 mm Hg, then pulse pressure is (120–80) which is about 40 mmHg.
- Thus, it suggests us about stroke volume and compliance of vessels.

Low-volume Pulse
- Volume of pulse decreases in—aortic stenosis, shock, pulmonary stenosis, etc.
- In all the above conditions, the pulse pressure gap shortens (i.e. less difference between systolic and diastolic).

- Low-volume pulse is known as a thready pulse or a pulse which is very weak to feel.

High-volume Pulse
- Volume of pulse increases in exercise, fever, thyrotoxicosis, etc.
- In all the above conditions, the pulse pressure gap widens (i.e. more difference between systolic and diastolic).
- High-volume pulse is also called as bounding pulse.

Q.4. What is the significance of examining pulse?
Examination of the pulse provides the following information:
- Working status of the heart
- Circulatory state of the body, e.g. blood pressure, blood volume, etc.
- State of the body's metabolism
- Temperature of the body
- Condition of the vessel wall

Q.5. What precautions are taken before the examination of the pulse?
Precautions
- Subject should relax and rest for a few minutes.
- Subject's forearm should be semi-pronated and wrist should be semi-flexed.
- Pulse must be examined for rate, rhythm, volume, character, tension, force, equality, and condition of the vessel wall.
- Pulse rate should be counted for the full 1 minute.
- Pulse must be examined and compared on both sides.

Q.6. What is the force of the pulse?
- Force is the amount of pressure applied to completely obliterate the pulse.
- Pressure is applied with the index finger (when you are examining the pulse with three fingers).
- Force should be expressed as moderate, i.e. moderate amount of pressure is applied to obliterate the pulse.
- Force of pulse corresponds approximately to systolic pressure.

Q.7. What is the tension of the pulse?
- Tension is the amount of pressure applied to feel the pulse best.
- Pressure is applied by the index finger (when you are examining a pulse with three fingers).
- Volume should be expressed as moderate, i.e. a moderate amount of pressure is applied to feel the pulse best.
- Tension of pulse corresponds approximately to diastolic blood pressure.

Q.8. What do you understand by radio femoral delay?
The pulse itself is a rise in pressure and distention of the vessel wall due to blood filling in the aorta

during ventricular systole, which is transmitted to any peripheral artery that we feel as a pulse. Thus for all practical purposes, the pulse should be felt at all arterial pulse sites simultaneously. As the name suggests, radio femoral delay is a delay in the appearance of a pulse in the radial artery and femoral artery. This is seen in coarctation of aorta mainly when constriction is present distal to the origin of the left subclavian artery.

Q.9. What are the different types of characters of pulse waves?

1. **Anacrotic pulse:** This pulse wave is slow to rise. It gives two upbeats. It is felt when there is prolonged ejection of stroke volume as in aortic stenosis.
2. **Dicrotic pulse:** It is called as twice beating pulse. It is felt in febrile states like typhoid fever.
3. **Water hammer pulse (collapsing pulse):** It is characterized by rapid upstroke and rapid downstroke of pulse wave. It is felt in aortic regurgitation (AR).
4. **Pulsus bisferiens:** It is a combination of low rising (Anacrotic) and collapsing pulse. It is seen in aortic stenosis which is associated with aortic incompetence.
5. **Pulsus alternans:** Alternate beats are strong and weak. Seen with left ventricular failure.

Q.10.Why pulse should be examined with three fingers?

- Clinical examination of the pulse is carried out always with the help of three fingers. The distal finger is used to obliterate retrograde palmar arch pulsations. The middle finger is used to feel the pulse.
- The proximal finger is used to adjust the pressure so that one can judge the force and tension of the pulse.

Q.11. What is sinus arrhythmia?

- Variation in pulse rate with respect to phases of respiration is called sinus arrhythmia.
- There is an increase in pulse rate with inspiration and a decrease in pulse rate with expiration.

Q.12. Pulse rate is less in athletes. Give physiological basis.

With regular exercise, cardiorespiratory endurance increases in athletes. There is functional hypertrophy of the myocardium and optimum sympathetic nervous system stimulation that results in increased cardiac output (as stroke volume increases). Hence, heart rate is reduced by the baroreceptor mechanism (increase in vagal tone).

Q.13. What is arterial pulse tracing?

- It is an instrumental record of pulse by Dudgeon's sphygmograph (Check in the Charts section).
- There is an **anacrotic/ascending limb** which is also called as percussion (tidal) wave, which is due to the ejection of blood during ventricular systole (that corresponds with the maximum ejection phase of the cardiac cycle).
- **Dicrotic/descending limb** occurs due to the rebound of blood from the closed aortic valve. The dicrotic notch seen on the descending limb corresponds with aortic valve closure and it indicates the end of ventricular systole and beginning of ventricular diastole.

Q.14. What is apex pulse deficit?

- Normally, pulse rate corresponds with heart rate.
- In cases of extrasystole, some heartbeats are not registered at the wrist at all, therefore pulse rate is less than the heart rate (as heard at the apex beat). This is known as **apex-pulse deficit** or pulse deficit (as extrasystole generated at the heart may not be of sufficient strength that they are carried to the peripheral artery). Please refer to the definition of pulse.

Arterial Pulse Examination

Observations

Name	Age	Sex
Pulse: Rate beats/min	*Rhythm:* Regular/Irregular	*Volume:* Good/Low/High
The character of pulse wave	Tension	Force
Condition of vessel wall	Equality on both sides	

Note: In a normal person when one examines– pulse rate is between 70 to 90 beats/min, with a regular rhythm, good volume, adequate force and tension, normal character of pulse wave (with smooth ascend and descend), equal on both sides and cannot be palpated as a rope-like structure as nature of vessel is elastic.

OBJECTIVE STRUCTURED CLINICAL EXAMINATION (OSCE)

Procedure station 1: Examine the radial pulse of a given subject.

S. No.	Assessment criteria	Marks assigned	Marks given
1.	Greet and stand on the right side of the subject		
2.	Ask the subject to sit comfortably and explains the procedure		
3.	Examine pulse with the correct position of the forearm of the patient with the use of three fingers		
4.	Record pulse rate, rhythm, volume, character of the pulse wave, force, tension, condition of the vessel wall and equality		
5.	Report and viva on clinical examination		
6.	Total		

COMMON STATIONS – SPOTS IN PRACTICAL EXAMINATION (2/3 MARKS)

Q.1. Diagram of arterial pulse recording. Identify and write the use of each finger in the examination of the pulse.

Q.2. Enumerate physiological/pathological conditions causing bradycardia.

Q.3. Enumerate physiological/pathological conditions causing tachycardia.

Q.4. Diagram of arterial pulse tracing—Label anacrotic and dicrotic limb. Write the significance of the dicrotic notch.

CASE-BASED SCENARIO/ PROBLEM-BASED (2/3 MARKS)

Case 1: 20-year-old comes to OPD with a fever. On examination, the pulse rate is 100 beats/min.
- Define pulse
- What can be the cause of the raised pulse rate in him?

Case 2: A 30-year-old female comes to a casualty with c/o weakness, and vomiting. On examination pulse was 95 beats/min, and was feeble/thready blood pressure 90/70 mm Hg.
- What is thready pulse? (clue-shock and low BP causing decreased pulse pressure)
- How do you normally judge the volume of the pulse?

Case 3: A 8-year-old boy comes to your clinic which is on the 5th floor by using stairs and the doctor examines his pulse and says it's a bounding pulse.
- What do you mean by bounding pulse (clue-more gap between systolic and diastolic BP)
- State the physiological reason for it in this case.

Case 4: A 22-year marathon runner for 10 years comes to a clinic for a routine check-up. His pulse is 58 beats/min.
- What is the cause of bradycardia in him?
- What do you mean by a high-volume pulse?

■ KEY POINTS TO REMEMBER

- Pulse is defined as a rise in pressure and distention of the vessel wall due to blood pumped in the aorta during ventricular systole, which is felt at any peripheral artery as a pulse.
- Normal pulse finding you describe as pulse rate is—beats/min, rhythm regular, volume and tension moderate, good volume, normal character, elastic consistency of vessel wall and equal on both sides.
- High-volume pulse is observed during exercise and a low-volume pulse in circulatory shock.
- Middle finger is used to feel the pulse. The ring finger is used to prevent retrograde pulsations coming from the palmar arch and the index finger is used to put pressure, to judge the force and tension of the pulse.
- Pulse helps us to detect the circulatory status of a person and the blood pressure and metabolism of a person (Hyperthyroidism– with excess thyroid secretions as metabolic rate is high, there is resting tachycardia).

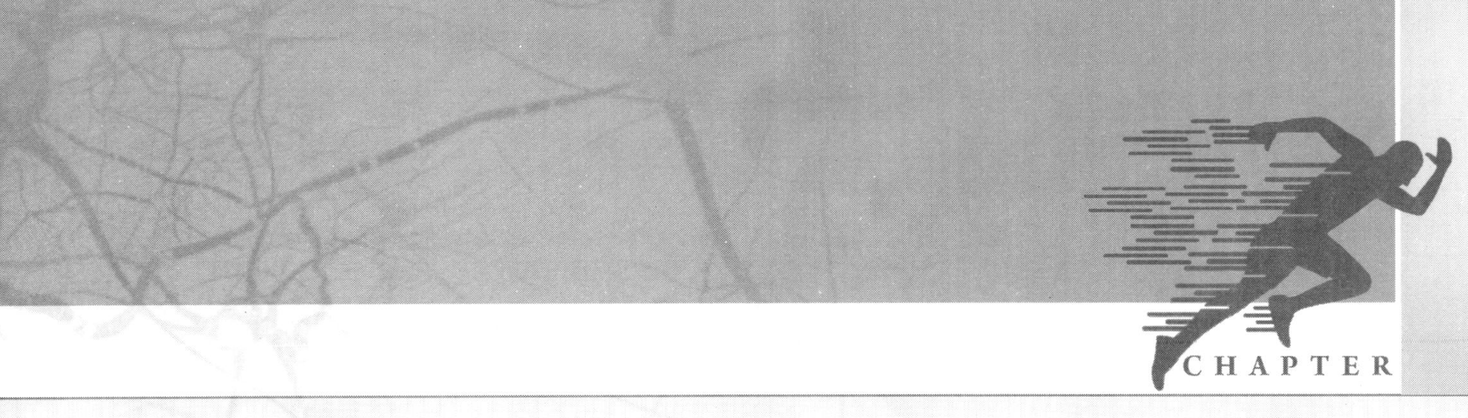

Recording of Blood Pressure

Competency:

PY 5.12: Record blood pressure and pulse at rest and in different grades of exercise and posture in volunteer or simulated environment.

Learning Objectives

After completion of this practical, students shall be able to:

- Record blood pressure by palpatory and auscultatory method
- Give the principle of the sphygmomanometer
- List physiological variations in blood pressure (BP)
- Give the importance of checking BP by palpatory method
- Explain the significance of the silent gap
- Give normal values of systolic, diastolic, pulse, and mean arterial pressure
- Define hypertension and hypotension

Aim

To record the arterial blood pressure of a given subject.

Apparatus

Sphygmomanometer and stethoscope.

Normal Blood Pressure

- Blood pressure is the lateral pressure exerted by a column of blood on the wall of the artery.
- Blood pressure is always expressed as systolic pressure/diastolic pressure. In a normal young adult person, BP is 120/80 ± 15 mm Hg. Pulse pressure is the difference between systolic and diastolic pressure normally it is 40 mm Hg. It indicates stroke volume.
- **Mean arterial BP** is calculated as 60% diastolic + 40% systolic BP. Thus, it is normally 100 mm Hg. It is the head pressure causing the flow of blood in circulation.
- There can be physiological variations in BP with exercise, emotions, age, sleep posture, etc. Blood pressure has to be regulated for proper tissue perfusion and oxygenation
- **Common symptoms**: If BP is higher, the patient might come with symptoms like fatigue, headache, palpitations (feeling of own heartbeat), chest pain, sweating, etc. With a fall in BP patient can come with symptoms of fatigue, lethargy and even fainting.
- A person can be brought in causality as an accident case with a lot of blood loss or with severe burns, excess water loss (dehydration, excess vomiting, diarrhoea) where BP may fall drastically and a person can go into a state of shock.

■ METHOD OF RECORDING

Arterial BP can be recorded by two methods:

Direct Method

By directly inserting a cannula in an artery and the other end of the cannula connected to the mercury column. As this method is not safe and carries an additional risk of infection, this method is mainly used for experimental purposes.

Indirect Method

Blood pressure is recorded with the help of a sphygmomanometer.

Principle

Balancing pressure in cuff against pressure in brachial artery, for details please refer (Question no 3).

Sphygmomanometer

Mercury manometer: It consists of:
- Rubber bag connected to manometer covered by cloth.
- A rubber pump with a valve.
- It is a U-shaped tube having one broad limb and another narrow limb.
- In the broader limb, there is mercury and the narrow limb is graduated from 0 mm to 300 mm, from downwards to upwards.
- Smallest division corresponding to 2 mm Hg.
- Mercury reservoir is connected to a rubber tube **(Fig. 19.1)**.

Cuff

- It is called Riva–Rocci cuff. It has an inflatable rubber bag covered by no distensible fabric.
- Two tubes are connected to the bag, one transmits air pressure to the mercury column and the other is connected to the air pump.
- The width of the cuff is about 12 cm (8 cm for children).

Rubber Pump

- It is a rubber hand bulb with a one-way valve at its free end and a leak valve arrangement at the other.
- Rubber bag is inflated by turning the screw clockwise and compressing the bulb.
- Deflation of the bag is achieved by turning the screw anticlockwise.

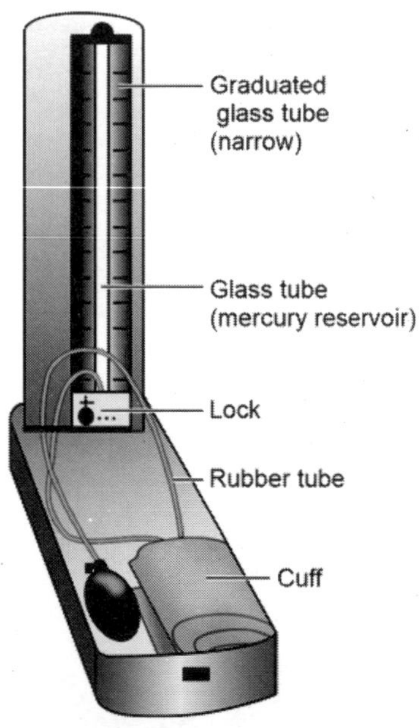

Fig. 19.1: Mercury manometer

Pre-requisites

- Subject should be physically and mentally relaxed.
- He/she should sit or lie comfortably.
- Zero of sphygmomanometer and cuff should be at the level of the heart.
- Blood pressure is measured first by palpatory and then auscultatory method.
- While taking a reading, the eye should be at the level of the mercury column (examiner's).
- The cuff should not be kept inflated for a long.

Recording of Blood Pressure

Palpatory Method

- After taking all the above-mentioned precautions, tie the cuff around the middle of the arm (1 inch above the cubital fossa).
- Palpate for radial artery at wrist (using three fingers).
- Hold the rubber tube in the other hand in such a way that the thumb and index finger are free to manipulate the leak valve screw.
- Raise pressure in the mercury column and continuously feel a radial pulse.
- Raise the mercury column about 10 mm Hg above the point of disappearance of the pulse
- Reduce pressure gradually and note mercury level, where pulse reappears. Note that pressure (systolic pressure).
- Reduce pressure level to zero rapidly.

Advantages of the Palpatory Method

- A stethoscope is not required for this method of recording BP.
- The palpatory method gives a rough idea about systolic BP.
- Auscultatory gap is not missed.

Auscultatory Method

- Record BP by palpatory method first as described above.
- Raise pressure about 30 mm Hg high at which radial pulsation is no longer felt (by palpatory method).
- The diaphragm of the stethoscope is put just medial to the tendon of the biceps (on the brachial artery).
- Gradually lower pressure and listen for the reappearance of sound, then change in the character of sound and finally disappearance of sound.
- The level at which sound is first heard is systolic BP and the disappearance of sound is diastolic BP.
- As the pressure in the cuff is lowered, sound undergoes a series of changes in intensity and quality. These sounds are called Korotkoff sounds **(Fig. 19.2)**.

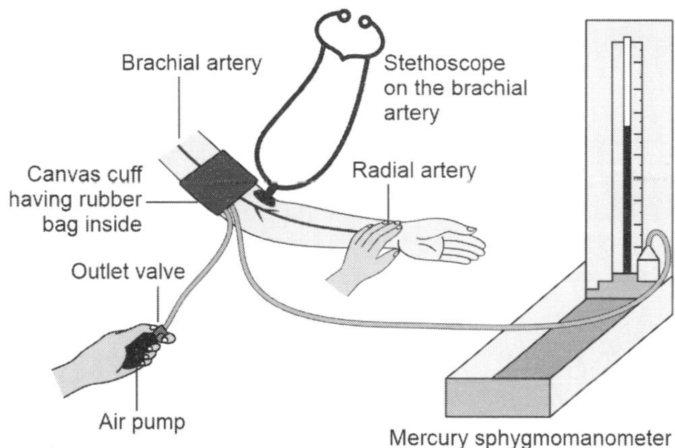

Fig. 19.2: Auscultatory method for measurement of BP

Advantages of the auscultatory method
- Gives us an accurate value of systolic pressure.
- Diastolic pressure is also detected.

Observations

Systolic BP—mm Hg   Diastolic BP—mm Hg

■ IMPORTANT QUESTIONS AND ANSWERS

Q.1. What is systolic blood pressure?
- It is the maximum pressure in arteries recorded during systole of the heart.
- Systolic BP depends on cardiac output. Thus, systolic BP indicates the force of contraction of the heart.

Q.2. What is diastolic blood pressure?
- It is the minimum pressure in arteries recorded during the diastole of the heart.
- It depends on peripheral resistance (load against which the heart pumps).

Q.3. What is the principle used in sphygmomanometer?
- Balancing air pressure in the cuff against pressure in the brachial artery.
- When the pressure in the cuff reaches just below arterial pressure, blood escapes beyond the occlusion in the peripheral part of the artery, and the pulse starts reappearing.
- This is recorded as systolic pressure (appearance of sounds in stethoscope).
- Subsequently, the quality of sound changes and then disappears. This is recorded as diastolic BP.

Q.4. What is the postural drop of BP?
- In a normal person, BP recorded in a standing position may drop as there is venous pooling of blood in lower limbs.
- However, it is immediately corrected by an efficient baroreceptor mechanism.

Q.5. What is auscultatory gap?
- In hypertensive people, when systolic BP is very high, as one lowers the pressure in the cuff, a faint tapping sound is heard which on further reducing the pressure, disappears and again reappears at a much lower level.
- This reading is wrongly taken as a systolic BP reading.
- The difference between this reading and a true systolic BP reading is called as auscultatory or silent gap.
- To avoid this always, BP is first recorded by the palpatory method.

Q.6. What are the physiological variations in BP?
Physiological variations in BP
- **Age**: Blood pressure increases with age.
- **Sex**: Blood pressure is less in females as compared to males of the same age (in females, progesterone relaxes smooth muscles of blood vessels).
- **Sleep**: Blood pressure decreases with sleep.
- **Emotions**: There is sympathetic stimulation, which increases BP.
- **Posture**: In the standing position, BP slightly falls but is immediately corrected via baroreceptor reflex.
- **Exercise:** With exercise due to sympathetic stimulation, systolic BP increases, and diastolic pressure remains unchanged, especially with mild-to-moderate exercise. With severe exercise, diastolic pressure falls due to vasodilatation.
- **Diurnal variation:** In the morning time, BP is slightly higher than evening time.

Q.7. What is hypertension? What is essential hypertension?
- **Hypertension**: It is defined as a sustained elevation of arterial pressure. To label a person as hypertensive, 3 successive readings that are recorded at 6 hourly intervals, show a reading of above 140/90 mm Hg pressure.
- Hypertension is broadly classified into essential hypertension and secondary hypertension.

- **Essential hypertension**: When the aetiology (cause) of hypertension is not known, it is labelled as essential hypertension. This is the most common variety of hypertension.

Q.8. What is hypotension?
- When BP goes below 90/60 mm Hg, it is labelled as hypotension.
- Common causes include circulatory shock and heart failure.

Q.9. What are the Korotkoff sounds?
Physiological basis of Korotkoff's sounds
- When we measure arterial blood pressure by auscultatory method and raise the pressure in the mercury column above 20 to 30 mm Hg (above the reading of the palpatory method).
- As one releases the valve and reduces pressure, blood starts flowing gradually in the brachial artery. Different sounds that are appreciated by stethoscopes due to the refilling of the artery with blood are called as Korotkoff's sounds.
- As blood flow increases gradually, the quality of sound changes. They are Grade I to IV.

Grade I	The sudden appearance of a clear tapping sound (recorded as systolic)
Grade II	After a further decrease in pressure in the cuff, the sound becomes softer
Grade III	With the further decrease in pressure in the cuff, sound becomes still softer than at Grade II
Grade IV	With a further decrease in pressure in the cuff, sound intensity reduces and becomes muffled. This is recorded as diastolic pressure

Q.10. What is mean arterial pressure and what is pulse pressure?
Please check above.

Q.11. What is the clinical significance of finding out BP?
- Blood pressure measurement is one of the important vital signs of the patient. A normal BP level is required to be maintained for normal tissue perfusion and oxygenation.
- Systolic pressure gives an idea about cardiac output and thus contractile capacity of the heart pump.
- Diastolic pressure gives an idea about peripheral resistance. It is an obstruction to the flow of blood. It may increase with advancing age with atherosclerosis.

Q.12. State different methods of recording/monitoring BP.
Methods of measurement of BP
- **Direct method**: Blood pressure is measured by placing a cannula in the lumen of the artery that is connected to a pressure transducer.
- **Indirect method**: This is a more commonly used method to record BP. Two methods are the sphygmomanometer method and the oscillometric method.
- **Automated machines**: Blood pressure nowadays is widely recorded by automated BP Monitors, especially in critically ill patients where 24-hour monitoring of BP is important.

Q.13. Enumerate causes of secondary hypertension.
- **Secondary hypertension**: It is a type of hypertension produced due to some underlying pathology.

Common causes of secondary hypertension:
- Renal disease, e.g. tumours of JG cells, glomerulonephritis
- Thyrotoxicosis
- Adrenal medullary tumour–pheochromocytoma

Q.14. What is prehypertension?
- **Prehypertension**: It is a state, where the patient is not on any of the antihypertensive drugs but has systolic BP in the range of 120–139 and diastolic BP in the range of 80 to 89 mm of Hg.
- Such people stand a high chance of getting hypertension in the near future if no corrective measures (lifestyle modifications) are taken.
- Obesity, unhealthy lifestyle, inadequate sleep, failure to cope with stress, physical inactivity hypercholesteremia are some of the common risk factors associated with prehypertensive state. This can make them prone to coronary heart disease and even renal failure in later stage of life
- Taking care of all the pillars of your life, that includes–(diet, sleep, exercise, social and mental health and addictions) simultaneously becomes the key factor for the prevention of such conditions).

OBJECTIVE STRUCTURED CLINICAL EXAMINATION (OSCE)

Procedure station 1: To record the blood pressure of a given subject in a supine/standing/sitting position.

S. No.	Assessment criteria	Marks assigned	Marks given
1.	Greet and stand on the right side of the subject		
2.	Ask the subject to lie down in a supine position comfortably and explain the procedure (ask the patient to sit or stand as per the question)		
3.	Check for zero readings on the mercury manometer		
4.	Check the normal functioning of the stethoscope		
5.	Expose the arm of the subject and ties the cuff about 2.5 cm above cubital fossa		

Contd....

Contd....

S. No.	Assessment criteria	Marks assigned	Marks given
6.	Keep the sphygmomanometer at the level of the heart of the subject and record BP first by palpatory and then auscultatory method		
7.	Report and viva on clinical examination		
8.	Total		

Procedure station 2: Record systolic BP only by the palpatory method.

S. No.	Assessment criteria	Marks assigned	Marks given
1.	Greet and stand on the right side of the subject		
2.	Ask the subject to lie down in a supine position comfortably and explains the procedure		
3.	Check for zero readings on the mercury manometer		
4.	Check the normal functioning of the stethoscope		
5.	Expose the arm of the subject and ties the cuff about 2.5 cm above cubital fossa		
6.	Keep the sphygmomanometer at the level of the heart of the subject and record systolic BP by palpatory method		
7.	Report and viva on clinical examination		
8.	Total		

■ COMMON STATIONS – SPOTS IN PRACTICAL EXAMINATION (2/3 MARKS)

Q.1. Enlist common symptoms patients come for checking BP.

Q.2. Sphygmomanometer: Identify the instrument. State principle used to measure BP by this instrument.

Q.3. Define mean arterial pressure and pulse pressure and state its significance.

Q.4. Sphygmomanometer: Identify and enumerate precautions taken before recording BP.

Q.5. Sphygmomanometer: Identify and write the importance of recording BP by palpatory method first and then auscultatory method.

Q.6. A person doing exercise, what do you expect his BP after 5 minutes of exercise? Give its physiological basis.

■ CASE-BASED SCENARIO/PROBLEM-BASED (2/3 MARKS)

Case 1: A 35-year-old male was brought to casualty after he met with an accident. There is quite a good amount of blood loss. On examination, the patient is conscious, pulse– 96 beats/min

- What do you expect his BP to be?
- Why do BP corrective measures have to be taken immediately? Give its physiological basis (to prevent a state like shock, one has to correct BP).

Case 2: A 28-year-old lady comes to a casualty in an absolutely afraid state of mind, as she hears about some bomb blast in the nearby area. She complains of sweating and palpitations. You record her BP and it is 150/80 mm Hg.

What can be the physiological basis of the rise in her systolic pressure level? (emotions and anxiety may increase BP).

Case 3: A 32-year-old male who is 98 kg weight. He is a manager with a desk-type job. His lifestyle is sedentary. He comes to complain of headaches on and off for the last 4 to 5 days. His BP is 140/90 mm Hg.

- What advice you will give to him? What are the risk factors he is associated with to be a future hypertensive candidate?
- What is pre-hypertension?

■ KEY POINTS TO REMEMBER

- Blood pressure is lateral pressure exerted by a column of blood on the walls of blood vessels.
- In young adult persons, BP is 120/80 ± 15 mm Hg.
- Mean arterial pressure is 100 mm Hg and pulse pressure is about 40 mm Hg.
- Always BP is recorded by the palpatory method first and then the auscultatory method in order to prevent an auscultatory gap.
- The pre-hypertensive stage has to be corrected by making healthy changes in lifestyle.

Examination of Cardiovascular System

PY 5.15: Demonstrate the correct clinical examination of the cardiovascular system in a normal volunteer or simulated environment.

■ LEARNING OBJECTIVES

At the end of this practical, the students shall be able to:

- List parameters to be examined in the clinical examination of the cardiovascular system
- Define precordium and define apex beat
- Enumerate different conditions where the apex beat is not palpable
- Localize apex beat
- Give the significance of the sternal angle
- Percuss the right and left border of the heart
- Locate different auscultatory areas on the precordium
- Auscultate for heart sounds
- List differences between first and second heart sound
- Give types and causes of heart sounds and their significance.

■ SYMPTOMS

The patient can come with c/o chest pain, nausea, vomiting, shoulder pain, palpitations, and difficulty in breathing (dyspnea). The pattern of cardiovascular disease has changed over the years, and today coronary artery disease has emerged as one of the common causes of premature death in the world. Thus good history and meticulous detailed clinical examination become important for patients with cardiovascular diseases.

The cardiovascular system should be examined under four headings:
1. Inspection
2. Palpation
3. Percussion
4. Auscultation

Examination of jugular venous pressure (JVP), arterial pulse, and recording of blood pressure completes cardiovascular system examination. Recording ECG of the patient is also one of the basic investigations that has to be done for a person with chest pain.

Inspection

- Precordium
- It is an area of the anterior chest wall overlying the heart

It is inspected for:

- Any bulging of precordium. Bulging of the precordium indicates enlargement of the heart.
- Size and shape of the chest is also observed for any obvious depression or bulging.

Inspection for Apex Beat

- Apex beat is the lowermost and lateralmost point of definite cardiac pulsation.
- For locating the apex beat, the precordium is inspected at more than one angle by tangential inspection of the precordium.
- Normally, the apex beat is located in the left fifth intercostal space 3.5 inches away from the midsternal line or 0.5 inches medial to the midclavicular line.

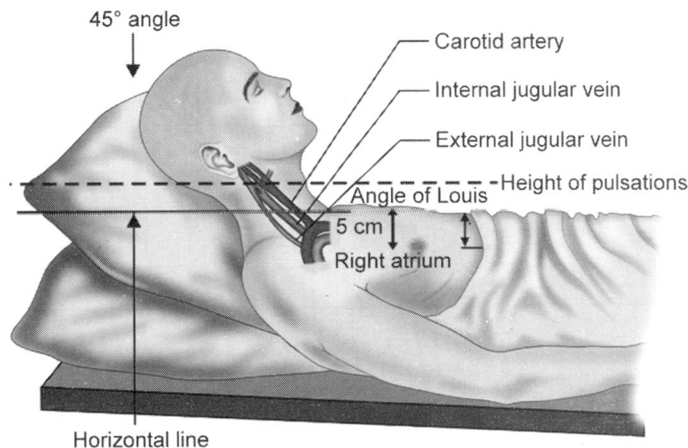

Fig. 20.1: Method of clinical assessment of jugular venous pressure (JVP). The vertical height of JVP above the clavicle with the patient reclining at 45°.

- Apex beat is invisible in many healthy adults due to a thick chest wall, pendulous breast, shift of mediastinum to right, obesity, etc.
- Any other pulsations - in precordium, if present, must be inspected and noted down.
- Epigastric pulsations are seen in normal thin people. They are aortic pulsations.

Jugular Venous Pressure

- Internal jugular vein communicates directly with the right atrium.
- Jugular venous pressure is pressure in internal jugular veins.
- Normally, it is 2.5 cm above the sternal angle with the subject reclining at an angle of 45°, so it is not visible **(Fig. 20.1)**. If pressure is higher only then it is visible in the neck.

Palpation

Palpation of Apex Beat

- First apex beat is felt by flat of the hand, then with ulnar border by keeping it over the intercostal space and then it is pointed out by the fingertip **(Fig. 20.2)**.
- During palpation, its location, duration, and extent is noted.
- Normally, it lies in the left fifth intercostal space 3.5 inches away from the midsternal line. The normal extent of the apex beat is less than 1 inch in diameter.
- Duration of apex beat is very small (felt only in early systole).

Tapping apex beat: Typically appreciated with mitral stenosis. Forceful and well-sustained apex beat, seen with left ventricular hypertrophy (seen with long-standing hypertensive patients).

Sternal Angle

- This is taken as reference point to find out intercostal spaces.

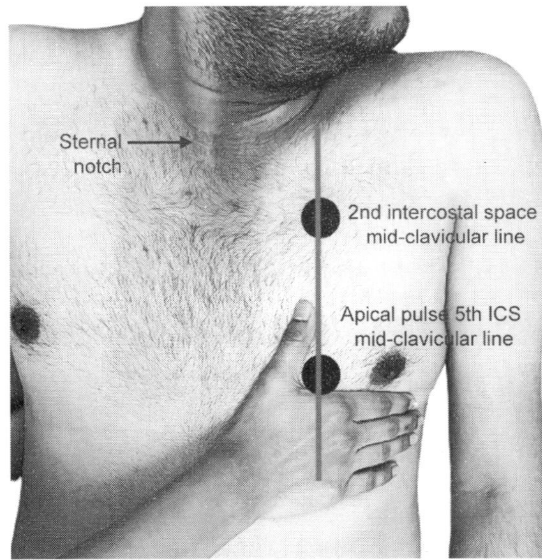

Fig. 20.2: Important landmarks for palpation of apex beat and percussion of the left border of the heart

- Sternal angle is the junction between body and manubrium of sternum.
- Along the sternal angle lies second costal cartilage.
- Thus, after finding the sternal angle, intercostal spaces are calculated.

■ PERCUSSION

Percussion of Left Border of Heart

- Before percussion of the left border of the heart, the position of apex beat is confirmed (normally, it lies in the left 5th intercostal space 0.5 inches medial to mid-clavicular line) as shown in **Fig. 20.3A**).
- From the same intercostal space from where apex beat is obtained, percussion is started from the midaxillary line toward the heart till a dull note is obtained.
- Percuss in the fourth and third intercostal spaces from the midaxillary line till you get a dull note.

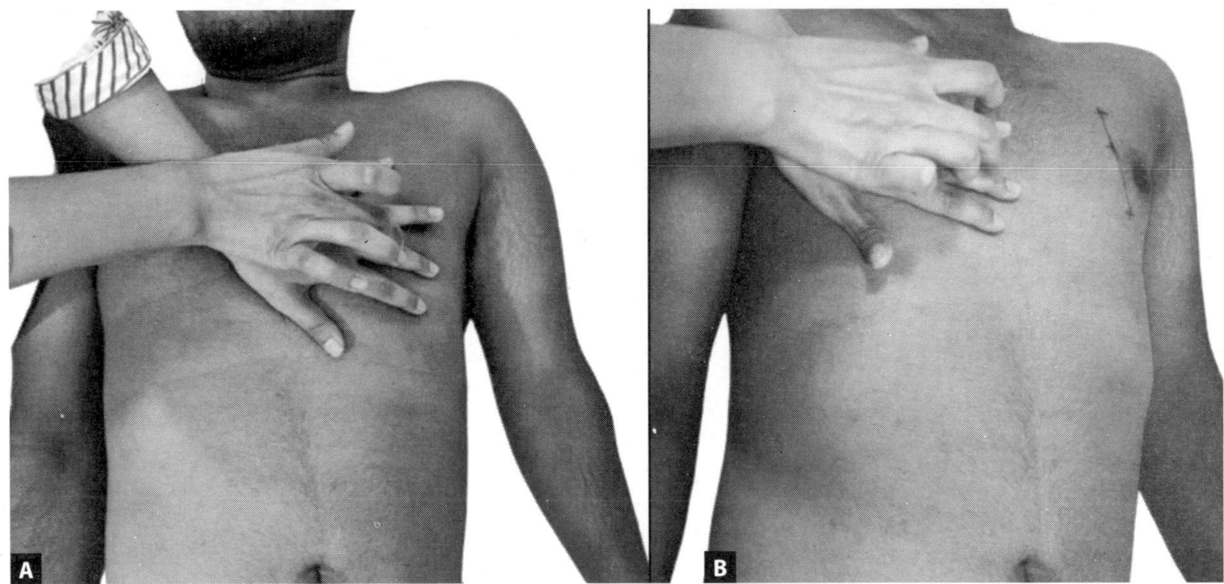

Figs. 20.3A and B: (A) Percussion of the left border of the heart;
(B) Percussion of right border of the heart.

- The left border of the heart, normally, lies in the left third, fourth, and fifth intercostal spaces approximately along the mid-clavicular line.
- Shift of the left border of the heart is seen with left ventricular hypertrophy.

Percussion of Right Border of Heart

- The upper border of the liver is first determined by percussing in the right mid-clavicular line in the first, second and third intercostal spaces. Liver dullness is usually obtained at the fifth or sixth right intercostal space **(Fig. 20.3B)**.
- Then in two or three spaces above, percussion is carried out from the midaxillary line towards right sternal margin.
- Normally, no dullness is obtained as right border of the heart is retrosternal therefore cannot be percussed.

AUSCULTATION: AUSCULTATORY AREA IN PRECORDIUM

- Heart sounds are produced due to vibrations set in the blood due to the closure of heart valves. They are heard by putting stethoscopes on various areas on the precordium.
- These areas are not named according to the anatomical position of different valves (sound produced by each valve is heard best over those respective areas) as shown in **Fig. 20.4**.

Four areas for auscultation are:
1. **Mitral area:** This area lies over the apex beat.
2. **Tricuspid area:** It lies at the lower end of the sternum to the left of the sternum.

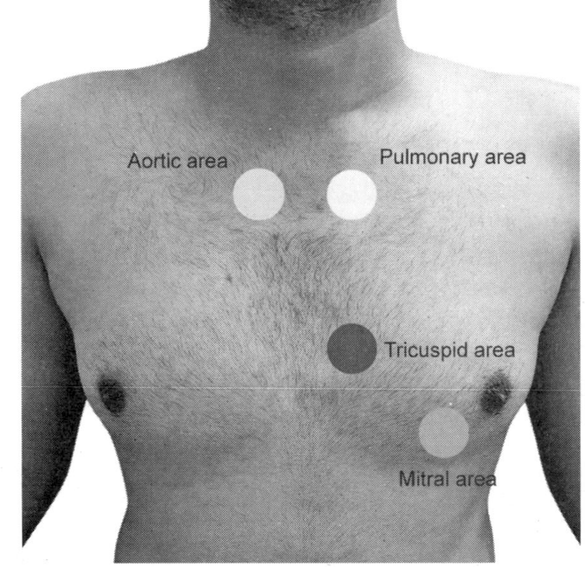

Fig. 20.4: Location of auscultatory areas on the precordium

3. **Pulmonary area:** It lies in left second intercostal space to the left of the sternum.
4. **Aortic area:** It lies in right second intercostal space to the right of the sternum.

Heart sounds: There are four heart sounds.
- **I heart sound:** It is heard due closure of AV valves (mitral and tricuspid) which sets in vibrations in surrounding blood which are conducted to chest wall and heard with the help of a stethoscope.
- **II heart sound:** It is heard due to the closure of semilunar valves (aortic and pulmonary) which sets in vibrations in surrounding blood which are conducted to the chest wall and heard with the help of a stethoscope.
- I heart sound is better heard in the mitral and tricuspid area as compared to aortic and pulmonary areas.

- **III heart sound:** It is heard due to vibrations appreciated in blood when blood flows from atria to the ventricles (during the rapid passive filling phase). The third heart sound (weak rumbling sound heard at the beginning of the middle third of diastole) is sometimes heard in the children with a stethoscope. Its duration is 0.04 seconds.
- **IV heart sound:** It is produced due to atrial systole. Atria contract and set in vibrations in blood appreciated as IV heart sound. It is not audible with a stethoscope (frequency is below 20 cycles/second).
- II heart sound is better heard in the aortic and pulmonary areas as compared to mitral and tricuspid areas.
- Third and fourth heart sounds are recorded with the help of a phonocardiogram as they are of very low frequency and thus cannot be heard with the help of a stethoscope.

Splitting of the second sound

- It is heard in a pulmonary area normally during inspiration.
- This is due to the separation of the aortic (A2) and pulmonary (P2) components of the second heart sound.

Observations – Examination of Cardiovascular System Proforma

Systemic examination of CVS: Any systemic examination is to be done after complete general examination as shown in the Chapter 1 General examination.

Inspection
Size and shape Symmetrical/Asymmetrical Movements with respiration Type of breathing Respiratory rate
Precordium - Apex Beat - Seen/Not seen Position -
Visible Pulsations Neck Veins - Distended/Not Distended
Surgical Scars- Present/Absent
Palpation
Confirm all points mentioned above in inspection by palpation
Apex Beat - Position Character Rhythm Rate Force and extent If any other visible pulsations -
Percussion: Find out notes on the right and left and upper border of the heart (taking the sternal angle as reference point to calculate intercostal spaces)
Left border of the heart Right border of the heart Upper border of heart
Auscultation
Mitral   Aortic   Pulmonary   Tricuspid
Any Abnormal Sounds

■ IMPORTANT QUESTIONS AND ANSWERS

Q.1. Enumerate common risk factors for a cardiovascular disease.

Common risk factors include:

- Diabetes, family h/o premature vascular disease, smoking, obesity, hypertension, hypercholesterolemia. Following a healthy lifestyle helps in the prevention or reduced risks of all such conditions.
- Past medical history of stroke, renal impairment, rheumatic fever.

Q.2. In general examination which are important signs especially with respect to cardiovascular system?

Important signs with respect to cardiovascular system

- **Pallor:** Pallor has to be carefully assessed as anaemia is known to exacerbate heart failure or symptoms of angina.
- **Cyanosis:** Peripheral and central cyanosis sign becomes important for patients suffering from heart failure, pulmonary edema.
- **Clubbing:** It is rare, but is observed with congenital cyanotic heart disease when child is in his/ her infancy.
- **Coldness of extremities:** This is common sign observed with heart failure due to reduced cardiac output (reflex vasoconstriction of cutaneous bed).
- **Oedema:** Subcutaneous pitting oedema is common with congestive heart failure and even with salt and water retention by kidneys.
- **Arterial pulse:** There has to be a thorough assessment of pulse for rate, rhythm, character, volume, force, tension, and equality of both sides as all the normal features that are assessed may change with respect to underlying cardiovascular disease.
- **Measurement of BP:** Accurate measurement of arterial blood pressure becomes very important for cardiovascular system assessment and is one of the important vital signs in a patient with general examination.
- **Jugular venous pressure:** Details of measurement of JVP is described above. Normal upper limit is 4 cm, which becomes 9 cm from right atria (check above description of JVP for details) and that becomes about 6 mm Hg. Elevated JVP is seen with congestive heart failure, pulmonary embolism.
- **Jugular venous pulse:** Fluctuations in right atrial pressure during the cardiac cycle do generate a pulse which is transmitted to jugular veins. (Refer Chapter 52 Charts section).

Q.3. Define apex beat. Where does it lie normally?

- Apex beat is defined as lowermost and outermost point of definite cardiac pulsation. Normally, it is located 0.5 inches medial to mid-clavicular line in 5th intercostal space (or 3.5 inches away from midsternal line). However, there can be variations normally and apex beat can be present in left 4th or 6th intercostal space also.

Q.4. What conditions apex beat shift from a normal position?

- Apex beat normally lies in left 5th intercostal space 3.5 inches away from midsternal line.
- However, conditions like enlargement/hypertrophy of myocardium, mediastinal shift, and lung pathologies can cause shift of apex beat from normal position.
- With enlargement of left ventricle apex beat is abnormally forceful and sustained.
- Slapping/tapping apex beat is appreciated with mitral stenosis (stenosis of the mitral valve)

Q.5. Enumerate causes of impalpable apex beat.

Causes:

- Thick chest wall (obesity)
- Apex beat lying under the rib
- Pneumothorax
- Left-sided pleural effusion
- Dextrocardia (heart situated on the right side)

Q.6. Compare and contrast first and second heart sound.

First heart sound	Second heart sound
First heart sound is produced due to the closure of atrioventricular (AV) valves	Second heart sound is produced due to the closure of semilunar valves
It corresponds with a carotid pulse	It follows the carotid pulse
The first heart sound is low-pitched and prolonged and resembles the utterance of the word LUB	The second heart sound resembles the utterance of the word DUB second heart sound
It is soft, low-pitched, and prolonged with a duration of 0.14 seconds	It is shorter, sharp, and high pitched and with a duration is 0.11 seconds
It is better heard over mitral and tricuspid areas (as compared to aortic and pulmonary areas)	It is better heard over pulmonary and aortic areas (as compared to mitral and tricuspid area)

Q.7. How do you differentiate between first and second heart sounds clinically?

- Even though we know various characteristic features of first and second heart sounds, all these features are difficult to appreciate clinically. Clinically first heart sound corresponds with a carotid pulse and the second heart sound follows it. When one is auscultating for heart sounds, simultaneously should feel for a carotid pulse as shown in **Fig. 20.5**.
- The time interval between the first and second heart sound is lesser (systole) as compared to the interval between the second heart sound and the next first heart sound (diastole).

Q.8. What is the splitting of the second heart sound?

- Splitting of second heart sound is heard in a pulmonary area normally during inspiration. This is

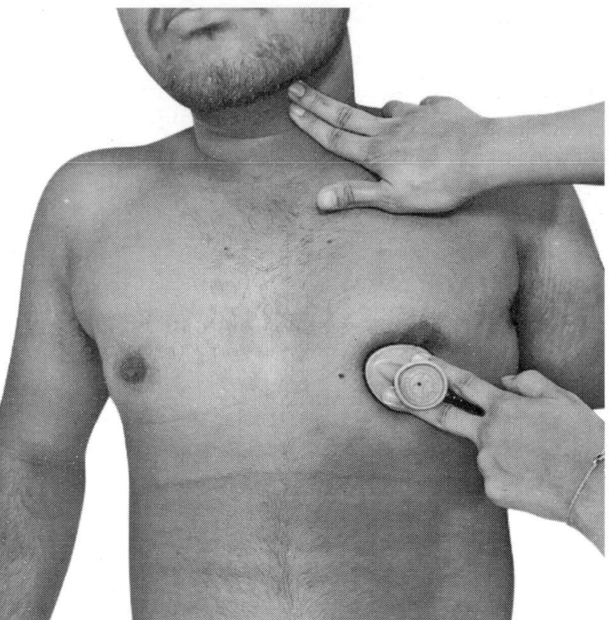

Fig. 20.5: Feeling carotid pulse to differentiate first heart sound from second heart sound

due to the separation of the aortic (A2) and pulmonary (P2) components of the sound.

- When the second heart sound is single, the split can be produced by asking the person to take deep inspiration. With deep inspiration, venous return and right ventricular filling are increased and its ejection time is prolonged. This prolongs the occurrence of P2.
- However, same time left ventricular filling time is decreased and its ejection time is shortened causing A2 to appear early. The separation of A2 and P2 gives rise to the splitting of the second heart sound during inspiration.

Q.9. What is the significance of sternal angle?

- Sternal angle is fixed at a distance of 5.0 cm from the centre of the right atrium in any position of the subject. This serves as a convenient reference point for expressing jugular venous pressure.
- This pressure is clinically expressed as the vertical height (cm of blood) of jugular venous distention above the sternal angle.

Q.10. Why internal jugular veins are preferred over external jugular veins while examining neck veins?

Internal jugular veins directly communicate with the right atrium and reflect the pressure changes in the chamber.

Q.11. What is jugular venous pressure? How is it estimated?

- The term jugular venous pressure denotes mean pressure in the internal jugular veins during the cardiac cycle. Clinically, it is estimated by noting the upper limit of distension and pulsation of internal jugular vein with reference to sternal angle. This is an indirect method of estimation of jugular venous pressure (Sir Thomas Lewis method).

- Upper limit of normal jugular venous pressure is 2.5 cm above the sternal angle with subject reclining at an angle of 45° (this comes just below the clavicle and thus normally is not visible) as shown in **Fig. 20.1**.
- Direct method of estimation of jugular venous pressure is by passing a catheter in right atrium and connecting it to the manometer.

Q.12. How to percuss left and right border of the heart?

- In order to percuss the left border of heart first find out apex beat and then percuss from same intercostal space from midaxillary line (for details see above).
- For right border of heart one has to find liver dull note on right side and then percuss above in right intercostal spaces. Normally, right border of the heart lies behind the sternum and hence cannot be percussed (for details please refer above).

Q.13. What are areas for auscultation of heart sounds?

- Four areas for auscultation of heart sounds are mitral, tricuspid, pulmonary and aortic. Details of their anatomical locations are provided above.
- These are the areas where sound produced by those respective valves are heard best. They do not denote the anatomical position of the valves.

Q.14. What are murmurs?

- **Murmurs:** Heart murmurs indicate the turbulence of blood flow in the heart and great vessels.
- Rarely they are heard without any pathology (innocent murmurs). Usually, they indicate presence of valvular heart disease or atrial or ventricular septal defects.
- Heat murmurs are defined by four characteristics which include loudness, quality, location, and timing with respect to cardiac cycle.
- Accordingly, they can be mid-systolic, early diastolic, mid-diastolic or pan systolic (heard throughout systole), etc.

Thrills: These are palpable murmurs that are mainly appreciated when a person holds a breath in expiration. They are appreciated with valvular heart diseases.

Q.15. What is the normal extent of the left border of the heart? Enumerate conditions where it can shift to more left or right.

- Normally, left border of the heart extends from left 3rd, 4th and 5th intercostal spaces approximately in mid-clavicular line
- Common cause of shift of the apex beat more to left is left ventricular hypertrophy.

Q.16. What conditions can cause percussable right border of the heart?

- Normally, right border of the heart lies posterior to the sternum (retrosternal) and thus cannot be percussed.
- Enlargement of right or left or both atria may show with percussable right border.

Q.17. What is friction rub?

- It is a high-pitched scratching sound that is heard in any part of the cardiac cycle especially during expiration (with the patient leaning forward) on the left pericardium.
- It is classically recorded with pericarditis.

Q.18. What one can see on a normal chest X-ray with respect to cardiovascular examination?

- A normal chest X-ray of a person is shown in **Fig. 20.6**.

Q.19. What is echocardiography?

- Echocardiography is a commonly done noninvasive imaging technique to understand the working of the heart.
- It does not use ionizing radiation, and hence can be done for pregnant females as well.
- The relationships of the cardiac chambers and their connections with the great vessels are readily determined. Valvular abnormalities and septal defects can also be recognized
- It also helps to assess the contractile function of the heart, dilatation and hypertrophy of the myocardium.
- M mode echocardiogram helps to measure chamber dimensions and left ventricle wall thickness.
- Intra-cardiac tumours or thrombi can be visualized with echocardiography.
- In the pediatric age group combination of 2D echo and colour flow Doppler is one of the common noninvasive tools to assess congenital heart defects.

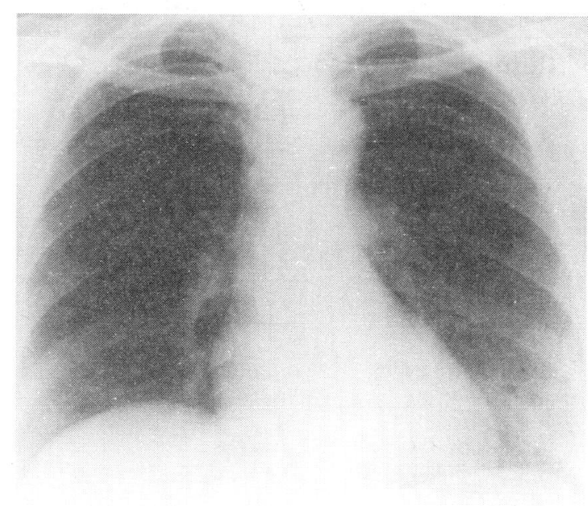

Fig. 20.6: Normal chest X-ray: Posteroanterior projection. Note the heart is not enlarged. Cardiothoracic ratio <50% and the lung fields are clear.

Stress echocardiography: It is used to assess myocardial ischemia in a suspected case of coronary artery disease.
Doppler echocardiography: Helps to assess the direction and velocity of blood flow and thus can be helpful to understand the severity of valvular heart diseases.

Q.20. Enumerate other techniques/investigations to assess cardiac functions.

Techniques/investigations include:

- Various techniques like cardiac MRI, CT scan, PET scan, cardiac angiography, and pulmonary angiography are routinely performed to diagnose various clinical conditions, as well as to assess differences in function post-treatment or surgery.
- **Cardiac markers**: Enzymes and structural proteins are released from necrosed myocytes following a myocardial infarction which reflect biochemical markers of injury. **MB isoenzyme** of **creatine kinase (CK)** is the specific marker of cardiac injury. Nowadays, even highly specific troponin T and troponin I do indicate myocardial injury. Raised circulating troponin levels are indicators of it.
- **Raised BNP level**: With chronic left ventricular stress or heart failure, there is release of natriuretic peptide from the heart (brain natriuretic peptide) that stimulates natriuresis and can worsen symptoms and even progress of the disease.
- **Renal function tests**: Renal dysfunction is very common with long standing hypertension or cardiac conditions.
- **Lipid profile**: Regular assessment of triglycerides, cholesterol levels, HDL and LDL are also to be done routinely as raised levels of TG, cholesterol and LDL are independent risk factors for cardiac function.

◼ OSCE—CARDIOVASCULAR SYSTEM

Procedure station 1: Inspect precordium.

S. No.	Assessment criteria	Marks assigned	Marks given
1.	Greet and stands on the right side of the subject		
2.	Ask the subject to lie down in a supine position comfortably and explains the procedure		
3.	Stand and observes precordium from the right side/foot end of the patient		
4.	Try to observe apex beat and any other visible pulsation on precordium		
5.	Look for distended veins in neck		
6.	Report and viva on clinical examination		
7.	Total		

Procedure station 2: Inspect chest for apex beat.

S. No.	Assessment criteria	Marks assigned	Marks given
1.	Greet and stands on the right side of the subject		
2.	Ask the subject to lie down in supine position comfortably and explains the procedure		
3.	Inspect apex beat		
4.	Give his/her findings on inspection of apex beat		
5.	Report and viva on clinical examination		
6.	Total		

Procedure station 3: Palpate precordium for apex beat.

S. No.	Assessment criteria	Marks assigned	Marks given
1.	Greet and stand on the right side of the subject		
2.	Ask the subject to lie down in supine position comfortably and explains the procedure		
3.	Inspect apex beat		
4.	Feel for the apex beat first with the palm then with ulnar border and then locate it with the index finger of the right hand (keeps a finger on apex beat)		
5.	With left hand feel the sternal notch and then the sternal angle and taking that as a reference counts intercostal spaces and confirms position of the apex beat		
6.	Report and viva on clinical examination		
7.	Total		

Procedure station 4: Percuss left border of the heart.

S. No.	Assessment criteria	Marks assigned	Marks given
1.	Greet and stands on the right side of the subject		
2.	Ask the subject to lie down in supine position comfortably and explains the procedure		
3.	Inspect apex beat		
4.	Feel for the apex beat first with the palm then with ulnar border and then locate it with the index finger of right hand (keeps finger on apex beat)		
5.	With left hand feel sternal notch and then sternal angle, taking that as reference count intercostal spaces and confirm position of apex beat		

Contd...

Contd...

S. No.	Assessment criteria	Marks assigned	Marks given
6.	Same intercostal space where he/ she feel for apex beat moves till midaxillary line and start percussing till dull note of apex beat is appreciated		
7.	Similarly, repeat the procedure in the above three intercostal spaces going up and percuss from the midaxillary line of the next above intercostal space till a dull note is appreciated due to heart		
8.	Report and viva on clinical examination		
9.	Total		

Procedure station 5: Percuss the right border of the heart.

S. No.	Assessment criteria	Marks assigned	Marks given
1.	Greet and stands on the right side of the subject		
2.	Ask the subject to lie down in supine position comfortably and explains the procedure		
3.	Start percussion from right 2nd intercostal space downwards in mid-clavicular line till he/she gets dullness of liver		
4.	Confirm liver dullness by counting intercostal spaces taking the sternal angle as a reference point		
5.	Go in above intercostal spaces and starts percussion from lateral to medial side in the above intercostal spaces over the sternum in the right side		
6.	Confirm and reports the right border of the heart		
7.	Report and viva on clinical examination		
8.	Total		

Procedure station 6: Auscultate mitral area.

S. No.	Assessment criteria	Marks assigned	Marks given
1.	Greet and stands on the right side of the subject		
2.	Ask the subject to lie down in supine position comfortably and explains the procedure		
3.	Inspect apex beat		
4.	Feel for the apex beat first with the palm then with ulnar border and then locates it with the index finger of the right hand (keeps a finger on apex beat)		

Contd...

Contd...

S. No.	Assessment criteria	Marks assigned	Marks given
5.	With the left hand feel the sternal notch and then sternal angle and taking that as a reference count intercostal spaces and confirm position of the apex beat		
6.	Check for the normal functioning of the stethoscope and place the earpiece comfortably into the ears along the direction of the ear canals		
7.	Keep stethoscope on the apex beat and simultaneously feel for a carotid pulse		
8.	Report and viva on clinical examination		
9.	Total		

Procedure station 7: Auscultate tricuspid area.

S. No.	Assessment criteria	Marks assigned	Marks given
1.	Greet and stand on the right side of the subject		
2.	Ask the subject to lie down in supine position comfortably and explains the procedure		
3.	Check for the normal functioning of the stethoscope and places the ear piece comfortably in to the ears along the direction of the ear canals		
4.	Place the diaphragm of the stethoscope just lateral to lower end of sternal border in the left side after the proper counting of intercostal spaces (taking sternal angle as a reference point)		
5.	Simultaneously feel for carotid pulse		
6.	Report and viva on clinical examination		
7.	Total		

Procedure station 8: Auscultate pulmonary area.

S. No.	Assessment criteria	Marks assigned	Marks given
1.	Greet and stands on the right side of the subject		
2.	Ask the subject to lie down in a supine position comfortably and explains the procedure		
3.	Check for the normal functioning of the stethoscope and places the earpiece comfortably into the ears along the direction of the ear canals		

Contd...

Contd...

S. No.	Assessment criteria	Marks assigned	Marks given
4.	Place the diaphragm of the stethoscope 2 cm lateral to sternal border on the pulmonary area on the left side of the chest after proper counting of intercostal space (taking sternal angle as a reference point)		
5.	Simultaneously feels for a carotid pulse		
6.	Report and viva on clinical examination		
7.	Total		

Procedure station 9: Auscultate aortic area.

S. No.	Assessment criteria	Marks assigned	Marks given
1.	Greet and stand on the right side of the subject		
2.	Ask the subject to lie down in a supine position comfortably and explains the procedure		
3.	Check for the normal functioning of the stethoscope and places the earpiece comfortably into the ears along the direction of the ear canals		
4.	Place the diaphragm of the stethoscope 2 cm lateral to sternal border on the aortic area on the right side of the chest after the proper counting of intercostal space (taking sternal angle as a reference point)		
5.	Simultaneously feel for a carotid pulse		
6.	Report and viva on clinical examination		
7.	Total		

COMMON STATIONS – SPOTS IN PRACTICAL EXAMINATION (2/3 MARKS)

Q.1. Enlist common symptoms patients come with cardiovascular disease.

Q.2. Figure of physician palpating apex beat, percussing right or left or upper border of the heart, auscultating for heart sounds in any of the four areas (mitral, tricuspid, aortic, pulmonary): Identify the picture and answer anyone or two questions related to it (as given above).

Q.3. Diagram of auscultation areas and name the areas and write their anatomical landmarks.

Q.4. Figure of manubrium and body of sternum: Label or write anatomical landmark to count intercostal space.

Q.5. Diagram of JVP measurement: Identify and write two conditions that can increase JVP.

Q.6. Diagram of jugular venous pulse tracing: Identify, label and describe any of the waveforms refer Chapter 52 charts section.

Q.7. Normal diagram of heart sounds: Identify and enumerate characteristics of any of the heart sound.

Q.8. Fill cardiovascular system proforma for a normal person: (Please check above).

Q.9. For spots in the examination of the arterial pulse, refer to chapter 18.

Q.10. For spots in examination of arterial blood pressure, Refer to chapter 19.

CASE-BASED SCENARIO/PROBLEM-BASED (2/3 MARKS)

Case 1: 75-year-old male comes for his routine checkup. He is a known hypertensive for the last 25 years. On examination, the apex beat is found to be displaced more laterally than normal. Trachea is centrally placed. BP is 160/100 mm Hg

- What is the probable cause of the shift of position of the apex beat? (clue- left ventricular hypertrophy due to long-standing hypertension).
- Write the normal location of the apex beat.

Case 2: A 28-year-old male person, weighing 90 kg comes for a corporate checkup. On examination, pulse– 78 beats/min, BP– 110/80 mm Hg. Apex beat is not palpable in the supine position

- What can be the probable cause of the apex beat not being palpable in the supine position?
- Do you suggest any change in the position of the subject to make the apex beat palpable?
- Enumerate common conditions where the apex beat is not palpable.

IMPORTANT POINTS TO REMEMBER

- Apex beat is the lowermost and outermost point of definite cardiac pulsation.
- Heart sounds can be auscultated in four areas on the chest.
- First heart sound is produced due to the closure of AV valves (soft pitched and long duration).
- Second heart sound is produced due to the closure of semilunar valves (high-pitched and short duration).
- The clinical way to differentiate between first and second heart sound is by palpating the carotid pulse while auscultating for heart sounds.
- First heart sound corresponds with and the second heart sound follows the carotid pulse.

Examination of Respiratory System

Competency:

PY 6.9: Demonstrate the correct clinical examination of the respiratory system in a normal volunteer or simulated environment.

Learning Objectives

After completion of this practical, students shall be able to:

- List headings under which the respiratory system is examined
- List points for inspection of the respiratory system
- Describe the principle of tactile vocal fremitus and enumerate common conditions, that alter it
- List rules of percussion
- List differences between bronchial and vesicular breathing

■ SYMPTOMS

Patients can come with c/o cough, hemoptysis (blood in cough/sputum) cold, difficulty in breathing, etc. Respiratory accounts for about more than 1/3rd mortality/morbidity diseases in most countries.

Clinical examination of the respiratory system should be carried out with the subject lying down, supine or sitting position. It is examined under four headings:

1. Inspection
2. Palpation
3. Percussion
4. Auscultation

■ INSPECTION

Under the inspection of the chest, one should inspect for:

Shape of the Chest

- In normal individuals, the shape is bilaterally symmetrical.
- Transverse diameter is more than anteroposterior diameter.
- One should look for chest abnormalities (e.g. funnel-shaped chest, barrel-shaped chest, etc.).

Funnel-shaped chest: Anteroposterior diameter is reduced. Seen in rickets.

Barrel-shaped chest: Increased anteroposterior diameter of chest, ribs are horizontal with excess concavity of the spine. Seen in emphysema of the lungs.

Spine abnormalities like kyphosis, and scoliosis can cause abnormal shape of the chest.

Symmetry of the Chest

- Usually, the chest is bilaterally symmetrical. Kyphosis (forward bending) or scoliosis (lateral bending) of the spine can lead to chest asymmetry and even can restrict lung movement if severe.
- If the chest is bulged (bulging is associated with pleural effusion, pneumothorax) or depressed that should be noted (depression is associated with fibrosis or collapse of lungs).

Movement of the Chest

While inspecting the movements of respiration, it is seen that the chest moves bilaterally equally, symmetrically, and simultaneously with respiration.

Respiratory Movements

Respiratory movements should be inspected for rate, rhythm, depth, and type of breathing.

- Normal rate of respiration is 12–14 min. The rhythm of respiration is normally regular.
- In women, respiratory movements involve the upper part of the thorax (intercostals play an important role). The type of breathing described is thoracic or thoracoabdominal.
- In men, breathing is abdominal as it is dependent on the diaphragm. Therefore, it is described as abdominal or abdominothoracic.

Use of Accessory Muscles of Respiration

With normal breathing, accessory muscles of respiration are not used.

Position of Trachea

Inspect the trachea for any obvious shift.

Position of Apex Beat

- Position of apex beat is seen.
- Normally, the apex beat lies in the left fifth intercostal space along the mid-clavicular line.

■ PALPATION

Position of Trachea

The trachea can be palpated in the following ways:

First Method
- Place the index finger firmly in the suprasternal notch and try to locate the trachea.
- See if the trachea is placed centrally or deviated to one side or other by its relation to the suprasternal notch and insertion of sternomastoid muscle.

Second Method
- Find space between the anterior border of the sternomastoid muscle and trachea.
- If the trachea is deviated to any one side, the space will become narrow on that side.
- That means if the finger goes equally deep on both sides, it indicates that normally the trachea is centrally placed **(Fig. 21.1)**.

Position of Apex Beat

Confirm the position of the apex beat on palpation (the apex beat normally lies in the left 5th intercostal space 0.5 inches medial to midclavicular line).

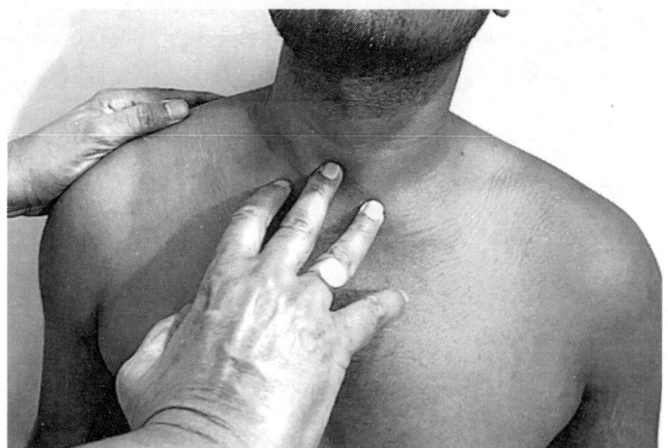

Fig. 21.1: Palpation of trachea

Displacement of the apex beat or trachea or both suggests that the position of the mediastinum is altered (due to disease of the lung or pleura).

Mediastinal shift: The mediastinum if pushed away from the affected side is called as a **contralateral deviation**. It is seen with pleural effusion and pneumothorax.

In contrast, **ipsilateral deviation** is one where the mediastinum is pushed towards the affected side. It is seen with fibrosis, and collapse of the lungs.

Palpation for Respiratory Movements

Chest is palpated in upper, middle, and lower zones for respiratory movements.

Palpation in the Upper Zone (or Apical Region)

- For palpation of the upper zone, the subject sits on the stool.
- Two hands are placed on apical regions from behind in the supraclavicular fossa; thumbs are approximated in the midline at the back.
- Excursions of thumbs from the midline, as the subject breathes indicate the degree of expansion on two sides. If one thumb remains closer to the midline, this suggests diminished expansion on that side **(Figs. 21.2A and B)**.

Palpation of Middle and Lower Zones

- Two hands are placed symmetrically on either side of the subject's chest.
- Thumbs are stretched so that they just meet in the midline.
- Excursion of each thumb from the midline judges the degree of expansion of that side.
  (Palpation of chest for respiratory movements is done on anterior and posterior chest wall).

Palpation for Tactile Vocal Fremitus

Detection of vibrations, which are communicated to the chest wall from the larynx via the bronchi and lungs during the act of phonation by tactile perception, is termed as tactile vocal fremitus **(Fig. 21.3)**.

Steps

- The ulnar border of the hand is placed in intercostal spaces of the chest wall, while the subject is made to repeat some suitable phrase such as "ninety-nine" or "one, one, one" with the same pitch and intensity.
- It is necessary to compare tactile vocal fremitus on two sides of the chest in corresponding intercostal spaces.
- One should proceed systematically downwards from apices to the base of the lungs first anteriorly then in the midaxillary region and finally posteriorly.
- Tactile vocal fremitus is increased in lung consolidation and decreased in pleural effusion, pneumothorax, collapse, fibrosis of the lung, etc.

■ PERCUSSION

Percussion of lungs is done for:
- Determining the condition of underlying tissue (lungs, pleura, etc.)
- Determining the borders of the lung.

Procedure for Percussion

- The middle finger of the left hand is placed firmly on the part to be percussed. This finger is called a pleximeter.
- Other fingers of the examiner's left hand are lifted away from the patient's chest.
- The middle finger of the right hand (plexor finger) is used to strike the middle phalanx of the pleximeter finger.

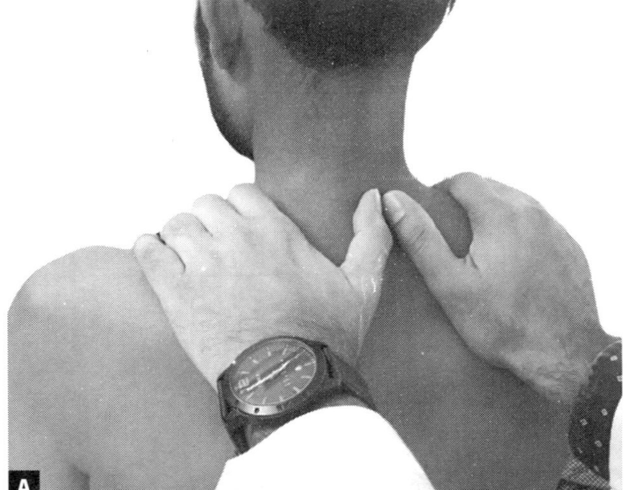

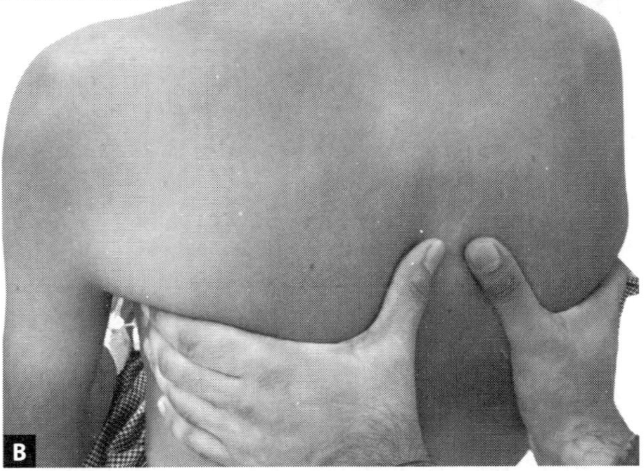

Figs. 21.2A and B: (A) Upper thoracic expansion; (B) Posterior thorax expansion

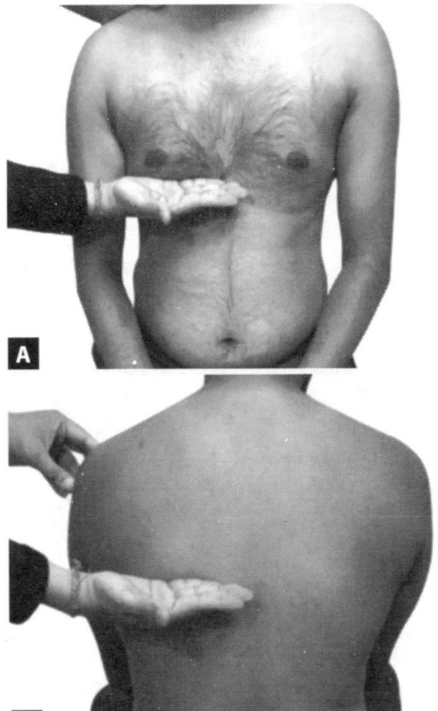

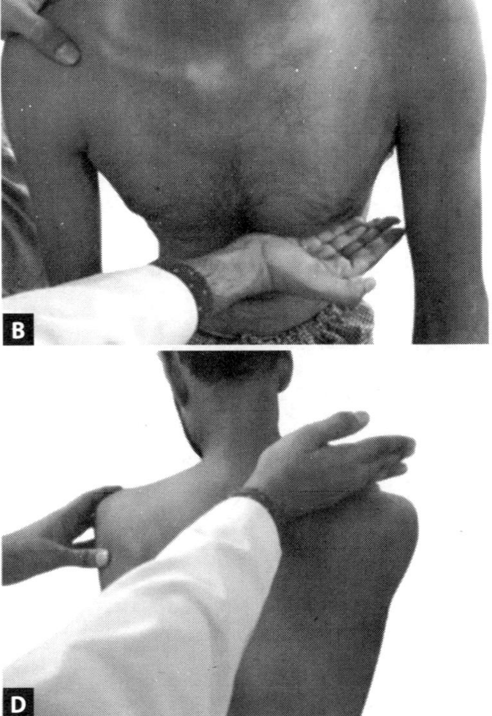

Figs. 21.3A to D: Palpation for tactile vocal fremitus

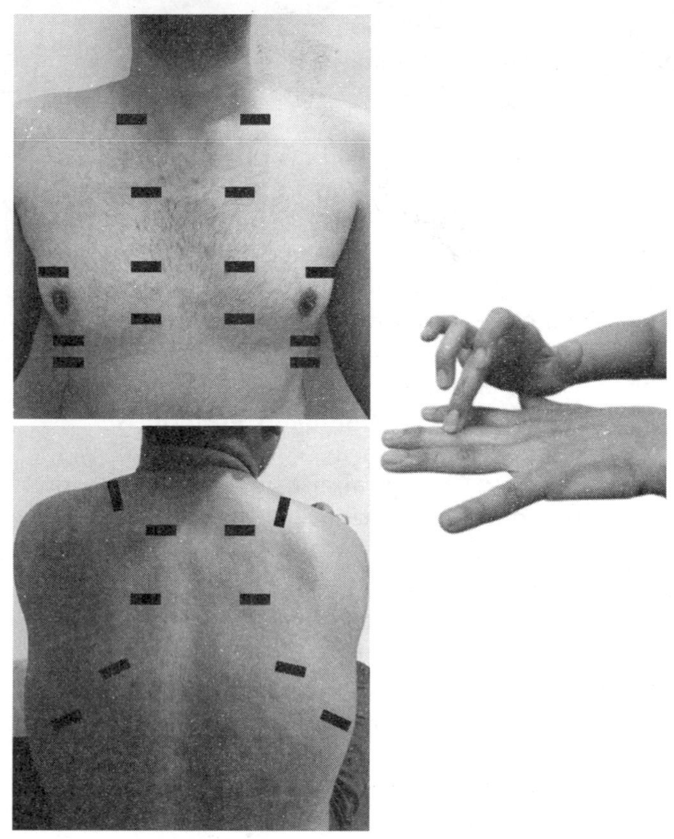

Fig. 21.4: Areas for percussion of lungs on anterior and posterior chest wall

- Stroke should be delivered from the wrist, and finger joints, and not from the elbow or shoulder.
- Plexor finger should strike the pleximeter finger perpendicularly **(Fig. 21.4)**.
- Effective percussion requires practice.

Rules for Percussion

- When boundaries of organs are to be defined, percussion is carried out from the resonant area to the dull area or from more resonant to less resonant areas.
- The long axis of the pleximeter finger should be parallel to the edge of the organ.
- The direction of percussion should be perpendicular to the edge of the organ.
- In order to define the boundaries of the lung, apical percussion and basal percussion should be carried out.
- On percussion of lungs, the normally resonant note is obtained. The degree of resonance does vary with individuals and even in one person at different regions of the chest.

Apical Percussion

- The upper border of the lung is determined by percussing in supraclavicular fossae.
- Normally, the upper border is 3–5 cm above the clavicle.

Basal Percussion

- This is done to determine the lower boundary of the lung.
- The lower border of the right lung lies in the mammary line along the 6th rib; in the midaxillary line along the 8th rib; and in the scapular line along the 10th rib.
- Lower border of left lung overlaps stomach. Posteriorly besides splenic dullness, the resonant note is observed.

■ AUSCULTATION

Auscultation of Lungs

- The ideal position of the patient for auscultation of the lungs is upright (either sitting or standing).
- The person is asked to do deep breathing (through the mouth) for hearing proper auscultatory sounds.
- Auscultation is done in various regions of the lungs (anterior, posterior, and axillary regions as shown in **Fig. 21.5**.
- Corresponding regions on two sides of the chest are compared on auscultation for:
  1. Character and type of breath sounds.
  2. Presence of adventitious sounds.

Auscultation of Trachea

- By auscultating over the trachea, bronchial breathing is heard.
- Bronchial breath sounds are produced by the passage of air through the tubes (trachea and large bronchus) as shown in **Figs. 21.6A to C**.

Auscultation of Lungs for Vocal Resonance

- Vocal resonance means hearing of sounds over various parts of the chest during the act of speech or phonation.
- Vibrations initiated by speech are transmitted along the air passage and through the lungs to the chest wall.
- Patient is asked to say "ninety-nine" or "one-one-one".
- Vocal resonance should be heard on the anterior, posterior, and axillary surfaces of the chest and

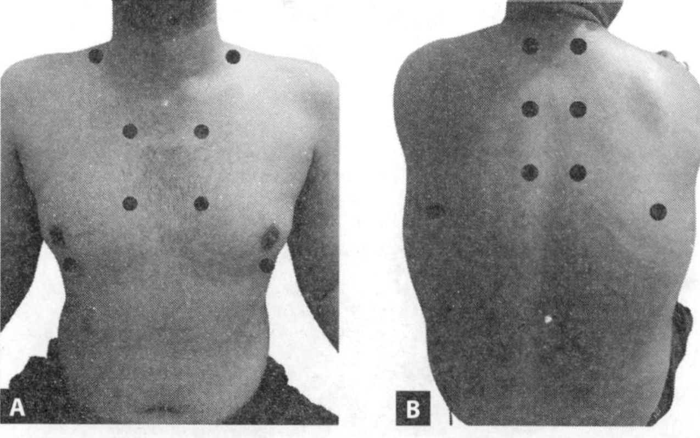

Figs. 21.5A and B: Auscultation areas on the lungs

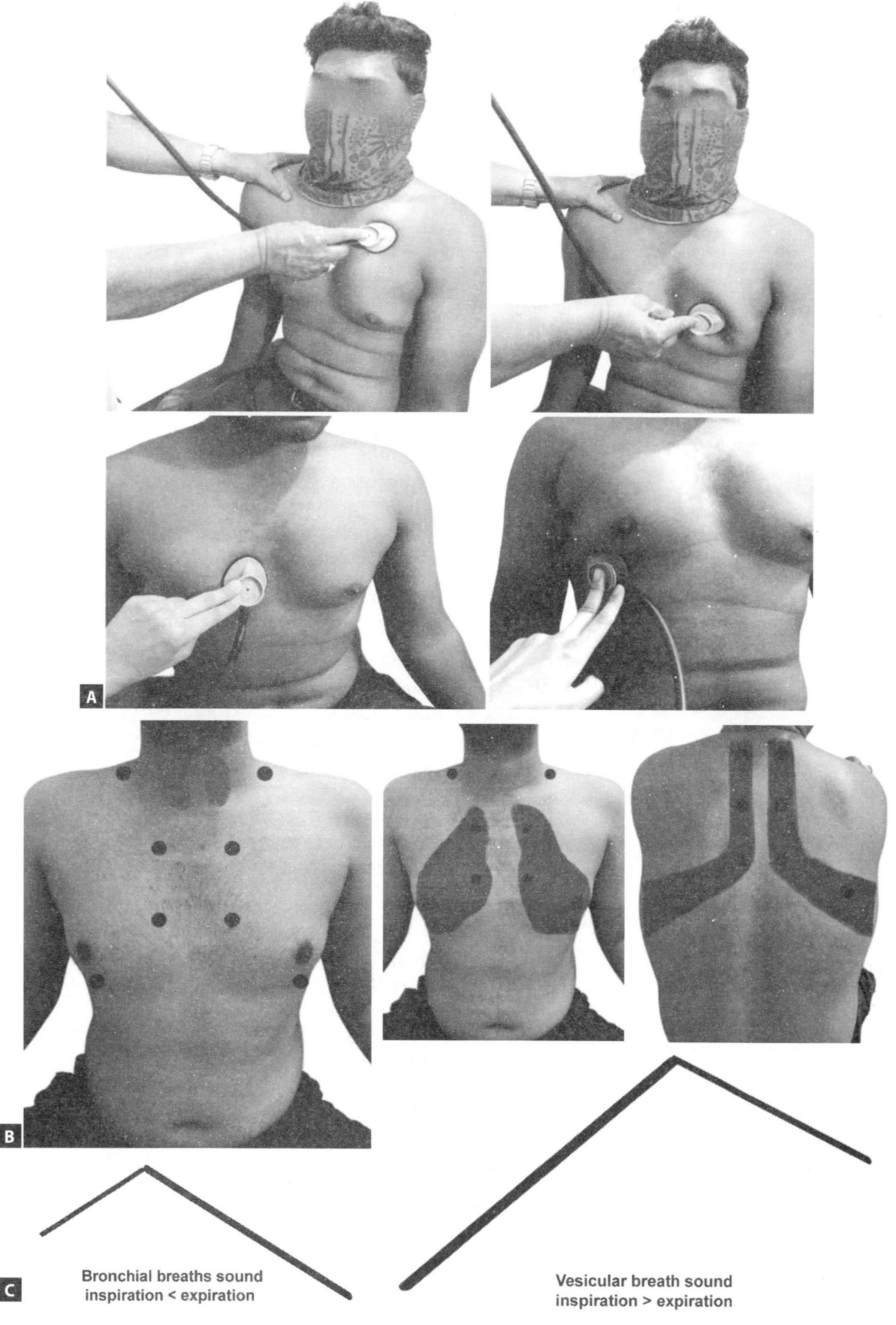

Figs. 21.6A to C: (A) Auscultation of lungs; (B) Bronchial breath sounds; (C) Vesicular breath sounds

compared with the corresponding area on the other side.

Observations: Examination of respiratory system proforma.

Systemic examination of RS: Any systemic examination is to be done after a complete general examination as shown in Chapter 1 General Examination.

Inspection
Chest wall–(size and shape)   Symmetrical/Asymmetrical
AP diameter   Transverse diameter
Chest wall movement with respiration-   Resp. rate Rhythm
Type of breathing- Abdominothoracic/Thoracoabdominal Apex beat position-
Trachea position—central/right/left   Accessory muscle of respiration– used/not used
Neck veins – distended/ not distended Surgical scars – present/absent

Palpation
Confirm all points mentioned above in the inspection of RS by palpation
Tactile vocal fremitus (for right and left lung – corresponding intercostal spaces on both sides to be palpated and compared simultaneously)
Anterior chest wall– Apices   Supramammary   Mammary Inframammary
Posterior chest wall– Suprascapular   Intrascapular Infrascapular
Axillary region
Percussion– Find out notes on right and left lung in the following areas, in corresponding intercostal spaces
Anterior chest wall–   Apices   Supramammary Mammary   Inframammary
Posterior chest wall– Suprascapular   Intrascapular Infrascapular
Axillary region

Auscultation
Air entry – On both sides   Trachea- Auscultate   Anterior chest wall   Posterior chest wall   Axilla
Type of breathing–   Trachea   Lungs
Any abnormal sounds   Heard/ not heard
Vocal resonance for right and left lung–corresponding intercostal spaces on both sides to be auscultated and compared simultaneously
Anterior chest wall Apices   Supramammary   Mammary Inframammary
Posterior chest wall Suprascapular   Intrascapular Infrascapular
Axillary region

■ IMPORTANT QUESTIONS AND ANSWERS

Q.1. Define the following terms.
- **Tachypnea:** An increased respiratory rate that is observed by a doctor
- **Dyspnea:** It is breathlessness that the patient experiences.
- **Apnea:** Cessation (stoppage) of respiration. It is of two types
  1. **Central apnea:** Respiratory efforts are not seen in a person with stoppage of breathing (apnea).
  2. **Obstructive apnea:** Respiratory efforts are seen with stoppage of breathing (apnea). It is due to obstruction of the upper airways.

Q.2. What is a thoracoabdominal and abdominothoracic type of breathing?
- **Thoracoabdominal breathing:** In females, intercostal muscles play a dominant role in respiration and involve movement of the upper part of the thorax and is described as thoracoabdominal breathing.
- **Abdominothoracic breathing:** In males, breathing is abdominal as it is mainly dependent on the diaphragm and is described as abdominothoracic breathing.

Q.3. Enumerate physiological and pathological conditions causing tachypnea and bradypnea.

Tachypnea	*Bradypnea*
Physiological conditions	Physiologically– Rare
Newborn, children, exercise excitement	Pathological conditions
Pathological conditions	CNS depression (as the respiratory centre is placed in the medulla)
Any condition that causes hypoxia (lung or cardiac pathologies)	

Q.4. Enumerate causes of unilateral and bilateral restriction/reduced/absent respiratory movements.

Causes of unilateral reduced respiratory movements	*Causes of bilateral reduced respiratory movements*
• Pleural effusion • Pneumothorax • Fibrosis of lung • Collapse of lung	• Emphysema • Bilateral consolidation • Bilateral pleural effusion

Q.5. What is Cheyne-Stokes breathing?
- **Cheyne-Stokes breathing:** There are alternate periods of increased rate and depth of respiration followed by diminished respiratory rate and effort. It is seen in patients with heart failure, and neurological diseases.
- Biot's respiration is observed with meningitis. There is an irregular rate and depth of respiration.

Q.6. How trachea is palpated?
The trachea can be palpated by any of the two methods described above.

Q.7. What is the principle of percussion and enumerate the rules of percussion.

Explained above.

Q.8. What are the causes of the shift of mediastinum?

Common causes of shift of mediastinum

- *Due to lung pathology:* Pleural effusion, pneumothorax (shifts to opposite side), atelectasis
- *Due to cardiac pathology:* Left ventricular hypertrophy
- *Other causes:* Scoliosis

Q.9. What is tactile vocal fremitus and how is it tested?

- **Tactile vocal fremitus** is a vibratory sensation that is appreciated on palpation. (while the person is saying ninety – nine or one-one) Detailed steps and areas of TVF are described above.
- TVF has to be compared on corresponding intercostal spaces for equality.
- **Conditions altering TVF**: TVF is decreased/absent in pleural effusion and pneumothorax. Increased TVF is observed with lung consolidation (As with consolidation, sound conducted is better than air conducted in the lungs).

Q.10. What is vocal resonance and how is it tested?

- Vocal resonance is an **auscultatory counterpart of TVF.** The procedure remains the same, only thing is instead of palpating with an ulnar border of the hand, the stethoscope is put in intercostal spaces to appreciate vibrations.
- All clinical conditions that alter TVF do alter vocal resonance.

Q.11. What are the differences between bronchial and vesicular breathing?

S. No.	Characteristics of vesicular breath sounds	Characteristics of bronchial breath sounds
1.	Are produced by passage of air in and out of normal lung tissue	Are produced by the passage of air through the trachea and large bronchi
2.	They are heard all over the chest under normal conditions	They are heard by listening over the trachea and not heard over normal lung tissue
3.	Duration of inspiration is more than expiration	Duration of expiration is more than inspiration
4.	Inspiratory sound is more intense than expiratory sound (rustling sound)	Expiratory sound is more intense than inspiratory sound
5.	There is no gap between inspiration and expiration	There is a gap between inspiration and expiration

Q.12. What is physiological basis of breath sounds?

- Breath sounds do originate from turbulence mainly in upper airways. We hear a sound that is filtered by lung tissue, till it is conducted to lung area where we have kept our stethoscope.

- Lung tissue normally filters high frequencies and make breath sounds quieter. These are normal vesicular breath sounds heard on lungs.

Q.13. What conditions can alter vocal resonance?

- When there is a consolidation of the lung, vocal resonance is increased.
- Vocal resonance is entirely abolished or diminished in pleural effusion, thickened pleura, emphysema of lungs.

Q.14. What are adventitious sounds?

Adventitious Sounds

- **Wheezes** (initially called Ronchi) are continuous sounds produced by partial obstruction of the respiratory passages. They are heard in bronchitis and bronchial asthma. Wheezes are more pronounced during expiration (when there is airway narrowing)
- **Stridor:** One should not confuse with wheezes. As wheezes involve obstruction of smaller airways, stridor involves larger airway obstruction. Heard mainly on trachea and are heard with inspiration as well as expiration.
- **Rales** (moist sounds and crepitations/**crackles**) are discontinuous cracking sound produced either in alveoli, bronchi, or bronchioles. They indicate presence of fluid secretions in air sacs. They are classified as fine, medium, and coarse. Localized, loud and coarse crackles are heard with bronchiectasis.
- **Pleural rub**: It is characteristic of pleural inflammation. It is accompanied with pleural pain.

Do not confuse pleural rub with movement of stethoscope on patient's skin/clothes.

Q.15. Why neck inspection becomes important part while examining respiratory system?

- While we do examine respiratory system of patient, in general examination, examination of neck for neck veins becomes important part.
- A raised jugular venous pulse can be seen in patients with pulmonary hypertension with chronic obstructive pulmonary diseases (COPD).

Q.16. Which lymph node palpation becomes important with respect to respiratory system?

- Lymph nodes especially in supraclavicular fossae, cervical, axillary region and behind sternocleidomastoid muscles, if are enlarged, can be secondary to spread of malignancy from the chest.
- For better palpation of lymph nodes patient should be seated and examining him/her from behind.

Q.17. Why taking occupational history and family history is very significant while examining the respiratory system?

- Lungs in one of the susceptible objects to working environment/conditions. Many substances are responsible for occupational asthma, e.g. asbestos exposure is common with thermal and fire insulation, mining, aircraft manufacturing, electricians, carpenters, etc.

- There can be strong susceptibility for asthma in families and thus has to be carefully enquired.

Q.18. Enlist common respiratory conditions causing clubbing.

Respiratory causes of clubbing include carcinoma of the bronchus, pulmonary fibrosis, bronchiectasis, lung abscess.

Q.19. What are the other tests that can be done for understanding lung functions?

- **Pulmonary function tests:** These include a variety of tests where one can estimate various lung volumes and capacities. It is measured with the help of a spirometer (Refer to chapter 28, 29 and 30).
- **Assessment of gas exchange function of lungs:** Normal gas exchange consists of the uptake of oxygen into the pulmonary capillary blood and the release of carbon dioxide into the alveoli. It can be tested by using a small amount of carbon monoxide A person inspires as much as possible (to his/her TLC) and holds breath for about 10 seconds and then expires completely. The difference between inspired air CO concentration and expired air CO concentration is a measure of the efficiency of gas exchange.
- **Arterial blood sampling:** Here partial pressure of O_2 (PaO_2), partial pressure of CO_2 ($PaCO_2$) and pH can be measured. PaO_2 reflects effective ventilation of alveoli that are perfused with adequate blood for proper gas exchange. Any condition that reduces alveolar ventilation $PaCO_2$ rises. Arterial blood sampling is important for a variety of clinical conditions including respiratory failure.

Q.20. How one can do imaging of the chest and lungs?

- **Chest X-ray:** It is one of the important investigations that is done after a thorough clinical examination of the respiratory or cardiovascular system.

One has to look for lung fields, bony skeleton, outline of heart and mediastinum, and name of patient.

- **Computed tomography scan:** Here X-rays are passed through different angles and this information is processed in a computer to get a series of cross-sectional images. One of the important diseases in which it is used is the staging of lung cancer.
- **Radioisotope imaging:** A ventilation-perfusion scan is obtained to identify the distribution of radioactivity which can alter with different clinical conditions.
- **Magnetic resonance imaging, and ultrasound:** These are other techniques that can be used to diagnose various clinical conditions.

- **Fositron emission tomography (PET) scan:** A particular radiolabeled molecule is administered which is specifically picked by highly metabolic active tissues as cancer.
- **Flexible bronchoscopy and endobronchial ultrasound:** This investigation is useful to diagnose a variety of conditions. Even a forcep can be passed through a bronchoscope to get a biopsy of a tissue or even fine needle aspiration for lymph nodes can be done.
- **Pleural aspiration and biopsy**
- **Immunological tests:** These tests are particularly useful for asthma patients to find out allergens.

OBJECTIVE STRUCTURED CLINICAL EXAMINATION (OSCE)

Procedure station 1: Inspect the chest for the anterior chest wall for respiratory system examination and give your findings.

S. No.	Assessment criteria	Marks assigned	Marks given
1.	Greet and stands on the right side of the subject		
2.	Ask the subject to sit comfortably and explains the procedure		
3.	Inspect the chest for shape and symmetry		
4.	Inspect the chest for respiratory movements		
5.	Inspection chest for respiratory rate, respiratory rhythm, and type of respiration		
6.	Report and viva on clinical examination		
7.	Total		

Procedure station 2: Palpate apices of lungs for respiratory movements and give your findings.

S. No.	Assessment criteria	Marks assigned	Marks given
1.	Greet and stands on the right side of the subject		
2.	Ask the subject to sit comfortably and explains the procedure		
3.	For apical zone expansion, stand behind the subject		
4.	Place both the hands on the shoulder with four fingers of each hand in the supra-clavicular fossae with thumbs approximated in midline (behind the neck)		
5.	Observe and appreciates equal movement of fingers placed in right and left supraclavicular fossae		
6.	Report and viva on clinical examination		
7.	Total		

Procedure station 3: Palpate the chest in the upper, middle, and lower zones for respiratory movements and give your findings.

S. No.	Assessment criteria	Marks assigned	Marks given
1.	Greet and stands on the right side of the subject		
2.	Ask the subject to sit comfortably and explains the procedure		
3.	For apical zone expansion – stands behind the subject		
4.	Ask person to take deep breaths		
5.	Place both the hand on the shoulder with four fingers of each hand in the supraclavicular fossae with thumbs approximated in midline (behind the neck)		
6.	Observe and appreciates equal movement of fingers placed in right and left supraclavicular fossae		
7.	Place palms of both hands on anterior chest wall grabbing chest wall with both hands and thumbs approximated in midline		
8.	Check for equality of movement on the posterior chest wall in suprascapular, intrascapular and infrascapular regions with thumbs approximated in midline		
9.	With steps 5,6,7 and 8 observe for equal away movement of thumbs from the midline		
10.	Report and viva on clinical examination		
11.	Total		

Procedure station 4: Palpate trachea and give your findings.

S. No.	Assessment criteria	Marks assigned	Marks given
1.	Greet and stands on the right side of the subject		
2.	Ask the subject to sit comfortably and explains the procedure		
3.	Place index finger and ring finger of the right hand on sternoclavicular joints on either side		
4.	Place the middle finger in the suprasternal notch		
5.	Gently pushe middle finger forward to feel the tracheal ring		
6.	Appreciate the space between the sternocleidomastoid muscle and the trachea by insulating the finger between the trachea and sternocleidomastoid muscle		
7.	Report and viva on clinical examination		
8.	Total		

Procedure station 5: Palpate chest for tactile vocal fremitus and give your findings.

S. No.	Assessment criteria	Marks assigned	Marks given
1.	Greet and stands on the right side of the subject		
2.	Ask the subject to sit comfortably and explains the procedure		
3.	Find sternal angle as a landmark to count intercostal spaces		
4.	Ask the person to say ninety-nine or one-one repeatedly in the same intensity of voice. For steps 5 to 8		
5.	Place the ulnar border of the hand in the supraclavicular fosse on both sides to feel for vibrations		
6.	Place the ulnar border of the hand on the anterior chest wall and in corresponding intercostal spaces (supra mammary, mammary and infra-mammary regions) to feel for vibrations		
7.	Place the ulnar border of the hand on the posterior chest wall and in corresponding intercostal spaces (suprascapular, intrascapular and infra-scapular regions) to feel for vibrations (asking person/subject to bend forward and cross his hands on his shoulders)		
8.	Place the ulnar border of the hand in axilla in corresponding intercostal spaces to feel for vibrations (asking the person/subject to keep his hands on his head)		
9.	Report and answers viva on clinical examination		
10.	Total		

Procedure station 6: Percuss the lung to determine the condition of underlying tissue and give your findings.

S. No.	Assessment criteria	Marks assigned	Marks given
1.	Greet and stands on the right side of the subject		
2.	Ask the subject to sit comfortably and explains the procedure		
3.	Follow all the rules of percussion		
4.	Percuss apices of lungs, anterior chest wall (three regions) on corresponding intercostal spaces		
5.	Percuss posterior chest wall and axilla on corresponding intercostal spaces		
6.	Report and answers viva on clinical examination		
7.	Total		

Procedure station 7: Auscultate chest for breath sounds and give your findings.

S. No.	Assessment criteria	Marks assigned	Marks given
1.	Greet and stands on the right side of the subject		
2.	Ask the subject to sit comfortably and explains the procedure		
3.	Place the diaphragm of the stethoscope in corresponding right and left supraclavicular fossae (for apices of lungs)		
4.	Ask the person/subject to take deep breaths and listen for breath sounds		
5.	Place stethoscope on trachea		
6.	Place diaphragm of stethoscope in corresponding intercostal spaces on anterior chest wall – in supramammary, mammary and inframammary regions		
7.	Place the diaphragm of stethoscope in corresponding intercostal spaces on posterior chest wall– in the suprascapular, intrascapular and infrascapular region (with asking the person to bend forward and cross his hands on shoulders		
8.	Place the diaphragm of the stethoscope in corresponding intercostal spaces on the axilla– on the right and left side (asking the subject to keep his hands on his head		
9.	Report and answers viva on clinical examination		
10.	Total		

Procedure station 8: Auscultate chest for vocal resonance and give your findings.

S. No.	Assessment criteria	Marks assigned	Marks given
1.	Greet and stands on the right side of the subject		
2.	Ask the subject to sit comfortably and explains the procedure		
3.	Instruct the subject to say one-one or ninety-nine-ninety-nine repeatedly with same tone while doing steps 4, 5 and 6 and 7		
4.	Place the diaphragm of the stethoscope in corresponding right and left supraclavicular fossae (for apices of lungs)		
5.	Place diaphragm of the stethoscope in corresponding intercostal spaces on the anterior chest wall– in supramammary, mammary and inframammary regions		

Contd...

Contd...

S. No.	Assessment criteria	Marks assigned	Marks given
6.	Place the diaphragm of the stethoscope in corresponding intercostal spaces on the posterior chest wall– in the suprascapular, intrascapular and infrascapular region (asking the person/subject to bend forward and cross his hands on shoulders)		
7.	Place the diaphragm of the stethoscope in corresponding intercostal spaces on the axilla– on the right and left side (asking the subject to keep his hands on his head)		
8.	Report and answers viva on clinical examination		
9.	Total		

COMMON STATIONS– SPOTS IN PRACTICAL EXAMINATION (2/3 MARKS)

Q.1. Enlist common symptoms patient comes with respiratory diseases.

Q.2. Figure of physician palpating trachea, apex beat, tactile vocal fremitus, auscultating, percussing lungs: Identify the picture and one or two questions related to it (as given above).

Q.3. Figure of vesicular or bronchial breathing: Identify and enumerate its features, and write areas where they are heard.

Q.4. Figure of manubrium and body of sternum: Label or write anatomical landmark to count intercostal space.

Q.5. Figure showing a person bending forward and crossing his hands while the post-chest wall is examined: Give a reason for the peculiar position of the patient.

Q.6. X-ray chest film: Identify and write what you see in the X-ray.

Q.7. Fill respiratory proforma for a normal person (please check above for a proforma).

CASE-BASED SCENARIO/PROBLEM-BASED (2/3 MARKS)

Case 1: An 18-year-old boy comes with c/o breathlessness and on auscultation of chest wheezing is present.
- What is wheezing?
- What type of breathing does one hear on auscultation of lungs normally?

Case 2: 60-year-old male, with a known case of heart failure, complains of breathing difficulty. The physician observed that his breathing has a typical waxing and waning pattern.

- What type of breathing probably this patient have?
- Define tachypnea.

Case 3: 48-year-old female comes with complaints of breathlessness. On examination, pulse– 90 beats/min, BP– 120/60 mm Hg. Hb was found to be 5.2 g/dl
- What probably patient is suffering from?
- What do you expect from a morphological picture of RBCs in this lady?

Case 4: A person comes with h/o fever for 5 days and c/o cough. On percussion of lungs, TVF on the right side in the mammary region was more compared to the left side.
- What is the principle of TVF?
- Which conditions TVF is raised?

Case 5: A person c/o difficulty in breathing. On examination, the right side of the chest wall shows decreased respiratory movements. On auscultation breath sounds are not heard and vocal resonance is absent and percussion notes are dull.

- Enumerate causes of decreased or absent vocal resonance.
- What could be his O_2 saturation normal/less or more? Give its physiological basis.

■ KEY POINTS TO REMEMBER

- Chest has to be inspected for respiratory rate, rhythm type of movement, and equality of chest expansion on both sides with respiration.
- For palpation and percussion of lungs, start first with supraclavicular region for apices of the lung, on the anterior chest wall in supramammary, mammary, and inframammary regions and on the posterior chest wall supra-, intra- and infrascapular.
- Tactile vocal fremitus is palpatory and vocal resonance is its auscultatory counterpart of vocal resonance.

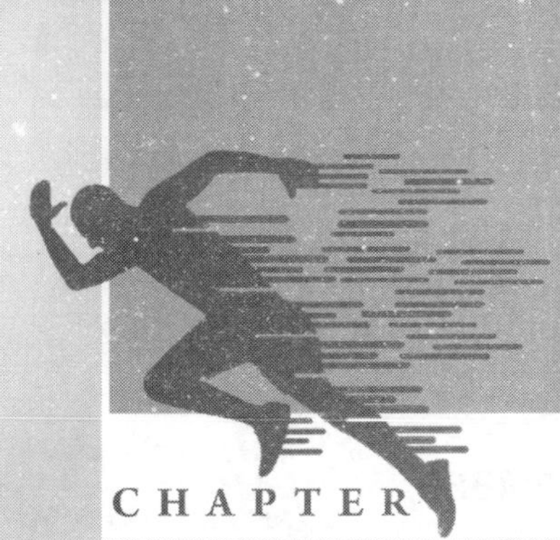

22

Effect of Exercise on Posture and Blood Pressure

Learning Objectives

At the end of this practical, students shall be able to:
- Record blood pressure (BP) in different postures (sitting, standing, and supine positions)
- List physiological changes in BP on standing
- List physiological changes in BP with exercise

■ EFFECT OF POSTURE

Introduction

- Change in body posture does affect functions of the cardiovascular system, which can be detected by various tests.
- Changes achieved are due to the action of the autonomic nervous system (reflex activity, e.g. baroreceptor reflex).
- Changes in systolic as well as diastolic BP are common with changes in posture. In a standing position due to venous pooling of blood systolic BP may fall which is corrected by baroreceptors in 1 to 2 minutes. Even there can be a slight increase in diastolic BP in a standing position which again is corrected in a few minutes by intact baroreceptors.
- These tests help to detect the efficiency of the cardiovascular system and autonomic functions.

Apparatus

Sphygmomanometer and stethoscope.

TABLE 22.1: BP recorded in supine, sitting, and standing positions

Systolic BP (mm Hg)	Diastolic BP (mm Hg)	Position of person
		Supine
		Standing
		Sitting

Method

Heart rate and BP are recorded in supine, sitting, and standing positions. Enter observation in the table given below **(Table 22.1)**.

Precautions

- As BP changes with a change in posture only for a short period, BP should be recorded immediately after a change in position.
- It is better not to remove the cuff while we record BP in various postures.

Procedure

- Ask the subject to lie down in a supine position.
- Record BP and check the pulse of the subject in the supine position.
- Do not remove the cuff and ask the subject to sit and record his/her pulse and BP.
- Do not remove the cuff and ask the subject to stand up and record pulse and BP.
- Compare the pulse and BP. Record in all three positions and enter observations.

Physiological Changes in BP on Standing

- When a person stands in an erect posture, blood is pulled in the lower parts of the body due to the effect of gravity.
- This decreases venous return and cardiac output. This in turn decreases the BP. This is immediately corrected through the baroreceptor reflex. The baroreceptor reflex is a very effective mechanism that prevents changes in BP that may happen with a change in body positions with day-to-day activities.

■ EFFECT WITH EXERCISE

Principle

Cardiovascular functions change with exercise. Pulse rate and BP are recorded before and after the exercise. Results are compared to study the effects of exercise.

Procedure

- After relaxing for 5 minutes, record the pulse and blood pressure of a given subject.
- Various forms of physical activity such as hopping, climbing upstairs, jumping, etc. can be given for a period of about 5 minutes.
- Common test done is the Master's step test where a person walks on the Master's step test for 5 minutes.
- Record pulse, and BP immediately, after 2 minutes, after 4 minutes, 6 minutes, 8 minutes and after 10 minutes. Calculate pulse pressure and mean pressure.
- Enter all findings in a table and find out the effects of exercise **(Table 22.2)**.

Observation

- Heart rate and systolic BP rise after exercise.
- Diastolic pressure may or may not change. Pulse pressure changes accordingly. As pulse pressure is the difference between systolic and diastolic pressure when systolic increases and diastolic remains the same, pulse pressure rises.
- After 5 to 10 minutes BP and heart rate return back to normal.

Precautions

- Pre- and post-exercise, BP must be recorded in the same position.
- Subject should exercise for 5 minutes.
- Immediately after exercise, BP and pulse must be recorded.

Cardiovascular Changes with Exercise

- Heart rate increases with the degree of exercise.
- There is an increase in stroke volume (stroke volume is the amount of blood pumped by the ventricle with each beat, normally it is 75 ml).
- Cardiac output increases with an increase in heart rate and stroke volume. Systolic pressure increases.
- Diastolic pressure does not change or might decrease with severe exercise (vasodilatation).
- Blood flow to exercising muscles increases.
- There is an increase in the coronary blood flow (normal coronary blood flow is about 225 ml/min).
- Due to sympathetic stimulation (vasoconstriction), there is decreased blood flow in the kidneys and gastrointestinal (GI) tract.

Respiratory Changes with Exercise

- There is increased O_2 supply to tissues.
- Lung volumes and capacities increase.
- Hyperventilation and increased respiratory minute volume (normal respiratory minute volume is respiratory rate tidal volume, i.e. about 6 litres/min).
- With the increase in pulmonary blood flow, there is an increase in perfusion of alveoli.
- Diffusing capacity of lungs increases.
- There is a shift of the O_2-dissociation curve to the right which causes O_2 release from hemoglobin (Hb) at tissue level.

Other Changes

- Body basal metabolic rate (BMR) increases.
- Body temperature increases (it depends on the intensity and duration of exercise).
- Lipolysis occurs with prolonged aerobic exercise.

TABLE 22.2: Observation of the effect of exercise on blood pressure (BP)

	Heart rate (bpm)	Systolic BP (mm Hg)	Diastolic BP (mm Hg)	Pulse pressure
At rest				
Immediately after 4–5 minutes of exercise				
Recovery:				
2 minute after exercise				
4 minutes after exercise				
6 minutes after exercise				
8 minutes after exercise				
10 minutes after exercise				

■ IMPORTANT QUESTIONS AND ANSWERS

Q.1. Explain the physiological basis of changes in cardiovascular system parameters with exercise.

- Exercise is a physiological stress to the body. To maintain homeostasis in such a situation. There are changes in various parameters of the body especially in the cardiorespiratory system.
- With exercise due to activation of the sympathetic nervous system, an increase in heart rate, cardiac output, stroke volume, and systolic BP are observed. To fulfil the demands of tissues, vasodilatation is observed (in active or exercising muscles) which decreases peripheral resistance. Therefore, with prolonged exercise, there may be a decrease in diastolic BP. As the myocardium works more, there is an increase in coronary blood flow. Changes in these parameters vary with type, intensity and duration of exercise. After exercise, all these parameters come back to normal within a few minutes.

Q.2. Explain the physiological basis of changes in respiratory system parameters with exercise.

- The main function of the respiratory system is to supply oxygen and to remove metabolic end products from tissues. When a person exercises in order to fulfil the demands of exercising muscles, the respiratory rate increases and all lung volumes and capacities rise. There is an increase in minute ventilation.
- Oxygen dissociation curve shifts to the right. This right shift means decreased affinity of Hb with oxygen which helps easy liberation of oxygen to tissues.

Q.3. What is postural hypotension?

It is a fall in BP with a sudden change in posture (commonly from a supine to a standing position).

■ OBJECTIVE STRUCTURED PRACTICAL EXAMINATION (OSPE)

Procedure station 1: Record the BP of a subject in supine and standing position.

S. No.	Assessment criteria	Marks assigned	Marks given
1.	Greet and stands on the right side of the subject		
2.	Ask the subject to sit comfortably and explains the procedure		
3.	Record BP in the supine position as explained above		
4.	Record BP in standing position as explained above.		
5.	Report and viva on clinical examination		
6.	Total		

■ COMMON STATIONS– SPOTS IN PRACTICAL EXAMINATION (2/3 MARKS)

Q.1. In a person BP is recorded in the supine position. BP was 120/80 mm Hg. On standing immediately BP was recorded and it was 110/78 mm Hg. Why there is a fall in BP after standing? Give a physiological basis.

Clinical Examination of Higher Functions

Competency:

PY 10.11: Demonstrate correct clinical examination of the nervous system: Higher functions, sensory system, motor system, reflexes, and cranial nerves in a normal volunteer or simulated environment.

Learning Objectives

At the end of this practical, the students shall be able to:
- Enlist all parameters that are assessed while examining higher functions
- Enumerate different higher functions
- Enumerate different levels of consciousness
- Enumerate different types of aphasia

■ SYMPTOMS

Unconsciousness, altered consciousness, speech defects, loss of memory, illusion, hallucinations

■ EXAMINATION OF HIGHER FUNCTIONS

1. **Level of Consciousness**: It can be judged by the response of the patient to painful stimuli. Various levels of consciousness are:
   - **Fully conscious state**: Patient is completely alert and responds to all stimuli, attentive, and cooperative.
   - **Somnolence:** Patient can be aroused by various stimuli, and able to make appropriate motor responses on verbal command.
   - **Stupor:** The patient can be aroused by painful stimuli and may respond for a short period to verbal commands.
   - **Semi-coma:** On painful stimuli or repeated stimuli may cause withdrawal and then with removal of stimulus returns to normal position.
   - **Coma**: The patient is deeply unconscious and does not respond to any stimulus or may respond to a very painful stimulus (pressure on the supraorbital ridge). The Glasgow coma scale is used to assess the level of consciousness in the patient.

2. **General Behaviour and Mental State**

   Evaluation of mental state is an integral part of neurological examination. It includes:
   - **Appearance and behaviour**: Look for the general appearance of the patient. His/her gait, sense of dressing, personal hygiene, way of talking, etc.
   - **Emotional state**: Mood, facial expression, depression, and euphoria, etc.
   - **Delusions and hallucinations:**
     - ⊙ **Delusions:** They are false beliefs which continue to be held despite evidence to the contrary.
     - ⊙ **Hallucinations:** They are false impressions referring to organs of special sense (hearing, vision, etc.)
     - ⊙ **Illusion:** Optical phenomenon in which the image is distorted or different from the object.
   - **Orientation in time and space:** Judged by asking the patient his name, day, and time of the day, etc.
   - **Sleep**: Ask for the duration of sleep and any disturbance in sleep
   - **Intelligence**: It can be judged by educational status, the way he/she is answering etc.

- **Memory**: It can be judged by examining recent memory and past or remote memory.
- **Speech**: Find out whether speech is normal or abnormal. Try to observe the fluency of speech and the content of it. Speech has motor and sensory components. In clinical examination one has to assess naming, comprehension, repetition, reading and writing.

OBSERVATIONS – PROFORMA FOR ASSESSMENT OF HIGHER FUNCTIONS IN CNS

Name	*Age*	*Sex*
Level of consciousness	Hallucination Delusion Illusion	
Sleep	Memory (past and recent), speech	
Intelligence	Orientation to time, place and person	

■ IMPORTANT QUESTIONS AND ANSWERS

Q.1. What are the different levels of consciousness?
Please refer above.

Q.2. Define illusion, delusion, and hallucination.
Please refer above.

Q.3. What is aphasia?
Aphasia: It is a disturbance of the ability to use language in speaking, writing and comprehension. Aphasia results from injury to higher centres.

Q.4. What is sensory aphasia?
- **Sensory aphasia:** It is the inability to understand spoken or written words of others.
- **Pure word deafness:** Inability to understand spoken words writing and talking are normal. This is seen with lesions in the auditory association area of the cortex.
- **Pure word blindness (Visual aphasia):** Inability to understand written words only. This is seen with lesions in the visual association area of the cortex.
- **Global aphasia:** All aspects of language and speech are impaired. The patient cannot read, write or repeat. He/she has poor auditory comprehension. It results from the combined dysfunction of Wernicke's and Broca's areas.

Q.5. What is the gait of the person?
- The gait of the person is defined as how the person is walking. It can be observed right from the patient enters in room.
- The physician has to assess if the patient can walk, can walk in a straight line or if he/she is falling in any particular direction and any difference with the eyes of the patient open and closed.

- Different clinical conditions can give rise to different types of gaits, e.g. spastic gait, hemiplegic gait, ataxic gait (wide base gait), high stepping gate (Please refer to Chapter on general examination).

Q.6. What is intelligence quotient (IQ)? Enumerate different grades of intelligence.
IQ: It can be found by dividing mental age by chronological age and then multiplying it by 100.

Grades of IQ

Below 20	Very severe mental retardation
21–34	Severe mental retardation
50–70	Mild mental retardation
70–130	Average
131 and above	Genius

■ OSCE–CNS HIGHER FUNCTIONS

Procedure station 1: Assess higher functions in a subject.

S. No.	Assessment criteria	Marks assigned	Marks given
1.	Greet and stand on the right side of the subject		
2.	Asses the subject under all the headings mentioned above		
3.	Report and answers viva on clinical examination		
4.	Total		

COMMON STATIONS – SPOTS IN PRACTICAL EXAMINATION (2/3 MARKS)

Q.1. Enumerate various levels of consciousness.

Q.2. Pictures of different gates: Identify and describe the importance of examining the gait of a patient.

CASE-BASED SCENARIO/PROBLEM-BASED (2/3 MARKS)

Case 1: A patient 65-year-old male, known as hypertensive is brought to the emergency department by a relative. There was h/o sudden collapse of the patient while he was walking towards the kitchen.

On examination, it was found that the patient was not responding to verbal commands, however, was responding to painful stimuli, rest vitals were normal.
- What level of consciousness, does the patient look to be?
- Enumerate different levels of consciousness.

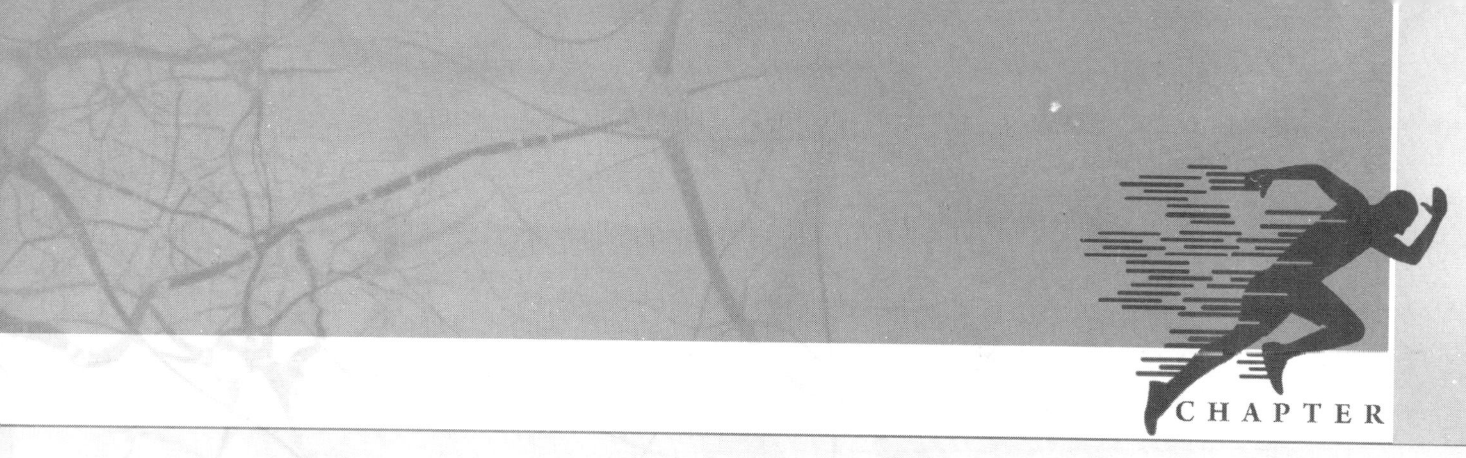

Clinical Examination of Cranial Nerves I to VI

Competency:

PY 10.11: Demonstrate correct clinical examination of nervous system: Higher functions, sensory system, motor system, reflexes, and cranial nerves in a normal volunteer or simulated environment.

Learning Objectives

At the end of this practical session, students shall be able to:

- Enumerate all cranial nerves
- Demonstrate assessment and integrity of cranial nerves I and enumerate abnormalities in smell perception
- Demonstrate integrity of optic nerve, demonstrate test for acuity of vision, field of vision, colour vision
- Demonstrate integrity of oculomotor, trochlear and abducent nerves. Demonstrate conjugate movements of the eyeball, define ptosis and nystagmus, and extraocular muscles with their actions
- Demonstrate integrity of trigeminal nerve. Assess its motor and sensory function

■ INTRODUCTION

- There are 12 pairs of cranial nerves. Some cranial nerves are purely sensory, some are purely motor, and some have mixed functions as sensory and motor.
- Systematic examination of cranial nerves is an important part of the evaluation of patients with neurological deficits. Cranial nerves can be affected by primary disease of cranial nerves, or by disease of the brain, and meninges.

■ CRANIAL NERVE I OLFACTORY

- **Introduction**: This nerve carries sense of smell. Olfactory nerve is pure sensory nerve. Olfactory receptor cells are bipolar sensory neurons situated under nasal epithelium.
- Central axons of these neurons project via cribriform plate into olfactory bulb which project via olfactory tract to frontal and temporal lobe.

Apparatus

Small bottles of clove oil, camphor, peppermint, etc. **(Fig. 23B.1)**.

Procedure

- Each nostril is tested separately with closed eyes by holding bottles near each nostril which are not labeled (clove oil, oil of peppermint, oil of eucalyptus, etc.)
- Both nostrils smell sensation with different substances is compared.
- *Note the result:* Normal smell sense/reduced/altered.

Precautions

- Subject should close the eyes.
- Must be familiar with the odour.
- Both nostrils should be examined separately.
- The substance with which one is testing should not be irritating to the nose.

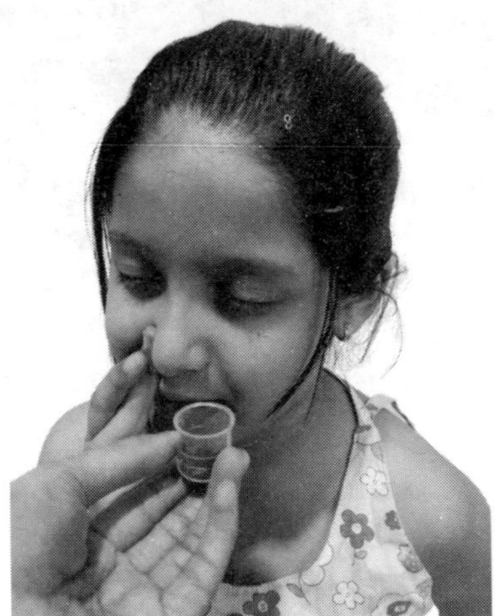

Fig. 23B.1: Test of the integrity of cranial nerve I (Olfactory) (cover eyes to prevent identity)

■ CRANIAL NERVE II OPTIC

- **Introduction:** It carries the sensation of vision. The optic nerve is pure sensory.
- The optic nerve runs from the posterior side of the globe of the eyeball to the apex of the orbit into the skull via the optic canal to optic chiasma where it is also joined by the optic nerve of the other and then via lateral geniculate body to the visual cortex (for details check visual pathway).
- Optic nerve has to be tested for:
  - Acuity of vision
  - Field of vision
  - Colour vision

Apparatus

Snellen's chart, pencil torch, Jaeger's chart, Ishihara chart.

Acuity of Vision

- It is defined as the power or ability of an eye to resolve two stimuli separately in space.
- It is checked by testing perception of light, hand movements and finger-counting test (these tests are done when vision is severely affected).
- Snellen's chart is used to test distant vision. Jaeger's chart is used to test near vision.

Snellen's chart: It has eight letters of different fonts black colour. The topmost line can be read by a person with a normal distant vision from 60 meters and followed by rows downwards from 36, 24, 18,12,6 and 5 meters lastly (for young children based on Snellen's principle, pictures are used).

■ DISTANT VISION- SNELLEN'S CHART

Procedure

- Proper instructions are given to the subject.
- Subject sits at a distance of 6 meters from the chart.

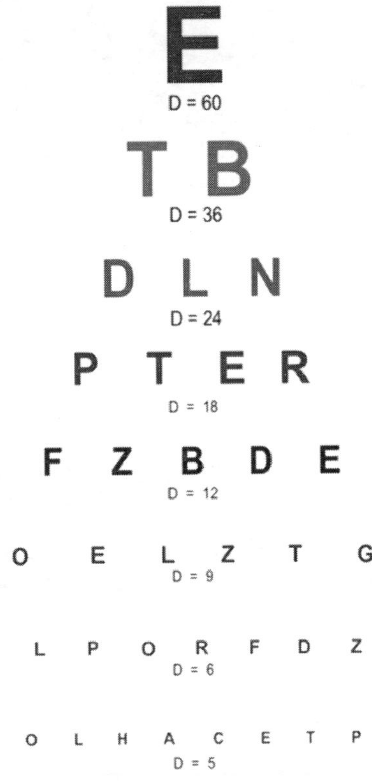

Fig. 23B.2: Snellen's chart

- Each eye is to be tested separately (one eye at a time).
- Note till what line the subject can read comfortably **(Fig. 23B.2)**.

Precautions

- Instructions to the subject must be proper.
- Confirm that the subject knows the language in which letters are written.
- Snellen's chart should be well-lighted.
- If the subject wears glasses visual acuity should be tested with and without glasses.

Observations

- Normal visual acuity is 6/6.
- Visual acuity is expressed as 6/6, 6/9, 6/12, 6/18, 6/24, 6/36, 6/60.
- Numerator 6 is fix as it is distance between subject and the chart.
- When we say 6/9 that means person with normal acuity of vision can read the line from 9 meters of distance which subject is able to read from 6 meters.
- Thus, acuity of vision for both eyes is tested and report is noted. If visual acuity of a person is less than 6/60 then finger counting/perception of hand movements should be tested.

■ NEAR VISION-JAEGER'S CHART

This chart has letters of various sizes. The smallest point is N5 and the largest point is N36 **(Fig. 23B.3)**.

READING TEST TYPES

as approved by

THE FACULTY OF OPHTHALMOLOGISTS,

LONDON, ENGLAND

N. 5

He moved forward a few steps: the house was so dark behind him, the world so dim and uncertain in front of him, that for a moment his heart failed him. He might have to search the whole garden for the dog. Then he heard a sniff, felt something wet against his leg — he had almost stepped upon the animal. He bent down and stroked its wet coat. The dog stood quite still, then moved forward towards the house, sniffed at the steps, at last walked calmly through the open door as though the house belonged to him. Jeremy followed, closed the door behind them; then there they were in the little dark passage with the boy's heart beating like a drum, his teeth chattering, and a terrible temptation to sneeze hovering around him. Let him reach the nursery and establish the animal there and all might be well, but let them be discovered, cold and shivering, in the passage, and out the dog would be flung. He knew so exactly what would happen.

(From "Jeremy" by Hugh Walpole).

wire sons vain error unwise cream remove

N. 6

The camp stood where, until quite lately, has been pasture and ploughland; the farm house still stood in a fold of the hill and had served us for battalion offices; ivy still supported part of what had once been the walls of a fruit garden; half an acre of mutilated old trees behind the wash-houses survived of an orchard. The place had been marked for destruction before the army came to it. Had there been another year of peace, there would have been no farmhouse, no wall, no apple trees. Already half a mile of concrete road lay between bare clay banks, and on either side a chequer of open ditches showed where the municipal contractors had designed a system of drainage. Another year of peace would have made the place part of the neighbouring suburb. Now the huts where we had wintered waited their turn for destruction.

(From "Brideshead Revisited" by Evelyn Waugh)

nervous manner immune over unanimous wear

N. 8

And another image came to me, of an arctic hut and a trapper alone with his furs and oil lamp and log fire; the remains of supper on the table, a few books, skis in the corner; everything dry and neat and warm inside and outside the last blizzard of winter raging and the snow piling up against the door. Quite silently a great weight forming against the timber; the bolt straining in its socket; minute by minute in the darkness outside the white heap sealing the door, until quite soon when the wind dropped and the sun came out on the ice slopes and the thaw set in a block would move, slide and tumble high above, gather way, gather weight, till the whole hillside seemed to be falling, and the little lighted place would crash open and splinter and disappear, rolling with the avalanche into the ravine.   *(From "Brideshead Revisited" by Evelyn Waugh)*

immense snow came near arrow use.

Fig. 23B.3: Jaeger's chart

Procedure

- Proper instructions are given to the subject.
- Subject should sit comfortably.
- Jaeger's chart to be held at 10–12 inches (about 25 cm) from subject's eyes.
- Smallest type of letter that subject can read is noted.
- Each eye is tested separately, while testing one eye, other eye should be closed. Test is also does with both eyes open.

Precautions

- Confirm that subject knows the language in which letters are written.
- Room should have adequate light.
- Chart to be kept at distance of 12 inches (about 25 cm) from subject's eyes.

Observations

Result is expressed by noting the lowest size of letters that subject can read.

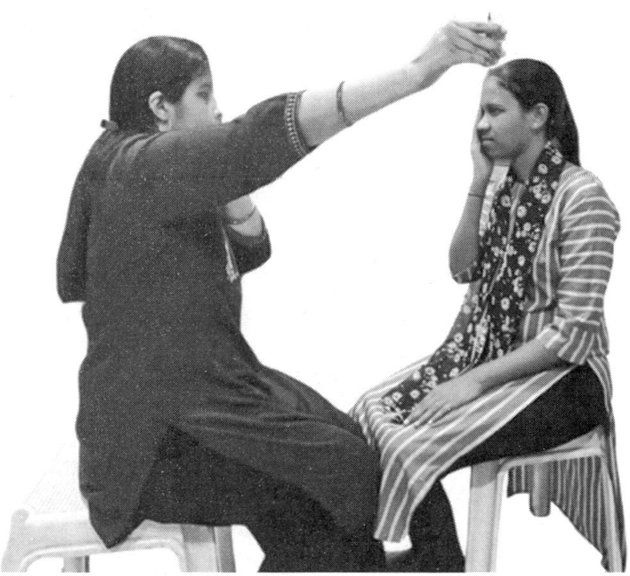

Fig. 23B.4: Confrontation test

Field of Vision

Field of vision is defined as a part of external world which can be seen by that eye at any given moment. It is tested by two methods:

1. Confrontation method.
2. Perimetry

■ CONFRONTATION METHOD

Procedure

- Subject is asked to sit on the stool.
- The examiner should sit on the stool in front such that his eyes and subject' eyes remain at same level (distance of 3 m).
- Subject is asked to close one of his eyes and examiner closes the opposite eye.
- Examiner should move the finger midway between subject and himself to test the field of vision in all four quadrants (nasal, temporal, maxillary and frontal) as shown in **Fig. 23B.4**.
- Subject should not move his neck while following the moving finger.
- Procedure is repeated for the second eye.
- Examiner compares his field of vision (which is supposed to be normal) with that of subject's for both eyes.

Perimetry

- It is more accurate test to detect field of vision than the confrontation test.
- It is process of mapping of uniocular field of vision done with the help of instrument called as the perimeter. Please check in human experiments section for details.

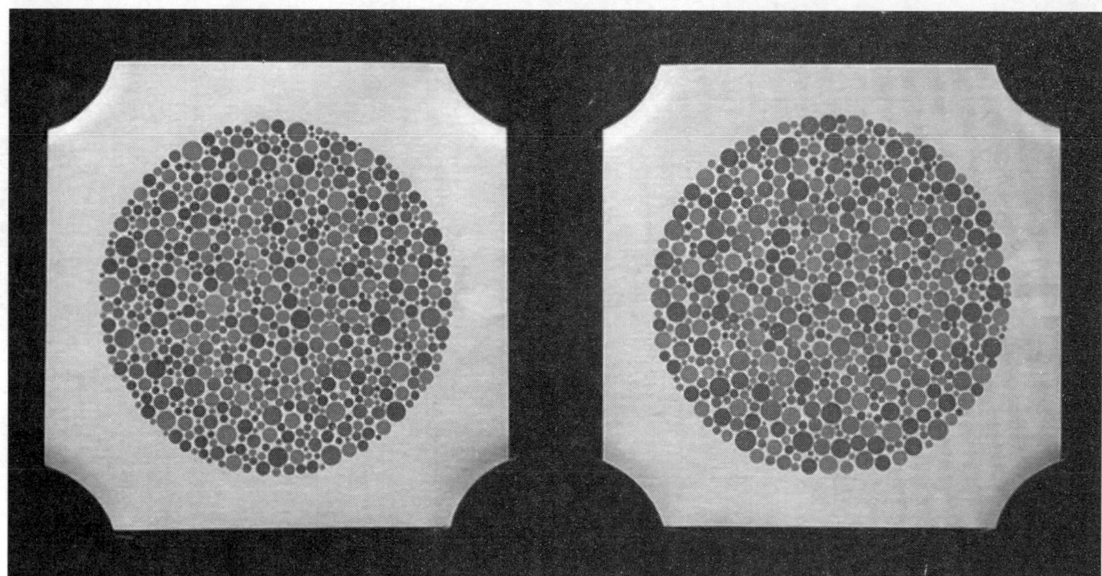

Fig. 23B.5: Ishihara colour vision test

■ COLOUR VISION

Colour vision is tested with the help of the Ishihara chart, Edridge–Green Lantern test, and Holmgren's wool matching test. Testing colour vision is important as even optic neuropathy many times can lead to acquired unilateral loss of colour vision.

Physiological basis of colour vision: The human eye is sensitive to wavelengths of light from 400 to 700 nm. Red, green and blue are the three types of cones that are responsible for colour vision. Due to the stimulation of different colour cones in different percentage we can perceive different colours.

■ TESTING OF COLOUR VISION

Ishihara Chart (Fig. 23B.5)

- It consists of lithographic plates in which numerals or alphabets are printed with coloured dots with backgrounds of different coloured dots.
- A person with a colour vision defect will read a different number than a normal person (result is also given in the appendix so that a colour-blind person can also carry out the test).

Instructions

- Give proper instructions to subject and ask him to sit comfortably in room with good illumination.
- Instruct subject to read numbers and note the result.

Edridge–Green Lantern Test

In this test, different colours are shown by lantern and the subject is asked to name the colour. It contains red, yellow, green, purple and blue colour. The subject is asked to sit about 6 meters away from the lantern and name the colours. Result is noted.

Holmgren Wool Matching Test

Subject is asked to perform colour matching from the collection of wool pieces of different colours. They are available in sets of different colours. The subject tries to match different colours in all the sets.

Colour Blindness

It is defect in the perception of colour. Colour blindness is inherited as X linked recessive disorder. Red and green colour blindness is common.

Pupillary Reflexes and Accommodation Reflex

Examination of the pupils and their responses to light and accommodation provides information not only about specific neurological syndromes that affect the pupils but also the integrity of optic nerves, brainstem and efferent parasympathetic and sympathetic pathways to the pupillary sphincter and dilator muscles, respectively. It is tested by:

- Light reflex
- Consensual light reflex
- Accommodation reflex

Light Reflex

- Powerful light beam is thrown in each eye.
- Pupillary contraction is noted **(Fig. 23B.6)**.

Consensual (Indirect Light Reflex)

- Light is thrown on one eye.

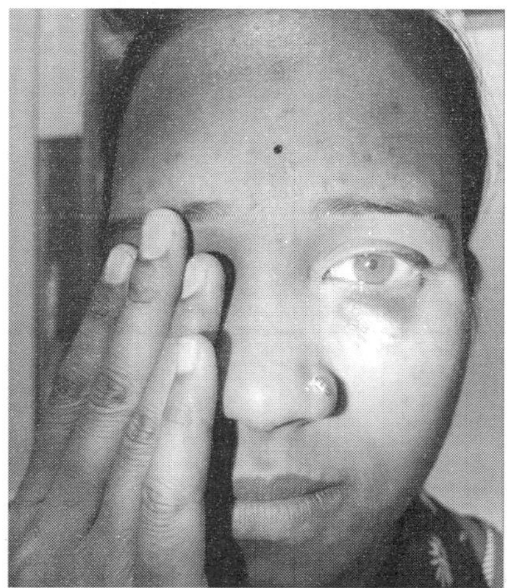

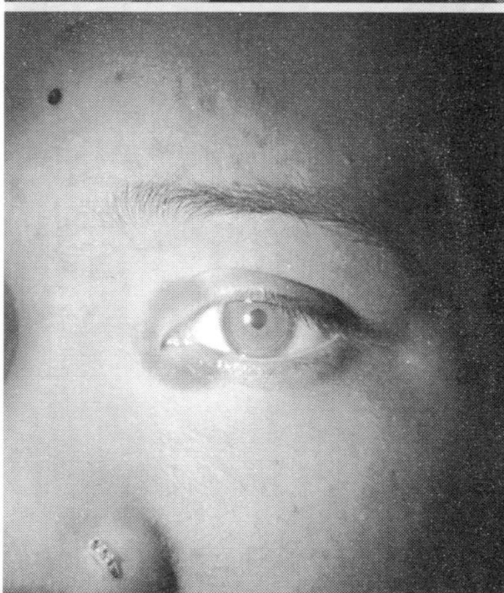

Fig. 23B.6: Direct light reflex

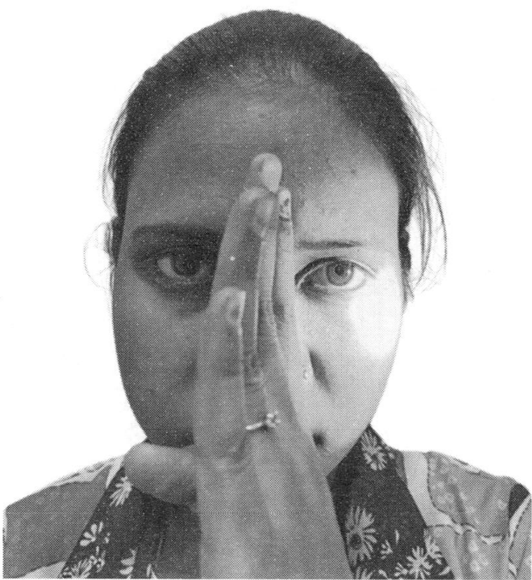

Fig. 23B.7: Indirect/consensual light reflex

- There is constriction of the pupil of the other eye (non-stimulated eye).
- This is due to the crossing over of nerve fibres in the visual pathway **(Fig. 23B.7)**.

Accommodation for near vision

- The person is asked to look at a distance.
- Then suddenly asked to fix his eyes on the tip of his nose or examiner's fingers (which is about 9 inches from the subject's nose).
- This results in the convergence of the eyeball and constriction of the pupil.

CRANIAL NERVES III, IV AND VI OCULOMOTOR, TROCHLEAR AND ABDUCENS

Introduction

- Third, fourth, and sixth nerves are always tested together as they innervate all extraocular muscles **(Fig. 23B.8)**. The nucleus of IIIrd cranial nerve is in the midbrain, IVth cranial nerve nucleus is caudal to IIIrd cranial nerve nucleus. VIth nerve nucleus lies on the floor of the fourth ventricle in the pons.
- Eyeball moves in different directions (by contraction of different muscles) and movements are named accordingly.

Procedure

- Subject is asked to sit comfortably on the stool.
- The examiner sits in front of the subject.
- Proper instructions to the subject are given.
- The examiner holds his index finger at a distance of about 12 inches from the subject's eyes and finger is moved in different directions.
- Subject is asked to follow the finger (without moving neck).
- At each position finger should be held for at least 5 seconds.
- Movement of the eyes of the subject are observed.

Precautions

- The distance between examiner's finger and subject's eyes must be 12 inches.
- Finger should be moved in all directions (all quadrants). That includes up down, in out, upwards, and downwards. One eye at a time and then simultaneously for both eyes.

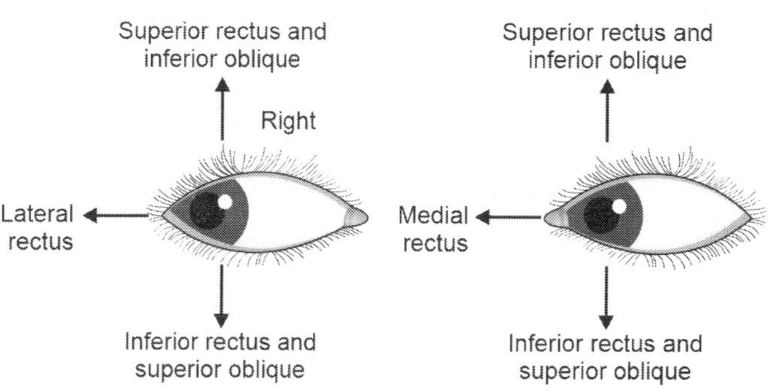

Fig. 23B.8: Actions of different extraocular muscles

- At each position finger must be held for 5 seconds.
- One should look for ptosis, lagging of one or other eye, squint or strabismus and nystagmus.

Different terminologies for eye movements

Abduction: It is horizontal movement of the eyeball outwards (laterally)

Adduction: It is horizontal movement of the eyeball inwards (medially)

Elevation and depression: Vertical movement upwards and downwards respectively

Rotatory movements: Eyes twist on the anteroposterior axis.

Intorsion: Intorsion is rotation such that the upper part of the eye moves medially and the lower part of the eye moves laterally.

Extorsion: Extorsion is rotation such that upper part of the eye moves laterally and lower part of the eye moves medially

Convergence: It is adduction of both eyes to focus on a specific thing

Cranial nerve V Trigeminal

- It supplies muscles of mastication and carries sensation from face. It is formed of ophthalmic, maxillary, and mandibular divisions.
- It is a mixed nerve; motor as well as sensory function is tested. Trigeminal nerve emerges from pons as sensory and motor roots.

Apparatus

Cotton wool, pin, glass tubes with warm and cold water, hammer.

Procedure

- Proper instructions are given to the subject.
- Subject sits comfortably on the stool.
- All sensations on the face are tested with the help of cotton wool, pinprick, and hot and cold test tubes (testing for touch, pain, and temperature, respectively).
- Sensations are compared on both sides at strictly corresponding areas as shown in **Figs. 23B.9A and B**.
- Subject is asked to clench his teeth and prominence of temporalis and masseter is palpated.
- Subject is asked to open the jaw, there should not be any deviation normally.
- Pterygoid muscle is checked by asking subject to do side-to-side movements of the jaw.
- **Jaw jerk:** With mouth partially open, index finger is placed below the lower lip and is tapped with a hammer. The response is observed (jaw closes) as shown in **Fig. 23B.10**.
- **Corneal reflex**: Cornea is gently touched with the wisp of cotton wool and blinking of eyes is observed **(Fig. 23B.11)**.

Precautions

- Instructions to subject should be given properly.

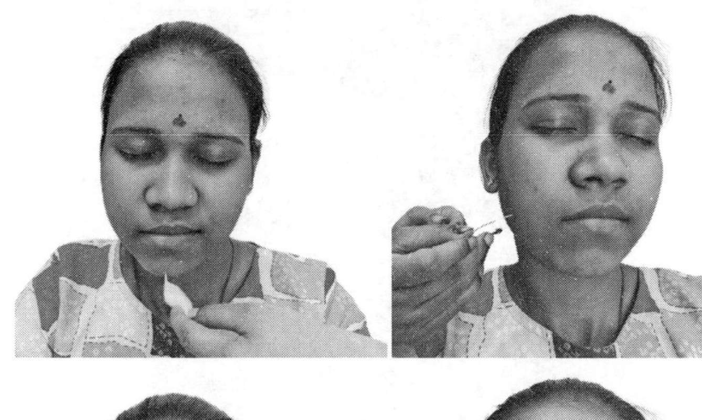

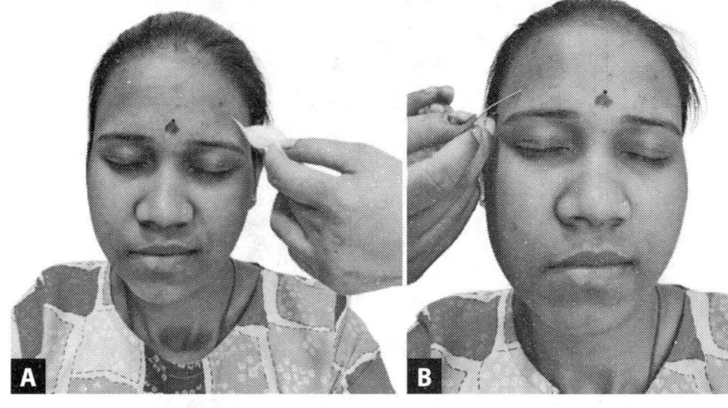

Figs. 23B.9A and B: Sensations are compared on both sides at strictly corresponding areas

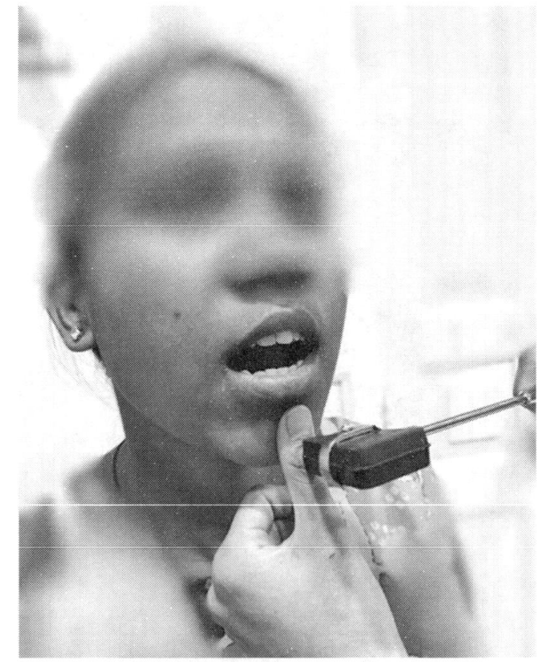

Fig. 23B.10: Jaw jerk

- All sensations elicited on face according to distributions of three divisions of the trigeminal nerve.
- Masseter and temporalis should be tested and compared on both sides simultaneously.

Observations: Examination of cranial nerves I to VI proforma: Any systemic examination is to be done after a complete general examination as shown in

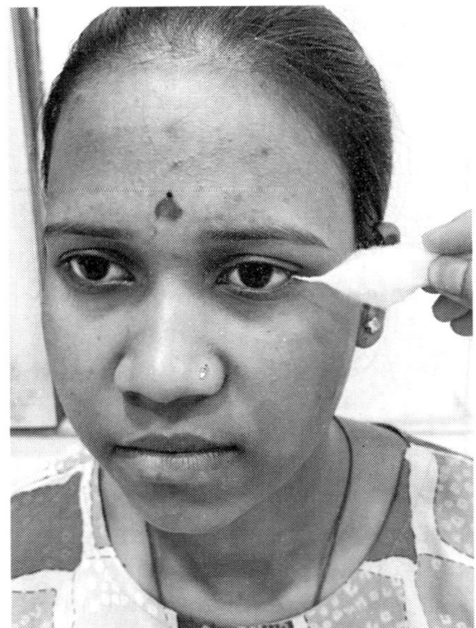

Fig. 23B.11: Corneal reflex

Chapter 1–General Examination) The proforma is given below:

■ IMPORTANT QUESTIONS AND ANSWERS

Cranial Nerve I-Olfactory

Q.1. What is significance of cranial nerve examination?
- Cranial nerve examination is one of the important parts of neurological assessment of a patient.
- Cranial nerves can get affected by primary disease of the cranial nerve or by diseases of brain or meninges.
- Any cranial nerves can get affected in its individual intracranial or extracranial course.
- Cranial nerve nuclei are lower motor neurons as their activity is controlled by higher centers.

Q.2. How do you test the olfactory nerve? Enlist the precautions before testing the olfactory nerve.

Refer above

I Olfactory nerve

Right nostril	Left nostril		Name of the smell perceived

II Optic nerve

Acuity of vision	Field of vision	Colour vision	Pupillary reflexes	
Distant vision:	Snellen's chart	With glasses	Right eye	Left eye
		Without glasses	Right eye	Left eye
Near vision	Jaeger's chart	With glasses	Right eye	Left eye
		Without glasses	Right eye	Left eye
Field of vision	Confrontation test	Temporal Nasal	Frontal	Maxillary
Perimetry	**Blind spot**	**Temporal Nasal**	**Frontal**	**Maxillary**

If vision is less than 6/60   Check-   Hand movements   Light perception-

Colour vision- Ishihara chart -

III, IV and VI (Oculomotor, trigeminal and abducent) nerve

Conjugate movements of eyeball	Right eye	Left eye	Both eyes

Pupillary reflexes	Direct light reflex	Indirect light reflex

Accommodation reflex   Present/Absent

V (Trigeminal) nerve

Sensory functions	**Right side**	**Left side**
Touch		
Pain		
Temperature		
Motor functions	**Right side**	**Left side**
Temporalis		
Masseter		
Pterygoids		
Reflexes	**Right side**	**Left side**
Conjunctival		
Corneal		
Jaw jerk		

Q.3. Enumerate abnormalities of smell sensation.

Abnormalities of Smell Sensation

- **Anosmia**: Loss of olfactory sense. It can be unilateral or bilateral
- **Hyposmia:** Diminished sense of smell
- **Parosmia:** Perverted sense of smell
- **Hypersomnia**: The threshold for sensitivity to smell is altered

Sub-frontal meningioma may cause unilateral or bilateral anosmia.

Cranial Nerve II – Optic

Q.4. How optic nerve is tested?

Headings under which optic nerve is tested:

- Acuity of vision
- Field of vision
- Colour vision

Q.5. Define the field of vision. Enumerate two methods to test it.

Field of vision: It is defined as a part of the external world which can be seen by that eye at any given moment. It is tested by two methods.

- Confrontation method
- Perimetry

Q.6. What are the different areas of the visual field?

There are four main areas of field of vision.

- **Nasal field:** The area of nasal side of vision (it represents temporal part of retina)
- **Temporal field**: The area of lateral side of vision (it represents nasal part of retina)
- **Superior field**: The area of inferior part of retina
- **Inferior field**: The area of superior part of retina

Q.7. What is physiological blind spot? What is its normal location?

- At the entry of optic nerve into the eye, receptors (rods, cones) are absent. This is called as blind spot.
- In the field of vision, this spot lies 15° lateral to centre as optic nerve enters the eye through an area lying little to medial pole.

Q.8. What is clinical significance of examining visual fields?

- Assessment of visual fields is one of the important parts in neurological examination of the patient.
- **One eye affected:** When only one eye visual field is affected it indicates retinal or optic nerve disorder.
- **Both eyes affected:** Lesion in optic chiasma, behind optic chiasma in optic tract, visual radiations in pathway and occipital cortex can cause visual field defects in both eyes.

Goldman perimeter or, automated Humphrey fields are used to detect field defects.

Q.9. What is clinical significance of examining pupils?

Examination of pupils helps to find specific pupil defects, the integrity of optic nerves, intact parasympathetic supply to the pupillary sphincter and sympathetic supply to dilator muscle. It also helps to understand integrity of brain stem (for pupillary reflexes please check cranial nerve examination of IIIrd, IVth and VIth nerve).

Q.10. What is colour vision? How is it tested?

Refer above.

Q.11. Give the physiological basis of colour vision.

Refer above.

Q.12. What is a pathway for colour vision?

Colour-sensitive ganglion cells, do pass via optic nerve and then optic tract to reach to lateral geniculate body (in thalamus) from where they project to visual cortex area 18 and visual association area of cortex.

Q.13. Classify types of colour blindness.

- **Deuteranopia**: A person is green blind as green cones are absent. Person is called deuteranope.
- **Protanopia:** A person is red blind as red cones are absent. Person is called protanope. Thus, person with red green colour blindness (which is commonest blindness) is a deuteranope and protanope.
- **Tritanopia:** A person is blue blind as blue cones are absent. Person is called tritanope.

If instead of absent cones, it is a weakness for perception of that particular colour it is called as deuteranomaly (green colour weakness), protanomaly (red colour weakness) and tritanomaly (blue colour weakness).

Q.14. Enumerate steps for the testing field of vision by confrontation method.

Refer above.

Q.15. Enumerate precautions taken for the confrontation test.

Refer above

Q.16. Which chart is used to test distant vision.

Snellen's chart is used to test distant vision. For details refer above.

Q.17. How do you interpret when we say vision of right eye of a patient is 6/24?

- Normal distant vision is 6/6 (details given above)
- When we say vision is 6/24, that means this person is able to read a line at a distance of 6 meters which a normal person can read from a distance of 24 metres.

Q.18. Enumerate factors affecting visual acuity. What is its clinical significance?

Factors affecting visual acuity are:

- 1-size of the object, 2- illumination, 3- spherical and chromatic aberrations, 4- size of pupil, 5-colour of the object (better for white objects than coloured objects). Visual acuity is maximum at the fovea and decreases towards periphery of retina.

- Visual acuity is directly proportional to visual angle. Visual angle is a ratio of the size of the object/distance of the object from the eye.
- **Clinical significance**: Testing visual acuity is important neurologically as well as ophthalmologically. Optic nerve damage also affects visual acuity.

Q.19. Define myopia and hypermetropia.

- **Myopia**: Parallel rays coming from a distant object are focused in front of retina. It is also called as short-sightedness. It is corrected by concave lens.
- **Hypermetropia**: Parallel rays coming from a distant object are focused behind the retina. It is also called as long-sightedness. It is corrected using a convex lens.

Q.20. Define following terms.

- **Far point:** It is the farthest point that can be focused sharply on retina without accommodation
- **Near point** It is the nearest point that can be focused sharply on retina without accommodation.

Cranial Nerve III, IV and VI- Oculomotor, Trochlear and Abducent

Q.21. Enumerate points under which one should examine movements of eyeball.

One should look for:

- Ptosis
- Lagging of one or other eye while testing eye movements in different quadrants
- Squint/strabismus
- Nystagmus

Q.22. What is ptosis?

Ptosis

- It is drooping of upper eyelid.
- It is observed with impairment in function of oculomotor nerve which paralyses levator palpebrae superioris muscle. Ptosis can also be seen in myasthenia gravis **(Fig. 23B.12)**.

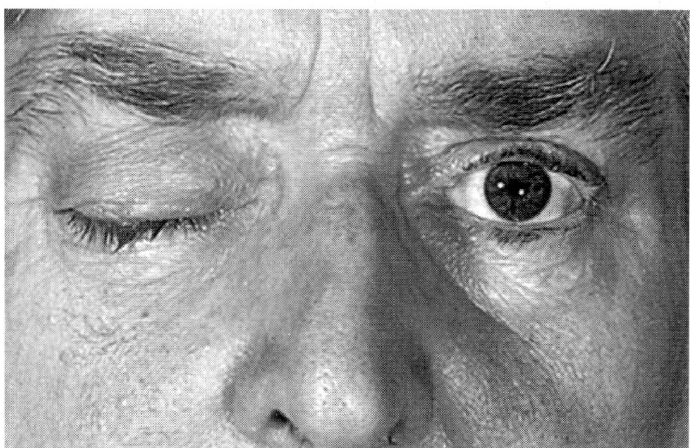

Fig. 23B.12: Ptosis

Trochlear nerve damage causes paresis of superior oblique muscle and abducent nerve damage will cause paresis of lateral rectus muscle.
Unilateral third nerve damage is associated with ptosis and laterally deviated eye.

Q.23. Define strabismus. Enumerate its types.

Strabismus (Squint)

- It is defined as lack of fusion of eyes in one or more coordinates.
- Strabismus can be horizontal, vertical, or torsional.

Q.24. What is nystagmus?

Nystagmus

- It is involuntary, rhythmic, and jerky movements of the eyeball when gaze is fixed in one direction.
- It can be due to visual defects, vestibular lesions, and cerebellar diseases.
- In pendular nystagmus movement is slow in both directions and in jerky nystagmus slow phase in one direction and fast phase in opposite direction is seen.

Q.25. Test for conjugate movements of eyeball. Test integrity of IIIrd, IVth and VIth cranial nerve.

Refer above.

Q.26. Enumerate conditions that can cause abnormal eye movements.

- Lesion of IIIrd, IVth and VIth cranial nerve
- Disorders of brainstem, cerebral hemispheres, cerebellum
- Neuromuscular junction affected between oculomotor nerve and eye muscles
- Defect in eye muscles
- Lesions affecting content of orbit.

Q.27. Enumerate actions of different ocular muscles with help of diagram.

Refer to **Fig. 23B.8**. The following table illustrates the nerve that supplies the muscle of the eye and its action **(Table 23B.1)**.

Nerve	Muscle	Action
Abducens; VI	Lateral rectus	Abduction
Oculomotor; III	Inferior rectus	Depression
Oculomotor; III	Inferior oblique	Extorsion; elevation
Oculomotor; III	Medial rectus	Adduction
Oculomotor; III	Superior rectus	Elevation
Trochlear; IV	Superior oblique	Intorsion; depression

TABLE 23B.1: Specific cranial nerves, their corresponding muscles, and the actions controlled by each muscle

Q.28. What is direct and indirect light reflex?

Refer above.

Q.29. Write light reflex pathway.

Light reflex pathway

From retina→optic nerve→optic chiasma→optic tract→pretectal nucleus→Edinger–Westphal nuclei of both sides→oculomotor nerves→ciliary ganglia→ciliary nerves→sphincter pupillae muscles.

Q.30. Write pathway of accommodation reflex.

Accommodation reflex-pathway

Retina→optic nerve→optic chiasma optic tract lateral geniculate body→geniculocalcarine tract-visual cortex (area 17)→frontal eye fields (area 8)→Edinger-Westphal nucleus of opposite side oculomotor nerve→ciliary ganglion ciliary nerves constrictor pupillae of the eye.

Q.31. Enumerate changes taking place in eye when eye accommodates for near and far vision.

Changes for near vision	Changes for far vision
• With the contraction of ciliary muscles, refractive power of lens increases (up to + 29D)	• With the relaxation of ciliary muscles, refractive power of lens decreases (up to + 15D)
• Constriction of pupil	• Dilatation of pupil
• Convergence of eyeballs	• Divergence of eyeballs

Q.32. What is Argyll Robertson pupil?

Argyll Robertson pupil

- It is a condition where the accommodation reflex is present in a person while the light reflex is absent.
- Pupils are small, irregular, and unequal pupils
- It is seen in neurosyphilis.

Q.33. What is physiological anisocoria?

It is a physiological condition where pupil size is not equal. However, reaction to light and accommodation is normal.

Q.34. What is ciliospinal reflex?

Ciliospinal reflex: By pinching the skin of the neck, there is dilatation of the pupil. This is due to reflex excitation of dilator pupillae muscle in the cervical sympathetic.

With cervical and upper thoracic cord lesions, this reflex is abolished.

Q.35. Define Horner's syndrome. Enumerate its characteristics.

- With damage to the cervical sympathetic chain, sympathetic nerves supplying eyes are interrupted and this condition leads to Horner's syndrome.
- A lesion of the sympathetic supply to the pupil at any point between the hypothalamus and the orbit is responsible for two features of Horner's syndrome: constriction of the pupil (which will still react to light by further constricting) and ptosis (drooping of the upper eyelid).
- Damage to the hypothalamus can cause unilateral Horner's syndrome.

Characteristic features include:
- Partial ptosis on the corresponding side
- Loss of ciliospinal reflex
- Permanent constriction of the pupil on the affected side
- Blood vessels on affected side are dilated
- Impaired sweating on ipsilateral side

■ CRANIAL NERVE V TRIGEMINAL

Q.36. How to test integrity of Vth cranial nerve?

Refer above

Q.37. What is trigeminal neuralgia?

- Severe pain experienced over one side of face along the path of sensory distribution area of Vth cranial nerve is called as trigeminal neuralgia.
- Painful attacks can be triggered by chewing, touching the face, etc.

■ OSPE FOR I TO VI CRANIAL NERVES

Procedure station 1: Test the sensation of olfaction. Demonstrate integrity of first cranial nerve.

S. No.	Assessment criteria	Marks assigned	Marks given
1.	Greet and stands on the right side of the subject		
2.	Ask the subject to sit comfortably and explains the procedure		
3.	Make sure both the nostrils are patent		
4.	Make sure that the subject is familiar with the odours used for test		
5.	Ask the subject to close the eyes and one nostril		
6.	Ask the subject whether subjects correctly perceive the smell		
7.	Compare the responses on the other side		
8.	Report and viva on clinical examination		
9.	Total		

Procedure station 2: Test the far vision/distant vision.

S. No.	Assessment criteria	Marks assigned	Marks given
1.	Greet and stands on the right side of the subject		
2.	Ask the subject to sit comfortably at 6 meters from the Snellen's chart and explains the procedure		
3.	Ask the subject to close one of the eyes		
4.	Ask the subject to read the chart from top to bottom with the open eye		
5.	Observe the line up to which subject can read comfortably		
6.	Compare the responses on the other side		
7.	Report and viva on clinical examination		
8.	Total		

Procedure station 3: Test the near vision.

S. No.	Assessment criteria	Marks assigned	Marks given
1.	Greet and stands on the right side of the subject		
2.	Ask the subject to sit comfortably and holds the Jaeger's chart at 10–12 inches from subjects' eye and explains the procedure		
3.	Ask the subject to read the chart from top to bottom with each eye separately		
4.	Observe the lineup to which subject can read comfortably		
5.	Compare the responses on the other side		
6.	Report and viva on clinical examination		
7.	Total		

Procedure station 4: Test the field of vision using finger confrontation test.

S. No.	Assessment criteria	Marks assigned	Marks given
1.	Greet and stands on the right side of the subject		
2.	Ask the subject to sit comfortably and explains the procedure. Sits at a distance of 3 feet from the patient taking care that examiner's eye level remains at the eye level of the subject		
3.	Ask him/her to close one of the eyes and close his or her opposite eye		
4.	Ask the subject to fix the gaze at the tip of his/her nose and instructs the subject to say "yes" when he/she sees the tip of a finger in the field of vision		
5.	Move finger midway between him or her and the patient from the periphery to the centre of four quadrants (temporal, nasal, upper and lower)		
6.	Compare the field of vision of the subject with his or her own field of vision		
7.	Report and viva on clinical examination		
8.	Total		

Procedure station 5: Test the colour vision.

S. No.	Assessment criteria	Marks assigned	Marks given
1.	Greet and stands on the right side of the subject		
2.	Ask the subject to sit comfortably and explains the procedure		
3.	Hold Ishihara chart at a distance of 25 centimeters from the subjects' eyes. Test each eye separately by closing one eye at a time. (Time spent at each line /letter of minimum 10 seconds)		

Contd...

Contd...

S. No.	Assessment criteria	Marks assigned	Marks given
4.	Note down the observation		
5.	Repeat the procedure for the other eye		
6.	Report and viva on clinical examination		
7.	Total		

Procedure station 6: Test the direct and indirect light reflex.

S. No.	Assessment criteria	Marks assigned	Marks given
1.	Greet and stands on the right side of the subject		
2.	Ask the subject to sit comfortably and explains the procedure		
3.	**Direct light reflex**: Shine the light with a torch into the patient's pupil and observe for pupillary constriction in the ipsilateral eye		
4.	Assess the **consensual pupillary reflex:** Shine the light with the help of a torch into the same pupil, but this time observe for pupillary constriction in the contralateral eye		
5.	Compare the responses on the other side		
6.	Report and viva on clinical examination		
7.	Total		

Procedure station 7: Test the accommodation reflex.

S. No.	Assessment criteria	Marks assigned	Marks given
1.	Greet and stands on the right side of the subject		
2.	Ask the subject to sit comfortably and explains the procedure		
3.	Ask the subject to focus on a distant object (clock on the wall/light switch)		
4.	Examiner should place a finger approximately 20–30 cm in front of the subject's eyes		
5.	Ask the subject to switch from looking at the distant object to the nearby finger		
6.	Interpretation of results		
7.	Report and viva on clinical examination		
8.	Total		

Procedure station 8: Test cranial nerves III, IV and VI (Oculomotor, Trochlear and Abducent).

S. No.	Assessment criteria	Marks assigned	Marks given
1.	Greet and stands on the right side of the subject		
2.	Ask the subject to sit comfortably and explains the procedure. Observe for the presence of ptosis, squint or nystagmus in any of the eyes or in both		
3.	Sit at the same eye level in front of the subject. Instruct the subject to look at the tip of the finger (25 cm from the patient's eye) and follow the movement of the finger only by eyeball (no movement at head and neck)		
4.	Move the finger lateral, vertical (up and down), medial, and oblique all quadrants to test the movement of each eye muscle, with each eye separately and together		
5.	Report and viva on clinical examination		
6.	Total		

Procedure station 9: Test the 5th cranial nerve in the subject.

S. No.	Assessment criteria	Marks assigned	Marks given
1.	Greet and stands on the right side of the subject		
2.	Make the subject sit on a stool and explain the procedure		
3.	Ask the subject to look at a distance and touches his/her conjunctiva with a wisp of cotton and notes the response		
4.	Test the sensations of touch and pain with a wisp of cotton and a pin on identical points on the two sides of the face		
5.	Ask the subject to show his/her teeth and then to clench his/her teeth. Watches and feels the masseter and temporalis muscles contracting		
6.	Ask the subject to open his/her mouth and move the mandible from side to side		
7.	Test the jaw jerk		
8.	Report and viva on clinical examination		
9.	Total		

(A question can be tested for motor/sensory component of the trigeminal nerve).

COMMON STATIONS– SPOTS IN PRACTICAL EXAMINATION (2/3 MARKS)

Q.1. Enlist precautions taken while testing the integrity of I cranial nerve.

Q.2. Figure of ptosis, conjugate movements of eyeball, jaw jerk, Snellen's chart, Jaeger's chart, Ishihara's chart, perimeter, light reflex to identify and one or two questions related to it (as given above).

Q.3. Diagram of one eye adduction and other eye abduction and label different eye muscles acting with the movement.

Q.4. Enlist the number of tests to test the integrity of the Vth cranial nerve.

Q.5. Enlist precautions to perform the confrontation test.

Q.6. Fill proforma for a normal person for examination of I to VI cranial nerves (please check above for a proforma).

Q.7. Enumerate changes seen when a person accommodates the eye for near vision.

(Any of the questions discussed in the section of the important questions and answers can be asked as spots).

CASE-BASED SCENARIO/PROBLEM-BASED (2/3 MARKS)

Case 1: A 12-year-old boy comes with a complaint of not being able to read from backbench things written on the board.

- What test you will do using what? (Snellen's chart)
- What is 6/6 vision numerator and denominator
- If in his right eye vision is normal but his left eye vision is 6/18, how do you interpret it?

Case 2: A 25-year-old male is sent to OPD for eye testing before joining a duty as driver in a company

- Among all the tests which test will be very important for him?
- What is red-green colour blindness?

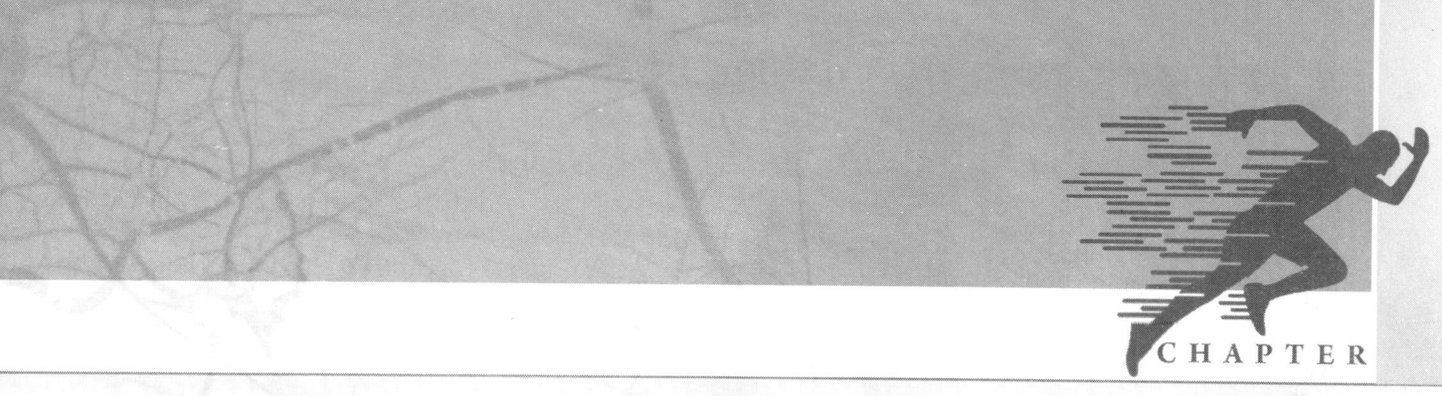

Clinical Examination of Cranial Nerves VII to XII

Competency:

PY 10.11: Demonstrate clinical examination of the nervous system: Higher functions, sensory system, motor system, reflexes, and cranial nerves in a normal volunteer or simulated environment.

Learning Objectives

At the end of this practical session, students should be able to:

- Enumerate all cranial nerves
- Demonstrate assessment and integrity of the VIIth cranial nerve
- Differentiate between supranuclear and intranuclear facial palsy
- Demonstrate integrity of VIIIth cranial nerve
- Demonstrate Rinne's test and Weber's test on a volunteer, enlist precautions taken for the tests
- Demonstrate integrity of IXth cranial nerve
- Demonstrate integrity of Xth cranial nerve
- Demonstrate integrity of XIIth cranial nerve, enumerate effects of lesion of the XIIth cranial nerve and give its physiological basis.

■ CRANIAL NERVE VII FACIAL

Facial Nerve (VII Nerve)

- It is mainly a motor nerve and it supplies muscles of the face of one side.
- It also has small general somatic sensory and major gustatory components and parasympathetic functions.

It carries taste sensation from the anterior two-thirds of the tongue.

- The nucleus of the facial nerve is in the caudal pons and receives upper motor neuron input from both cerebral hemispheres. Lower motor neuron fibres from the fascial nucleus emerge via pons to form the facial nerve.

Symptoms

Facial asymmetry, drooping of mouth, drooping of saliva, and sounds heard louder than normal (hyperacusis).

Apparatus

Small bottles with sugar, lemon juice, salt, chloroquine, cotton wool.

Procedure

Motor Functions—Upper Face

- Subject is asked to look upwards and wrinkling at forehead is observed.
- Normally, it is symmetrical on both sides (**frontalis muscle**).
- The subject is asked to close his eyes tightly and the examiner tries to open them against the resistance.
- Normally, eyes cannot be opened against resistance (**orbicularis oculi muscle**)
- In nerve weakness, eyes cannot be closed properly (Bell's phenomenon).

Motor Functions—Lower Face

- Subject is asked to smile or show his teeth.
- Face normally remains symmetrical and there is no deviation of the angle of the mouth (**orbicularis oris muscle**).
- Nasolabial folds on both sides are observed. Normally, they are symmetrical.
- Subject is asked to inflate his mouth; cheeks are tapped lightly (**buccinator muscles).**
- Air escapes from the mouth on the paralyzed side due to paralysis of buccinators.
- Subject is asked to whistle (orbicularis oris and buccinator).
- Subject is asked to clench his teeth and observe for the prominence of the **platysma** muscle in the neck **(Fig. 23C.1).**

Sensory Function

Anterior two thirds part of the tongue is tested for all primary taste sensations.

Ask the subject to protrude the tongue, dip the cotton for various taste solutions.

Precautions

- Subject should be properly instructed.
- Both sides of facial muscles are to be checked simultaneously and compared
- Subject should rinse mouth after testing for each taste.

■ CRANIAL NERVE VIII VESTIBULOCOCHLEAR

Vestibulocochlear Nerve (VIII Nerve)

- VIII nerve is a sensory nerve and it is responsible for hearing as well as maintaining balance and equilibrium.

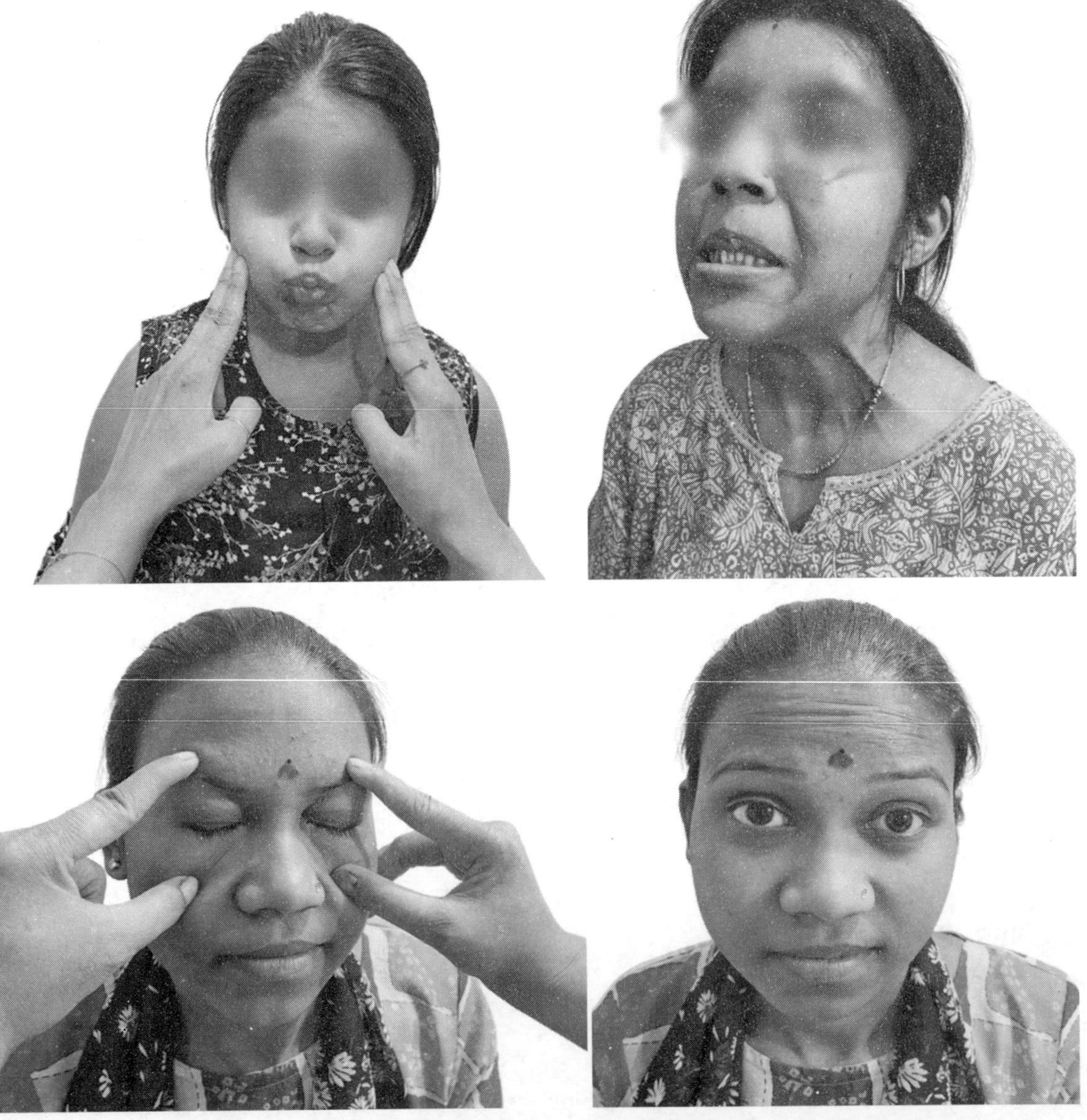

Fig. 23C.1: Testing various facial muscles–Examination of VIIth cranial nerve

- Cochlear and vestibular nerve convey afferents from cochlea and vestibular apparatus via internal auditory meatus reach cochlear and vestibular nuclei in the brainstem.
- Vestibular nerve supplies semicircular canals and labyrinth and is responsible for equilibrium and balance.
- Cochlear nerve supplies cochlea and is responsible for hearing.

Symptoms: Impaired or loss of hearing sense, tinnitus (perception of sound without any stimulus), vertigo.

Apparatus: Watch, Tuning fork 256Hz or 512 Hz, audiometer.

Cochlear Part Tests

Auditory Acuity Test

- The auditory acuity of the patient is compared with that of the physician (considering he/she has normal auditory acuity).
- Find out the distance at which a loud talk is heard by the patient and compare that with the examiner (physician).
- Evaluate the distance at which the tick of the watch is appreciated by the patient when it moves away and when brought near. Compare that with the examiner.
- Evaluate the whisper heard by the patient and compare it with the examiner (type of hearing loss cannot be detected with this test. It is just a crude test to detect hearing impairment).

Deafness Tests

Rinne's Test

- Ask the subject to sit comfortably and explain the procedure.
- A vibrated tuning fork (256 cps) is placed on the mastoid process on one side of the subject.
- Once the subject stops hearing, hold the prongs of the tuning fork parallel to the external ear and ask if he/she can hear the sound.
- Repeat the procedure for another ear **(Fig. 23C.2)**.
- Normally, he can hear the sound as air conduction is better than bone conduction.

Precautions

- Proper instructions should be given to the subject.
- Hold the stem of tuning fork in such a way that it does not touch the blades of tuning fork.
- Check for both ears.

Significance of Test

- **Rinne's test positive**: Normally, air conduction is better (that means hearing for longer time) than bone conduction.

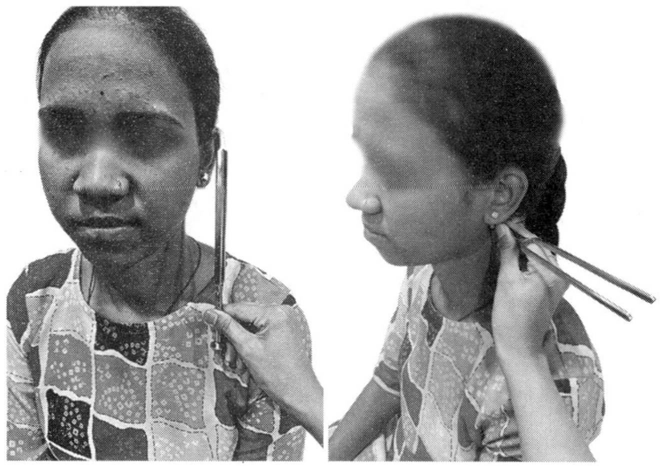

Fig. 23C.2: Rinne's test

- **Rinne's test negative**: In middle ear diseases bone conduction becomes better than air conduction.
- In nerve deafness both air and bone conductions are diminished.

Weber's Test

- Ask the subject to sit comfortably and explain him the procedure
- A vibrated tuning fork (256 cps) is kept on the center of vertex or on the forehead of the subject. This test is done to differentiate between nerve deafness and conduction deafness.
- Normally, sound should be heard equally on both sides **(Fig. 23C.3)**.
- When sound is heard better in one ear, it is called as lateralization of sound.

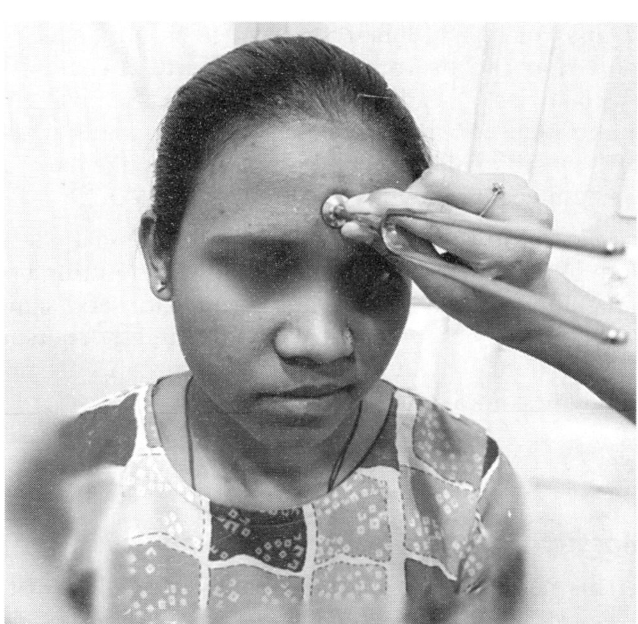

Fig. 23C.3: Weber's test

Precautions

- Proper instructions should be given to the subject.
- Hold the stem of the tuning fork in such a way that it does not touch the blades of the tuning fork.
- Check for both ears.

Significance of Test

- This test is done to differentiate between nerve deafness and conduction deafness.
- Normally, sound should be heard equally on both sides.
- When sound is heard better in one ear it is called as lateralization of sound.
- In conduction deafness sound is heard better on the affected side (e.g. right ear conduction deafness-sound better heard in right ear).
- In nerve deafness sound is better heard in the normal ear (e.g. right ear nerve deafness sound is better heard in the left ear).

Audiometry

- It is an objective and accurate method to assess degree of deafness.
- It is done using an audiometer. Test is conducted in soundproof room. At different frequencies threshold intensity is estimated and plotted as percentage of normal hearing. Graph is called as audiogram. Audiometer can test frequencies in the range of 250 to 8000Hz.

Brainstem auditory evoked potentials is an objective hearing test. Please refer to the Chapter on. It is an accurate method to assess hearing loss.

Vestibular Part Tests

Barany chair test: Subject is asked to sit on a specific chair that can be rotated at a definite speed with which subject's head can be tilted to specific positions to stimulate a particular pair of semicircular canals. Effect of stimulation of semicircular canals like nausea, nystagmus, vomiting, feeling of fall are noted.

Barany calorie test: Test is like the Barany chair test. Here semicircular canals are stimulated by putting hot and cold water via external auditory meatus and same symptoms are observed as that in the chair test. A person with vestibular dysfunctions, these symptoms are not seen with stimulation of semicircular canals.

Cranial nerve IX, X and XI glossopharyngeal and vagus and spinal accessory nerve.

Glossopharyngeal Nerve (IX Nerve)

- This nerve (mixed) carries general as well as taste sensations from posterior two-thirds of tongue and mucous membrane of pharynx.
- It also supplies motor fibres to middle constrictor of pharynx and stylopharyngeus muscle. It also carries sensation from the carotid sinus.
- IXth nerve is involved in palatal reflex, pharyngeal reflex and secretion of saliva
- IXth cranial nerve is one of the buffer nerves and is on of the afferents involved in baroreceptor reflex (short-term regulation of BP).

Symptoms: Nasal regurgitation, dysphagia (difficulty in swallowing), hoarseness of voice.

Apparatus: Taste solutions (as req in fascial nerve), swab.

Procedure to Test Motor Function of IXth Cranial Nerve

- Subject sits comfortably on the stool.
- All primary taste sensations from posterior two-thirds of tongue are tested.
- **Pharyngeal reflex (gag reflex):** The subject is asked to open their mouth and examiner stimulates back of the throat with tongue depressor to see contraction of posterior pharyngeal wall **(Fig. 23C.4)**.
- **Palatal reflex:** Touching the soft palate, responds by elevation of soft palate.
- For **both gag reflex and palatal reflex,** afferent is 9th cranial nerve and efferent is Xth cranial nerve and center is medulla.

Procedure to Test Sensory Function of IXth Cranial Nerve

Sensation of the taste on posterior one-third of the tongue is tested.

Effects of Paralysis of IX Nerve

- Loss of taste sensation from posterior two-thirds of the tongue.

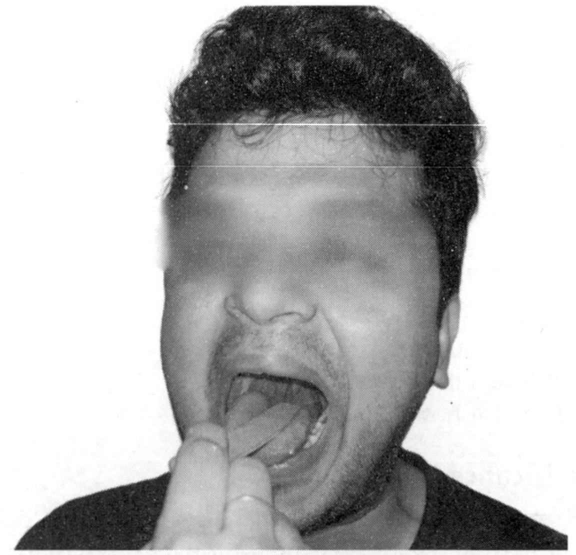

Fig. 23C.4: Gag reflex

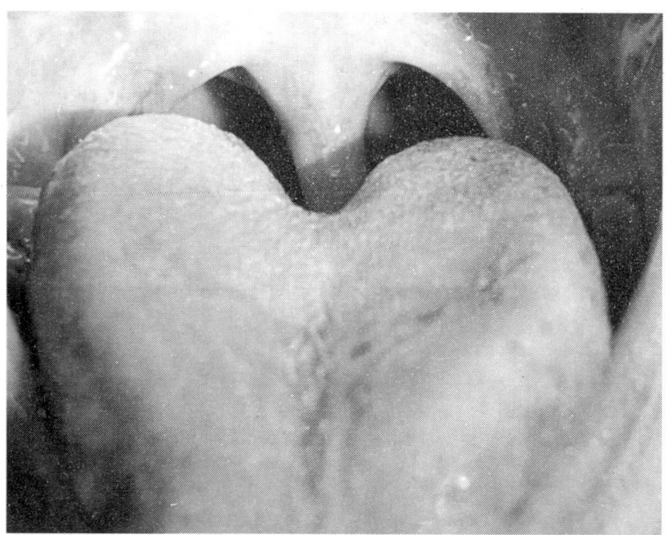

Fig. 23C.5: Symmetrical movement of palate

- Absence of gag reflex and difficulty in swallowing.
- Decreased secretion of saliva.

Vagus Nerve (X Nerve)

- It supplies motor fibres to the soft palate, pharynx, and larynx.
- It also innervates respiratory passage, most of the abdominal and thoracic viscera.

Apparatus: Swab

Procedure to Test Vagus Nerve

- It can be tested by—judging **position of uvula** and **movement of palate (Fig. 23C.5)**. After introducing tongue depressor, ask the subject to say 'ah'. Normal response is constriction of posterior pharyngeal wall and movement of uvula backwards.
- **Examining pharynx and gag reflex**—as explained above.
- **Examining vocal cords and movements of larynx**: With help of laryngoscopy vocal cord is examined. With deglutition, larynx moves upwards.

Effect of Paralysis of Xth Cranial Nerve

- With vagal nerve paralysis, uvula gets deflected to normal side (instead of the central position)
- Patient may give a history of regurgitation of food via nose due to paralysis of the vagus
- Damage to recurrent laryngeal nerve leads to hoarseness of voice.

■ CRANIAL NERVE XI SPINAL ACCESSORY

Spinal Accessory Nerve

- This nerve supplies sternomastoid and trapezius muscles.

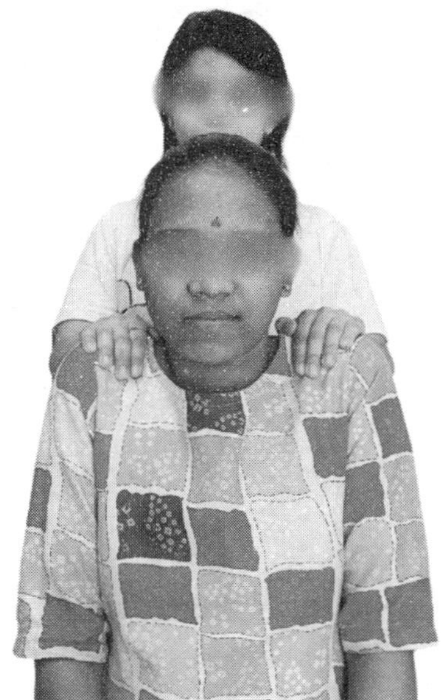

Fig. 23C.6: Testing trapezius muscle

- This nerve has only motor functions. Functions are tested by testing actions of the muscles.
- Cranial portion of the nerve is responsible for normal phonation and swallowing.

Procedure

- Subject sits comfortably on the stool.
- Proper instructions are given to subject.

To Assess Function of Trapezius (Fig. 23C.6)

- Subject is asked to shrug his shoulders against resistance.
- When trapezius of one side is weak shoulder on that side is weak and shrugging is weaker (Trapezius is supplied by spinal nerve).

To Assess Function of Sternomastoid (Fig. 23C.7)

- Ask subject to move his chin to one side.
- Try to prevent it by opposing movement.
- Note prominence of sternomastoid muscle on opposite side.
- Repeat procedure by asking him to move chin on opposite side with resistance.
- Lesions of accessory nerve can cause the inability to raise the shoulders and difficulty in turning the head.

■ CRANIAL NERVE XII HYPOGLOSSAL

Hypoglossal Nerve

- The hypoglossal nucleus in the medulla contains motor neurons which innervate tongue muscles. It is purely motor nerve that supplies the muscle of tongue.
- This nerve is tested by testing movements of tongue **(Fig. 23C.8)**.

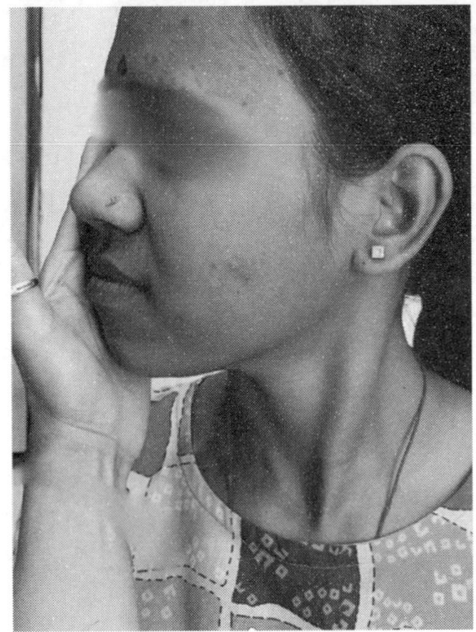

Fig. 23C.7: Testing sternocleidomastoid

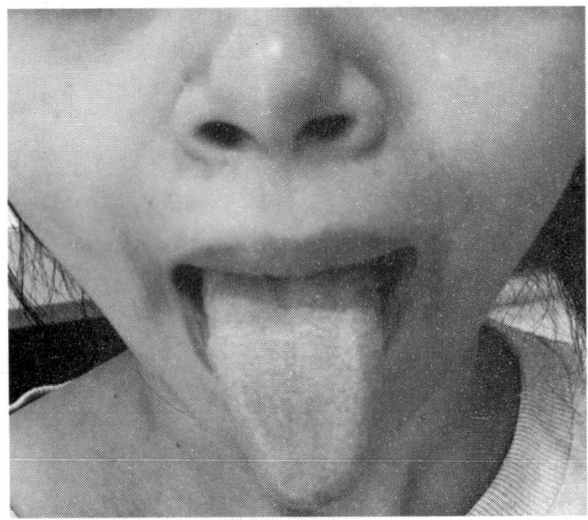

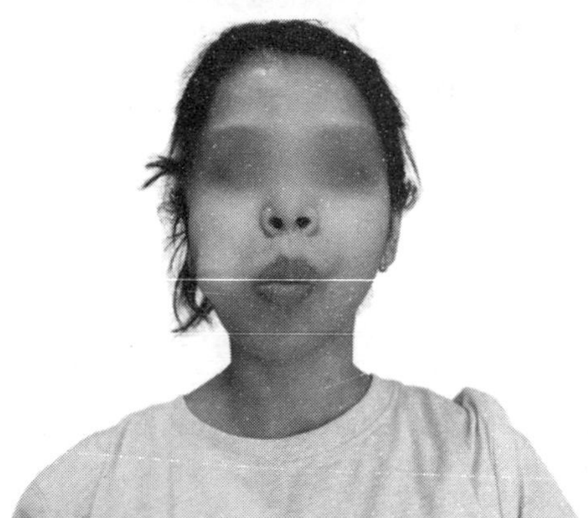

Fig. 23C.8: Movements of the tongue

Procedure

- Subject is asked to put out his tongue.
- Normally, tongue remains in the center.
- Subject is asked to move the tongue from side to side and push his cheek laterally from inside with the help of tongue.

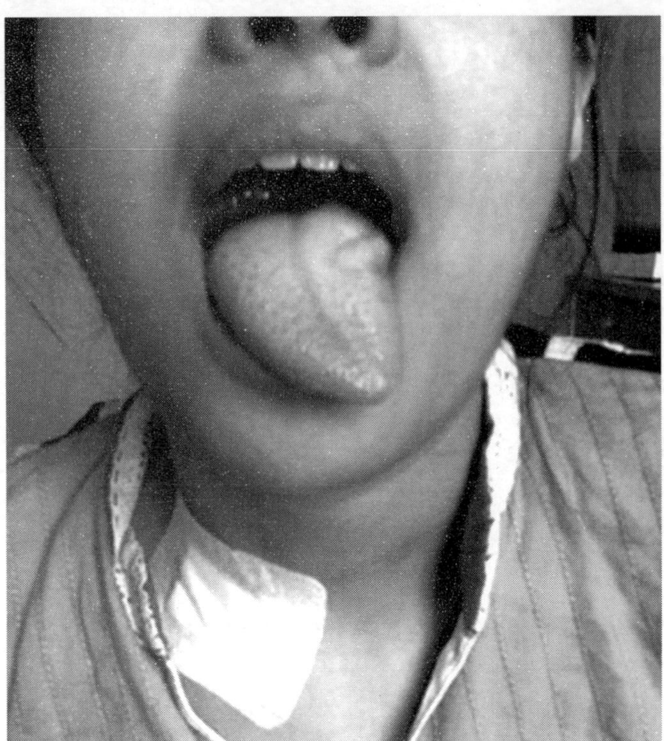

Fig. 23C.9: Acute left hypoglossal nerve lesion

- Strength of the muscles is tested by palpating from outside.
- Fibrillation or wasting of tongue muscles should be looked for (observed with LMN paralysis of the hypoglossal nerve) as shown in **Fig. 23C.9**.

Observations: Examination of cranial nerves VII to XII proforma. Any systemic examination is to be done after a complete general examination as shown in Chapter 1– General Examination.

■ IMPORTANT QUESTIONS AND ANSWERS

Cranial Nerve VII Facial

Q.1. How do you test the seventh cranial nerve?
- The seventh cranial nerve has to be examined for motor part integrity in the upper and lower face.
- For sensory part integrity taste sensation for anterior 2/3rd of the tongue (Details described above).

Q.2. Which all muscles are tested when we examine integrity of VIIth cranial nerve?

When you ask the subject to	One is testing
Lookup	Occipitofrontalis
Close his/her eyes tightly	Orbicularis oculi
Show his/her teeth and smile	Levator anguli oris muscle
Blow cheeks	Buccinator muscle
Depress the lower lip	Depressor labii inferioris
Frown	Nasociliaris
Taste identification	Chorda tympani
Listen to a whistle	Stapedius

VII facial nerve		
Motor functions – Power of the muscles		Sensory function– Anterior 2/3rd of the tongue for taste sense
Frontalis	Right side	Left side
Orbicularis oculi		
Buccinator		
Orbicularis oris		
Platysma		

VIII vestibulocochlear nerve	
Auditory acuity—	
Rinne's test – Right side	Left side
Weber's test – Right side	Left side

IX glossopharyngeal and X vagus nerve, cranial part of XIth nerve	
Nasal twang— Hoarseness of voice Nasal regurgitation—Present/Absent	Position of uvula Palate movement Pharyngeal reflex

XI spinal accessory nerve			
Motor function–Power of	Trapezius	Right side	Left side
	Sternocleidomastoid	Right side	Left side

XII hypoglossal nerve	
Position of tongue Central /deviated	Tongue movements

Q.3. Enumerate the effects of paralysis of the seventh cranial nerve.

Effects of paralysis

- The affected side of the face loses expression.
- Eye does not close properly on the affected side.
- Nasolabial fold is less prominent on the affected side.
- Deviation of the angle of the mouth is observed on the normal side.
- There is a loss of taste sensation from anterior two-thirds of the tongue.
- Facial nerve lesions may be supranuclear or infranuclear.

Q.4. Which part of the face will be affected in upper motor neuron (LMN) lesion or supranuclear palsy?

- Lesion above the fascial nucleus causes UMN or supranuclear palsy. In supranuclear palsy, the lower part of the face is mainly affected.
- Taste sensation may not be altered.
- Upper part of face is usually spared as fascial nuclei that innervates upper part of muscles are bilaterally innervated. Muscles that are responsible for voluntary movements of the face are affected. Emotional expression remains intact as these muscles are not affected.

Q.5. Which part of the face will be affected with unilateral UMN lesion?

- If there is a unilateral UMN lesion of right side then left side lower face muscles will be affected and vice versa.
- This is because, fascial nuclei supplying lower face are controlled by opposite side cerebral cortex.

Q.6. Which part of the face will be affected with (Lower motor neuron) LMN lesion?

- Lesion, distal to the nucleus causes lower motor neuron paralysis where both upper and lower part of face, on the side of the lesion is affected as final common pathway is damaged.
- Infranuclear fascial palsy is called as **Bell's palsy** and is the most common lesion of the fascial nerve. The cause is idiopathic (not known).
- There can be loss of taste sensation on the site of lesion and emotional component of the fascial muscle is not involved.

Q.7. What is hyperacusis?

- In infranuclear lesion, the stapedius muscle is paralysed. Stapedius muscle is responsible for damping of sound.
- The sound on the side of facial palsy is abnormally loud (due to paralysis of stapedius) This is called and hyperacusis.

Cranial Nerve VIII Vestibulocochlear

Q.7. Enlist procedure to demonstrate Rinne's test. Enlist precautions and significance of the Rinne's test.

Refer above.

Q.8. Enlist procedure to demonstrate Weber's test. Enlist precautions and significance of Weber's test.

Refer above.

Q.9. What do you mean by Rinne's test positive and negative?

Refer above.

Q.10. What is lateralisation of sound?

- In a normal person with Weber's test. Sound heard is equal in both ears.
- When sound is heard better in one ear than the other it is called as lateralisation of sound.
- In pure conduction deafness, sound is heard better on the side of conductive deficit. For example, in the right ear conductive deafness, sound is better heard on the right side (Due to masking effect).
- In nerve deafness, sound is heard louder on the normal side. For example, in the right ear nerve deafness, the sound is better heard on the left side.

Unilateral sensory neuronal deafness is one of the important features of cerebellopontine angle lesion like acoustic neuroma or meningioma

Q.11. How do you assess the function of the vestibular part of VIIIth nerve?

- Ask for h/o nystagmus, vertigo, dizziness.
- **Test for nystagmus:** It can be observed by asking the subject to look in different directions
- **Caloric test and Chair test:** Refer above

Q.12. How the gait can be assessed for testing vestibular component of VIIIth cranial nerve?

Stance and gait: In the presence of unilateral disturbance of vestibular functions, the patient tends to reel towards the affected side.

Q.13. What is optokinetic nystagmus?

- **Optokinetic nystagmus:** It is a physiological nystagmus that involves occipital cortex and frontal eye fields.
- It is observed when visual scene if it is moving continuously before the eyes, e.g. person looking at the landscape from a moving train. The slow phase of nystagmus occurs in the direction of movement of the object and fast or corrective component in the opposite direction.

Cranial Nerves IX, X and XI – Glossopharyngeal, Vagus and Spinal Accessory Nerve

Q.14. How do you test IXth, Xth and XI and XIIth cranial nerve?

Refer above.

Q.15. Which muscles are you testing when you ask subject to do different tongue movements?

When subject is told	You are testing
Show his/her tongue	Genioglossus
Touch tongue to the palate	Palatoglossus
Roll the tongue in the mouth	Extrinsic and intrinsic muscles of the tongue
Depress the tongue on floor of the mouth	Hyoglossus

Q.16. What are the effects of paralysis of the IXth cranial nerve?

Refer above.

Q.17. What is the effect of a lesion of the spinal accessory nerve?

With a lesion of XIth cranial nerve, person is not able to lift his/her shoulders. There can be dropping of shoulders. Person finds difficulty in turning the head.

Q.18. What is the effect of lower motor neuron (LMN) paralysis and upper motor neuron (UMN) paralysis on the XIIth cranial nerve?

- With UMN (bilateral paralysis) there can be difficulty in swallowing the food. Common symptoms are dysphagia and dysarthria. The tongue becomes spastic.
- With LMN (bilateral paralysis) tongue cannot be protruded out. Tongue muscle wasting and fasciculations are seen. With unilateral lesions, however atrophy or fasciculation is observed only on the affected side.

OSCE for Cranial Nerves VII to XII

Procedure station 1: To test the 7th cranial nerve in the subject.

S. No.	Assessment criteria	Marks assigned	Marks given
1.	Greet and stand on the right side of the subject		
2.	Explain the procedure to the subject		
3.	Test for all muscle powers of fascia; muscles (as explained above)		
4.	Examine the taste sensation in the anterior 2/3rd of the tongue		
5.	Report and viva on clinical examination		
6.	Total		

Procedure station 2: To demonstrate Rinne's test.

S. No.	Assessment criteria	Marks assigned	Marks given
1.	Greet and stand on the right side of the subject		
2.	Ask the subject to sit comfortably and explain the procedure		
3.	Select either 512 Hz or 256 Hz tuning fork and strikes one of the prongs on the heel of his/her hand		
4.	Follow the same procedure for Rinne's test as explained above		
5.	Check for air and bone conduction		
6.	Report and viva on clinical examination		
7.	Total		

Procedure station 3: To test the glossopharyngeal nerve of the subject.

S. No.	Assessment criteria	Marks assigned	Marks given
1.	Greet and stand on the right side of the subject		
2.	Ask the subject to sit comfortably and explain the procedure		
3.	Demonstrate sensory and motor integrity of ninth cranial nerve as explained above		
4.	Report and viva on clinical examination		
5.	Total		

Procedure station 4: To test the 11th cranial nerve of the subject.

S. No.	Assessment criteria	Marks assigned	Marks given
1.	Greet and stand on the right side of the subject		
2.	Ask the subject to sit comfortably and explain the procedure		
3.	Check for functions of trapezius and sternocleidomastoid on both sides (as explained above)		
4.	Observe the atrophy of the trapezius and sternocleidomastoid muscle		
5.	Report and viva on clinical examination		
6.	Total		

Procedure station 5: To test the 12th cranial nerve in the subject.

S. No.	Assessment criteria	Marks assigned	Marks given
1.	Greet and stand on the right side of the subject		
2.	Ask the subject to sit comfortably and explain the procedure		
3.	Ask the subject to push out his/her tongue as far as possible, then inspect its position, evidence of wasting and fasciculation		
4.	Ask the subject to move his/her tongue from side to side and in all directions, to palate as explained above		
5.	Report and viva on clinical examination		
6.	Total		

COMMON STATIONS – SPOTS IN PRACTICAL EXAMINATION (2/3 MARKS)

Q.1. Diagrams of testing different fascial muscles, diagram of Weber's test or Rinne's test, testing trapezius or sternocleidomastoid, movement of the uvula, movements of tongue, etc. to identify which nerve integrity is assessed with one or 2 questions on the same.

Q.2. Facial palsy picture affecting lower side of face (right/left): Identify and name its supranuclear or infranuclear lesion.

Q.3. Enumerate different muscles and their actions as one tries to test the integrity of the seventh cranial nerve.

Q.4. Enumerate different muscles and their actions as one tries to test the integrity of XIIth cranial nerve.

CASE-BASED SCENARIO/PROBLEM-BASED (2/3 MARKS)

Case 1: In OPD 56-year-old person is tested for Weber's test. On examination, there is lateralization of sound on the right side. He is diabetic for about 20 years and has poor glycemic control
- What is the significance of Weber's test?
- What is the probable cause of this finding? Give physiological basis.

Case 2: A 52-year known hypertensive comes with c/o weakness of facial muscles. He also complains of not being able to drink water properly.
- Which nerve integrity you would like to assess?
- What is the difference between supranuclear and infranuclear fascial palsy?

Case 3: A 75-year-old male person comes with c/o not able to hear and says that the intensity of this has increased in the last couple of years.
- Which type of deafness is common with old age?
- What is audiometry?

Clinical Examination of Sensory System

Competency:

PY 10.11: Demonstrate correct clinical examination of the nervous system: Higher functions, sensory system, motor system, reflexes, and cranial nerves in a normal volunteer or simulated environment.

Learning Objectives

After completion of this practical, students shall be able to:

- Describe the importance of assessment of the sensory system
- Classify various sensations and receptors
- Trace the pathway for all sensations
- Elicit all the tests to assess different types of sensations
- Enlist precautions taken while assessing various tests in sensory system examination

Common Symptoms

Tingling numbness in hands or legs, hyperesthesia, paresthesia, and pain.

Apparatus

Cotton, tuning fork, compass aesthesiometer, and von Frey's hair aesthesiometer.

Examination of the Sensory System

- All sensations depend upon impulses arising through the stimulation of receptors. They are conveyed to the CNS through afferent or sensory fibres.

- Disease of the sensory system may affect the nerve, nerve roots, brain stem, thalamus, and cortex. Lesions at different levels of the sensory system produce specific sensory deficits.
- Different sensory modalities are elicited from different receptors. Sensory fibres from each segment innervate a specific dermatome of the body. This dermatomal innervation makes the sensory map of the body. Dermatomes on both sides are compared to check the integrity of different segments of the spinal cord.

■ CLASSIFICATION OF SENSATION

Classification

- Sensations are classified as general, special and visceral.
- **General sensations** are-touch, pressure, pain, vibration, pressure, etc.
- **Special sensations** are-vision, hearing, smell, taste and equilibrium.
- **Visceral sensations** are-all the sensations originating from viscera, e.g. distension of the stomach, bladder, etc.

General sensory modalities to be tested are:

Superficial

- Touch-light touch, tactile localization, tactile discrimination.
- Pain
- Temperature

- Deep pressure
- Pain
- Position sense, appreciation of movement (proprioception)
- Vibration

■ FINE TOUCH
Procedure
- Give proper instructions to the subject (says "yes" when he feels the touch).
- The eyes of the subject must be closed.
- With the help of cotton lightly touch the skin on different body parts and compare corresponding opposite areas of the body. Observe if he feels the touch sensation.
- Elicit dermatome-wise sensation on both sides of the body.
- If there are areas of decreased sensation (hypo-aesthesia) or increased sensation (hyper-aesthesia) should be properly noted down.

Precautions
- Proper instructions should be given to the subject.
- The eyes of the subject should be closed.
- Sensations should be elicited according to different dermatomes of the body.
- The corresponding area of the opposite side must be checked and compared.
- If any sensation is altered, the area of alteration of sensation should be outlined properly.

Threshold for Light Touch
- It is tested with Von Frey's hair aesthesiometer **(Fig. 23D.1)**.
- Find out the maximum length of protruding hair from the hair aesthesiometer with which touch is felt.
- The longer the length of the hair, the lesser the intensity of the stimulus.

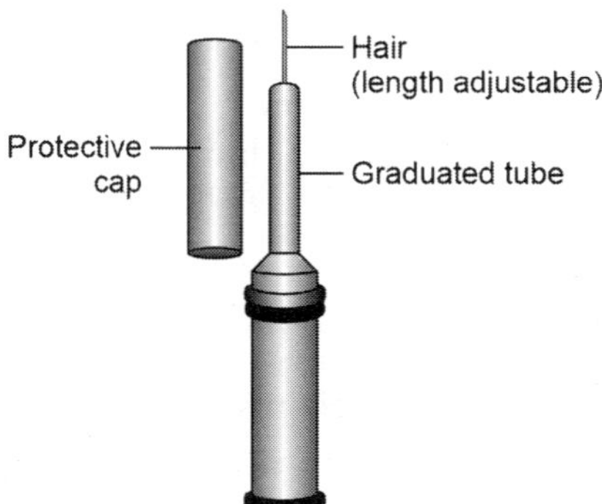

Fig. 23D.1: Von Frey's hair aesthesiometer

■ TACTILE LOCALIZATION
Procedure
- Give proper instructions to the subject.
- With the help of pain or cotton try to touch different body parts of the subject. Ask him immediately to localize the area where it was touched
- Subject should localize the body part that is touched.

Precautions
- Proper instructions should be given to the subject.
- Subject's eyes should be closed.
- Sensations are to be elicited according to the dermatomes of the body.
- With the help of cotton wool, lightly touch different parts of the body of the subject

■ TWO POINT DISCRIMINATION
Procedure
- For testing two-point discrimination, Weber's compass aesthesiometer is used. The subject is instructed properly.
- Subject is asked to close eyes.
- Separate two limbs of the aesthesiometer a little and touch that to the skin of the subject and ask if he is being touched at one point or two points.
- If the subject feels it is only at one point, then go on increasing the distance between two points and repeat the procedure.
- The minimum distance (between two limbs of the aesthesiometer) at which they are perceived as two separate points by the subject is called minimal separable distance.
- This distance varies in different body parts.
- It is about 2 mm on the fingertip, 30 mm on the back and so on.
- Record minimum separable distance on different body parts on both sides.

Precautions
- Same as described for tactile localization.
- Sensations should be elicited starting from the minimum distance between two limbs of the aesthesiometer **(Fig. 23D.2)**.
- Two points must be touched simultaneously.
- Corresponding body parts of opposite sides are to be tested simultaneously and compared.

■ TEMPERATURE
Procedure
- Proper instructions are given to the subject.
- Subject should close his eyes.
- Test tubes containing warm and cold saline are taken.
- Warm and cold saline tubes are applied randomly.

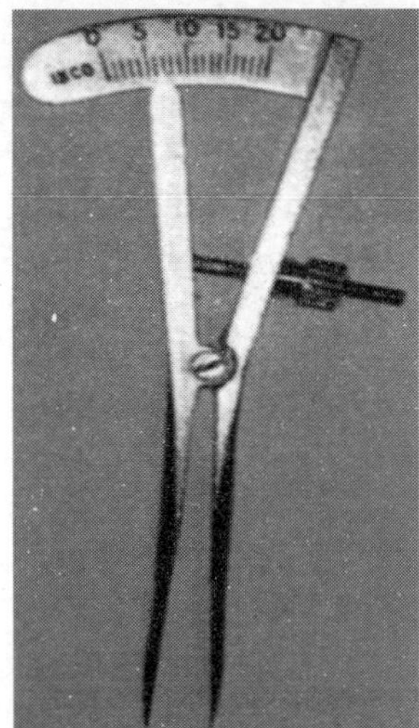

Fig. 23D.2: Weber's compass aesthesiometer

- Ask the subject to report if he feels the temperature is hot or cold.
- Compare symmetrical body parts.

Precautions

Same as that for fine touch.

■ PAIN

Superficial Pain

Procedure

- Pain sensation is elicited with the help of a pinprick.
- Give proper instructions to the subject.
- Compare symmetrical body parts.
- Outline the area of analgesia, hypoalgesia or hyper-algesia if present.

Precautions

Outline the area of analgesia, hypoalgesia or hyper-algesia if present.

Deep Pain

Procedure

- Proper instructions to the subject should be given.
- Subject is asked to close his eyes.
- Apply firm pressure on calf muscles or squeeze Achilles tendon between thumb and finger or,
- Use an algometer to press on the corresponding body parts to appreciate pressure pain **(Fig. 23D.3)**.

Precautions

Same as described for fine touch.

■ STEREOGNOSIS

Procedure

- Ask the subject to close the eyes.

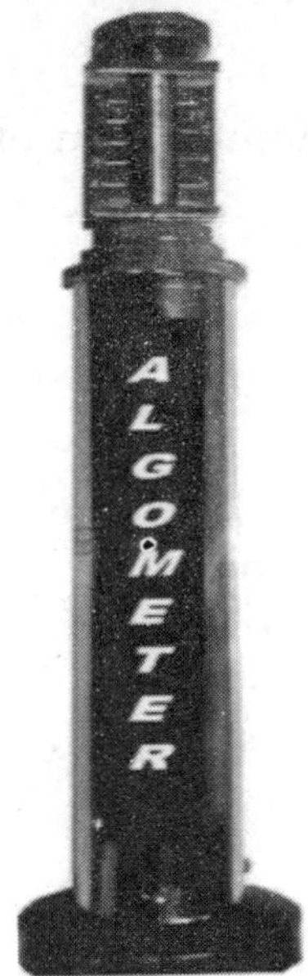

Fig. 23D.3: Algometer

- Place a suitable common object in his hand (e.g. pen chalk, etc.).
- Ask the subject to recognize the object by palpating it.

Precautions

- Proper instructions should be given to the subject.
- The eyes of the subject should be closed.
- Familiar objects should be given in hand.
- Test sensation should be elicited in one hand at a time.

■ SENSE OF POSITION AND JOINT MOVEMENT

Perception of movement is close to the sense of position, so both senses are tested together. Passively subject's limb is kept in a particular position and the subject is asked to recognize the position of the limb as described below.

Procedure

- Proper instructions are given to the subject.
- Subject is asked to close their eyes.
- The examiner passively moves the limbs of the subject to a particular position and the subject is asked to recognize the position of the limb.
- The subject's upper limb or lower limb is placed in a particular position and he is asked to keep the other limb in the same position.
- Procedure is repeated by changing the positions of all limbs.
- Movement is made at all joints and the subject is asked to recognize if he perceives movement at the joint.
- Movements of a minimum of 10 degrees are appreciated at all joints normally.

Precautions

- Explain the procedure clearly to the subject
- Subject has to close his eyes
- All possible movements of joints and position of limbs should be tested.

■ SENSE OF VIBRATION

Procedure

- Proper instructions should be given to the subject.
- In the case of upper limb, it is tested on the styloid process, olecranon. In the case of lower limbs, it is tested on malleoli, patella, lower end of tibia, etc.
- A vibrating tuning fork (128 cps) is kept on various bony prominences in the upper and lower limbs.
- Subject is asked to raise his finger when he stops feeling vibration.
- A tuning fork is placed on the corresponding bony prominence of the examiner's own body.

Precautions

- Subject should be instructed properly.
- The vibrating tuning fork should be kept on bony prominences.
- Sensations should be elicited from the corresponding bony prominence of the opposite side of the body.

Observations

Examination of sensory system proforma: Any systemic examination is to be done after a complete general examination as shown in Chapter 1– General Examination.

To Test the Nutrition of Muscles		
Nutrition		
Upper limbs	Right side	Left side
Lower limbs	Right side	Left side

Test –　　　　　　　All dermatomes of the body
Fine touch
Tactile localization
Tactile discrimination
Pain
Crude touch
Sense of vibration-　Upper limbs　　　Lower limbs
(On bony prominences)

■ IMPORTANT QUESTIONS AND ANSWERS

Q.1. How are the sensations classified?
Please check the above.

Q.2. Enumerate sensations carried by the posterior column tract and anterolateral pathway.
Sensations carried by the posterior column tract
- Fine touch
- Tactile localization
- Tactile discrimination
- Joint sense and sense of position (proprioception)
- Vibration

Sensations carried by the anterolateral tract
- Pain
- Temperature
- Crude touch
- Pressure
- Tickle and itch
- Sexual sensation

Q.3. What are receptors? Describe the classification of receptors.
Receptors are specialized afferent nerve endings that carry sensory information to the CNS. Receptors are capable of converting any form of energy into electrical energy and thus are capable of transmitting it to CNS. Receptors are therefore also called as transducers.

Classification of Receptors

- **Exteroceptors**: Receptors distributed on the surface of the body, e.g., Meissner's corpuscles, and Merkel's disc.
- **Interceptors**: Receptors that are present inside the body, e.g., osmoreceptors, chemoreceptors
- **Proprioceptors**: Receptors that are present in muscles, and joints, e.g., muscle spindle, Ruffini's end organs.
- **Tele receptors**: Receptors that are concerned with events away from the body, e.g., Receptors of eye and ear.

Q.4. What is a sensory map and what is its significance?
The segmental field of skin innervated by each spinal nerve is called a dermatome. Dermatomal innervation by sensory fibres constitutes a sensory map of the body. Different dermatomes are tested when we assess the sensory system which conforms intactness of a particular segment of the cord.

Q.5. How testing two-point discrimination can vary in different regions of the body?
- Two-point discrimination is the ability of the person to distinguish contact by two points at varying distances from each other. It is tested with the help of Weber's compass aesthesiometer (as explained above).
- Two points of compass are applied simultaneously to the skin. Distance between two points at which these points (of stimuli) are perceived as separate points is noted.
- **On the fingertips:** Minimum distance between two points of stimulation where stimuli, as perceived as 2 separate stimuli, is 2 to 5 mm on fingertips (this is minimum separable distance).

- **On the back**: Minimum distance between two points of stimulation where stimuli as perceived as 2 separate stimuli is about 30 mm.
- **Physiological basis:** This is because the density of receptors varies in different body parts.

Q.6. What is dissociated sensory loss? Give its physiological basis.

Dissociated sensory loss: Loss of pain and temperature sensation with preservation of touch and other forms of sensations is termed as dissociated sensory loss.

Physiological basis: Dissociated sensory loss is observed when there is damage to the grey matter of the spinal cord near the central canal. This is because fibres of the dorsal column pathway (that carry touch and other sensations), ascend in the dorsal column of the spinal cord and thus are spared. In contrast, fibres of the anterolateral pathway (carrying pain and temperature sensations) do cross opposite sides of the spinal cord at the same segment and lie very close to the central canal while crossing the other side. Thus, fibres of this pathway are damaged, sparing fibres of dorsal column path leading to dissociated sensory loss.

Q.7. What are the abnormal responses to pain sensations? What are its causes?

- **Analgesia:** Absence of sensibility to pain.
- **Hypoalgesia:** Partial loss of pain sensibility. A common cause is nerve compression.
- **Hyperalgesia:** Exaggerated pain sensibility. It is seen in tabes dorsalis, thalamic, and parietal lobe lesions, excess sensitivity of pain receptors.
- **Paresthesia:** Unusual pain sensation described as pricking, tingling, numbness, etc.
- **Allodynia:** Condition where the ordinarily painless stimulus is perceived as very painful.

Q.8. Enumerate abnormalities in sensation. Give their causes.

- **Anaesthesia:** It means loss of all sensations.
- **Dissociated anaesthesia:** Explained below.
- **Hyper-aesthesia:** Response to sensory stimulation is exaggerated. Seen with thalamic lesions.
- **Hemianaesthesia:** Loss of sensation that affects one side of the body. Seen in thalamic lesions.
- **Paresthesia:** Perverted touch sensation where a touch can cause pain, pricking, or numbness type of sensations. Seen in nerve compression and vitamin B12 deficiency (subacute combined degeneration of the spinal cord).

Q.9. What is anaesthesia? Enumerate its causes.

Anaesthesia: It is a complete loss of sensation.

Causes: Complete transection of the spinal cord (below the level of lesion), peripheral nerve lesions or lesions of nerve roots or compression of the nerves. Anaesthesia will be observed according to the distribution of nerve fibres. Common conditions where nerves are affected are uncontrolled diabetes and leprosy.

Q.10. Trace the pathway of the dorsal column tract and anterolateral pathway.

1. **Dorsal column pathway:** All afferents (from receptors) relay onto the dorsal root of the spinal cord (sensory root). **First-order neurons** are from receptors in spinal cord.
   - Each fibre from here divides into two branches medial and lateral. The medial branch runs upward and continues in the dorsal column path (the lateral branch relies on interneurons at the same level in the spinal cord and is responsible for forming the spinocerebellar tract).
   - Medial branch that runs upwards ascending in dorsal column relay in nucleus gracilis and nucleus cuneatous in the medulla. These fibres cross opposite sides as arcuate fibres and ascend in the brainstem as medial lemnisci. **Second-order neurons** from the spinal cord to the thalamus.
   - Fibres from medial lemnisci terminate in the ventrobasal nucleus of the thalamus. From the ventrobasal complex, third-order **neurons** project to the post-central gyrus of the cerebral cortex (somatic sensory areas I and II). Sensations carried by the tracts are mentioned above.

2. **Anterolateral pathway:** All afferents (from receptors) relay onto the dorsal root of the spinal cord (sensory root). Fibres cross the anterior commissure of the spinal cord to the opposite side and ascend as anterior spinothalamic (crude, tickle sensations) and lateral spinothalamic tract (pain, temperature sensations).
   - The anterolateral pathway terminates in two areas—reticular nuclei of the brain stem (majority of anterolateral path relays in the brainstem) and some fibres in ventrobasal nuclei of the thalamus from where some fibres go to the cortex (same areas as dorsal column path).

■ OSCE—SENSORY SYSTEM

Procedure station 1: Test the sensation of fine touch and tactile localization aspect of the subject's forearm.

S. No.	Assessment criteria	Marks assigned	Marks given
1.	Greet and stand on the right side of the subject		
2.	Ask the subject to sit comfortably and explain the procedure		
3.	Ask him/her to put forearms on the table. Tells her to close his/her eyes		

Contd...

Contd...

S. No.	Assessment criteria	Marks assigned	Marks given
4.	Take a piece of cotton and twist it into a pointed 'wisp'		
5.	Then lightly touch the skin on the fingertips, palms, and forearm of one hand		
6.	Ask the subject to localise the sensation and checks the responses occasionally without the stimulus		
7.	Compare the responses on the opposite forearm		
8.	Report and viva on clinical examination		
9.	Total		

Procedure station 2: Test two-point discrimination on the anterior forearm of the right side.

S. No.	Assessment criteria	Marks assigned	Marks given
1.	Greet and stand on the right side of the subject		
2.	Ask the subject to sit comfortably and explain the procedure		
3.	Explain the procedure to the subject and ask him to respond "one", "two", or "don't know" when touch his skin with the compass points		
4.	Ask him to close his eyes. Open the compass a little and lightly touch the fingertips, palm, back of fingers and hand, front and back of the forearm, one after another		
5.	If the response is "one" at any place, open the compass points and tests again, till he responds with "two"		
6.	In this way, note the discrimination between the two points at various places		
7.	Compare the responses on the opposite side		
8.	Report and viva on clinical examination		
9.	Total		

Procedure station 3: Test the sensation of vibration in the leg and arm of the subject provided.

S. No.	Assessment criteria	Marks assigned	Marks given
1.	Greet and stand on the right side of the subject		
2.	Ask the subject to sit comfortably and explain the procedure		
3.	Explain the procedure and assure him that no pain will be caused		

Contd...

Contd...

S. No.	Assessment criteria	Marks assigned	Marks given
4.	Select a tuning fork of 128 Hz, and strikes one prong against the edge of his/her hand to set it into vibration. Then places its base on his knuckle to familiarize him with the 'vibrating tremor'		
5.	Test the vibration on subject's knuckles, head of the radius, elbow, patella, and medial malleolus then asks "now". Examines occasionally test with a fingertip or a pencil		
6.	Note the response in each case with a "yes", "no", or "don't know", if the response is "no" or "don't know", the examiner should test on another bony prominence		
7.	Compare the responses on the other side		
8.	Report and viva on clinical examination		
9.	Total		

4. Procedure station: Test the sensation of proprioception, joint sensation upper and lower limb of the subject provided.

S. No.	Assessment criteria	Marks assigned	Marks given
1.	Greet and stand on the right side of the subject		
2.	Ask the subject to sit comfortably and explains the procedure		
3.	Explain the procedure and assure him that no pain will be caused		
4.	Examine the position sense Instructs the subject to imitate the movement done in one hand/leg with the opposite		
5.	Examine the joint sense, and instruct the subject to recognise the movement up or down. Holds the terminal phalanx of thumb/great toe and does the flexion or extension		
6.	Examine the Romberg sign. Instruct the subject to stand straight with feet closed together, and then to close eyes. Observe for swaying and reports		
7.	Compare the responses on the other side		
8.	Report and viva on clinical examination		
9.	Total		

Procedure station 5: Test the sensation of temperature of the subject provided.

S. No.	Assessment criteria	Marks assigned	Marks given
1.	Greet and stand on the right side of the subject		
2.	Ask the subject to sit comfortably and explain the procedure		
3.	Explain the procedure and assure him that no pain will be caused		
4.	Instruct the subject to say yes when he/she feels the sensation of cold or warm		
5.	Instruct the subject to close the eyes		
6.	Touch the various dermatomal areas of the upper limb alternatively, with the help of a test tube containing hot or cooled water		
7.	Elicit temperature sensations on the corresponding area of the opposite side		
8.	Report and viva on clinical examination		
9.	Total		

Procedure station 6: Test the sense of stereognosis on the subject provided.

S. No.	Assessment criteria	Marks assigned	Marks given
1.	Greet and stand on the right side of the subject		
2.	Ask the subject to sit comfortably and explains the procedure		
3.	Explain the procedure and assure him that no pain will be caused by them		
4.	Instruct this subject to identify the object by just palpating it		
5.	Instruct the subject to close their eyes		
6.	Place familiar objects in one hand of the subject and ask him or her to identify them		
7.	Repeat with two or three different familiar objects		
8.	Report and viva on clinical examination		
9.	Total		

▌ COMMON STATIONS – SPOTS IN PRACTICAL EXAMINATION (2/3 MARKS)

Q.1. Diagram or instrument: Algometer, Weber's aesthesiometer, tuning fork: Identify any one or two questions from above.

Q.2. Diagram of anterolateral or dorsal column pathway: Identify and enumerate sensations carried by them.

Q.3. Any of the figures shown above: Identify, and enumerate procedures, and precautions while performing the test.

Q.4. Diagram or photo of the person doing Romberg's test: Identify and describe the test and give its significance.

▌ CASE-BASED SCENARIO/PROBLEM-BASED (2/3 MARKS)

Case 1: Due to a spinal cord trauma, a 35-year-old male person has altered pain and temperature sensitivity.
- Which tract probably must be damaged?
- Write pathway of the same

Case 2: A physician was carrying out a CNS examination of the patient. While trying to assess various sensations. On pinprick to the lower limb, he observed that the person withdrew his leg.
- What type of reflex it is? (Withdrawal reflex)
- Name two pathways that carry pain sensation. (Neospinothalamic and paleospinothalamic tract).

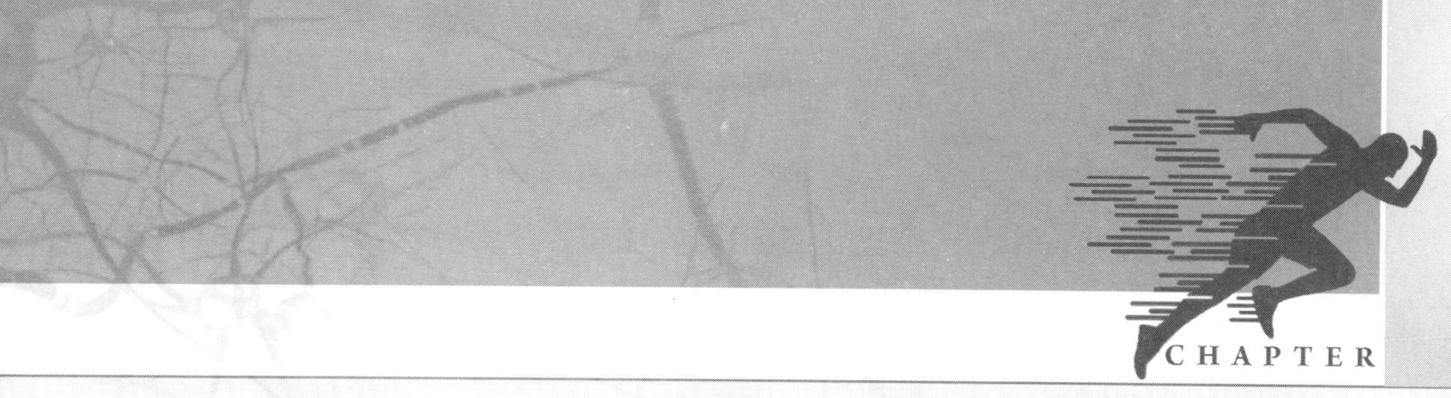

Clinical Examination of Motor System

Competency:

PY 10.11: Demonstrate correct clinical examination of the nervous system: Higher functions, sensory system, motor system, reflexes, and cranial nerves in a normal volunteer or simulated environment.

Learning Objectives

After completion of this practical, students should be able to:

- Assess the integrity of the motor system and the importance of checking it
- Check the nutrition of muscles in the upper and lower limbs
- Demonstrate normal tone of muscles and give its physiological basis
- To enumerate various common conditions causing hypertonia and hypotonia
- Grade and demonstrate the power of muscles in upper and lower limbs
- Demonstrate coordination of movements in upper and lower limbs.
- Name motor (descending) pathways and trace their course along with functions
- Enumerate different gates and postures in various clinical conditions
- Elicit superficial and deep reflexes
- Differentiate upper motor neuron lesion and lower motor neuron lesion features with its pathophysiological basis

Common symptoms: Difficulty in walking, weakness of a particular group of muscles, abnormal movements.

■ EXAMINATION OF MOTOR SYSTEM

- Integrity of the motor system can be assessed by examining—the nutrition of the muscle, tone and power of muscles, coordination, and involuntary movements.
- It also includes an assessment of various reflexes where the intact motor system is a part of the efferent arc of the reflex loop.

Nutrition of the Muscles

- **Bulk of muscles** on both sides of the body is tested (with the help of measuring tape). Mid-arm and mid-forearm circumference of upper limbs is measured.
- **Mid-thigh and mid-calf circumference** of lower limbs is measured (9 inches above knee joint and 6 inches below knee joint) and mid-arm and mid-forearm circumference of upper limbs.

Tone of the Muscles

- It is a state of partial contraction of a muscle. It is the resistance of a muscle to passive stretching.
- It is tested by passively moving different parts of the body.

Procedure

- Subject should relax completely.
- Tone is tested in the upper and lower extremities.
- Different body parts at various joints are tested passively.
- Degree, type of resistance, and range of movements (by doing flexion, extension, and rotation at each joint) is observed.
- The tone of muscles on both sides of the body is assessed and compared simultaneously.

Power of Muscle

- It is graded from grade 0 to grade 5. Normally, power is grade 5.
- Each muscle is tested. When a patient does a particular movement, the examiner tries to oppose the same with his strength. One has to test muscles of the upper limbs, lower limbs, and trunk and is tested bilaterally **(Table 23E.1)**.
- It is tested by active movement against the resistance.

Methods for Testing the Power of Muscle *(Fig. 23E.1)*

- The power of muscles can be tested in two ways as mentioned below.
- Subject is asked to perform movement of any part of the body and examiner opposes the movement actively (e.g. subject is asked to flex the arm and examiner tries to extend it).
- Muscle to be tested is put in its final position, e.g. ask the subject to hold the hand in flexion and the examiner tries to extend it and the subject tries to keep it in flexion.
- The strength of same group of muscles on the other side is compared simultaneously. The strength of

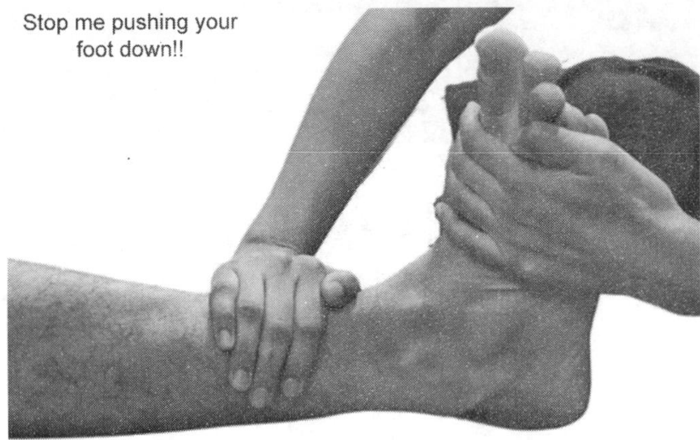

Ankle dorsiflexion and plantarflexion

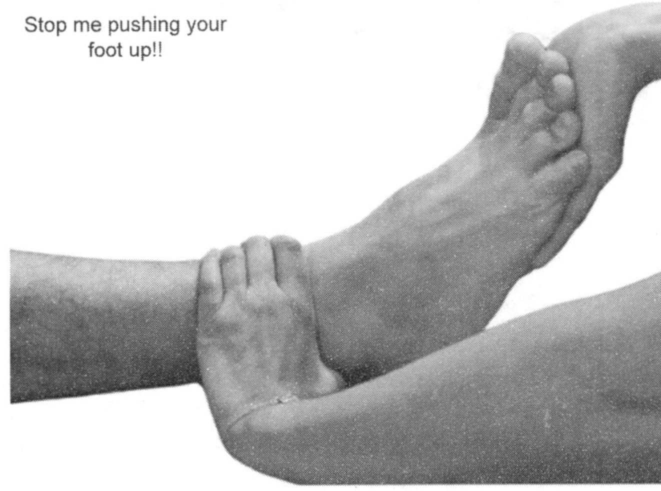

Fig. 23E.1: Testing power in lower limbs

muscles of the upper limbs, lower limbs and trunk of the body is tested.

- Each and every possible movement should be tested. Possible movements at various joints that have to be tested in upper limbs.

TABLE 23E.1: Grading power of muscle
Grade 0 – Complete paralysis
Grade 1 – A flicker of contraction
Grade 2 – Movement possible only on the elimination of gravity
Grade 3 – Movement possible against the gravity but not against the examiner's resistance
Grade 4 – Movement possible against gravity with moderate or subnormal resistance by examiner
Grade 5 – Movement possible against gravity with normal resistance by examiner

Power in Upper Limbs

Testing muscle power in upper limbs

I. Shoulder			
Muscle	**Nerve, nerve roots**	**Action**	**For testing power**
Supraspinatus	Suprascapular C5,C6	Abduction-	Subject lifts the arm at a right angle to his side against the resistance. First 30 degree movement is by supraspinatus and later 60 degrees by deltoid
Deltoid	Axillary C5,C6	Abduction and extension	Arms are abducted and the examiner tries to push down against resistance
Infraspinatus	Suprascapular C5,C6	External rotation	Subject is asked to tuck his elbow into his side with forearm flexed to right angle. Subject is asked to rotate limb outward against the resistance
Pectoralis major	Pectoral nerves C5, C6,C7,C8	Adduction of arms with flexion of shoulders	The subject is asked to stretch his arms out in front of him and then clasp his hands together while examiner tries to hold them apart
Serratus anterior	Long thoracic C5, C6, C7	Lateral and forward movement and fixation of scapula	Subject is asked to push forwards with his hands against the resistance such as wall
Latissimus dorsi		Adduction and lateral extension	Subject is asked to adduct horizontally and laterally extended arm against the resistance

Testing muscle power in upper limbs

II. Elbow			
Muscle	**Nerve, nerve roots**	**Action**	**For testing power**
Biceps	Musculocutaneous C5, C6	Flexion	The subject is asked to bend the forearm against the resistance with the forearm in full supination
Brachioradialis	Radial C5,C6	Flexion	Subject flexes the elbow midway between supination and pronation and examiner resists
Triceps	Radial C6,C7	Extension	Subject is asked to strengthen out his forearm against the resistance (by the examiner)

Testing muscle power in upper limbs

III. Wrist			
Muscle	**Nerve, nerve roots**	**Action**	**For testing power**
Extensor carpi radialis longus	Radial C6,C7	Extension and abduction	Subject is asked to make a fist and extend the wrist against resistance
Extensor carpi ulnaris	Posterior interosseous C7,C8	Extension and adduction	Subject is asked to make a fist and extend the wrist against resistance
Flexor carpi radialis	Median C6,C7	Flexion and abduction	Subject flexes supinated wrist against resistance, fingers relaxed
Flexor carpi ulnaris	Ulnar C7,C8,T1	Flexion and adduction	Subject flexes supinated wrist against resistance, fingers relaxed

Testing muscle power in upper limbs

IV. Fingers			
Muscle	**Nerve, nerve roots**	**Action**	**For testing power**
Extensor digitorum communis	Posterior interosseous C7, C8	Extension	Hand-prone, subject extends the fingers against the resistance

Contd...

Contd...

IV. Fingers

Muscle	Nerve, nerve roots	Action	For testing power
Flexor digitorum profundus	Anterior interosseous, C7, C8, T1 Ulnar C7,C8,T1	Flexion	Subject places hand on flat surface, examiner holds middle phalanx down, subject flexes distal phalanx against the resistance
Abductor pollicis brevis	Median C8,T1	Thumb abduction	Subject is asked to abduct his thumb in a plane at right angles to the palmar aspect of index finger against the resistance of the examiner's thumb. Muscles can be seen and felt
First dorsal interosseous muscle	Ulnar C8,T1	Abduction of index finger	Subject is asked to abduct his index finger against resistance
Abductor digiti minimi	Ulnar C8,T1	Abduction of the fifth finger	Subject is asked to abduct his fifth finger against resistance

Power in Lower Limbs

Testing muscle power in lower limbs

I. Hip

Muscle	Nerve, nerve roots	Action	For testing power
Iliopsoas	Lumbar plexus, femoral L1,L2,L3	Flexion	Subject flexes hip to 90 degrees and flexes knee, examiner tries to extend the hip and subject resists
Gluteus maximus	Inferior gluteal L5,S1,S2	Extension	Subject lies on the back and examiner tries to lift the leg, lifting the distal femur
Adductor magnus longus and brevis	Obturator L2,L3,L4	Adduction	Subject squeezes his legs together and examiner tries to place them apart
Gluteus medius and gluteus minimus	Superior gluteal L4,L5,S1	Abduction	Subject tries to separate the legs, examiner tries to get them close to each other

Testing muscle power in lower limbs

II. Knee

Muscle	Nerve, nerve roots	Action	For testing power
Quadriceps femoris	Femoral L2,L3,L4	Extension	Subject's knee is bent and is pressed to his chin by examiner and subject is asked to straighten it out against the resistance
Hamstrings	Sciatic L4,L5,S1,S2	Flexion	Subject's leg is raised from the bed supporting the thigh and holding ankle. Subject is asked to bend his knee against the resistance

Testing muscle power in lower limbs

III. Ankle

Muscle	Nerve, nerve roots	Action	For testing power
Tibialis anterior	Deep peroneal L4, L5	Dorsiflexion	Subject dorsiflexes ankle and examiner tries to extend it
Tibialis posterior	Tibial L5,S1	Inversion	Subject inverts the foot against resistance
Peroneus longus and brevis	Superficial peroneal L5,S1	Eversion	Subject everts the foot against resistance
Medial and lateral gastrocnemius, soleus	Tibial L5,S1,S2	Plantar flexion	Subject uses examiner's hands as accelerator or clutch pedal and examiner resists

Testing muscle power in lower limbs

IV. Toes

Muscle	Nerve, nerve roots	Action	For testing power
Extensor hallucis longus	Deep peroneal L5,S1	Big toe extension	Subject extends great toe against the resistance
Extensor digitorum longus and brevis	Deep peroneal L5,S1	Extension of other toes	Subject extends toes against the resistance
Flexor digitorum longus, flexor hallucis longus	Tibial L5,S1	Flexion	Subject flexes the toes against the resistance

By testing the power of muscles, one understands complete or partial loss of power in muscles of the body. Complete loss of power is paralysis and partial loss is called as paresis.

Coordination of Movements

- **Coordination of movements:** Harmonious activity and the correct sequence of action of appropriate muscles in order to accomplish a definite act is coordination. Coordination depends on three systems: The afferent system, the vestibular system, and the cerebellar system.
- It must be tested in both upper limbs and lower limbs.

In Upper Limbs

- **Finger nose test:** The subject is asked to touch tip of his nose with tip of his own index finger rapidly and repeatedly (with right and then left index finger). This is done first with eyes closed and then with eyes open.
- **Finger-to-finger test:** Subject touches his/her finger to that of examiner first with eyes open and then with eyes closed **(Fig. 23E.2)**.
- **Diadochokinesia:** Subject is asked to alternately carry out pronation and supination of forearm rapidly. Dysdiadochokinesia is the inability to carry out the above task.

In Lower Limbs

- **Knee heel test:** The subject lies in a supine position with eyes open first and then eyes closed, subject is asked to keep heel on the opposite knee and then slide the heel down the shin of his leg towards the ankle. He is asked to repeat it for the opposite limb **(Fig. 23E.3)**.
- **Romberg's test:** The subject is asked to stand with his feet close together with his eyes open and then eyes closed, if the patient sways or falls the **test is positive**. This test differentiates sensory ataxia from motor ataxia.
- **Walking along the straight line:** Walking along a straight-line keeping heel to toe (Tandem gait) initially with eyes open and then with eyes closed. This is used to check the balance of the patient. This test is done commonly to screen for neurologic and vestibular disorders **(Fig. 23E.4)**.

Involuntary Movements

- Normally, the body and limbs at rest do not move except voluntarily induced.
- Involuntary movements can be physiological or pathological and can be generalized or localized. (Refer Q No. 6).

Examination of Reflexes

Reflex: It is an involuntary motor response to a stimulus. Clinically reflexes are classified as superficial, deep and visceral. They are one of the important tests in neurological examination of a patient.

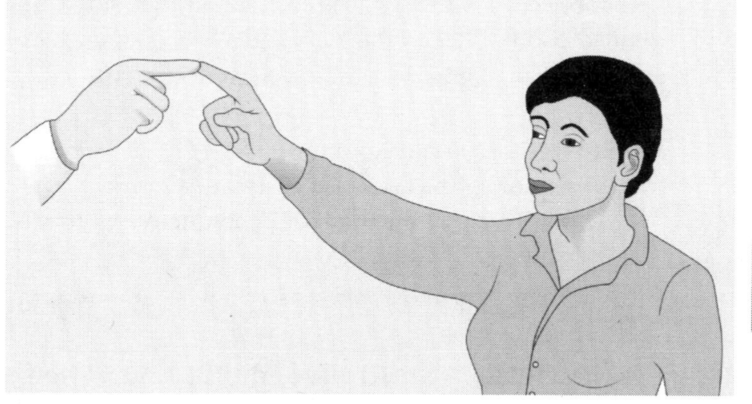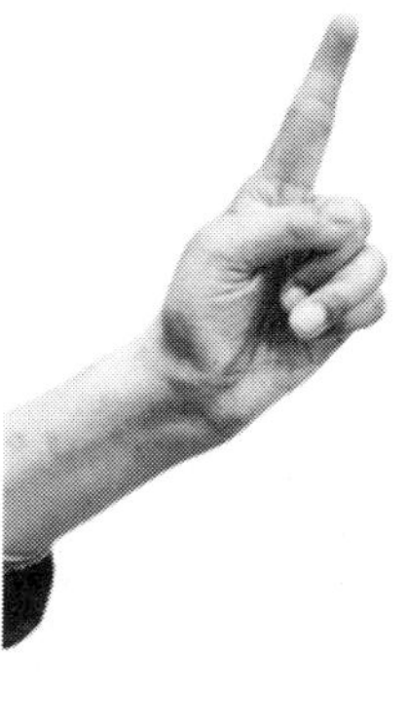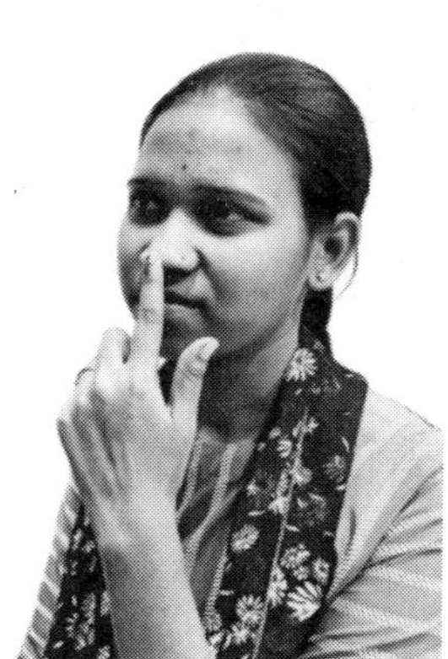

Fig. 23E.2: Finger-to-finger test and finger to nose test (coordination in upper limbs)

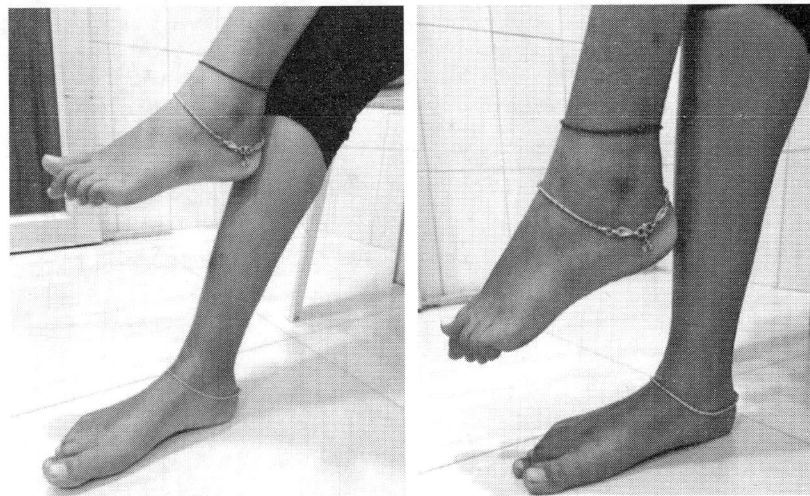

Fig. 23E.3: Knee heel test

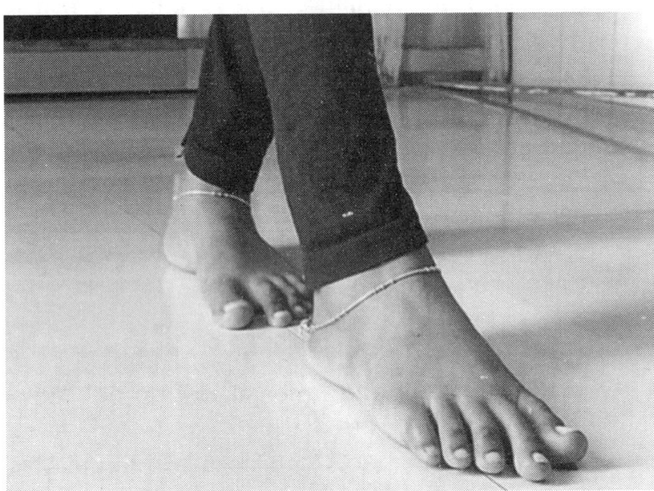

Fig. 23E.4: Walking in a straight line

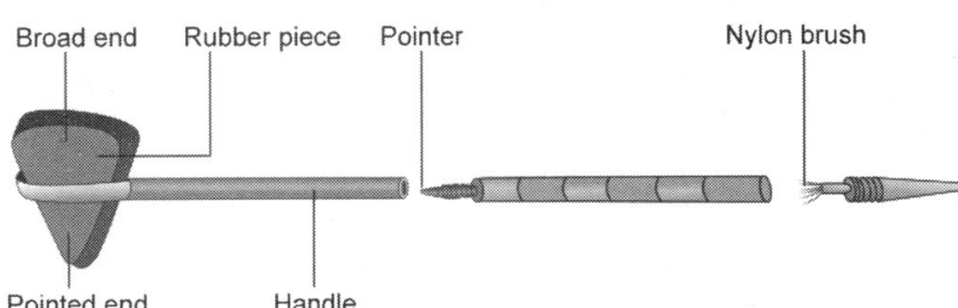

Fig. 23E.5: Hammer

Hammer

- It is required for eliciting various reflexes.
- It consists of a long metallic handle to which a triangular rubber piece is attached.
- The body of the handle is provided with a brush which is used during sensory system examination **(Fig. 23E.5)**.

■ SUPERFICIAL REFLEXES

They are elicited on stimulation of skin or mucous membranes.

Plantar Reflex (L5, S1)

- Subject lies in the supine position.
- With the help of a metallic portion of a hammer or pointer outer edge of the sole of the foot is scratched. from the heel towards the little toe and then medially towards the ball of the great toe **(Fig. 23E.6A)**.

Response: There is inversion and dorsiflexion of the ankle with flexion of all the toes at the metatarsals (this is flexor plantar response). Extensor plantar response

(Babinski's sign; **Fig. 23E.6B**) is found in upper motor neuron lesions (please see questions below).

Abdominal Reflex (T7–T12)

- Subject lies down in a supine position.
- Strike the abdominal wall with blunt objects at three regions (epigastrium, umbilical, hypogastrium) on both sides towards the umbilicus.

Response: Contraction of abdominal muscles on the same side in respective areas.

Cremasteric Reflex (L1, L2)

- This is elicited in male subjects.
- Expose the part (genitalia and upper thigh).
- Lightly scratches the inner aspect of the upper part of the thigh.

Response: Elevation of the testicle on that side due to contraction of the cremasteric muscle.

Conjunctival Reflex: (Nuclei of V and VIIth Cranial Nerves)

- Subjects sit on the stool.
- A wisp of cotton wool is twisted to a point.
- Approaching from the side, conjunctiva is touched with a wisp of cotton wool.

Response: Normal response consists of immediate closure of eyes.

Corneal Reflex: (Nuclei of V and VIIth Cranial Nerves)

- Subjects sit on the stool.

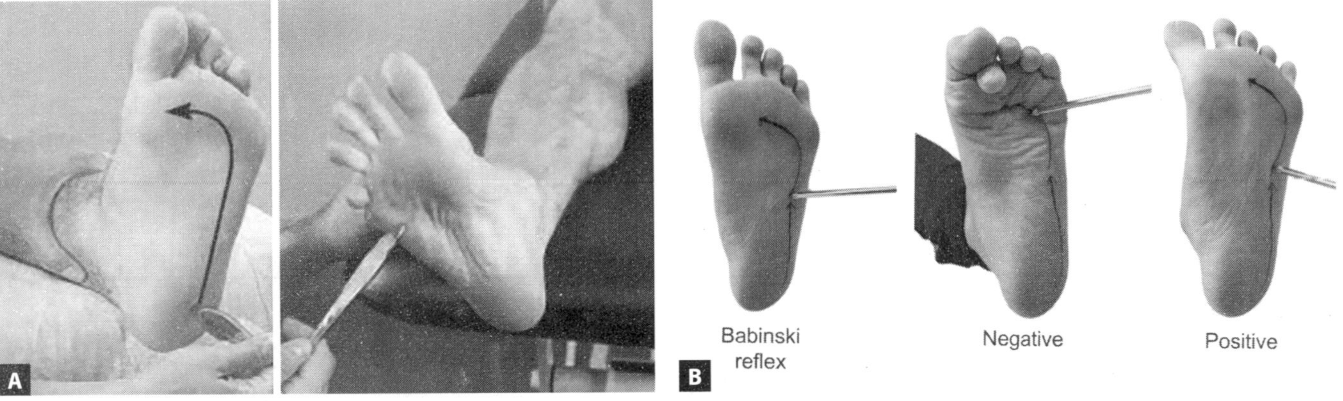

Figs. 23E.6A and B: (A) Plantar reflex; (B) Babinski sign

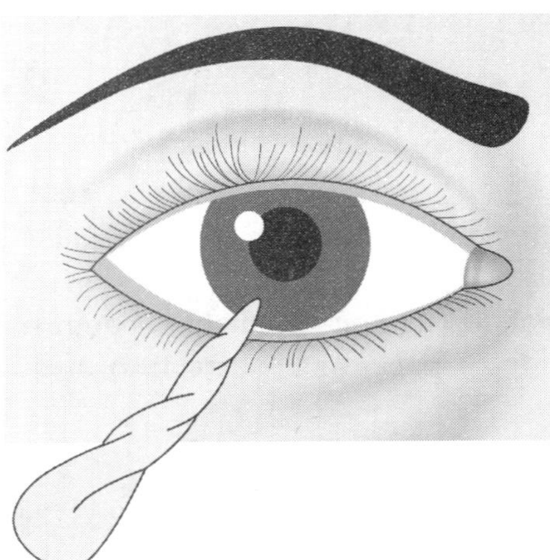

Fig. 23E.7: Corneal reflex

- A wisp of cotton wool is twisted to a point.
- Subject's lower lid is held down and is asked to look up.
- Approaching from the side, the cornea is touched with a wisp of cotton wool **(Fig. 23E.7)**.

Response: Normal response consists of immediate closure of eyes.

■ DEEP REFLEXES/TENDON JERKS

They are tendon reflexes that are elicited due to stretching of the muscle. Receptors are muscle spindles. With a stretch on the muscle spindle afferents fire which makes an excitatory monosynaptic connection with the alpha motor neurons of the same muscle. (Stretch reflex–The basic postural reflex). The normal response of eliciting tendon jerk is reflex contraction of the same muscle that is stretched. Reflexes can be graded from absent to exaggerated (see below).

Eliciting reflexes requires a practice. One has to be sure that the muscle you are testing, the tendon of the same muscle is effectively struck and accordingly sufficient force is to be applied while eliciting reflex.

Precautions

- Subject should be completely relaxed.
- Explain the procedure properly to the subject.
- Stand on right side of the subject.
- The subject's limb should be properly positioned (depending on which reflex one is eliciting).
- Tendon must be stroked briskly by sudden jerky movement at the wrist joint.
- Hammer to be held between thumb and index finger.
- For comparison reflex of opposite side must be tested.
- If reflex is not elicited reinforcement technique is used.

Biceps Jerk (C5, C6)

- Ask subject to relax.
- Subject's elbow is flexed at right angles and forearm is kept in semi-pronated position supported on examiner's forearm (or by placing on subject's abdomen).
- Place your thumb firmly on biceps tendon of subject.
- With the help of pointed end of hammer strike on the thumb (biceps tendon stretches by striking the thumb). Elicit biceps jerk on other limb and compare.

Response: There is contraction of biceps and flexion at the elbow **(Fig. 23E.8)**.

Abnormal response: Biceps jerk can be reduced or absent with lesion at C5 and C6 level.

Triceps Jerk (C6, C7)

- Subject's elbow is flexed at right angles and triceps tendon is tapped.
- Tendon is tapped just above olecranon process.
- Elicit triceps jerk on other side and compare.

Response: There is contraction of triceps muscle and extension of elbow **(Fig. 23E.9)**.

Abnormal response: Reduced or absent jerk in high radial nerve lesion or lesion at C6, C7 level.

Supinator/Brachioradialis Jerk (C5, C6)

- Hold the hand of the subject or allow it to rest on his abdomen.

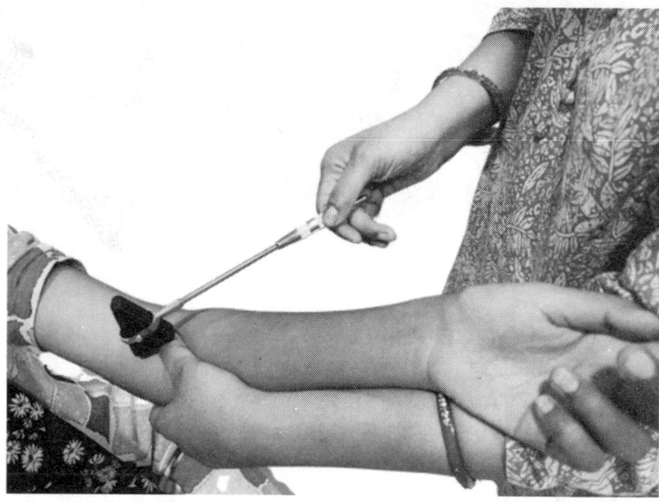

Fig. 23E.8: Biceps jerk

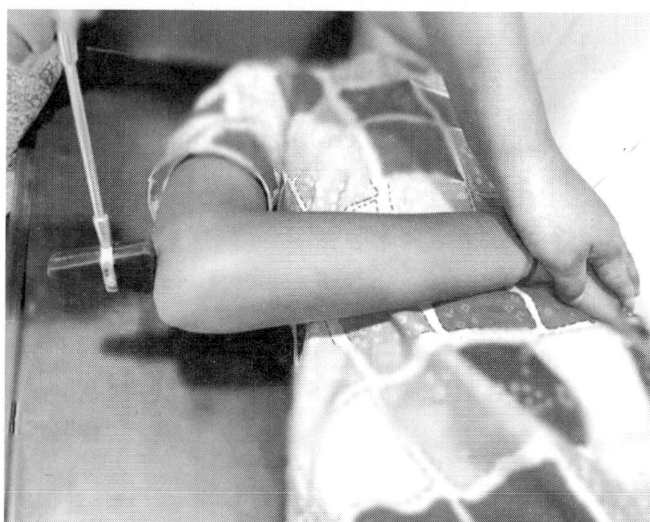

Fig. 23E.9: Triceps jerk

- With help of a hammer strike the radius 1–2 inches above the wrist over the styloid process.
- Elicit supinator jerk on the other side and compare **(Fig. 23E.10)**.

Response: There is flexion at the elbow and supination of the forearm.

Jaw Jerk (Mid Pons)
- Subject is asked to keep mouth open.
- Examiner places finger on chin of the subject.
- The finger is then strike with hammer.

Response: Closure of the jaw is observed.

Knee Jerk (L2, L3, L4)
It can be tested with subject in supine position as well as in sitting position.

In Supine Position
- Subject's leg is semi-flexed. Expose the portion of the leg to upper thigh region.

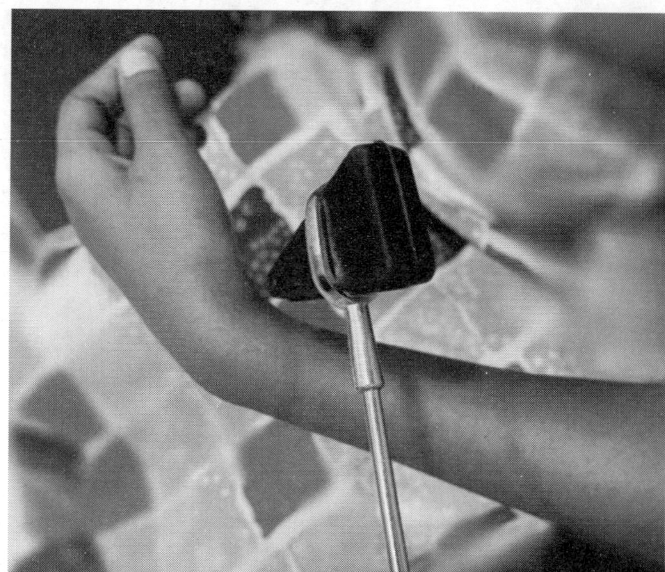

Fig. 23E.10: Supinator reflex

- Place the hand underneath subject's knee to raise it off the bed.
- Strike patellar tendon with help of hammer. Observe extension of knee and contraction of quadriceps muscle.
- Elicit knee jerk on opposite limb and compare.

Response: Contraction of quadriceps and extension of knee is observed.

In Sitting Position
- Subject is asked to sit at the edge of the table or chair so that his legs should be dangling freely.
- Subject is asked to cross one knee over the other.
- Elicit knee jerk on opposite limb and compare **(Fig. 23E.11)**.

Response: There is contraction of quadriceps muscle and extension at the knee.

Ankle Jerk (S1, S2)
This can be elicited in a supine as well as in a prone position **(Fig. 23E.12)**.

In Supine Position
- Hip and knee joints of the subject are partly flexed.
- Lower limb is placed in such a way that it lies everted and slightly flexed.
- With one hand slightly dorsiflex the foot so that there is stretch on the tendo-Achillis and tendon is tapped.

Response: There is contraction of calf muscles and plantar flexion of the foot.

In Prone Position
- Ask subject to kneel on the chair with feet projecting out.

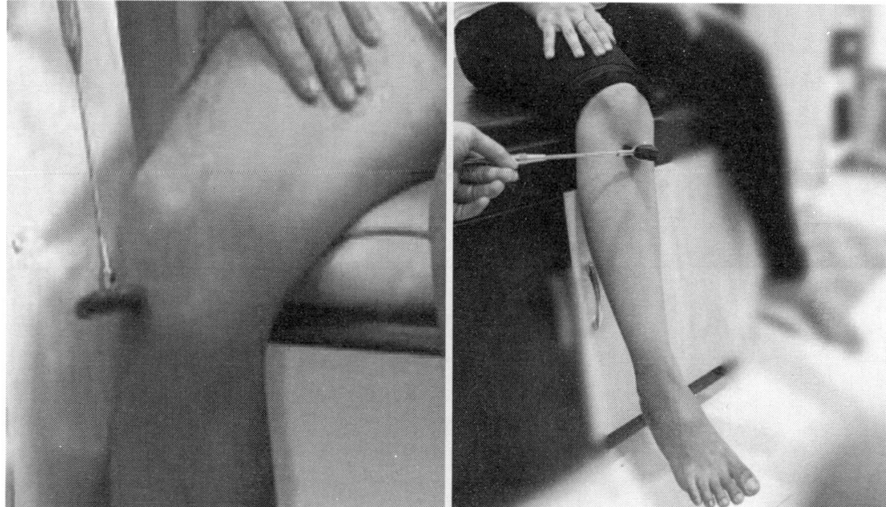

Fig. 23E.11: Knee jerk

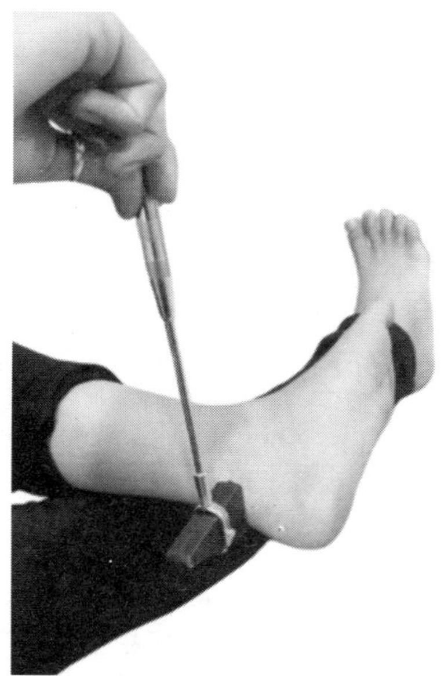

Fig. 23E.12: Ankle jerk

- Ankle of the subject is kept at right angles with slight dorsiflexion of the foot.
- Ankle is dorsi flexed to stretch tendo-Achillis and then tendon is tapped.

Response: There is a contraction of calf muscles and plantar flexion of the foot.

Visceral Reflexes

- This means reflexes which govern the process of respiration, deglutition, micturition and defecation.
- Observations – Examination of motor system proforma.
- Any systemic examination is to be done after a complete general examination as shown in the chapter on the examination of the nervous system.

■ PROFORMA TO TEST MOTOR SYSTEM

To Test Nutrition of Muscles				
Nutrition				
Upper limbs	Right side			Left side
Lower limbs	Right side			Left side

To test the tone of muscles					
Upper limbs	**Right side**	**Left side**	**Lower limbs**	**Right side**	**Left side**
Feel of muscle			Feel of muscle		
Degree of resistance			Degree of resistance		
Range of movements			Range of movements		
To test power of upper and lower limbs					

Contd...

Contd...

Upper limbs		Power grade	
Name of joint	Possible movements	Right side	Left side
Shoulder			
Forearm			
Wrist			
Fingers			

Lower limbs		Power grade	
Name of joint	Possible movements	Right side	Left side
Hip			
Knee			
Ankle			
Great toe			

Coordination in upper limbs and lower limbs

	Right side		Left side	
	Eyes open	Eyes closed	Eyes open	Eyes closed
Upper limbs • Finger nose test • Finger-to-finger test • Diadochokinesia				
Lower limbs • Heel knee test • Romberg's test • Tandem gait (walking in a straight line)				

■ IMPORTANT QUESTIONS AND ANSWERS

Q.1. Enumerate points under which examination of motor system is carried out?

Assessment of motor system:

- Nutrition of the muscle
- Tone of muscles
- Power of the muscles
- Coordination of muscle activity
- Abnormal movements

Q.2. How to test nutrition in upper and lower limbs and what is its significance?

Refer above.

Q.3. What is atrophy and hypertrophy, fasciculations of muscle?

- **Atrophy**: Decrease muscle mass due to a decrease in size of muscle fibres.
- **Conditions causing atrophy of muscles include**: Lesion of anterior horn cell, nerve roots, peripheral nerves, or muscle, e.g. poliomyelitis. **Disuse atrophy** is very common after prolonged immobilisation of the joint (plaster).
- **Hypertrophy**: It is increase in size of the muscle due to an increase in size of muscle Fibres. It can be seen with gigantism, acromegaly, muscular dystrophies. Functional hypertrophy of muscles is seen in athletes.
- **Fasciculations** are spontaneous contractions of muscle fibres of individual motor units within the muscle at rest which are seen as twitches in the muscle. Amyotrophic lateral sclerosis, peripheral neuropathies may show fasciculations of the muscle.

Q.4. Enumerate conditions causing hypertonia and hypotonia.

Hypertonia– Increased resting muscle tone	**Hypotonia**–Decreased resting muscle tone
Common causes of hypertonia • Upper motor neuron lesion • Parkinson's disease • Muscles across painful joints	**Common causes of hypotonia** • Lower motor neuron lesion • Sleep (in a normal person there is a decrease in tone of body muscles during sleep). • Cerebellar disease • Tabes dorsalis (lesion in afferent pathway)

Q.5. Define following terms.

- **Hemiplegia:** Paralysis of one side of the body
- **Paraplegia:** Paralysis of both legs/lower limbs
- **Quadriplegia:** Paralysis of all four limbs (upper limbs and lower limbs)

- **Monoplegia:** Paralysis of one arm or one leg.
- **Paresis:** Decreased power of contraction of the muscle due to weakness in the muscle
- **Paralysis:** Loss of power of muscle or muscle group.

Q.6. What are the types of abnormal movements?

Involuntary movements can be physiological or pathological and can be generalized or localized.

Localized involuntary movements	Other involuntary movements
• **Fibrillation:** It is contraction of single muscle fibre • **Fasciculation:** It is contraction of bundle of muscle fibres • **Myoclonus:** Sudden shock like contraction of group of muscles/single muscle • **Tremor:** Most common variety of involuntary movement. It is regular, rhythmic, purpose less to and from movements mainly of limbs	• **Chorea:** They are purposeless jerky, irregular movements • **Athetosis:** These movements are seen in small joints of the hands and wrist • **Hemiballismus:** They are violent, flinging abnormal movements of the extremities on one side of the body • **Tonic spasm:** Is observed with tetanus • **Clonic spasm:** Is observed with epilepsy

Q.7. Enumerate different types of tremors.

Common physiological conditions:

- Anxiety
- Cold
- Old age

Common pathological conditions:

- **Static tremors**: Parkinson's disease.
- **Intention tremors**: Cerebellar disease.
- **Hysterical tremors.**
- **Pill rolling tremors**: Parkinsonism.
- Tremors due to thyrotoxicosis
- Tremors due to alcoholism
- Tremors due to hypoglycaemia

Q.8. What is muscle tone? How is it tested?

- **Muscle tone**: It is a resistance offered by muscle during passive movements. Tone is just a partial state of contraction of the muscle under resting state. One should note for degree, type of resistance range of movements by doing flexion, extension, lateral and medial rotation at each joint.
- Tone may be normal, more (hypertonia) or less (hypotonia) as explained above.

Q.9. What is physiological basis of muscle tone?

- **Muscle tone:** It is resistance offered to passive stretch of muscle spindle, the peripheral contractile part (of N bag and N chain fibres) are continuously getting facilitatory inputs from gamma motor neurons of spinal cord.

- Due to continuous stimulation of these contractile parts, central non-contractile part of muscle spindle which is a receptor portion, gets stretched (due to which primary and secondary afferents coming from muscle spindle fire and as they make excitatory monosynaptic connection with alpha motor neuron of same muscle, there is some amount of contraction that is maintained in muscle even at rest. This is called as **muscle tone.**
- Thus, continuous stimulation of gamma motor neurons via gamma loop and stretch reflex does maintain normal tone of the muscles at rest.

Q.10. What is spasticity?

- **Spasticity** is a type of hypertonia following a upper motor neuron lesion.
- It affects upper limbs flexors more than extensors, thus causing more resistance to passive extension of the joints than flexion
- Resistance to stretch increases during applied stretch and then suddenly gives away like opening a pen knife. (**Clasp knife rigidity**) It is seen in pyramidal tract lesion.
- In leg spasticity adductors and extensors are affected more than flexors.

Q.11. What is rigidity?

- Rigidity is a type of hypertonia due to disease of basal ganglia (extrapyramidal)
- In this, resistance to passive movements is regularly or irregularly variable which is described as cog wheel rigidity. It is seen with substantia nigra involvement in disease of basal ganglia.
- Where resistance to passive movement is throughout it is called as lead pipe rigidity. It is common with Parkinson's disease, dementia. In advanced Parkinson's disease rigidity will affect all limbs, neck and trunk.

Q.12. What is sensory and motor ataxia?

- Ataxia is impaired coordination of body movements Ataxia is of two types – sensory and motor.
- With the help of Romberg's test one can differentiate between motor and sensory ataxia. With sensory ataxia, if visual input is present, person does not sway, but sways with eyes closed. In motor ataxia (with cerebellar damage) person sways/is unsteady with eyes open as well as eyes closed.

Q.13. What is Romberg's test. Give its physiological significance.

- **Romberg's test:** Subject is asked to stand erect with feets close together, once with eyes open and once with eyes closed. With sensory ataxia person will sway with eyes closed but not with eyes open. This is **Romberg's positive.** In this condition, standing cannot be maintained without visual fixation.

- Sensory ataxia indicates defective position sense (e.g. tabes dorsalis)

Q.14. How the power of muscles is tested? What are grades of power? What are the methods by which power can be tested?
Please refer above.

Q.15. How to test muscle power in upper limbs?
Please refer above.

Q.16. How to test muscle power in lower limbs?
Please refer above.

Q.17. Enumerate tests to assess coordination in upper and lower limbs.

For upper limbs	For lower limbs
Finger nose test	Knee heel test
Finger-to-finger test	Walking in a straight line
Diadochokinesia	Romberg test
	Tandem gait

Q.18. Define reflex. How do you classify reflexes?
- Reflex is the mechanism by which sensory impulse is automatically converted into motor effect through the involvement of CNS.
- There are various ways by which classification of reflex is done.
- Clinical classification of reflex–superficial reflexes and deep reflexes.

Q.19. What are precautions before eliciting tendon reflex?
Refer above.

Q.20. Enumerate various superficial and deep reflexes.

Superficial reflexes	Deep reflexes/Tendon jerks
• Plantar	• Jaw jerk
• Conjunctival	• Biceps jerk
• Corneal	• Triceps jerk
• Abdominal	• Brachioradialis jerk
• Cremasteric	• Knee jerk
	• Ankle jerk

Q.21. What is a reinforcement of reflexes? What is the Jendrassik maneuver?
Reinforcement of Reflexes
- If any particular jerk is not obtained (not elicited), it is reinforced through a voluntary act by (strong voluntary muscular efforts). This can be done by:
- Asking the subject to clench his teeth or,
- Asking to hook fingers of both hands and pull them apart tendon/deep reflexes. This muscle activity is supposed to increase gamma motor discharge from descending pathways that help to elicit reflexes **(Fig. 23E.13)**.

Q.22. What are tendon reflexes? What are the components of the reflex arc?
Tendon Reflexes/Deep Reflexes
- These reflexes are elicited by sudden stretching of the muscle with a sharp tap on a tendon. Thus, the

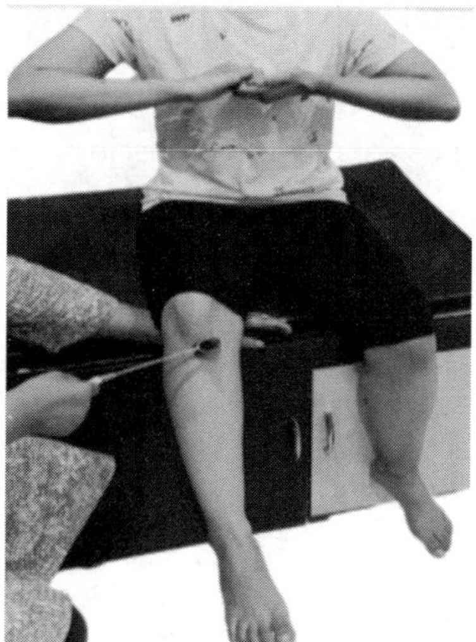

Fig. 23E.13: Jendrassik maneuver

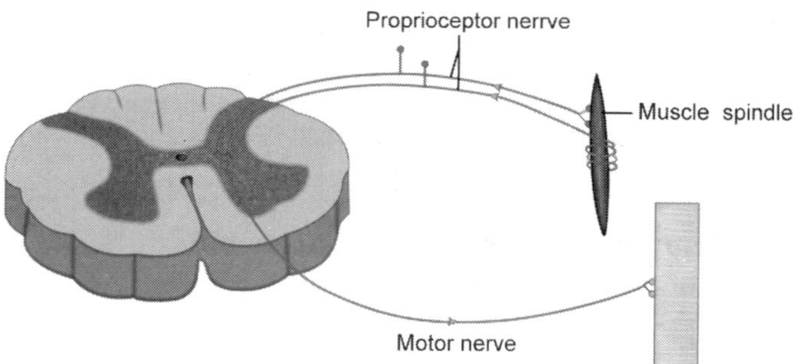

Fig. 23E.14: Components of reflex arc

contraction of muscle in response to sudden stretch produced by hammer is called as **tendon reflex.**
- These reflexes are monosynaptic.
- With tendon reflex one can assess integrity of afferent and efferent pathways and excitability of anterior horn cells in the spinal segment of the stretched muscle.

Components of reflex arc include the receptor (muscle spindle), afferent neuron, efferent neuron, and effector organ **(Fig. 23E.14)**.

Q.23. Define upper motor neuron (UMN) and lower motor neuron (LMN).
- **Upper motor neuron**: It consists of the cerebral cortex, and corticospinal tract till it descends and relay on alpha motor neurons of anterior horn of spinal cord. Clinically pure pyramidal tract lesion is rare. Along with the pyramidal tract, even extrapyramidal tracts are affected.
- **Lower motor neuron**: It consists of motor nuclei in the brain stem and alpha motor neuron along with its axon in the spinal cord, muscle fibres it innervates, neuromuscular junctions and muscles (skeletal) that contract. A lesion involving any of the above areas is called a lower motor neuron lesion

Q.24. Enumerate features of UMN lesion and LMN lesion

Features UMN lesion	Features LMN lesion
Exaggerated tone	Tone is decreased
Loss of power	Loss of power
Tendon reflexes are exaggerated	Tendon reflexes are diminished or absent
Superficial reflexes are absent	Superficial reflexes are absent
Babinski's sign is positive	Babinski's sign is not present
No muscle atrophy	Muscle atrophy seen
Muscles are affected in groups	Individual muscles are affected
Reaction of degeneration is absent	Reaction of degeneration is present

Q.25. How tendon reflexes can be graded?
Tendon Reflexes are graded as:
- Absent (seen with lower motor neuron lesion)
- Present (normal response)
- Brisk
- Exaggerated (seen with upper motor neuron lesion)
- Clonus (repetitive contraction of muscle through the mechanism of stretch reflex)

Q.26. What is the planter reflex? What is Babinski's sign?
- **Plantar reflex:** It is a superficial reflex. To elicit it, outer edge of the sole of the foot is stimulated from heel to the 5th toe laterally and then medially across the foot up to lateral border of second toe. It should not cross the medial border of first toe.
- Stimulation should be done with either pointed end of the hammer or key by gentle scratching.
- **Response:** Planter flexion of the toe is the normal response. The centre for reflex is S1, S2 segments of spinal cord.
- **Babinski's sign:** It is an abnormal response obtained when one elicits a planter reflex. **There is dorsiflexion of the toe and fanning of other toes**. This is a sign of pyramidal tract lesion. Otherwise Babinski's sign is positive physiologically up to one year of age (as tracts are not myelinated till that time).

Q.27. What will happen if painful stimulus is applied to elicit planter reflex?
When a painful stimulus is applied to elicit the plantar reflex, the response is as follows:
- Flexion of great toe
- Flexion and adduction of small toes
- Planter flexion of foot
- Inversion of foot
- Contraction of tensor fascia lata
- Adduction of thigh

■ OSCE—EXAMINATION OF MOTOR SYSTEM

Procedure station 1: To test the tone of the muscle on the upper limb of subject provided.

S. No.	Assessment criteria	Marks assigned	Marks given
1.	Greet and stand on the right side of the subject		
2.	Ask the subject to sit comfortably and explain the procedure		
3.	Make passive movements at various joints in the upper limb like the wrist joint, elbow joint, shoulder joint		
4.	Feel for the resistance offered by moving muscle		
5.	Compare the muscle tone in a similar fashion on the opposite side for individual muscle		
6.	Report and viva on clinical examination		
7.	Total		

Procedure station 2: To test the tone of the muscle on the lower limb of subject provided.

S. No.	Assessment criteria	Marks assigned	Marks given
1.	Greet and stand on the right side of the subject		
2.	Ask the subject to sit comfortably and explain the procedure		
3.	Make passive movements at various joints in the lower limb like ankle joint, knee joint and hip joint		
4.	Feel for the resistance offered by moving muscle		
5.	Compare the muscle tone in the similar fashion on the opposite side for individual muscle		
6.	Report and viva on clinical examination		
7.	Total		

Procedure station 3: To test and grades the power of the muscle on the upper limb of the subject provided.

S. No.	Assessment criteria	Marks assigned	Marks given
1.	Greet and stands on the right side of the subject		
2.	Ask the subject to sit comfortably and explain the procedure		
3.	Ask the subject to perform a movement of a muscle or group of muscles while he or she apply resistance to that movement. Wrist and fingers. Elbow muscles, shoulder muscles		

Contd...

Contd...

S. No.	Assessment criteria	Marks assigned	Marks given
4.	Compare the muscle tone in the similar fashion on the opposite side for individual muscle		
5.	Grade the power of a particular muscle group of upper limb		
6.	Report and viva on clinical examination		
7.	Total		

Procedure station 4: To test and grades the power of the muscle on the lower limb of subject provided.

S. No.	Assessment criteria	Marks assigned	Marks given
1.	Greet and stands on the right side of the subject		
2.	Ask the subject to sit comfortably and explain the procedure		
3.	Ask the subject to perform a movement of particular muscle group of muscle while he or she apply resistance to that movement (Ankle muscles, gastrocnemius muscles, thigh and hip muscles)		
4.	Compare the movement/strength of each muscle in a similar fashion on the opposite side		
5.	Grade the power of a particular muscle, group of lower limbs		
6.	Report and viva on clinical examination		
7.	Total		

Procedure station 5: To test for the coordination of movements of the upper limb of subject provided.

S. No.	Assessment criteria	Marks assigned	Marks given
1.	Greet and stand on the right side of the subject		
2.	Ask the subject to sit comfortably and explain the procedure		
3.	**Finger to nose test:** Test eyes open and then eyes closed for both hands separately		
4.	**Finger to finger test:** Test yes open and then eyes closed for both hands separately		
5.	**Diadochokinesia:** Alternate and rapid supination and pronation of the forearm. First with eyes open and then eyes closed of both hands separately		
6.	Report and viva on clinical examination		
7.	Total		

Procedure station 6: To test for the coordination of movements of the lower limb of subject provided.

S. No.	Assessment criteria	Marks assigned	Marks given
1.	Greet and stand on the right side of the subject		
2.	Ask the subject to sit comfortably and explain the procedure		
3.	**Knee-heel test:** Ask the subject to place heel on opposite knee and slide the heel down the shin towards ankle rapidly and repeatedly. First with eyes open and then eyes closed		
4.	**Knee-heel test:** Repeat with another leg		
5.	**Tandem walking test:** Ask the subject to walk in a straight line looking straight in erect posture		
6.	**Romberg's test:** Ask the subject to stand in an erect posture with feet's closed to each other looking front with eyes open		
7.	Ask the subject to close eyes and stand near the subject in supporting position		
8.	Report and viva on clinical examination		
9.	Total		

Procedure station 7: Elicit the bicep jerk.

S. No.	Assessment criteria	Marks assigned	Marks given
1.	Greet and stand near the subject		
2.	Ask the subject to sit comfortably and explain the procedure		
3.	Place the subject's one forearm in semi-flexed position supported by his/her arm in relaxed state		
4.	Place thumb on the tendon of bicep in cubital fossa		
5.	Tap on the thumb with the help of the percussion hammer		
6.	Elicit the jerk on the opposite side and compares		
7.	In case of failure to elicit perform the same with Jendrassik maneuver		
8.	Report and viva on clinical examination		
9.	Total		

Procedure station 8: Elicit the triceps jerk.

S. No.	Assessment criteria	Marks assigned	Marks given
1.	Greet and stand near the subject		
2.	Ask the subject to sit comfortably and explain the procedure		

Contd...

Contd...

S. No.	Assessment criteria	Marks assigned	Marks given
3.	Support the forearm of the subject on his/her arm at right angles		
4.	Strike the tendon of the triceps just above the olecranon process		
5.	Elicit the jerk on the opposite arm and compares		
6.	Observe and report the findings		
7.	In case of failure to elicit perform the same with Jendrassik Maneuver		
8.	Report and viva on clinical examination		
9.	Total		

Procedure station 9: Elicit the knee jerk.

S. No.	Assessment criteria	Marks assigned	Marks given
1.	Greet and stand near the subject		
2.	Ask the subject to sit comfortably on edge of chair legs dangling and not touching the ground or crossed legs, or in lying down position supporting the limb with one hand and explain the procedure		
3.	Expose the knee of the examining lower limb		
4.	Strike on the patellar tendon		
5.	Observe for the contraction of the quadriceps and extension of the knee		
6.	Elicit the jerk on the opposite side and compares		
7.	In case of failure to elicit perform the same with Jendrassik Maneuver		
8.	Report and viva on clinical examination		
9.	Total		

Procedure station 10: Elicit the jaw jerk.

S. No.	Assessment criteria	Marks assigned	Marks given
1.	Greet and stand near the subject		
2.	Ask the subject to partially open the mouth		
3.	Place a finger firmly on the chin		
4.	Tap over the finger with the help of the knee hammer		
5.	Observe the contraction of elevators of the jaw and closure of the mouth		
6.	Repeat the jerk and observe for contraction on the opposite side and compares		
7.	In case of failure to elicit perform the same with Jendrassik maneuver		
8.	Report and viva on clinical examination		
9.	Total		

Procedure station 11: Elicit the brachioradialis jerk.

S. No.	Assessment criteria	Marks assigned	Marks given
1.	Greet and stand near the subject		
2.	Ask the subject to sit down and relax completely		
3.	Hold the hand of the subject and laterally bend the forearm in the opposite direction		
4.	Strike the radius 1–2 inches above the wrist over the styloid process		
5.	Elicit the jerk on the opposite side and compares		
6.	Observe and report the findings		
7.	In case of failure to elicit perform the same with Jendrassik maneuver		
8.	Report and viva on clinical examination		
9.	Total		

Procedure station 12: Elicit the plantar reflex.

S. No.	Assessment criteria	Marks assigned	Marks given
1.	Greet and stand near the subject		
2.	Ask the subject to lie down with footwear removed and ask the subject to relax completely		
3.	With a blunt object strike the sole, from heel along the lateral border of foot towards greater toe		
4.	Observe the flexor response (Babinski sign)		
5.	Elicit the jerk on the opposite leg side and compares		
6.	In case of failure to elicit perform the same with Jendrassik maneuver		
7.	Report and viva on clinical examination		
8.	Total		

Procedure station 13: Elicit the abdominal reflex.

S. No.	Assessment criteria	Marks assigned	Marks given
1.	Greet and stand near the subject		
2.	Ask the subject to lie down in supine position exposing the abdomen and ask the subject to relax completely		
3.	With the help of blunt tip object, stroke parallel to costal margin on both below and above naval region		
4.	Observe for the contraction of the abdominal muscle		
5.	Elicit the jerk on the abdominal regions and compares		
6.	In case of failure to elicit perform the same with Jendrassik maneuver		
7.	Report and viva on clinical examination		
8.	Total		

Procedure station 14: Elicit the ankle jerk.

S. No.	Assessment criteria	Marks assigned	Marks given
1.	Greet and stand near the subject		
2.	Explain the procedure to the subject to and slightly dorsiflex the foot		
3.	Strike the tendon-Achillies with knee hammer		
4.	Observe the contraction of the calf muscle and plantar flexion of foot		
5.	Elicit the reflex on the opposite side and compares		
6.	In case of failure to elicit perform the same with Jendrassik maneuver		
7.	Report and viva on clinical examination		
8.	Total		

COMMON STATIONS–SPOTS IN PRACTICAL EXAMINATION (2/3 MARKS)

Q.1. Diagram or figure of eliciting various superficial / deep reflexes – identify, and write its root value, normal response, procedure and conditions where they are absent or exaggerated.

Q.2. Hammer, measuring tape – identify and write its use or any one or two questions from the above.

Q.3. Diagram/figure of finger nose, finger to finger, finger to nose test, knee heel test – identify and write its physiological basis and any conditions when they are altered.

Q.4. Diagram/figure of a person standing erect with eyes open and eyes closed. Identify the test. Write what is motor and sensory ataxia.

Q.5. Diagram of different gaits – identify and comment.

Q.6. Diagram testing tone of upper/lower limbs– Define hyper or hypotonia, enumerate conditions causing, the physiological basis of tone.

Q.7. Picture of Babinski's sign positive: Explain significance. Write normal response with a plantar reflex.

Q.8. Diagram/picture of any of the reflexes: Identify root value, normal response, etc. can be asked.

CASE-BASED SCENARIO/PROBLEM-BASED (2/3 MARKS)

Case 1: A physician is testing the power of the muscle a 60-year-old male who had a stroke last month and comes to OPD for follow-up. On examination, it was found that the patient is able to do all movements eliminating gravity and side-to-side movements but not able to perform the movements against the resistance offered by a physician

- What is the grade of power in him?
- How do you grade the power of the muscles?

Case 2: A 67-year-old know hypertensive developed sudden body weakness on the right side and he also noticed difficulty in speaking. He was brought to OPD by his relative. On examination- BP was 190/100 mm Hg. Babinski's sign was positive. Hypertonia was noted in the limbs.

- What is probably the person is suffering from?
- Enumerate features of UMN lesion.

Case 3: While eliciting reflex in a 20-year-old male person, the plantar reflex was elicited. The response was normal.

- What is a centre for plantar reflex?
- Enumerate various changes that you observe with the elicitation of the plantar reflex.

Case 4: A medical student was trying to elicit tendon jerks on a subject is a practical exam and was not able to elicit them. The student instructed the subject to clench his teeth. He also told him to hook his fingers and pull them apart.

- Name the procedure the student told the subject to do.
- What is the physiological basis of the same?

Case 5: A male person 25 years had a fractured radius of their right hand and his right hand was in plantar for about 6 weeks. After the removal of plaster after 6 weeks, on inspection, his right hand was looking thinner compared to his left hand

- What is this condition called? What is its physiological basis?
- What is functional hypertrophy of muscle?

Case 6: In a pediatric ward medical student was taking rounds. He found that a 9-month-old baby was admitted to the ward for fever. On reflexes examination, he found that Babinski's sign on plantar reflex is positive.

- What is Babinski's sign? What is the physiological basis of the sign positive in the patient?
- Enumerate other superficial reflexes you know.

Case 7: An old male of 65 years of age complains of inability to do movements of his fingers and complain that he is not able to play the piano which he used to play and this difficulty has progressively increasing since 7 to 10 months. When the physician tried to elicit Romberg's test, the patient was unsteady with eyes open as well as closed.

- What is the physiological basis of Romberg's test?
- What is the probable condition, the patient is suffering from?

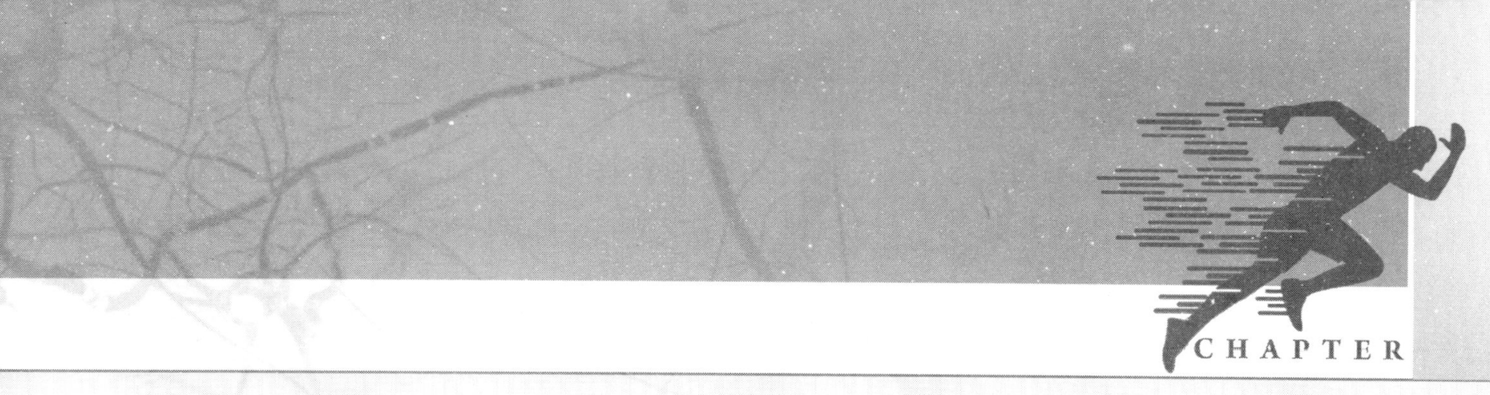

Auditory Evoked Potential

■ INTRODUCTION

The evoked potential is a recording of neural responses to external stimulation. By measuring different peak amplitudes and latencies these responses can be quantified. We can record visual as well as auditory evoked potentials from the eye and ear respectively by giving external stimuli. This is one of the effective methods to analyze CNS functions.

Brainstem Auditory Evoked Potential (BAEP)/Auditory Brain Response (ABR)

Recording BAEP is one of the important objective tests for the assessment of hearing. After the application of auditory stimulus recordings are done from the ear and scalp. When an auditory stimulus is given (receptors act as transducers) they convert acoustic stimulus to an electrical signal and action potential is generated in nerve fibres that in turn travel from the ear to the auditory cortex and we can trace these at many points throughout the auditory pathway.

Physiological Basis of BAEP

The potential is recorded in about 10 ms after the application of auditory stimulus. The waveform that is recorded does reflect the electrical activity of different landmarks in the auditory pathway (from cochlear nerve to inferior colliculi where complex integration of sound frequencies happens).

BAEP is a record of six waves and is named as wave I to wave VI. Each wave shows the activity of a particular region of the auditory pathway (Fig. 24.1).

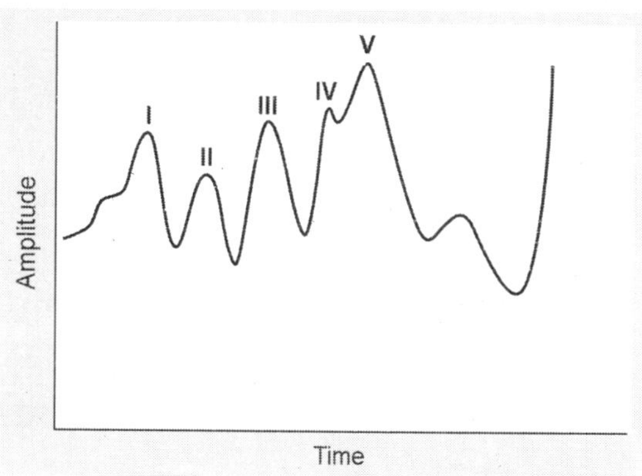

Fig. 24.1: Brainstem auditory evoked potential

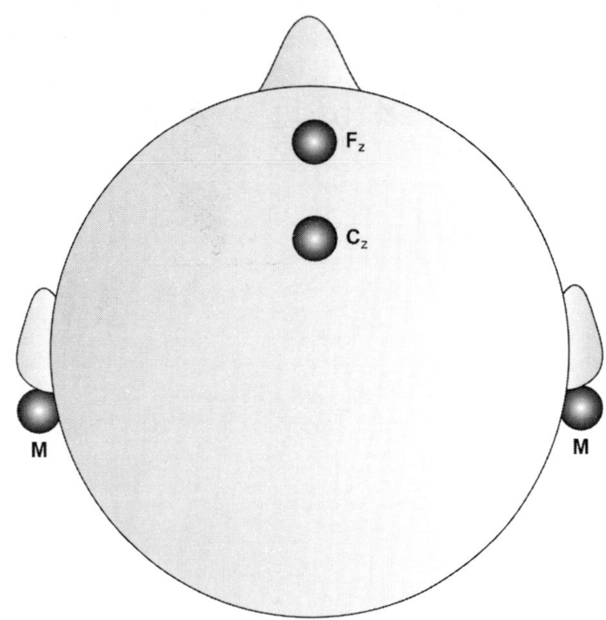

Fig. 24.2: Placement of electrodes for recording auditory evoked potential

Apparatus

Recording electrodes, earphones, evoked potential electromyogram machine, electrode paste/jelly.

Procedure

- Clean the area where electrodes are to be placed.
- Recording electrode is placed on the mastoid process or earlobes and reference electrode, in front of vertex and ground electrode in front of the reference electrode **(Fig. 24.2)**.
- Recording electrodes are connected to the amplifier and the filter setting is done properly.
- Stimulus of 0.1 ms duration is given and potentials from both ears are recorded (normally stimulus intensity is kept between 40 to 70 dB).

Precautions

- Instruct the subject properly and he should be relaxed.
- The room used should be quiet and comfortable.
- Proper placement of electrodes is required and amplification and filter settings must be checked before.
- Prevent all outside noises.
- Mask the opposite ear when stimulation is given to one ear.

Observation/Results

After a time, lapse of about 1.4 ms from the time of application of stimulus, electrical activity is recorded and can be traced throughout the auditory pathway. Normal BEAP shows five waves that are named as wave I, II, III, IV, V **(Table 24.1)**.

Auditory Pathway and Correlation of Waveforms of BAEP

About 5 to 7 vertex positive waves are evoked from the brainstem in response to an auditory stimulus. In most of the studies wave I, III and V are the most prominent.

■ IMPORTANT QUESTIONS AND ANSWERS

Q.1. Describe normal waveforms of BEAP.
Please refer to **Table 24.1** for describing normal waveforms of BEAP, their characteristics and corresponding regions in auditory pathway stimulation that cause it to record a particular wave **(Fig. 24.1)**.

Q.2. Enumerate factors affecting BEAP.
Factors affecting BEAP

- **Age:** Latency of BEAP varies with age. It has been found that is age-dependent up to 2 years of age. It is particularly less in premature infants. Older people

Important landmarks of the auditory pathway	Waveform correlation of BAEP	Characteristics of waveform
Electrical activity is picked up – From axons of spiral ganglion (that innervate hair cells) constitute cochlear nerve	Recorded as wave I and wave II	• Wave I is the first prominent upgoing peak • Wave II is poorly defined • Waves I and II appear about 1.4 ms after stimulus • Wave I and II can be reduced or absent with lesion /damage of the cochlear nerve
Then impulse passes from cochlear nerve fibres to dorsal and ventral cochlear nuclei	Recorded as wave III	• Wave III is recorded as a prominent upgoing peak and sometimes may show two peaks (bifid) • Wave III is reduced or absent in the lesion of the cochlear nucleus
Then impulse passes via the trapezoid body to the opposite side superior olivary complex	Recorded as wave IV	• Wave IV is very small and may appear as the upgoing slope of wave V • Wave IV is reduced or absent in lesion of the superior olivary nucleus
Then impulse travels to nuclei of the lateral lemniscus and inferior colliculi	Recorded as wave V	• Most prominent peak in BEAP recording (among all waves) • Appears about 5.5 ms after stimulus • Wave V can be absent with diseases of lateral lemniscus and inferior colliculi

TABLE 24.1: Auditory pathway and correlation of waveforms of BAEP

have been found to have longer latency compared to young people.

- **Sex:** Females have a higher amplitude of BEAP as compared to males and the latency period is shorter in them.
- **Hearing loss:** Conduction deafness does alter BEAP.
- **Temperature:** There is an inverse relationship between temperature and latency of BEAP. More is the temperature; less is the latency and vice versa.

Q.3. Give the clinical application of recording BEAP.

- BEAP or ABR is used clinically to detect neurological abnormalities. In neurological abnormalities, latency, inter-latency peaks, amplitude and wave V/I amplitude ratio helps to localize a lesion. It helps to diagnose conditions like brainstem tumours, and multiple sclerosis.
- When ABR is done in a series of intensities, it helps to detect audiological abnormalities. At all intensity levels smaller responses are obtained in conductive deafness and with sensorineural loss normal response is obtained especially at higher levels of intensity and smaller responses are obtained at low intensity levels.
- BEAP is used commonly in skull base surgeries mainly for posterior fossa lesions. BEAP is also helpful in cases of coma to differentiate metabolic and structural causes of coma.

Q.4. Enumerate various parameters of BEAP waveforms. How to interpret the results of BEAP?

BEAP waveforms have to be assessed for:

1. **Amplitude** (reflects the number of neurons firing). It is measured as the height from the peak of the wave to the trough of that wave.
2. **Latency, inter-peak latencies** (reflects the speed of transmission and time between two peaks). Interpeak latencies are measured are I-V and III-V. Different conditions are known to alter these inter-latency peaks.

I–V inter-peak latency	III–V inter-peak latency	I–III inter-peak latency
• Normal value 4.5 ms	• Normal value 2.4 ms	• Normal value 2.5 ms
• Reflects conduction time from the eighth nerve to the pons	• Reflects conduction time from lower pons to midbrain	• Reflects conduction time from the eighth nerve to the lower pons
• Prolonged values observed in degenerative diseases	• Isolated prolongation of this inter-peak latency is not significant clinically	• Prolonged values seen in diseases of the Ponto medullary junction

3. **Amplitude ratio of V/I**—We know that wave I is recorded due to the electrical activity of cochlear nerves (i.e. outside the brain) and wave V is recorded due to the electrical activity of lateral lemnisci and inferior colliculus (inside the brain). The normal range of the ratio varies from 50% to 33%.

Q.5. How one can differentiate between peripheral and central hearing impairment by recording BEAP?

For differentiating peripheral and central impairment in hearing, the amplitude ratio of V/I (as mentioned above is important).

When the ratio is less than 50 it reflects a small V wave, which originates in the brain region and thus indicates central impairment in hearing.

If the ratio is more than 33, it reflects a small amplitude of I wave which originates from cochlear nerves (outside the brain) indicating peripheral impairment in hearing.

Q.6. Enumerate common clinical conditions where the waveform of BEAP is altered.

Conductive hearing loss: In this wave I latency will be markedly delayed and there is a delay in the conduction of impulse till it reaches the cochlear nerve (which is responsible for wave I) interwove latencies are usually normal.

Sensory hearing loss: In this wave, I can be small or absent completely (damage to the cochlear nerve).

Neural hearing loss: This will show normal wave I, wave I–III and inter-wave latencies are delayed.

COMMON STATIONS – SPOTS IN PRACTICAL EXAMINATION (2/3 MARKS)

Q.1. Normal electrode placement diagram may be shown. Identify the procedure and give its application or any one or two questions from the above.

Q.2. Normal diagram of waveforms of BEAP. Identify, describe and comment.

Q.3. Diagram of recording of BEAP. Identify and comment.

CASE-BASED SCENARIO/PROBLEM-BASED (2/3 MARKS)

Case 1: A 5-month-old baby was brought to OPD by parents with c/o child not responding to verbal stimulation. She was suggested to get the auditory evoked potential test done.

- What is auditory evoked potential?
- Describe normal waveforms of the same.

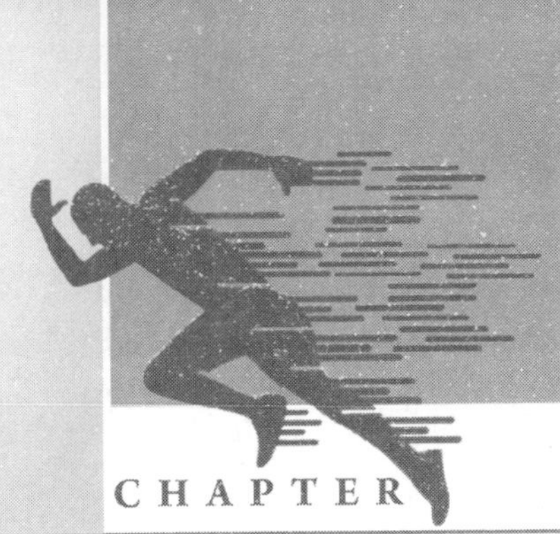

25

Visual Evoked Potential

Competency:

PY 10.19: Describe and discuss auditory and visual evoked potentials.

Learning Objectives

After completing this practical, students should be able to:
- Define visual evoked potential (VEP)
- Describe normal waveforms of VEP and enumerate factors that affect it
- Trace the visual pathway and correlate it with waves of VEP
- Alterations in waveforms with common clinical conditions

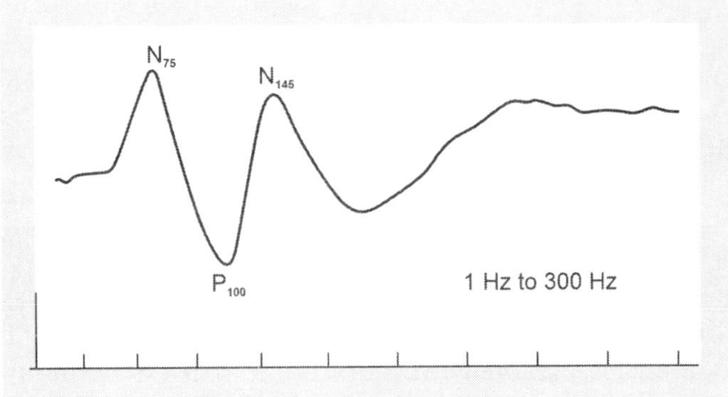

Fig. 25.1: Visual evoked potential

■ INTRODUCTION

The evoked potential is a recording of neural responses to external stimulation. By measuring different peak amplitudes and latencies these responses can be quantified. We can record visually evoked potentials from the eye by giving external stimuli. This is one of the effective methods to analyze CNS functions.

■ VISUAL EVOKED POTENTIAL (VEP)

Visual evoked potentials (VEP) are electrical potentials that are recorded when electrodes are placed on appropriate areas on the vertex in response to visual stimulus **(Fig. 25.1)**. It helps to assess the intactness of the visual pathway. It indicates the response of cortical and subcortical structures to visual stimulus. The tests assess the functional status of the visual system beyond ganglion cells. Abnormal responses of VEPs are obtained in different clinical conditions affecting the visual system.

Physiological basis of VEP: A visual stimulus applied, stimulates the visual pathway and generates activities in the visual cortex and response is recorded. When a visual stimulus is given, activities are generated in the visual cortex, association areas of the visual cortex and thalamocortical fibres and are recorded.

VEPs represent the macular region primarily as macular fibres project to the occipital lobe of the cortex (those from the peripheral retina project deep in the calcarine fissure) and over the course of the visual pathway macular field gets amplified as it reaches the cortex.

VEPs are recorded as a series of waveforms. A negative wave is denoted as N and a positive as P. These waves

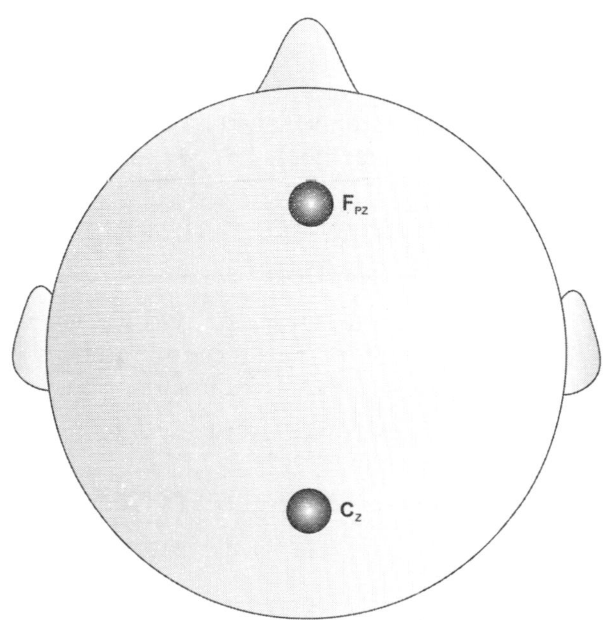

Fig. 25.2: Placement of electrodes while recording VEP

are elicited due to the activation of different areas in the visual pathway. Common waveforms that are recorded are N_{75}, P_{100} and N_{145}.

Apparatus

Recording electrodes, evoked potential machine, electrode paste/jelly.

Procedure

- Instruct the subject properly and he should be relaxed.
- The room used should be quiet and comfortable.
- Proper placement of electrodes (recording and reference) as shown in **Fig. 25.2**.
- Ground electrode is placed at the wrist with proper amplification and filter settings.
- Visual stimulus is presented to the subject for a specific number of times and the response obtained is recorded.

Precautions

- The subject should be explained in the detail procedure.
- Even though monocular stimulation is standard in children, binocular stimulation may be used.
- Ask the subject to wear glass/lens during the test if he/she is using it.
- Basic ophthalmic exam including the field of vision, pupillary reflexes, the field of vision, and visual acuity should be done beforehand.
- Any miotics or mydriatics should not be used 12 hrs. before the procedure (monocular undilated pupils).
- While performing flash VEP, the mechanical patch is applied to the unstimulated eye.

Observations/Results

Normal VEPs consist of a series of waveforms of opposite polarities and the main waves recorded are N_{75}, P_{100} and N_{145}. Peak latency and peak-to-peak amplitudes are recorded. The normal amplitude of VEPs is 3 to 25 microvolts.

Visual Pathway and Correlation of Waveforms of VEP

With the application of a visual stimulus, electrical activities are recorded in specific regions of the visual pathway. The evoked potential is triphasic (negative-positive and negative), with three peaks as seen in the **Fig. 25.1**.

N_{75}: It originates from the visual cortex (area 17) and is caused due to foveal stimulation.

P_{100}: It originates from area 19.

N_{145}: It originates from area 18.

Usually out of three waves peak latency, duration, and amplitude of P_{100} are measured. The normal latency of P_{100} is about 100 ms, with a duration of 60 ms and an amplitude of 11 microvolts.

■ IMPORTANT QUESTIONS AND ANSWERS

Q.1. What are the different ways in which VEP can be used?

Types of VEPs Stimuli

- **Pattern stimuli**: This is most used in clinical practice. These are represented in a checkerboard. Pattern onset/offset where the pattern is shown for a brief period of time and then replaced with a blank screen (of the same intensity). This is commonly done for patients with nystagmus.
- **Pattern reversal stimuli**: Here black and white checks reverse their orientation.
- **Flash stimuli**: VEP is evoked by either a flash of light or a pattern. This is used less commonly. They are used in children or non-cooperative patients. If flash stimuli are to be used, the examination room should be dimly illuminated.

Q.2. Enumerate factors affecting VEPs.

Factors affecting VEPs

- **Age**: The amplitude of waves can change with respect to age. P_{100} amplitude is high in children compared to adults. After 50 years of age, the amplitude of waves starts decreasing.
- **Visual acuity**: With the decrease in visual acuity amplitude of P_{100} decreases.
- **Sex**: Males (head size more in males) have a higher latency of P_{100} as compared to females.

- **Drugs:** Any miotic or mydriatic drug will reduce P_{100} latency.
- **Eye movements**: The amplitude of P_{100} is known to decrease with eye movement however there is no change observed in the latency of P_{100}.
- **Pupil size**: Pupillary constriction increases P_{100} latency.
- **Size of the stimulus**: The less the size of the stimulus the greater the amplitude of VEP.
- **Sedation/anaesthesia**: Will abolish VEPs.

Q.3. What are the properties of VEP?

Amplitude: It is the height of the wave (vertical) measured in microvolts from the preceding trough. Reduced amplitude represents axonal lesions.

Latency: It is measured in milliseconds and can vary from person to person. It is affected by pupil size, refractive error, and age of the person. Prolonged latency is seen with demyelinating diseases, (e.g. multiple sclerosis), and retinopathies.

Combined amplitude and latency abnormalities are common with optic nerve compression.

Q.4. Give the clinical application of VEPs.

Recording of VEPs is one of the noninvasive tests used to assess the intactness of the visual pathway. VEP helps to detect lesions like demyelination of optic nerves, optic neuropathy and cortical blindness by evaluating the amplitude and latency of the waveforms. VEPs also help to assess nutritional or toxic optic neuropathies.

Continuous monitoring of VEPs becomes important while performing surgeries to prevent optic nerve damage. One can get normal VEPs in unilateral lesions of optic chiasma with monocular stimulation as each eye projects to both occipital lobes.

COMMON STATIONS – SPOTS IN PRACTICAL EXAMINATION (2/3 MARKS)

Q.1. Normal electrode placement diagram may be shown: Identify the procedure and give its application or any one or two questions from above.

Q.2. Normal diagram of waveforms of VEP: Identify, describe and comment.

Q.3. Diagram of recording of VEPs: Identify and comment.

CASE-BASED SCENARIO/PROBLEM-BASED (2/3 MARKS)

Case 1: A 68-year-old patient with a known case of multiple sclerosis was referred to the electrophysiology lab to evaluate VEPs as he was complaining of impaired vision.

- What is visual evoked potential? Give its physiological basis.
- Describe normal waveforms of VEP.
- What abnormal finding do you expect in this patient?

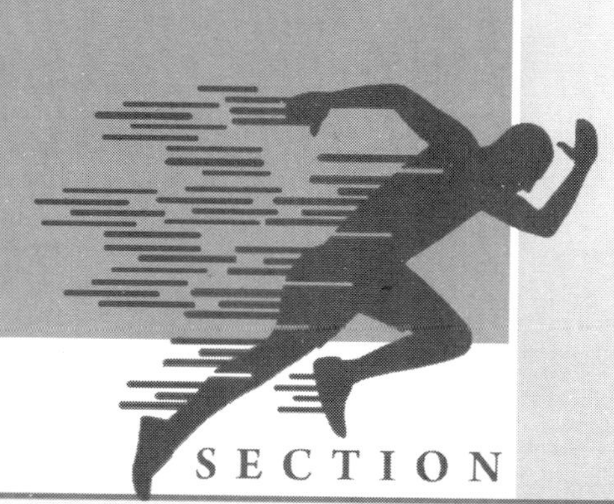

Human Experimental Physiology

Chapter Outline

- Ergography
- Stethography
- Spirometry
- Determination of Vital Capacity
- Peak Expiratory Flow Rate
- Electrocardiography (ECG)
- Tests for Physical Fitness
- Perimetry
- Measurement of Reaction Time to Visual and Auditory Stimulus

- Electromyography (EMG)
- Nerve Conduction Studies
- Electroencephalography (EEG)
- Test for Pregnancy Diagnosis
- Cardiopulmonary Cerebral Resuscitation
- Preparation of Diet Sheet
- Autonomic Function Tests
- Body Composition Analysis and Calculation of BMR

Ergography

■ INTRODUCTION

- Ergography is done to find out the work done by intact muscles.
- It was first introduced by Mosso, so it is called as Mosso's ergograph **(Fig. 26.1)**.
- It is a recording of voluntary contractions of skeletal muscle in human beings on a moving kymograph.
- It is performed to study the phenomenon of fatigue. In the ergograph, appropriate folders are available to

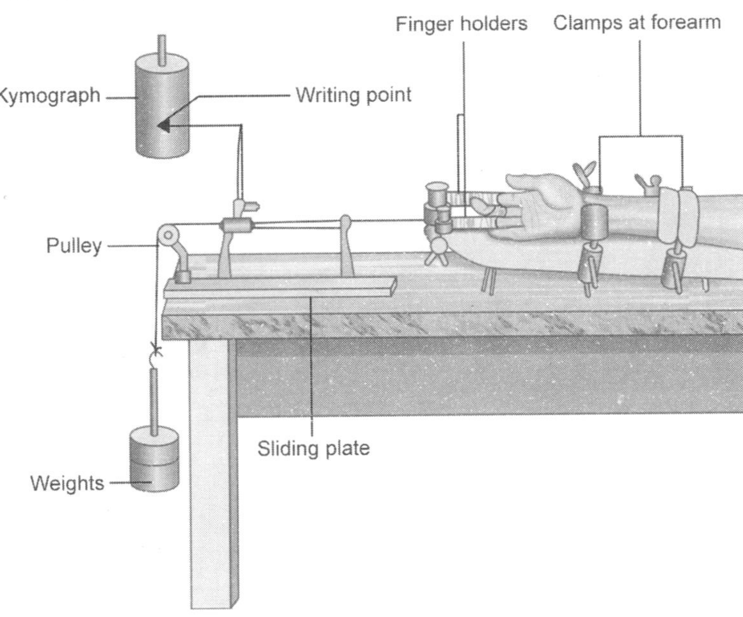

Fig. 26.1: Mosso's ergograph

place the forearm and fingers. One end of the sliding plate is attached to a cord passing over a pulley that carries a load of 3 kg. This sliding plate is connected through a sling to the finger metal plates are attached to a writing lever that records on a slow-moving drum. When the finger is placed, the load is lifted and the distance through which it is lifted gets marked on the drum.

Principle

The subject contracts flexors of the fingers against resistance till the finger is fatigued. Work done is calculated to assess the effect of various parameters on performance and time that fatigue sets in.

Procedure

- Proper instructions are given to the subject.
- The ergograph is kept at the edge of the table.
- 1–2 kg weight is attached to the cord.
- Subject is asked to insert index and ring fingers into fixed tube holders, and the middle finger pulls the load.
- Sling is connected to the middle finger.
- Metronome is started and the subject is asked to lift the load by maximal contraction of the flexors of the middle finger once every 2 seconds.
- Contractions are recorded on a slow-moving drum with a pencil or pen.
- Subject continues to work till fatigue.
- Fatigue time is recorded in seconds **(Fig. 26.2)**.

Effect of Rest-Pause

- Subject is asked to do the same work but short rest pauses are given after short intervals of work. Again, total fatigue is calculated.
- It is observed that fatigue is delayed.

Effect of Venous Occlusion

- Blood pressure cuff is tied around the arm and pressure is raised to 50 mm Hg.
- Subject is asked to flex the finger without rest pause.
- Fatigue time is noted.
- It is observed, that fatigue sets in earlier.

Effect of Arterial Occlusion

- A blood pressure cuff is tied around the arm and pressure is raised 10–20 mm Hg above the subject's systolic pressure (approximately between 160–200 mm Hg).
- Subject is asked to flex the finger without rest pause.
- Fatigue time is noted.
- It is observed that fatigue sets in earlier than with venous occlusion.

Effect of Median Nerve Stimulation

Even after fatigue, the median nerve is stimulated and the effect is recorded.

Precautions

- Subject should be instructed properly.
- Subject should continue to do work till he/she is unable to lift the load.

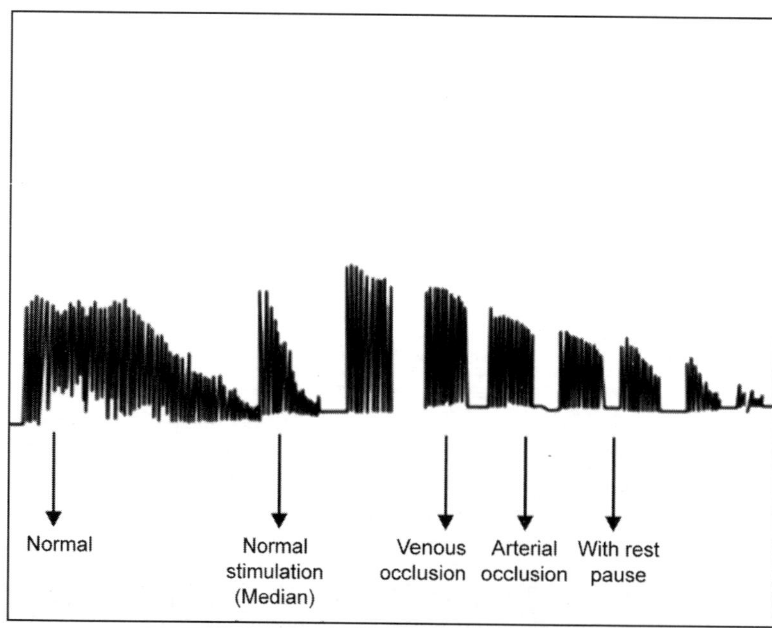

Fig. 26.2: Ergography

- Between all different procedures at least 12 to 15 minutes of gap has to be given to the subject.
- With performance with venous and arterial occlusion, BP cuff pressure of 40 and 200 mm of Hg must be raised respectively and maintained there throughout the performance.

Calculation of Work Done

- For finding out the average height of contractions, the record is divided into rectangles and triangles **(Fig. 26.3)**
- Average height = A +B/d

Where,
A = Area of rectangle (a × b)
B = Area of a triangle (a × c/2)
d = Total distance for which graph is recorded
Work done is calculated in grams centimetres.

Observations

- **Venous occlusion:** Decreases the amplitude of contraction and fatigue sets in earlier.
  Cause: With venous occlusion, there is an accumulation of metabolites, that decreases muscle performance.
- **Arterial occlusion:** Further decreases the amplitude of contraction and fatigue sets in still earlier.
  Cause: With arterial occlusion, there is not enough O_2 supply to muscles. O_2 is required for metabolic oxidation in tissues to provide adenosine triphosphate (ATP).
- **With rest pauses:** When the subject is asked to do the same work, with rest pauses in between, then fatigue time is calculated. It is observed that fatigue is delayed and the total amount of work done is more.
- **With median nerve stimulation:** Even after fatigue sets in when the median nerve is stimulated, muscle contraction is obtained. This indicates that the seat of fatigue is at the level of synapse in the intact body and not the neuromuscular junction (NM) junction.

■ IMPORTANT QUESTIONS AND ANSWERS

Q.1. What are the factors affecting the onset of fatigue?

Factors affecting fatigue are:

- O_2 and nutrients supply to muscle
- Training
- pH of body fluids
- Motivation
- Collection of waste products in muscle
- Degree and duration of work

Q.2. Enumerate other types of ergographs.

Other types of ergograph used are:

- Du-bois ergograph
- Weber's ergograph
- Bicycle ergograph
- Treadmill

Q.3. What is the application of ergography in industries?

One can determine the physical fitness of the subject by xerography. This is done by adding more load or stress. This experiment shows that when rest pauses are given, more work is done and even the fatigue is delayed. Rest pauses with recreation facilities will show better and longer performance of the work.

Proper encouragement can overcome fatigue. It indicates that fatigue does possess a cortical component and the actual duration of the work (without getting fatigue) is decided mostly by the psychological setup of a person. The efficiency of the work can be easily increased by motivation and encouragement.

Q.4. What is the seat of fatigue in an intact body?

The seat of fatigue in the intact body is at the level of synapse. Motivation and encouragement can prolong fatigue.

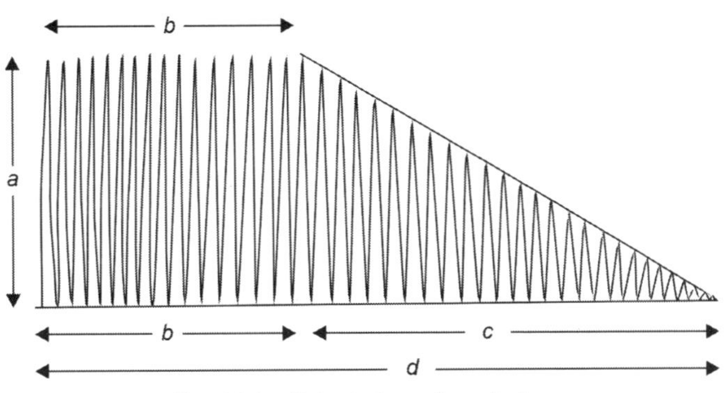

Fig. 26.3: Calculation of work done

OBJECTIVE STRUCTURED PRACTICAL EXAMINATION (OSPE)

Procedure station 1: To find the effect of venous occlusion on work done.

S. No.	Assessment criteria	Marks assigned	Marks given
1.	Explain the procedure to a given subject		
2.	Give proper instructions		
3.	Make sure the blood pressure (BP) cuff is tied around the arm and pressure is raised up to 50 mm of Hg		
4.	Do record till the subject is not able to flex the finger anymore and calculate the work done		
5.	Report and viva on clinical examination		
6.	Total		

Similar steps of OSPEs can be prepared to see the effect with arterial occlusion, median nerve stimulation, rest-pause, etc. (check above for details).

COMMON STATIONS – SPOTS IN PRACTICAL EXAMINATION (2/3 MARKS)

Q.1. Ergograph instrument/diagram: Identify and answer any one or two questions from the above.

KEY POINTS TO REMEMBER

- Fatigue is defined as the inability of the muscle to maintain muscle twitch tension due to repeated stimulation of the muscle.
- The seat of fatigue is at the level of synapse in the central nervous system (CNS). Fatigue is a completely reversible phenomenon.
- O_2 supply, training, motivation, and amount of waste products collected in muscle, are the factors that affect fatigue.

Stethography

Learning Objectives
After completing this practical, the students shall be able to:
- Define stethography
- Record respiratory movements normally after tying the stethograph around the chest of the subject
- Enumerate precautions taken while performing the experiment
- Give the physiological basis of deglutition apnea, the effect of pre- and post-exercise, breath holding and hyperventilation on respiration

■ INTRODUCTION

Stethography is a method in which respiratory movements are recorded by using a stethograph. This is one method by which pulmonary fitness is assessed. The stethograph consists of a corrugated rubber tubing having a side tube and chain attached. The side tube is connected to a rubber tube which connects it to Marey's tambour which has a lever with the pointer. The pointer records the movement on the recording drum. The recording drum rotates at a slow speed with a pully connection 4:1 and slow gear.

Principle

A stethograph is tied around the chest of the subject and the respiratory movements are recorded on the drum.

Apparatus

Stethograph, Marey's tambour, water, rubber tube, and kymograph.

Precautions

- Subject should sit comfortably on the stool.
- Tambour should be at the level of about 4th intercostal space, where maximum breathing movements are recorded **(Fig. 27.1)**.
- Before and after each procedure, normal respiration is recorded.
- While a person is exercising, the tambour should be disconnected and then attached again to record the effect after exercise.

Procedure

- Ask the subject to sit comfortably on the stool with his/her back towards the recording apparatus.
- Tie the stethograph around the chest at the level where respiratory movements are maximum.
- Connect Marey's tambour to the stethograph.

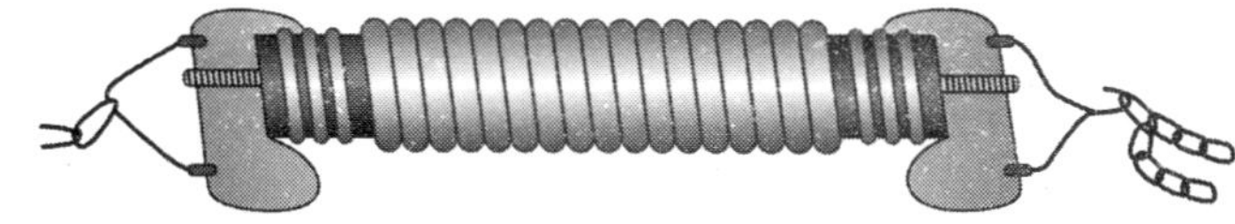

Fig. 27.1: Stethograph (Tambour)

- Record normal respiration. Upward stroke corresponds to expiration and downward stroke corresponds to inspiration.
- Ask the subject to hyperventilate for 2 minutes and record its effect.
- Again, record normal respirations and now ask the subject to drink water and record the effect.
- Again, after normal respiration ask the subject to do exercise for 3 minutes and record the respirations.
- Again, after normal respiration, ask the subject to talk and record the findings.
- Again, after normal respiration, record breath holding after quiet inspiration and expiration.
- Again, after normal respiration, ask the subject to hold their breath after the deepest possible inspiration. Record the finding and after breaking point record the respiration.

Observation/Results

- **Normal respiration:** Upstroke is expiration and downstroke is inspiration **(Fig. 27.2)**.
- **On voluntary hyperventilation:** There is an increased rate and force of respiration that is recorded.
- **On drinking water:** When the subject drinks water, there is a temporary stoppage of breathing recorded. This is called as deglutition apnea.
- **After exercise:** After exercise, an increase in rate and depth of breathing is recorded for some time.
- **Breath-holding:** During breath-holding, a straight line is recorded (as the person stops breathing) and after the breaking point, an increase in rate and depth of respiration is recorded for some time.

■ IMPORTANT QUESTIONS AND ANSWERS

Q.1. Define the terms—eupnea, hyperpnea, hypercapnia and apnea.

Eupnea: Normal quiet breathing is termed as eupnea.

Hyperapnea: It is an increase in the rate of respiration.

Hypercapnia: Increase in CO_2 concentration in body fluids is hypercapnia.

Apnea: It is a temporary stoppage of breathing.

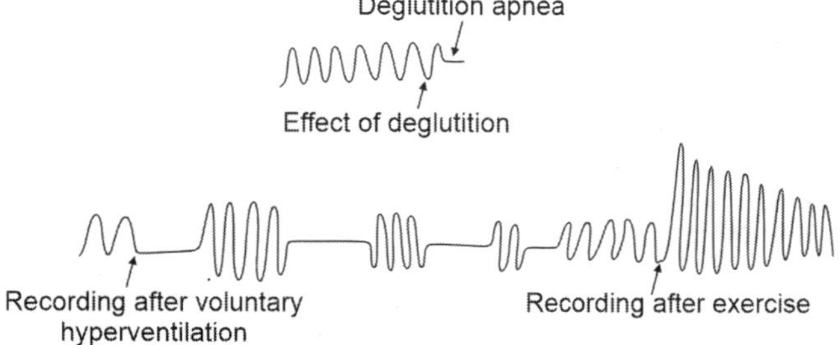

Fig. 27.2: Stethography normal recording

Q.2. What is deglutition apnea?
During deglutition (pharyngeal stage) respiration stops for some time, this is called as deglutition apnea. This happens due to the closure of the glottis which prevents entry of food in respiratory passage.

Q.3. What is breath-holding time?
Breath holding time is the maximum time for which a subject can hold his/her breath followed by inspiration as well as expiration. Normally, inspiratory breath holding time is longer than expiratory breath holding time.

Q.4. What is the breaking point?
After a person holds breath, voluntarily, there comes one point at which he/she cannot hold breath, this is called as breaking point.

Physiological basis: When a person holds breath, there is a rise in arterial pCO_2 and a fall in pO_2. This stimulates central and peripheral chemoreceptors which in turn stimulate respiration. Even the proprioceptive impulses from respiratory muscles are responsible for this breaking point. Normal breaking point reaches when alveolar pO_2 falls below 55 mm of Hg. If one inspires 100% O_2, (this will increase alveolar pO_2) or hyperventilates (which helps in washing out of CO_2) before holding breath then the breaking point is delayed.

Q.5. Explain the mechanism of hyperventilation in exercise.
Before a person starts doing exercise, the cortex sends impulses to contracting muscles and via collaterals sends impulses to the respiratory centre. This causes activation of the respiratory centre to increase ventilation even before the start of exercise. Once the exercise starts, movements of joints and, the activity of muscles send afferent impulses to activate the respiratory centre (in medulla) and keep pulmonary ventilation high. Normally this increase in ventilation is sufficient to supply the exact amount of extra O_2 required during exercise (as well as to remove excess CO_2 produced).

This helps to maintain partial pressure of respiratory gases (O_2 and CO_2) to maintain in the blood (especially in a trained person). With intense exercise CO_2 directly acts on central and O_2 (drop) on peripheral chemoreceptors and does final adjustment in ventilation.

Q.6. What is the cause of hyperventilation after exercise?
During exercise, muscles use an anaerobic mechanism of formation of energy from glucose. During this mechanism, lactic acid is formed from glucose anaerobically (without using O_2). This causes muscles to go out in O_2 debt. This O_2 is to be supplied after exercise and in order to fulfil that O_2 debt created during exercise, there is

hyperventilation observed in a person in the recovery period (following exercise).

▮ COMMON STATIONS – SPOTS IN PRACTICAL EXAMINATION (2/3 MARKS)

Q.1. Identify and comment on various recordings of respiration during normal reparation, drinking water, breath holding, etc.

Q.2. Stethography machine: Identify and write a procedure or write precautions before the experiment or any one or two questions from the above.

Q.3. Demonstrate the effect of various manoeuvres on the respiration of a person/subject using a stethograph.

▮ CASE-BASED SCENARIO/PROBLEM-BASED (2/3 MARKS)

Case 1: In a 30-year-old healthy adult male, stethography was done in MBBS practical exam. On drinking water, by the person, apnea was observed.

- State the physiological basis of deglutition apnea.
- Enlist precautions for stethography.

Case 2: A 25-year-old male person was made to use the Harvard step test for 3 minutes and then immediately with the help of stethography respiration was recorded.

- What can be the likely record of respiration post-exercise?
- Give the physiological mechanism of hyperventilation before exercise.

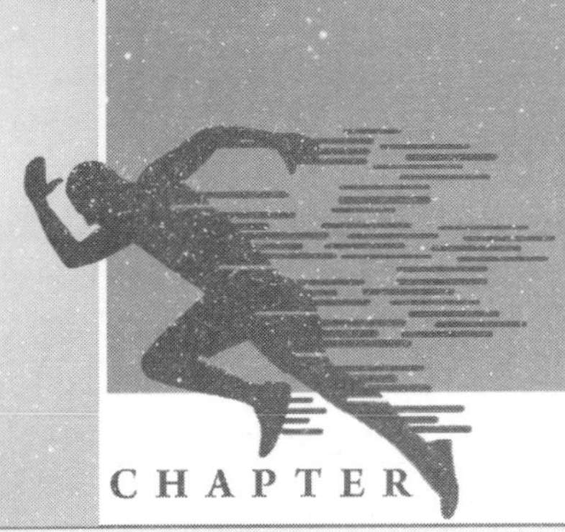

28

Spirometry

Competency:

PY 6.8: Demonstrate the correct technique to perform and interpret spirometry.

Learning Objectives

After completion of this practical, the students shall be able to:
- Define different volumes and capacities of the lung with their physiological significance
- List volumes and capacities of lungs that can be calculated by spirometer
- Differentiate between static and dynamic lung capacities
- Define peak expiratory flow rate and explain the physiological significance of the same
- Define timed vital capacity and give its significance

■ INTRODUCTION

- Lung volumes and capacities are measured with the help of an instrument called as spirometer.
- Various lung volumes and capacities assess ventilation, which is one of the important parameters of lung function tests. Residual volume, functional residual capacity (FRC), and total lung capacity are not recorded by spirometer.
- Functional residual capacity is measured by the helium dilution method or nitrogen washout method and from that residual volume and total lung capacity are calculated.
- Nowadays computerized spirometers with various functions are used to record lung volumes and capacities.
- With these non-invasive lung function tests one can assess lung working, and diagnose some lung disorders.

Hutchinson's Spirometer

- It consists of two light metal cylinder jars.
- The bigger one contains water in which smaller one (which is airtight due to the water seal) fits in an inverted position.
- It is counterbalanced by weight passing over the pulley.
- Central tubing inside the bigger jar, which rises above the level of water, is connected outside with a mouthpiece.
- When the subject breaths out of the mouthpiece, the rise of pressure within the airtight smaller jar will raise it.
- Rise in level is graduated in such a way, that it gives a reading for amount of air.
- Counter balance carries a pen for writing on kymograph paper **(Fig. 28.1)**.

Procedure

- Space between the outer and inner cylinder is filled three-fourths with water. Ask the subject to sit comfortably and relax. Check that the spirometer is airtight.

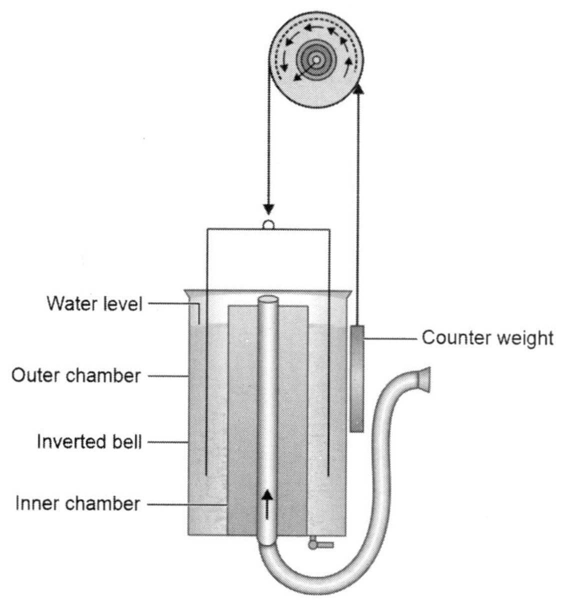

Fig. 28.1: Spirometer

- Use a sterile mouthpiece and connect it to a spirometer.
- Close nostrils with the help of a nose clip.
- Ask the subject to breathe in and out by mouth (tidal volume). Simultaneously graphic record is obtained. The horizontal line indicates time, the vertical line indicates volume and upstroke (inspiration) and downstroke (expiration) are recorded. (1 cm = 200 ml)
- Ask the subject to breathe in as much as possible after normal expiration [inspiratory reserve volume (IRV)].
- Ask the subject to exhale as much as he/she can after normal inspiration [expiratory reserve volume

(ERV)]. For recording expiratory volumes, empty the spirometer completely.
- Ask the subject to breathe out forcefully with the maximum possible effort after deep inspiration [that gives vital capacity (VC)].
- Adjust the dial with the pointer at zero mark for each recording.
- Different volumes and capacities are thus recorded. Different volumes and capacities recorded are shown in **Fig. 28.2**.

■ IMPORTANT QUESTIONS AND ANSWERS

Q.1. Define tidal volume (TV).
It is the volume of air taken in or given out during normal tidal respiration. It is 500 ml.

Q.2. Define inspiratory reserve volume (IRV) and inspiratory capacity (IC).
- **Inspiratory reserve volume**: It is the maximum volume of air that can be inspired over and above the tidal volume. It is 3,000 ml.
- **Inspiratory capacity**: It is the maximum volume of air that can be inspired after normal tidal expiration. It is equal to inspiratory reserve volume + tidal volume. It is 3,500 ml.

Q.3. Define expiratory reserve volume (ERV) and expiratory capacity (EC).
- **Expiratory reserve volume**: It is the maximum volume of air that can be expired over and above normal tidal expiration. It is 1,100 ml.
- **Expiratory capacity:** It is maximum volume of air that can be expired after normal tidal inspiration. It is equal to expiratory reserve volume + tidal volume. It is 1,600 ml.

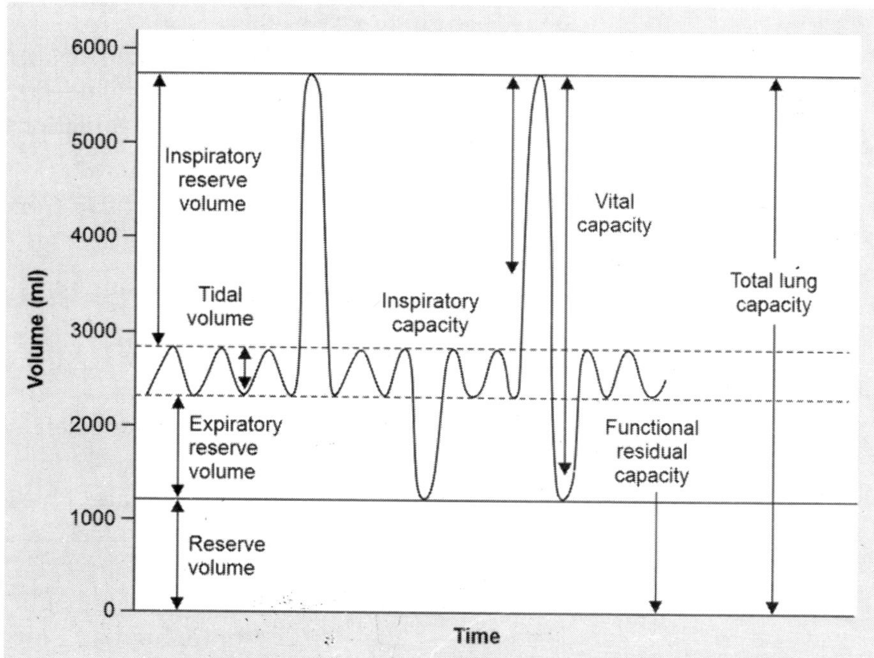

Fig. 28.2: Normal lung volumes and capacities

Q.4. Define vital capacity. Enumerate factors affecting it.

- **Vital capacity**: It is the maximum volume of air that can expire after filling the lungs by maximal inspiratory effort. It is equal to inspiratory capacity + expiratory reserve volume. It is 4,600 ml.

Factors affecting VC

- VC is more in males compared to females due to its large chest size and more power in muscles.
- With loss of elasticity in lungs, VC decreases with age.
- VC is more in standing than sitting position as with standing position, the diaphragm moves down, and more space available for inspiration. In pregnancy, VC decreases.
- VC decreases with various lung diseases like pleural effusion and emphysema.

Q.5. Define residual volume (RV).

Residual volume: It is the volume of air that remains in the lungs after forceful expiration. It is 1,200 ml.

Q.6. Define functional residual capacity (FRC).

- **Functional residual capacity**: It is the volume of air that remains in the lungs after normal tidal expiration. It is expiratory reserve volume + residual volume. It is 2,300 ml.
- **Significance of FRC**: It is the volume of air present in the lungs after tidal expiration.

Q.7. Define total lung capacity (TLC).

- **Total lung capacity**: It is the volume of air present in the lungs after maximum inspiration. It is 5,800 ml.

- **All lung volumes and capacities**: These values are for normal adult males.
- Values can change with respect to weight, age, sex, and height of a person.
- Predicted normograms are available. Deviation of about 20% from normal for that age, sex, and height are observed in normal subjects.

Q.8. What is respiratory minute volume? (RMV).

Respiratory minute volume:

- It is the volume of air breathed in and out in 1 minute.
- Tidal volume × respiratory rate = 500 × 12 = 6 litres/min.

Q.9. What is maximum breathing capacity and maximum ventilatory volume (MVV)?

Maximum breathing capacity or maximum ventilatory volume (MVV):

- It is the maximum volume of air that can be taken in and given out in 1 minute
- Subject breaths as rapidly and as deeply as possible for 15 seconds
- Normal MVV is 100 liters/min.

Q.10. What is breathing reserve?

Breathing reserve:

There is a difference between MVV and RMV.

- Percentage of breathing reserve $= \dfrac{MVV - RMV}{MVV} \times 100$

- Normal breathing reserve is $100 - 6 = 94$ litres/min.

Q.11. Enlist precautions taken while recording lung volumes and capacities on the spirometer.

Precautions

- The person in whom the recording is done should not face the spirometer.
- All volumes and capacities are measured from the end of expiration.

Q.12. Enumerate which volumes and capacities can not be measured by spirometry.

Residual volume, functional residual capacity (FRC), and total lung capacity are not recorded by spirometer.

Q.13. What are pulmonary function tests?

Various tests that assess different aspects of the functions of the lungs are collectively called as pulmonary function tests.

- **Tests to assess ventilatory function**: This can be done by finding out all lung volumes and capacities of the lung in a person. Measuring dead space, compliance and airway resistance also helps to assess the ventilatory function of the lungs.

- **Tests to assess gas exchange across lungs**: Besides CO diffusion test, pH and blood gases can be analyzed from arterial blood samples. Medical gas analyzer, Douglas bag, is used to collect inspired and expired air gas samples.

- **Tests for assessing perfusion across lungs**: Some tests to assess this function include X-ray chest, CT or CAT scan, MRI, lung, and ventilation scan.

Q.14: What is dead space air?

It is the amount/volume of air from a single breath that does not take part in the exchange of gases.

Q.15. What is anatomical and physiological dead space air?

- **Anatomical dead space**: It is the volume of air present from the nose to terminal bronchioles (with each breath) that does not take part in gaseous exchange. Normal value–150 ml.

- **Physiological dead space**: Physiological dead space air is the sum of anatomical dead space and alveolar dead space (in a normal person it is not present). If in some alveoli the amount of blood supplied is less, the VA/Q ratio is high and alveolar dead space is then formed.

Q.16. What are static and dynamic lung volumes and capacities?

- **Static lung volumes and capacities**: Static lung volumes are tidal volume, inspiratory reserve volume, and expiratory reserve volume. The time factor is not taken into consideration while recording these lung volumes and capacities.
- **Static lung capacities**: These are inspiratory capacity, functional residual capacity, vital capacity, and total lung capacity. All static lung volumes and capacities are expressed in ml or litre.
- **Dynamic lung volumes and capacities**: The time factor is taken into consideration when recording these lung volumes and capacities. **Dynamic lung volumes** are minute ventilation, and maximum voluntary ventilation. **Dynamic lung capacities** are timed vital capacity, and maximum mid expiratory flow rate. All dynamic lung volumes and capacities are expressed in ml or litre per second/minute.

Q.17. What is a dyspneic index?

Dyspneic index = MVV-RMV/MVV × 100

- MVV: Maximum voluntary volume, RMV: Resting minute volume
- Normal dyspneic index is 90% and when it falls below 70%, the person experiences dyspnea (difficulty in breathing).

Q.18. Enumerate various uses of PFT.

Uses of PFT:

- Helps to evaluate the respiratory fitness of patients.
- PFT helps to assess if treatment is effective or not.
- Helps in monitoring and diagnosing the progress of the disease.

▌OBJECTIVE STRUCTURED PRACTICAL EXAMINATION (OSPE)

Procedure station 1: Record tidal volume and inspiratory capacity in a given subject.

S. No.	Assessment criteria	Marks assigned	Marks given
1.	Greet and stand on the right side of the subject		
2.	Explain the complete procedure to the subject and keep reading at zero on the spirometer		
3.	Give proper instructions to the subject (as explained in the procedure) and sit		
4.	Record normal inspiration and expiration		
5.	Then ask the subject to breathe in max after normal tidal expiration to record inspiratory capacity		
6.	Report and viva on clinical examination		
7.	Total		

▌COMMON STATIONS– SPOTS IN PRACTICAL EXAMINATION (2/3 MARKS)

Q.1. Lung volumes and capacities diagram—To identify, label and answer any one or two questions from the above.

Q.2. Calculate alveolar ventilation, breathing reserve, MVV, and dead space from the given data. (refer to calculation section).

▌KEY POINTS TO REMEMBER

- With a spirometer one can measure different lung volumes and capacities.
- Residual volume and FRC cannot be measured with spirometer. FRC can be measured with help of helium dilution technique.

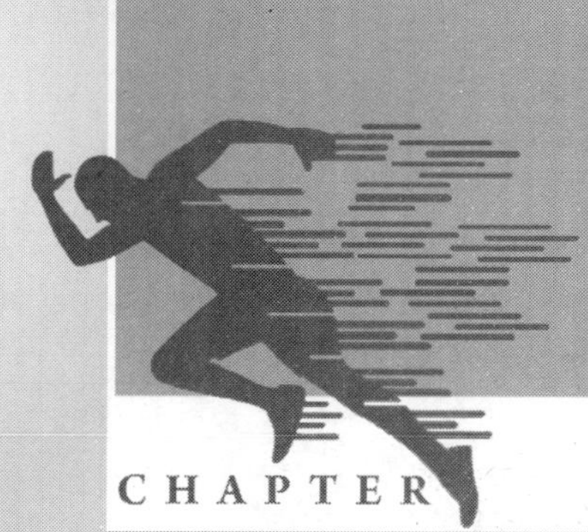

Determination of Vital Capacity

Competency:

PY 6.7: Describe and discuss lung function tests and their clinical significance.

Learning Objectives

At the end of the practical, the students shall be able to:
- Define vital capacity (VC)
- List the precautions taken while recording
- Give normal values of vital capacity
- List physiological and pathological factors that affect VC

■ INTRODUCTION

- Vital capacity is the maximum volume of air that can expire after filling the lungs by maximal effort. The average value of VC is 4.5 litres in males and 3.3 litres in females.
- Vital capacity indicates strength of respiratory muscles. It also helps to assess the ventilatory function of the lungs in health and disease states.

Apparatus

Hutchinson's spirometer and mouthpiece.

Procedure

- Adjust the pointer to the zero mark.
- Let the subject lie comfortably.
- Connect mouthpiece to subject's mouth.
- Ask the subject to take deep inspiration and then exhale forcefully to the maximum. Record vital capacity. This method is a standard method to measure vital capacity.
- Ask the subject to sit and record the same procedure. Ask the subject to stand and record the same procedure. Compare VCs in all three positions.

■ IMPORTANT QUESTIONS AND ANSWERS

Q.1. Enumerate physiological and pathological factors affecting vital capacity.

Factors affecting vital capacity

Physiological factors

- **Posture**
  - VC is more in a standing position than a sitting and supine position.

  Reason
  - In erect posture, the diaphragm descends and the capacity of the thoracic cage increases.
  - In contrast in the supine position, the diaphragm is pushed upwards, so the capacity of the thoracic cage decreases.
  - VC is more in young adults and low in old age and children (with age, there is a decrease in compliance of lungs and chest wall).

- **Sex**
  - VC is more in males as compared to females.

- **Pregnancy**
  - VC is low during pregnancy as the uterus becomes an abdominal organ (especially in the third trimester) chest expansion decreases.

- **Body built**
  - VC is high in well-built person as compared to obese and thin person.
  - VC is higher in athletes, and swimmers as they have stronger and better strength in their muscles.
- **Age**

  VC decreases with age due to loss of elasticity of lungs and weak compression forces.

  Pathological Factors
  - Loss of functional lung tissue, e.g. thick pleura, interstitial lung fibrosis
  - Loss of distensibility of lungs, e.g. pulmonary oedema and atelectasis.

Q.2. What is timed vital capacity?

Timed Vital Capacity

- It is VC expressed with respect to time. One has to calculate the amount of air coming out after the 1st, 2nd, and 3rd second (after inspiring maximally).
- The amount of air coming out at the end of 1st second (FEV1) is normally 80 to 85%, it is about 95% at the end of 2 seconds (FEV2) and almost 100% at the end of the third second (FEV3).
- FEV1 is the most useful test to detect airway obstruction. FEV1 decreases to drastic low levels in obstructive lung diseases. The ratio of FEV1/FVC, i.e. (forced vital capacity) is a more sensitive indicator of airway obstruction. The ratio of FEV1/FVC above 80% is normal and below that is considered as abnormal. There is no reduction of TLC (total lung capacity).
- In restrictive lung disease ratio of FEV1/FVC is normal or increased (as total lung capacity may get reduced). In restrictive lung diseases, there is a problem with lung expansion and there is no obstruction to the outflow of air from the lungs **(Fig. 29.1)**.

Q.3. What is the effect of posture on vital capacity?

- Vital capacity is maximum in the standing position and least in the supine position.

- In sitting and supine positions, muscle force of muscle of inspiration is less effective than in standing position.
- In the supine position, abdomen contents push the diaphragm up and affect the mobility of the chest.

Q.4. What is the clinical significance of the estimation of vital capacity?

Vital capacity helps us to assess the ventilatory function of the lungs as well as helps to assess the strength of respiratory muscles. It also helps us to understand if there is abnormal ventilation due to airway obstruction or difficulty in chest expansion. For differentiating obstructive and restrictive lung diseases timed vital capacity is a good test.

Q.5. What is the effect on lung volumes and capacities in obstructive and restrictive lung diseases?

The effect on lung volumes and capacities in obstructive and restrictive lung diseases is shown in **Fig. 29.2**. Further key differences in lung function tests between obstructive and restrictive lung diseases, which can aid in their diagnosis and management are listed below:

Lung parameter	Obstructive lung diseases	Restrictive lung diseases
Total lung capacity (TLC)	Normal/increased (air trapping)	Reduced
Residual volume (RV)	Increased (air trapping)	Decreased
Vital capacity	Frequently decreased (due to increased RV)	Decreased
FEV1/FVC	Decreased	Normal/increased

OBJECTIVE STRUCTURED PRACTICAL EXAMINATION (OSPE)

Procedure station 1: Record the vital capacity of a given subject.

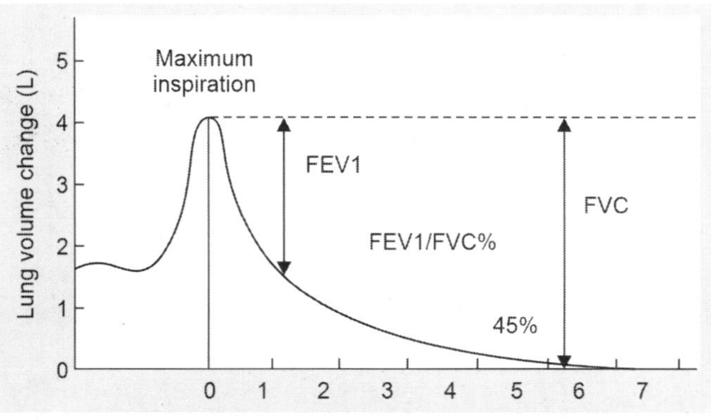

Fig. 29.1: Timed vital capacity

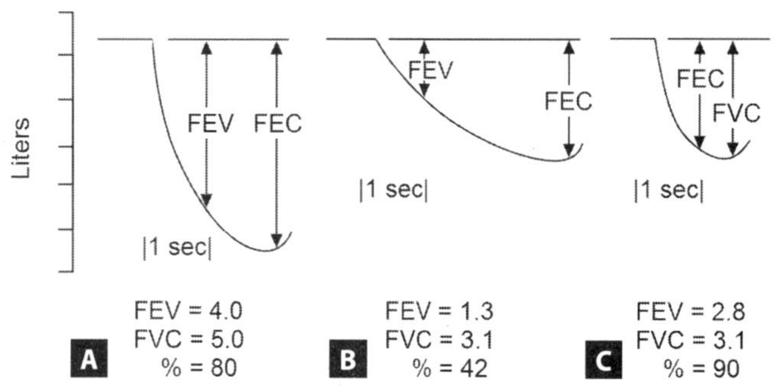

Figs. 29.2A to C: Comparison of vital capacity in normal person, obstructive and restrictive lung diseases: (A) Normal; (B) Obstructive; (C) Restrictive

S. No.	Assessment criteria	Marks assigned	Marks given
1.	Greet and stand on the right side of the subject		
2.	Explain the complete procedure to the subject and keep reading at zero on the spirometer		
3.	Give proper instructions to the subject (as explained in the procedure) and sit		
4.	Instruct the subject to repeat the same procedure three times and take the best reading from that		
5.	Report and viva on clinical examination		
6.	Total		

Procedure station 2: Record the vital capacity of the subject in supine, sitting and lying down positions and give the findings.

COMMON STATIONS – SPOTS IN PRACTICAL EXAMINATION (2/3 MARKS)

Q.1. Graph of timed vital capacity: To identify, and answer any one or two questions from the above.

Q.2. Graph showing reduced FEV1: To identify and enumerate two conditions causing obstructive lung diseases.

CASE-BASED SCENARIO/PROBLEM-BASED (2/3 MARKS)

Case 1: A 10-year-old comes to OPD with difficulty in breathing since morning O/E respiratory rate was 30/min vital capacity – 2.7 l and FEV1– 60%

- What is the probable diagnosis?
- How to find out timed vital capacity?

KEY POINTS TO REMEMBER

- Various physiological and pathological factors affect vital capacity.
- Timed vital capacity helps to differentiate obstructive and restrictive lung diseases.

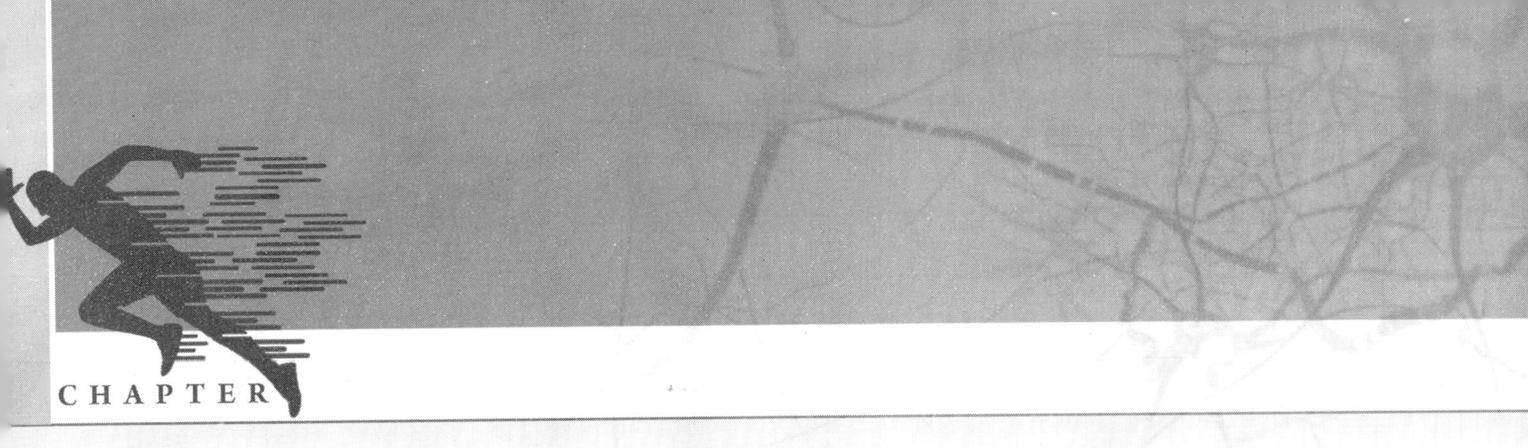

30

Peak Expiratory Flow Rate

Competency:

PY 6.10: Demonstrate the correct technique to measure peak expiratory flow rate in a normal volunteer or simulated environment.

Learning Objectives

At the end of this practical session, one should be able to:
- Define peak expiratory flow rate and tell its physiological significance
- Describe Wright's peak flow meter
- Enlist precautions to be taken before finding out the peak expiratory flow rate

■ INTRODUCTION

Peak expiratory flow rate is clinically significant in distinguishing reversible and irreversible lung conditions. Peak expiratory flow rate is found with the help of Wright's expiratory flowmeter.

Wright's Peak Flowmeter

- The peak flow meter is made up of plastic
- It is a simple and portable device to measure PEFR
- There is a pointer that moves in a slot which is parallel to the scale with numbers calibrated in L/minute
- Endways of the mouthpiece have holes provided for air escape **(Fig. 30.1)**.

Procedure

- Instruct the person to hold the flowmeter in such a way that fingers are not obstructing holes at the end

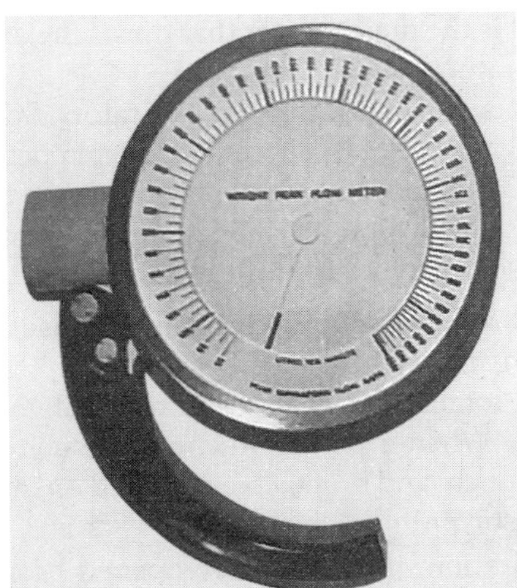

Fig. 30.1: Wright's peak flowmeter

of the apparatus and even not obstructing the scale provided on the flowmeter.
- Ask the person to stand and take a deep breath.
- Place mouth mouthpiece of the flowmeter around the person's mouth.
- Ask the person to blow and exhale rapidly and forcibly.
- There should be no leaks between the mouthpiece and his/her lips when a person is expiring.
- Note the reading on the scale.

Bring the indicator back to zero and record three such readings at one-minute intervals. The maximum value is reported.

Observation/Result

S. No.	PEFR (L/min)
1.	
2.	
3.	

■ IMPORTANT QUESTIONS AND ANSWERS

Q.1. Define peak expiratory flow rate.
Peak expiratory flow rate: It is the maximum flow rate of air with a single forced expiration. Normal PEFR is about 400–550 L/min and in females about 350–480 L/min.

Q.2. Why PEFR cannot go beyond when it reaches a certain maximum value?
- After deepest inspiration, when one expires with great force, the expiratory flow rate reaches its maximum. There is compression of the lungs and alveoli which increases expiratory flow rate and pressure. At the same time, bronchioles also collapse (due to increased outside pressure). This increases airway resistance.
- These opposing forces can no further increase the expiratory flow rate beyond a particular value once it reaches its maximum

Q.3. What is the major factor that limits the expiratory flow rate?
The major factor that limits the expiratory flow rate is the narrowing of small airways (as explained above). Therefore, PEFR reflects lung volume (thus used to assess ventilatory function) and is independent of effort. Thus, PEFR is also called as effort-independent flow.

Q.4. PEFR reduces constrictive lung diseases. Justify.
- With constrictive lung disease, lung volumes become smaller. Total lung capacity and residual volume are reduced. When a person inspires, in such patients, lungs bronchi and bronchioles are held open partially with elastic pull.
- On expiration, these partially opened bronchi and bronchioles do collapse easily by external pressure. This causes a reduction in PEFR.

Q.5. PEFR reduces more with obstructive lung disease. Justify.
- In obstructive lung diseases, it is difficult to expire as there is a tendency for bronchi and bronchioles to collapse. During inspiration, bronchi and bronchioles get distended due to elastic pull caused by negative pleural pressure. Therefore, PEFR is lesser than normal.
- With long-standing obstructive disease, there is the dissolution of alveolar septa causing the development of a larger alveolar sac (emphysema). In such patients even though TLC and RV are more than normal PEFR reduces, as explained above **(Fig. 30.2)**.

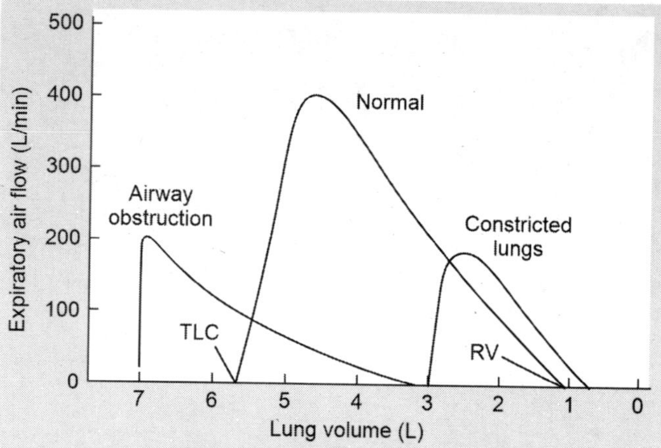

Fig. 30.2: Peak expiratory flow rate

Q.6. What is the significance of measuring PEFR in understanding the prognosis of patients with obstructive lung diseases?
PEFR can be checked in individuals who are on bronchodilators, to assess if PEFR has increased as compared to before the start of bronchodilator treatment (e.g. In a patient, If PEFR is about 150 L/min and with bronchodilators it is about say 300 L/min).

Q.7. What are the precautions that have to be taken while recording PEFR?
Precautions:
- There should be no leakage from the mouthpiece
- Subject has to be instructed to expire rapidly, forcefully, and completely in mouth mouthpiece.
- Results are affected by an individual's motivation and muscle power.

■ OBJECTIVE STRUCTURED PRACTICAL EXAMINATION (OSPE)

Procedure station 1: Record PEFR using wright's peak flow meter.

S. No.	Assessment criteria	Marks assigned	Marks given
1.	Check out the apparatus and pointer		
2.	Explain the procedure to the patient regarding how to operate the instrument		
3.	Explain the significance of avoiding air leaks from the mouthpiece		
4.	Make sure the subject holds the apparatus correctly in hand (explained above)		
5.	Instruct the subject on how to inhale maximum and how to exhale rapidly, forcefully and completely through a mouthpiece		
6.	Report findings and viva on clinical examination		
7.	Total		

COMMON STATIONS – SPOTS IN PRACTICAL EXAMINATION (2/3 MARKS)

- **Instrument:** Identify and answer any one or two questions as given above.
- Write the physiological significance of doing this test.

CASE-BASED SCENARIO/PROBLEM-BASED (2/3 MARKS)

Case 1: A patient comes with breathlessness. His Peak expiratory flow rate was found to be 200 L/min.

- Comment on the finding. Write normal level of PEFR in healthy males.
- What are the causes of reduced PEFR?

Case 2: A person comes to OPD for a follow-up. He is on prescribed bronchodilators for about 15 days. His PEFR done before treatment was 150 L/min and now after 15 days, you find his PEFR to be 300 L/min.

- Why does PEFR reduce asthma? What is its physiological basis?
- What is the physiological basis behind giving bronchodilators?

Electrocardiography (ECG)

Competency:
PY 5.13: Record and interpret normal ECG in a volunteer or simulated environment.

Learning Objectives
After completion of the practical, the students shall be able to:
- Define electrocardiography (ECG)
- List uses of ECG
- Identify different waves and intervals of ECG with their physiological basis
- Calculate heart rate from the ECG
- Classify different ECG leads
- List precautions required before recording ECG

■ INTRODUCTION
It is a method of recording the electrocardiogram (ECG). An electrocardiogram is the machine with which one records ECG. It is one of the important diagnostic tests. It is a graphic recording of the electrical activities of the heart. Electrical changes occurring in the heart are conducted all over the body and are picked up if electrodes are placed at appropriate positions.

Principle
Electrical activities generated within the heart are conducted from heart to body surface, which are picked up by electrodes and recorded as ECG.

Apparatus
ECG machine, ECG paper, leads, and cardiac jelly

ECG Machine
- ECG machine records electrical activities of heart.
- It has cathode ray tube which is amplifier recording system.
- Machine has got main switch, lead selection switch, calibration switch, and start or stop switch that regulates paper speed.

ECG Paper
- ECG paper has surface that is coated with wax and has big and small squares.
- Each small square is 1 mm × 1 mm. Every 5th line is heavily marked forming large squares.
- ECG is recorded at paper speed of 25 mm/second. Each smallest square vertically measures 0.1 mV. Each smallest square horizontally measures 0.04 seconds.
- Recording stylus gets heated automatically and this melts the coating of the wax on the ECG paper. So, black line is recorded across the paper **(Fig. 31.1)**.

Limb Electrodes
Limb electrodes are metal plates which are flat and can be fixed to body surface by clip type of clamps. Red, green, black, and yellow are the colours of the electrodes. Chest electrodes are metal cups that are fixed to body surface by suction produced by rubber bulbs.

Cardiac Jelly
This helps in establishing proper contact between electrode plates and body. Cardiac jelly helps to decrease resistance between skin and electrodes.

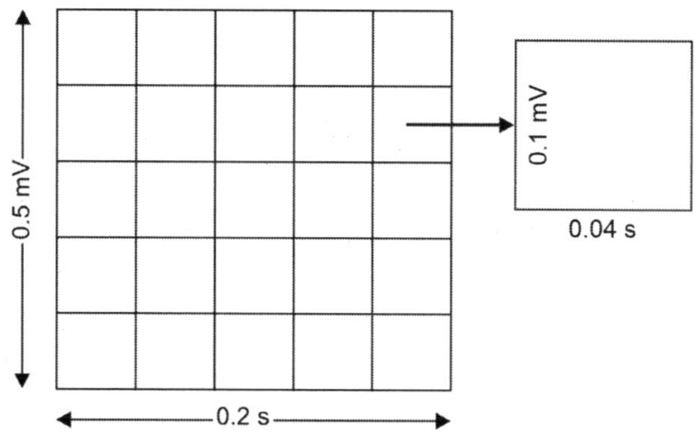

Fig. 31.1: ECG paper

ECG Leads

ECG is recorded normally in:
- Unipolar limb leads
- Bipolar limb leads
- Chest leads/precordial leads

Bipolar Limb Leads

Bipolar limb leads are lead I, lead II, and lead III **(Fig. 31.2)**.

Lead I

For recording ECG in lead I, the negative terminal of the electrocardiograph is connected to the right arm (RA) and positive terminal to the left arm (LA). A positive wave is recorded in ECG when RA is negative with respect to LA.

Lead II

For recording ECG in lead II, the negative terminal of the electrocardiograph is connected to the right arm and positive terminal to the left leg (LL). A positive wave is recorded in ECG when RA is negative with respect to LL.

Lead III

For recording ECG in lead III, the negative terminal of the electrocardiograph is connected to the left arm and the positive terminal to the left leg. A positive wave is recorded in ECG when LA is negative with respect to LL.

Einthoven's Triangle

Einthoven's triangle is a diagrammatic way of illustrating that the two arms and left leg form apices of a triangle surrounding the heart. It is the equilateral triangle with right and left shoulders and left leg as three apices. The right leg serves as a ground connector. All four electrodes must be attached to the extremities **(Fig. 31.2)**.

Unipolar Limb Leads

- Two electrodes are used for recording purposes. One is active (exploring electrode) placed on the body surface and the other is an indifferent electrode, which is kept at zero potential.
- Unipolar limb leads are augmented vector right (aVR), augmented vector left (aVL), and augmented vector foot (aVF).
- V stands for vector and R, L, and F indicate that the exploring or active electrode is on the right arm, left arm, and left foot, respectively.

Unipolar Chest/Precordial Leads

- There are six chest leads named from V1 to V6
- Chest leads employ an exploring electrode on the chest surface
- Position of exploring electrode in different leads are:
  - Lead V1 in the right fourth intercostal space near the sternum
  - Lead V2 in left fourth intercostal space near the sternum
  - Lead V3 halfway between V2 and V4
  - Lead V4 in left fifth intercostal space in the midclavicular line
  - Lead V5 in left fifth intercostal space at anterior axillary line
  - Lead V6 in left fifth intercostal space in midaxillary line **(Fig. 31.3)**.

Precautions before Recording ECG

- Subject should be relaxed.
- Right foot should be connected for grounding.
- Ensure proper application of leads at their places and good contact with the body surface.
- Jelly must be applied at the placement of electrodes to decrease resistance.
- Standardization and position of stylus must be checked before recording ECG.

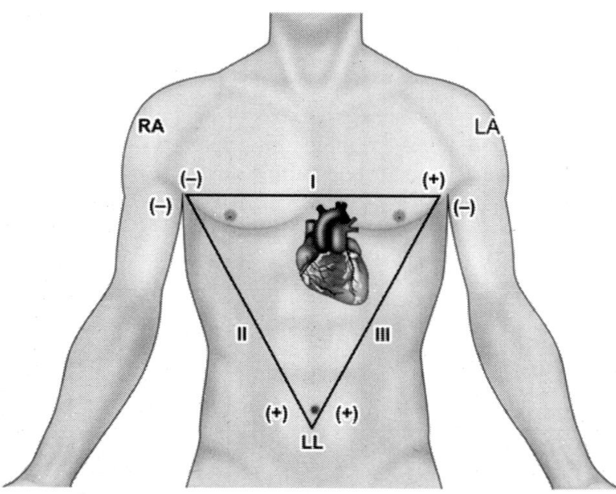

Fig. 31.2: Bipolar limb leads

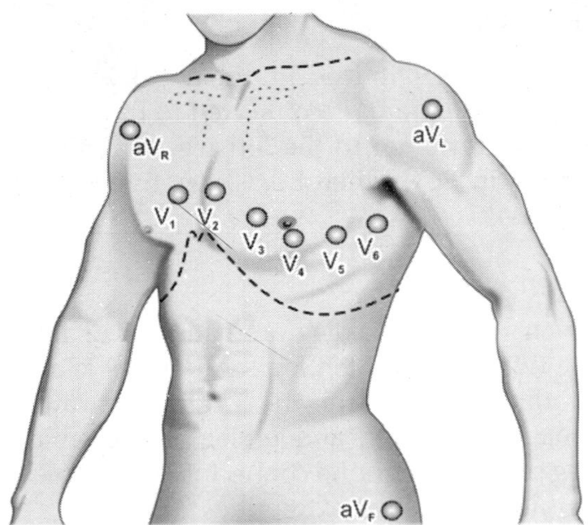

Fig. 31.3: Unipolar chest leads

Procedure

- Subject should relax and should lie down.
- Check that the instrument is satisfactorily earthed.
- Apply jelly around the left and right wrist, left leg, and right leg. Connect electrodes in position.
- Switch on the machine and keep the stylus at the centre of the paper.

- Record ECG in different leads. Study and interpret ECG
- Characteristic features of ECG waves are shown in **Table 31.1**.

■ IMPORTANT QUESTIONS AND ANSWERS

Q.1. What are different waves and intervals in ECG?
Please refer to **Fig. 31.4** and **Table 31.1**.

Q.2. Enumerate the uses of ECG.
Uses of ECG

- It provides information about the position of the heart in the chest and also the relative size of different chambers of the heart.
- It helps to detect ischemia of the myocardium.
- It helps to know the location, extent, and progress of myocardial infarction.
- It helps to diagnose various degrees of heart blocks.
- It helps to analyze abnormal rhythms and electrolyte abnormalities of the heart.

Q.3. How can one calculate heart rate from ECG?

- When the rhythm of the heart is regular, the heart rate can be calculated in two ways from the ECG. Usually, heart rate means ventricular heart rate.

TABLE 31.1: Normal waves and intervals in ECG

ECG component	Cause	Duration	Remarks
P-wave	Atrial depolarization	0.8–0.1 second	Normally inverted in aVR P wave absent or low amplitude in atrial fibrillation
Isoelectric period	-	0.04 second	-
QRS complex (ventricular complex)	Ventricular depolarization	0.08–0.12 second	Q-wave indicates septal depolarization R-wave indicates depolarization of ventricles S-wave indicates depolarization of basal parts of ventricles Broad or long QRS complex observed in ventricular hypertrophy, bundle branch blocks
ST segment	-	0.04–0.08 second	Measured from end of the S-wave to the beginning of the T-wave At the beginning of the ST segment lies J point
T-wave	Ventricular repolarization	0.27 second	T wave changes were observed with myocardial infarction, and ischemia
U-wave	Slow repolarization of papillary muscle	0.08 second	-
Intervals in ECG			
PR interval	Atrial depolarization and conduction in bundle of HIS	0.13–0.16 second	Measured from beginning of P-wave to beginning of R-wave (As Q wave is small, instead of PQ, PR interval is preferred.) PR interval is prolonged in different degrees of heart block
QT interval	Ventricular depolarization and repolarization	0.40–0.43 second	Measured from beginning of Q-wave to end of T-wave
RR interval	time interval during successive ORS complexes	0.83 second	It helps to measure ventricular rate (heart rate)
PP interval	Time interval between successive P waves	-	It helps to measure atrial rate
ST interval	Ventricular repolarization	0.32 second	Measured from end of S-wave to end of T-wave
J point	Point between end of S wave and beginning of ST segment	-	Point of no electrical activity

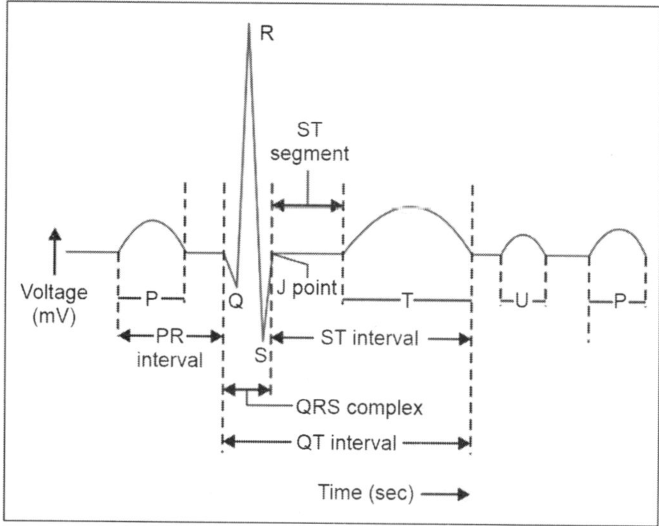

Fig. 31.4: Normal waves and intervals in ECG

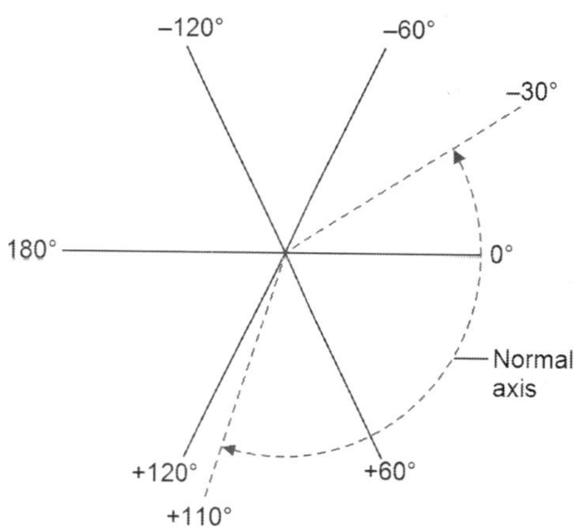

Fig. 31.5: Right and left axis deviation

- Heart rate per minute is 1500/number of small squares between two successive R waves. This is because 1500 small squares represent one minute (1 small square = 0.04 s)
- RR interval is measured in a number of small squares and by multiplying these squares by 0.04s, the time duration of the RR interval is found out.
- Thus, heart rate = 60 seconds (one minute)/duration of RR intervals in seconds. Normal heart rate varies from 60 to 100 beats/minute.

Q.4. Enumerate precautions taken before recording ECG.

Please refer above.

Q.5. Enumerate common conditions that alter normal waves and intervals in ECG.

- **P wave:**
  - P wave can be absent in atrial fibrillation, atrial flutter, hyperkalemia
  - With left atrial enlargement P wave can be wide and notched
  - A tall and peaked p wave is recorded with right atrial enlargement.
- **QRS complex:**
  - Wide and bizarre QRS complexes are recorded with ventricular fibrillation
  - With hypertrophy of the left ventricle QRS complex may be wide
  - High voltage QRS complex seen with ventricular hypertrophy
  - Low voltage QRS complex is noted with pericardial effusion, myxedema
- **Pathological Q waves:** They are recorded with a height almost close to R waves and are a sign of old myocardial infarction or unstable angina.
- **T waves:** Tall T waves indicate acute myocardial infarction and hyperkalemia. Inverted T waves can be

physiological in young children. Otherwise, they are seen with bundle branch block, myocardial ischemia
- **Abnormalities of ST segment:** ST segment elevation is seen with acute myocardial infarction and ST segment depression is a sign of myocardial ischemia
- **Prolonged QT interval:** It is seen if a person is on antiarrhythmic drugs, hypokalemia

Q.6. Enumerate common conditions causing sinus bradycardia and sinus tachycardia.

- Physiological variations in heart rate are discussed in the chapter Examination of Arterial Pulse
- **Sinus bradycardia**: It is seen in athlete (vagal tone), heart block, drugs (beta-blockers)
- **Sinus tachycardia**: It is seen with fever, anxiety, cardiac failure.

Q.7. What is the right and left axis deviation?

- **Right axis deviation:** When QRS complex in lead I is predominantly negative (dominant S in lead I) and ORS complex in aVF is predominantly positive (dominant R in aVF). It is said to be a right axis deviation **(Fig. 31.5)**.
- **Left axis deviation:** When QRS complex in lead I is predominantly positive and negative in aVF then it is left axis deviation.
- Normal axis of the heart lies in the direction of the mean QRS vector, i.e. between -30 to +110 degrees. Any deviation that falls to the left of -30 degrees is left axis deviation and any axis that falls to the right of +110 degrees it is right axis deviation.

COMMON STATIONS – SPOTS IN PRACTICAL EXAMINATION (2/3 MARKS)

Q.1. ECG instrument: Identify and enumerate its clinical uses.

Q.2. ECG leads: Identify and define lead. What are bipolar limb leads?

Q.3. ECG paper: Identify and write its use.

Q.4. ECG showing PR interval, how much is the duration of PR interval in a given ECG? Write its physiological significance.

Q.5. ECG recording: Measure heart rate from given ECG. What is sinus arrhythmia? (clue-increase heart rate with inspiration and decrease with expiration).

Q.6. Diagram of chest leads. Write the anatomical location of lead V4.

Q.7. ECG diagram. Ask to show J point. Write its physiological significance. (clue-J point is isoelectric even if a current of injury is present).

Q.8. Identify the rhythm in ECG. What is a pacemaker of the heart? What is its physiological basis? (clue-normally when the SA node is a pacemaker it is the P wave which is followed by the QRS complex which is followed by the T wave).

▌ CASE-BASED SCENARIO/PROBLEM-BASED (2/3 MARKS)

Case 1: A 69-year-old obese male patient comes with c/o chest pain which is radiating to left shoulder. On examination, pulse– 90/minute and BP– 150/90 mm of Hg. On recording ECG, ST segment elevation is seen.

- What is your probable diagnosis?
- What is the cause of the raised ST segment?
- What can be the reason for the pain radiating to the left arm?

Case 2: Mr ABC comes for a regular checkup. He has been known hypertensive for the last 20 years and takes medicine regularly, when ECG was taken:

- Comment on the axis of the heart.
- What can be the probable cause of left axis deviation? (clue-left ventricular hypertrophy as a consequence of long-standing hypertension).

▌ KEY POINTS TO REMEMBER

- ECG records the electrical activity of the heart with the help of ECG machine.
- ECG is recorded in different leads.
- With the SA node as a pacemaker, we get a normal waveform in a sequence of P wave followed by QRS complex and followed by T wave.
- J point is always isoelectric.
- Various abnormalities in waves and intervals of ECG can be noticed in various clinical conditions.

Tests for Physical Fitness

Competency:

PY 3.15: Demonstrate the effect of mild, moderate and severe exercise and record changes in cardiorespiratory parameters.

PY 3.16: Demonstrate the Harvard step test and describe the impact on induced physiologic parameters in a simulated environment.

Learning Objectives

At the end of the practical, the students shall be able to:

- Describe the importance of studying changes in physiological parameters with exercise
- Describe the effect of exercise on different body systems and apply a physiological basis to the changes observed
- List indications and contraindications for cardio-pulmonary efficiency tests
- List various degrees of exercise and differentiate between isotonic and isometric exercises

■ INTRODUCTION

Physical activity and exercise have proven role in imparting health benefits. It is very important for a would be doctor to understand the fundamentals of exercise, the grading of exercise and how different energy systems work depending upon type, grade, intensity and duration of exercise.

It is also important to understand the difference between physical activity and exercise. Various body systems work together when the body is subjected to exercise. Various acute and long-term changes happen in the body, especially with respect to the cardiorespiratory system with exercise. Cardiorespiratory fitness becomes one of the most important parameters of physical fitness. The cardiorespiratory response of a person who is trained (to do exercise) is different than untrained person.

Physical Activity and Exercise

Physical activity: It is defined as any bodily movement produced by skeletal muscles that requires energy expenditure.

Exercise: It is defined as a structured, planned, repetitive and purposeful activity performed in order to maintain or improve one or more components of physical fitness. Depending on the rate of O_2 consumption, increase in heart rate, work done exercise is classified into mild, moderate and severe grades (WHO grading of exercise).

Physical fitness: It is defined as the set of attributes that people have or achieve and physical fitness is defined as the ability to carry out daily tasks with vigour, alertness without undue fatigue with ample energy to enjoy leisure time pursuits and to meet unforeseen emergencies. It comprises cardiorespiratory endurance, muscle endurance, muscle strength, flexibility, balance, agility and coordination.

Exercise

I. Mild, moderate, and severe exercise – (WHO grading of Exercise)

Grade/level of exercise	Heart rate/min	O₂ consumption (L/min)	Relative load index (% of max O₂ consumption)	Metabolic equivalent task (MET)
Mild	Less than 100	0.4–0.8	Less than 25	Less than 3 METs
Moderate	100–125	0.8–1.6	25–50	3.0 to 4.5METs
Heavy	125–150	1.6–2.4	51–75	4.6–7 METs
Severe	More than 150	More than 2.4	More than 75	More than 7 METs

VO₂ max: Maximum O_2 consumption.

RLI: Relative load index- O_2 consumption as a percentage VO₂ maximum.

MET: O_2 consumption in multiples of basal O_2 consumption.

List of common exercises that are graded as mild, moderate and severe		
Mild	**Moderate**	**Severe**
• Leisure cycling • Sitting while using the computer • Light work with standing • Playing instruments • Walking at 2 miles/hr	• Cycling at 10 to 12 miles/hr • Brisk walking at 3 miles/hr • Badminton • Climbing 2 flights of stairs	• Basketball • Carrying heavy loads • Tennis singles • Soccer game • Running at 6 miles/hr • Cycling at more than 16 miles/hr

II. Types of exercise - Isotonic and isometric (different way response of cardiovascular system)

Isotonic exercise: In this type of exercise there is a change in the length of the muscle with no change in muscle tension, e.g. walking, or jogging.

Systolic BP increases and diastolic BP does not change much and with moderate to severe exercise diastolic BP falls (as blood flow to exercising muscles increases).

Isometric exercise: In this type of exercise, there is no change in muscle length but muscle tension increases, e.g. pushing against the wall. In this type of exercise, exercising muscle remains contracted throughout. In this type of exercise initially heart rate increases. Both systolic and diastolic BP increases. As muscle remains in a contracted state throughout, there is no increase in blood flow to exercising muscles, which increases the peripheral resistance and hence diastolic BP.

▌ BASIC TESTS FOR TESTING CARDIOPULMONARY EFFICIENCY

Apparatus: Stopwatch, Harvard's steps, stethoscope, BP apparatus.

1. Measurement of pulse rate, respiratory rate and blood pressure– In different body positions:
Change in posture does affect the function of the cardio-respiratory system, i.e. pulse rate, BP and respiratory rate are measured when the person is supine (lying down), standing changes in all three parameters are noted down.

Procedure

- Ask the subject to lie down in a supine position for about 5 minutes.
- Record pulse rate, respiratory rate and BP of the subject in a lying down position.
- Ask the subject to stand (do not remove the BP cuff) and immediately record the pulse rate, BP and respiratory rate of the subject.
- Record findings of pulse rate, respiratory rate and BP after 2 minutes after standing, and after 5 minutes of standing. (Refer to chapter 22).

Observations

Posture	Pulse rate (beats/ minute)	Respiratory rate (breath/ minute)	Blood pressure (mm Hg)
Supine (lying down)			
Immediately on standing			
2 minutes after standing			
5 minutes after standing			

2. Breath-holding test: One can test inspiratory breath-holding. Breath-holding time can vary from person to person and can vary with practice, respiratory muscle endurance and the psychology of a person.

Procedure

- Ask the subject to sit and explain the procedure
- Ask him to take expire maximum and then take maximum inspiration and hold the breath as much as he/she can hold the breath (without discomfort) count the period with the help of stop watch. Normal inspiratory breath holding is 45 to 55 seconds.

3. Harvard step test: This is a simple test to estimate and analyze person's cardiorespiratory efficiency and general fitness of the person.

Procedure

- Subject (male) is made the step up and down on a 20-inch-high (51 cm) bench (step) 20 times per minute for about 5 minutes

- Subject (female) is made the step up or down on 18 inches high (41 cm) bench (step) 20 times/minute for about 5 minutes
- At the end of 5 minutes ask the subject to sit. Count the pulse rate immediately.
- Then record pulse rate for one to one and half minutes, two to two and half minutes and three to three and half minutes, i.e for 30 seconds
- Calculate the **Harvard fatigue index** which gives us an idea about the fitness level of the person
- If the subject is not able to perform exercise for 5 minutes, note the duration till which he/she can do exercise.

$$\text{Harvard fatigue index} = \frac{\text{Duration of exercise in seconds}}{2 \times (\text{sum of pulse count during recovery})} \times 100$$

Normal recovery time is 5 minutes in a normal person after exercise.

Harvard fatigue index	Fitness level
Below 55	Poor
55–84	Low average
65–69	Average
80–89	Good
90 and above	Good

Observations

Name	Age	Sex
Height in cm	Breath holding time	
	Pulse BP	Respiratory rate
Posture -		
Lying down Sitting Standing		
Exercise		
Mild	Immediate after 5 minutes	
Moderate	Immediate after 5 minutes	
Severe	Immediate after 5 minutes	

■ IMPORTANT QUESTIONS AND ANSWERS

Q.1. What is the Harvard step test? How much is the normal Harvard fatigue index?

The Harvard step test is explained above. The normal Harvard fatigue index is 100%.

Q.2. What is the Master's step test?

Master's step test

- The basal pulse rate of the subject is noted.

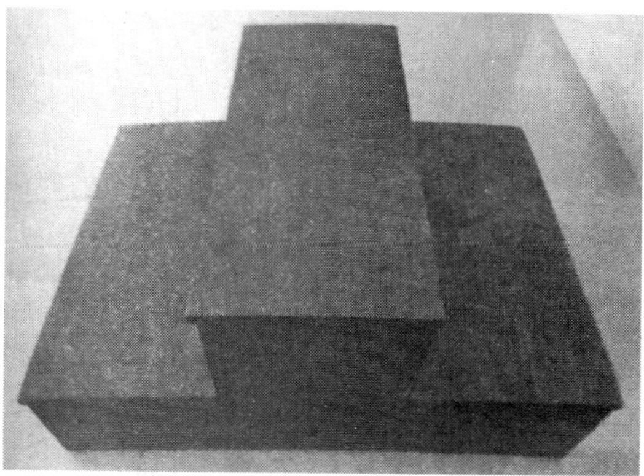

Fig. 32.1: Master's step test

- Subject is asked to step up and down on a platform of 9 inches in height, 12 times/minute.
- Pulse rate is noted immediately after exercise. The recovery time for the pulse rate to come to a normal level is noted.
- The experiment is repeated by increasing the frequency of steps to 18, 24, and 30 per minute. The amount of work is standardized for age, weight and sex. The pulse rate is noted after each time and the recovery time for the pulse rate to come to normal is also recorded. In a normal person, the pulse rate comes to normal (initial values) within 5 minutes **(Fig. 32.1)**.

Q.3. Enumerate the effects of acute and regular exercise in the body.

System	Effect of acute exercise	Effect of regular exercise
Cardiovascular system		
Heart rate	Increases with the severity of exercise	• Heart rate falls due to (parasympathetic predominance in trained people)
Stroke volume	Increases	• Increase in cardiac output is a product of an increase in stroke volume, precise sympathetic stimulation, and functional hypertrophy of myocardium
Cardiac output	Increase even up to 25 L/min (from normal of 5 L/min)	
Systolic BP	Rises	
Diastolic BP	Does not change/fall	
Pulse pressure	Increases	
Peripheral resistance	No change/increase or decrease depending on the type of exercise	• Cardiac output can go beyond 35 L/min (with not much change in heart rate)
Effect on skeletal system and circulations		
Muscle blood flow	Blood flow to skeletal muscle increases Decrease in cutaneous and splanchnic circulation	• Increase in the number of mitochondria • Increase in enzymes of oxidative metabolism

Contd...

Contd...

System	Effect of acute exercise	Effect of regular exercise
		• Increase in size of muscles • Increased number of capillaries • Better efficient extraction of O_2 from tissues • Effective disposal of metabolic end products

Effect on respiratory system

	• Increase in respiratory rate (hyperventilation) • More removal of metabolic end products • Increase in respiratory minute volume and work done • Better perfusion of alveoli	• Due to training, there is an increase in respiratory endurance which overall increases breathing capacity and VO_2 max • There is better cardiac output, better O_2 extraction from tissues and better work efficiency of respiratory muscles

Besides the effect on the cardiorespiratory system, in a trained individual there is a better increase in metabolism and body temperature. Response of the autonomic nervous system, endocrine system and efficient utilization of energy by carbohydrates, fats and proteins in a trained person than an untrained individual.

Q.4. What is the clinical significance of doing exercise?

• Exercise or any form of physical activity has proven health effects and is considered one of the important lifestyle interventions by a physician when it comes to dealing with various lifestyle-inflicted diseases.
• Exercise has a key role in health as well as disease. It has got its multiple benefits on various body systems right from cardiovascular and respiratory to CNS, gut health, and immune system to cardiometabolic health to sleep and much beyond.
• Exercise has its benefits at all levels of prevention (primary, secondary, and tertiary levels).
• Exercise helps to keep away from a lifestyle disease by controlling various risk factors like obesity, hyperlipidemia, hypertension, insulin resistance, etc. This is the **primary level of prevention**.
• If a person is having a particular disease, then exercise as prescribed by physician helps an individual to keep control of the progress of the disease and prevent its secondary complications, e.g. good glycemic control with proper diet and exercise helps to prevent kidney damage. This is **a secondary level of prevention.**

• Exercise does play an important role as it helps limit morbidity and mortality from a disease (due to multiple health benefits) and helps people avoid the tertiary level of treatment in hospitals. **This is the tertiary level of prevention.**

Till today there is no pharmacological alternative available for exercise.

Q.5. Enumerate modern cardiopulmonary efficiency tests.

Modern cardiopulmonary efficiency tests are:

• **Treadmill test**: A person is made to exercise to his/her 90% of maximal heart rate, which is calculated from the person's age sex, and physical training. Complete assessment of a person and basic lab tests are required before performing the test.
  – **With computerized treadmill testing** even simultaneous recording ECG is possible while graded exercise is performed by a person. And VO_2 max can be estimated by assessing cardiorespiratory fitness.
  – Most used is **Bruce protocol**, where a change in speed and inclination of the treadmill with respect to the grade of exercise is assessed.
  – Monitoring of ECG continues for about 6 to 8 minutes after the testing is over. The person's return of heart rate and BP to baseline is assessed, as ECG changes (if any e.g. ST segment) and their return to baseline and time taken to come to normal is recorded.
• **Bicycle ergometer:** This test is used when a person is not able to use the treadmill.
• **Colour Doppler test:** It can be done to assess vessels and the heart. It can test any blockage in vessels, functioning of valves of veins, heart, etc.

Q.6. Enumerate indications and contraindications to exercise testing.

Indications for exercise testing	Contraindications to exercise testing
• Evaluation of physical fitness • Evaluation of functional capacity of the heart • Screening test for coronary artery disease	• Unstable angina • Uncontrolled hypertension • Acute myocardial infarction • Congestive cardiac failure

Q.7. What is VO_2 max?

VO_2 max is the maximum oxygen a person's body can utilize during exercise. It indicates the aerobic power of an individual. VO_2 max is thus a good predictor of athletic performance. VO_2 max may vary with the age, gender and fitness level of the person.

Q.8. Enumerate other tests for pulmonary efficiency.

Other tests to assess pulmonary efficiency include vital capacity, timed vital capacity, % of breathing reserve and maximum voluntary ventilation.

Q.9. Define MET.

Metabolic equivalent of task (MET) is an objective measure of a ratio of the rate at which a person expends energy relative to the mass of that person, set by convention at 3.5 ml of O_2 per kg per minute.

Q.10. List down criteria to terminate exercise testing in a person.

Criteria to terminate exercise test:

- Symptoms of angina
- Excess rise in BP
- Shortness of breath/difficulty in breathing
- Any bodily discomfort/subject requests to stop
- Lightheadedness, nausea
- Technical issues with the treadmill machine.

▌COMMON STATIONS – SPOTS IN PRACTICAL EXAMINATION (2/3 MARKS)

Q.1. Treadmill/bicycle ergometer: Identify and write its use.

Q.2. Harvard step test: Identify/write its procedure and the significance of finding it.

Q.3. Harvard step test and subject can be given: Find out Harvard fatigue index in him.

Q.4. Enumerate acute changes with exercise.

Q.5. With isotonic exercise peripheral resistance increases. Give the physiological basis.

▌CASE-BASED SCENARIO/PROBLEM-BASED (2/3 MARKS)

Case 1: An MBBS student was made to do a step test for 5 minutes. His systolic BP changed from 110 mm Hg at rest to 140 mm Hg post-exercise. There was a slight drop in his diastolic BP.

- What are the changes in the cardiovascular system with acute exercise?
- Enumerate another test to assess cardiorespiratory fitness.

Case 2: A 30-year-old male weighing 90 kg and with a BMI of 32 came for a computerized treadmill test.

- What are the things that you would like him to do before you give him an appointment for exercise testing?
- Enumerate the health benefits of exercise.

33

Perimetry

Learning Objectives

At the end of the practical students should be able to:
- Describe the perimeter chart
- Define and determine the field of vision
- Enumerate various factors affecting the field of vision
- Trace visual pathways and name the physiological basis of vision loss at various levels
- List precautions for performing perimetry

■ INTRODUCTION

The part of an external world that can be seen with one eye at any given instance is the field of vision of the eye. The process of charting the monocular field of vision is called perimetry. Clinically field of vision is tested by the confrontation method (please refer to Chapter Examination of Cranial Nerves I to VI). There can be different defects that are noticed in the field of vision due to lesions in various areas of the visual pathway.

Perimeter (Fig. 33.1)

The perimeter consists of the following parts:
- **Stand**: Stand helps to give stability to the instrument. It does support the arc. Its vertical limb is broad.
- **Chin rest**: Patient's head is supported on chin rest. It is adjustable. The right-hand cup of chin rest is used when one is examining the left eye and vice-versa.

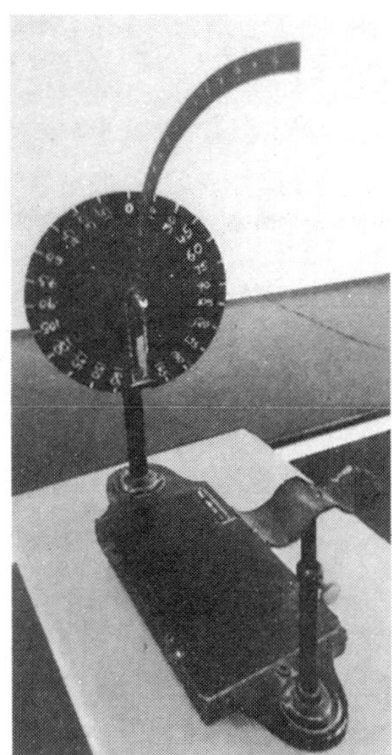

Fig. 33.1: Perimeter

- **Arc of the circle**: A metal arc is shaped in a large arc of a circle with concavity towards the patient. Arc (which is movable and calibrated in degrees and scale is marked on a convex surface) is pivoted in the centre so that it can rotate through each meridian.
  Irrespective of the placement of the object at any point on the arc the angle it subtends with the fixation axis at the eye may be read. The arc may be rotated about a horizontal axis into any required meridian.
- **Perimeter chart**: On this chart field of vision of each eye is plotted. The field of vision is depicted by a circle which is divided into a number of segments by

meridians. The concentric circle denotes the degree of each meridian. The chart is fixed to a wooden disc which is attached to the handle of the arc and it moves with it. From the chart meridian on which the arc is positioned can be made out.

Procedure

- Ask the subject to sit on the stool with chin resting on a chin rest.
- Adjust the chin rest in such a way that the line joining the fixating eye and centre of the arc is horizontal. The distance between the centre of the arc and the fixating eye is 33 cm.
- Position the arc in the frontal plane on zero meridian and fix the chart on the disc.
- Move 5 mm size white object from periphery towards the centre till the person perceives the object.
- At this point note recording in degrees on arc and mark on chart in that specific meridian
- Repeat the procedure to take 7 more readings, i.e. 45°, 90°, 135°, 180°, etc. on the temporal and nasal sides respectively **(Fig. 33.2)**.
- Join plotted eight points to get the field of vision for a particular eye. In the same way plot field of vision of another eye. By using different colours, the field of vision of different colours can also be plotted.

- Keep the arc at 100° meridian in the temporal side to mark the blind spot. Move the object from periphery to centre. When an object disappears from his/her visual field mark that area on the chart.
- Then the object is still moved towards the centre by about 10° the person starts seeing the object again. Mark this point as well on the chart.
- Join two points to make a circle which indicates a blind spot for a particular eye.

Precautions

- Test one eye at a time and cover the other eye while testing one.
- Confirm adequate illumination in the room.
- Explain procedure to the person whose eye are being tested.
- Person if wears glass, they should be removed as they affect the field of vision.
- Do mapping in the clockwise direction.

■ IMPORTANT QUESTIONS AND ANSWERS

Q.1. Define the field of vision. Describe the extent of the normal field of vision.

Field of vision: It is an area seen by an eye at a given instant.

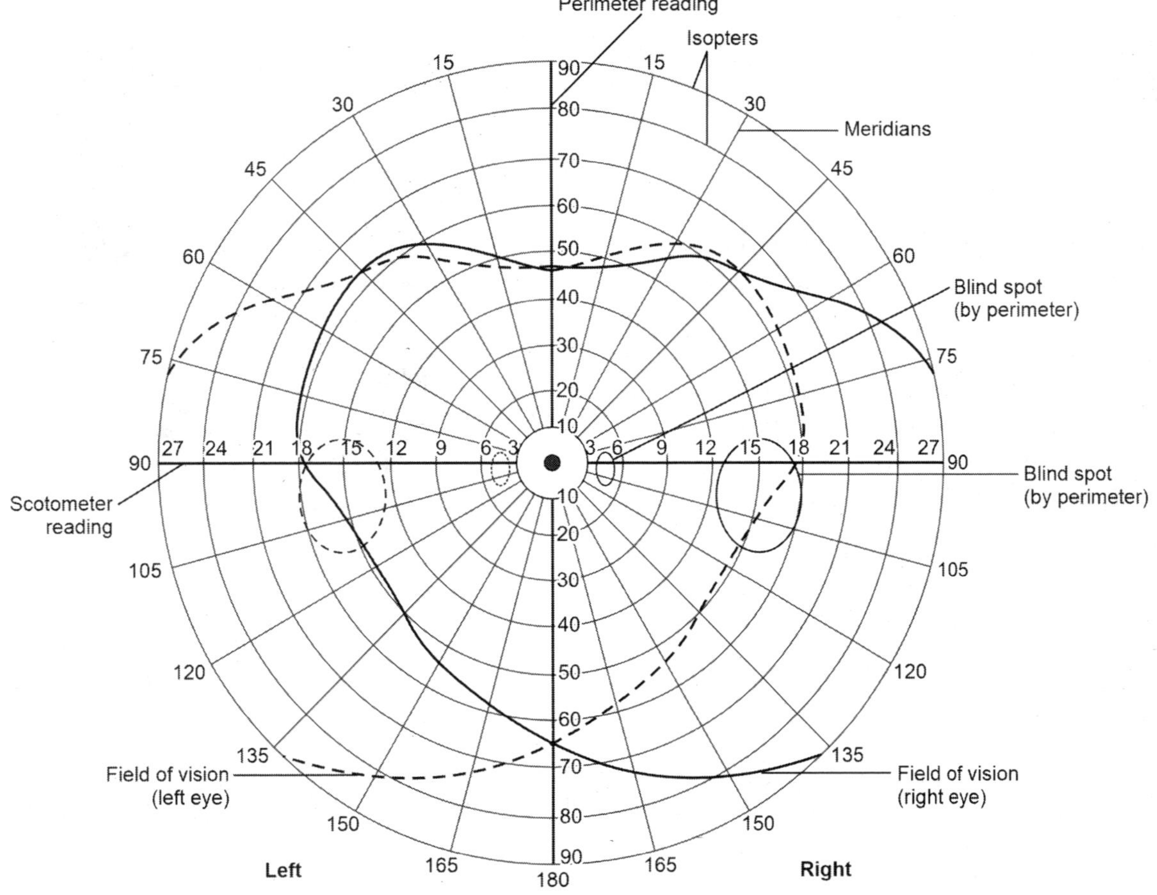

Fig. 33.2: Perimeter chart

Normal field of vision for white objects extends up to 100°, 56°, 60° and 75° on temporal, superior, nasal, and inferior sides respectively.

Q.2. Enumerate other methods to determine the field of vision.

The field of vision can also be determined by the confrontation method. It provides a rough estimate of the field of vision.

Q.3. What is a physiological blind spot? What is its significance?

Physiologic blind spot, do exist in every normal person. It corresponds to the entry of the optic nerve in the eye. In this area, there is complete absence of photoreceptors. Along with the optic nerve, even blood vessels enter the eye via this region.

Thus, the optic disc is the area which is located 3 mm medial and slightly above the posterior pole of the eye through which optic nerve and blood vessels enter the eye. Any image falling on optic disc is not visible as there are no rods and cones in the optic disc. The centre of the chart does correspond with the visual axis.

Q.4. Describe the visual pathway.

Visual pathway: Neurons (from bipolar and ganglion cell layer of retina) travel as optic nerves then carried in optic chiasma (where there is crossing over of fibres). Fibres coming from temporal side of retina (that receives information from nasal side of visual field) do cross and fibres from nasal side of each retina (that carries information from temporal half of visual field) do not cross to form optic tract **(Fig. 33.3)**. Thus, each optic tract contains temporal field of same side and nasal field of opposite side. Most of the fibres in optic tract terminate in lateral geniculate body of thalamus. From here via geniculocalcarine tract they reach visual cortex.

Q.5. Which region of the retina is not tested with perimetry?

The macular region which contains fovea centralis cannot be tested with perimetry. This region contains only cones and is a region of most acute vision.

Q.6. What is homonymous hemianopia?

Hemianopia means loss of sight in one half of the visual field. When the same half of both the fields is lost is called homonymous hemianopia. Lesion of the optic tract/optic radiation especially produces homonymous hemianopia. This type of hemianopia is also seen with tumours of the parietal or temporal lobes **(Fig. 33.4)**.

Lesion on right side produces left homonymous hemianopia and lesion on left side produces right homonymous hemianopia (homonymous- means right half of field of one eye and right half of field of another eye).

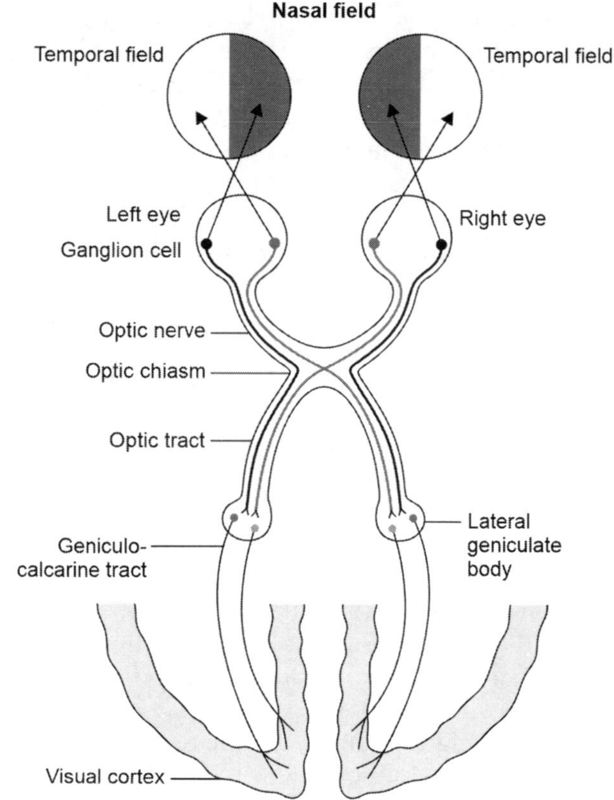

Fig. 33.3: Visual pathway

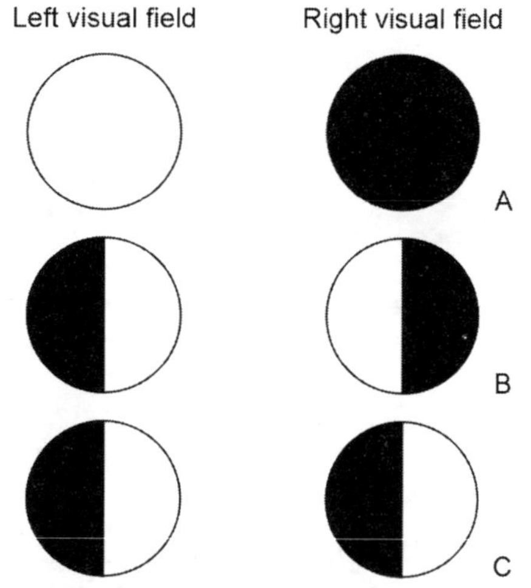

Fig. 33.4: Defects in visual pathway

Q.7. What is heteronymous hemianopia?

Hemianopia means loss of sight in one half of the visual field. When opposite sides of the visual field are lost it is called as heteronymous hemianopia.

Q.8. What is bitemporal hemianopia?

Bitemporal hemianopia: There is loss of loss of vision in the temporal halves (outer) of both fields.

Cause: Loss of function of the nasal half of each retina. This is seen with lesions of optic chiasma involving crossed fibres (e.g. pituitary gland tumour).

Q.9. What is binasal hemianopia?

Binasal hemianopia: There is loss of vision in the nasal halves (inner) of both fields.

Cause: Loss of function of the temporal half of each retina. This is seen with bilateral lesions of uncrossed fibres in optic chiasma.

Q.10. What is scotoma?

Any blind spot on the retina except a normal blind spot is called a scotoma.

Q.11. Enumerate factors affecting the field of vision.

Factors affecting the field of vision are:

- Size of the object
- Brightness of the object
- **Colour of the object:** It is best for white colours compared to other colours. It goes on decreasing for blue, yellow, red and green in the same order.
- **Illumination:** Poor illumination can decrease the visual field.

OBJECTIVE STRUCTURED PRACTICAL EXAMINATION (OSPE)

Procedure station 1: Determine field of vision of right/left eye.

S. No.	Assessment criteria	Marks assigned	Marks given
1.	Greet and stand on the right side of the subject		
2.	Explain the complete procedure to the subject		
3.	Follow all precautions (as given above)		
4.	Give proper instructions to the subject (as explained in the procedure) and make him/her sit		
5.	Report and viva on clinical examination		
6.	Total		

COMMON STATIONS – SPOTS IN PRACTICAL EXAMINATION (2/3 MARKS)

Q.1. Diagram/instrument of perimeter and perimetry chart: To identify and comment. Answer any one or two questions from the above.

Measurement of Reaction Time to Visual and Auditory Stimulus

Learning Objectives

After completing this practical, the students shall be able to:
- Demonstrate measurement of auditory and visual reaction time
- Explain the procedure to demonstrate the same
- Enlist factors affecting reaction time

■ INTRODUCTION

We do react to changes in the environment. Any change in the environment is perceived by sense organs. Reaction time is the time interval between the application of a stimulus and the appearance of the response. In the experiment, auditory and visual reaction time is determined. It also helps assess the pathway, i.e. afferents and efferents of the reaction path.

Principle

Reaction time helps to judge the ability of the person to concentrate and coordinate. Repeated practice can reduce the reaction time.

Procedure

An electric bell or bulb is connected to the circuit. Two keys are put in the circuit, one is operated by the observer and the other by the subject. When both keys are closed (by the observer) circuit is completed and the bulb is lighted or the bell rings.

The subject opens the key as soon as he/she sees the light or hears the bell. Both these points, i.e. lighting of the bulb (closing of the circuit) and light becoming off (due to opening of the key by the subject) are marked by the time marker. The time interval between these two points is the reaction time of the person.
- Procedure is explained properly to the subject
- Practice trials are given and final readings are taken. Normally, 3 to 4 readings are taken and the average is calculated
- Time interval is measured with the help of a tuning fork of 100 cps.

Observation and Calculation (Fig. 34.1)

Tuning fork = 100 cps

1 cycle = 0.01 seconds

Therefore, the reaction time in the graph
$$= 12 \times 0.01$$
$$= 0.12 \text{ seconds}$$

Computerized testing of reaction time: Nowadays a computer can help in the assessment of reaction time. Subjects sit in front of the keyboard and on the screen, one understands if it is an auditory or visual stimulus. With the visual mode change in the colour of the box and with auditory mode buzzer will be sounded and the subject is supposed to press with the change in colour and hearing of buzzer.

■ IMPORTANT QUESTIONS AND ANSWERS

Q.1. What is the difference between reaction time and reflex time?

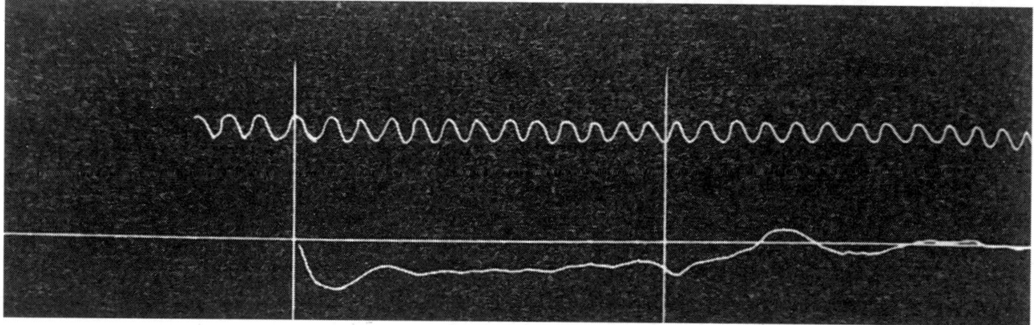

Fig. 34.1: Measurement of reaction time

Reaction time is the time interval between the application of stimulus and the appearance of response. It depends on the emotional state and concentration of a person.

Reflex time is not dependent on a person's ability to concentrate and thus not affected by stress or emotional state reflex time is always less than reaction time.

Q.2. What are the factors affecting reaction time?
Factors affecting reaction time are:

- **Emotional state**: Ability of a person to concentrate and focus and coordinate. Any emotional upset or stress thus can reduce reaction time.
- **Length and type of nerve fibre**: Reaction time does include conduction time via afferents and efferents. Thus, it depends on the type and length of the afferent and efferent nerve fibres.
- **Number of synapses**: Reaction time depends on number of synapses involved. More the number of synapses involved more is the reaction type.
- **Number of sense organs stimulated**: The more the number of sense organs stimulated, the lesser the reaction time.

- **Type of stimulation of sensory modality**: Reaction time is shorter when auditory stimulus is used (normal 0.12 to 0.18 seconds) than visual reaction time (normal 0.19 to 0.22 seconds).
- **Fatigue**: Reaction time is prolonged if a person is fatigued.
- **Intensity of stimulus**: An increase in intensity of stimulus may reduce reaction time to some extent.
- **Number of receptors stimulated**: The greater the number of receptors stimulated, the shorter is latent period and thus shorter is reaction time.
- **Practice**: Repeated practice does reduce the reaction time.

COMMON STATIONS – SPOTS IN PRACTICAL EXAMINATION (2/3 MARKS)

Q.1. Identify the graph. Calculate reaction time. Enumerate factors affecting reaction time.

Q.2. Measure auditory and visual reaction time in a given subject and write your findings.

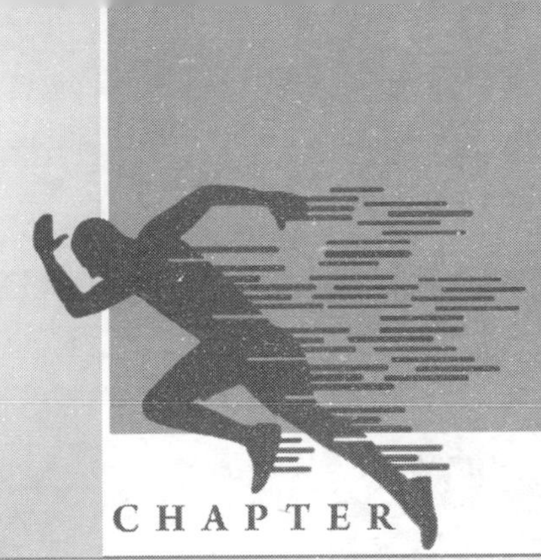

35

Electromyography (EMG)

Learning Objectives

At the end of this practical, the students shall be able to:
- Define EMG
- Describe the physiological basis of studying electro-myography
- Enumerate indications of EMG
- Define motor unit
- Enumerate factors affecting motor end plate potential

■ INTRODUCTION

With the help of electromyography, we can record the electrical activity generated by muscle fibers and motor units with muscles at rest and during muscle contraction. This record can be obtained by placing electrodes on the surface of the muscle or by inserting needle electrodes in the muscles. EMG is useful in the diagnosis of various clinical conditions. Abnormal EMG can be recorded in denervation, disorders of NM junction, and disorders of muscle (different types of myopathies).

Apparatus

Cathode ray oscilloscope (CRO), recording electrodes, electrode paste/jelly, spirit, amplifier and oscilloscope.

Electrodes

Needle electrodes, surface electrodes.

Procedure

- EMG can be recorded with the subject lying in a supine position on a couch.
- If you are recording EMG using surface electrodes, the skin overlying has to be cleaned first and then using electrode paste, electrodes are placed on specific areas of the muscle.
- Usually, one electrode is active, one is the reference electrode and the third electrode is for grounding. Recording of different muscles in different positions (e.g. flexion, extension, supination, pronation, etc.) and with gradual increase in force of contraction of muscles.
- If you are recording EMG by inserting a needle in muscles, inform the patient accordingly and then go on inserting the needle in the depth of muscle in a stepwise manner.
- Activity evoked in muscle by insertion/movement of the needle and with different strength of muscle contraction are recorded.

Precautions

- The subject should be given proper instructions and he/she should be asked to relax completely
- Subject should be grounded properly.

Observation/Result

- At rest no electrical activity is recorded from muscle.
- When a muscle contracts changes in potential can be recorded.

- A burst of electrical activity is observed with the insertion of a needle in the muscle.
- Miniature end plate potential is recorded when the needle reaches near end plate region. These are monophasic negative waves of about 100 mV and for not more than 2 m sec duration.
- As the strength of contraction increases, more and more motor unit potential (MEU) is recorded (as with the increase in muscle contraction, more motor units get recruited).

■ IMPORTANT QUESTIONS AND ANSWERS

Q.1. Define motor unit.
Motor unit: It is defined as an alpha motor neuron along with its axon and the number of muscle fibres it innervates. This constitutes one motor unit. Each motor unit is the functional unit of skeletal muscle. Each muscle is made of a number of motor units **(Fig. 35.1)**.

Q.2. What is motor unit potential? Give its characteristics.

Motor unit potential: It is a potential change that is produced by the excitation of muscle fibres of a motor unit **(Fig. 35.2)**.

Characteristics

- When we insert the needle in muscle, many muscle fibres do fire simultaneously and thus MUP has higher amplitude and long duration.
- **Strength of contraction**: A strength of contraction increases, more and more motor units get recruited and accordingly MUP frequency increases from mild to severe muscle contraction.
- **Normal duration** of MUP is 5 to 10 msec. Duration of MUP depends on the conduction velocity of nerve

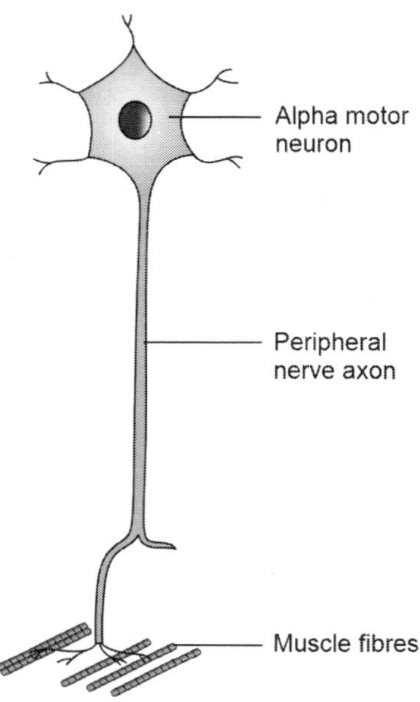

Fig. 35.1: Motor unit

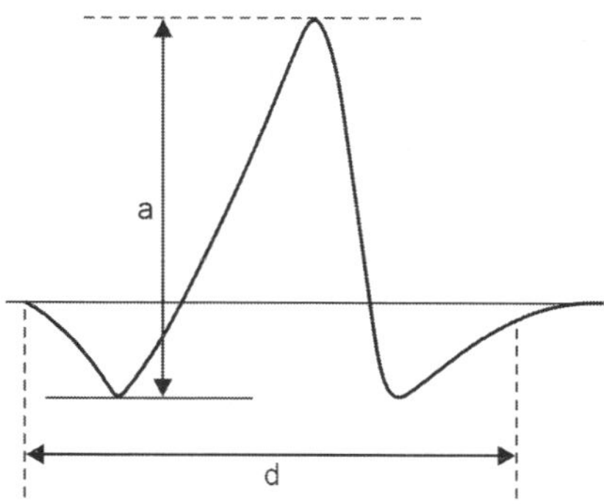

Fig. 35.2: Normal motor unit potential (a-Amplitude and d-Duration)

fibres, length of muscle fibres, and excitability of membrane. Therefore, MUP can vary in different clinical conditions as well.
- **Normal amplitude** of MUP is about 0.5 to 2 mV. It can vary with the age of a person, temperature of muscle and type of muscle fibres.
- **Phases of MEU**: With needle electrode when we record MUP it shows triphasic action potential (positive- negative- positive sequence). If more than three potentials are recorded it indicates some myopathies.

Q.3. Enumerate factors affecting motor unit potential.
Factors affecting MUP:
- **Age:** With more age, the amplitude, and duration of MUP do increase however firing rate decreases.
- **Type of needle** used and its location affect MEU. The amplitude of MUP is smaller when it is superficial and it goes on increasing as one goes deep in the muscle
- **Equipment settings:** MUPs can vary with respect to equipment settings and method of recording EMG.

Q.4. Resting muscles are electrically silent. Give physiological basis.
When muscle is at rest, all muscle fibres are at the resting membrane potential. This is why when you place recording electrode on surface of muscle there is no potential difference recorded as muscles are electrically silent.

When muscles receive signals from nerves which then travels across the neuromuscular junction leading to spread of signal to interior of muscle and muscle contraction.

Q.5. What are the different types of motor unit potentials (MUP)?
Types of MUPs:
- **Long-duration MUPs:** Long-duration MUP is associated with high amplitude. It is seen in neuropathies, and motor nerve damage/diseases.

- **Short-duration MUPs**: Short-duration MUPs are associated with low amplitude. They are seen in neuromuscular junction disorder and myopathies.
- **Mixed pattern MUPs**: They show a combination of short as well long duration MUPs.

Q.6. What is spontaneous activity in muscles?

Normally, muscles at rest do not show any electrical activity. However as mentioned above, with the insertion of a needle and miniature end plate potential is recorded in the end plate zone. Besides this otherwise spontaneous activity may be recorded with fibrillations or fasciculations of the muscle.

Q.7. What are fibrillations?

This is spontaneous muscle activity that is recorded from a single muscle fibre. They are commonly observed with diseases of neuromuscular junction or anterior horn cell diseases. A single fibre may fire at a rate of 1 to 15 Hz and amplitude even going to 22 microvolts.

Q.8. What are fasciculations?

These are spontaneous muscle activities that are recorded from a number of muscle fibres innervated by a motor unit. The motor unit is the functional unit of skeletal muscle.

Fasciculations can happen randomly and depending on the number of motor units involved its size and shape can vary. Fasciculations many times can be benign (physiological) or can be seen with amyotrophic lateral sclerosis.

COMMON STATIONS – SPOTS IN PRACTICAL EXAMINATION (2/3 MARKS)

Q.1. Diagram of normal motor unit potential—Identify and describe it. Write its characteristics.

Q.2. Enumerate different types of MUPs.

Q.3. Normal duration of MUPs is a measure of what?

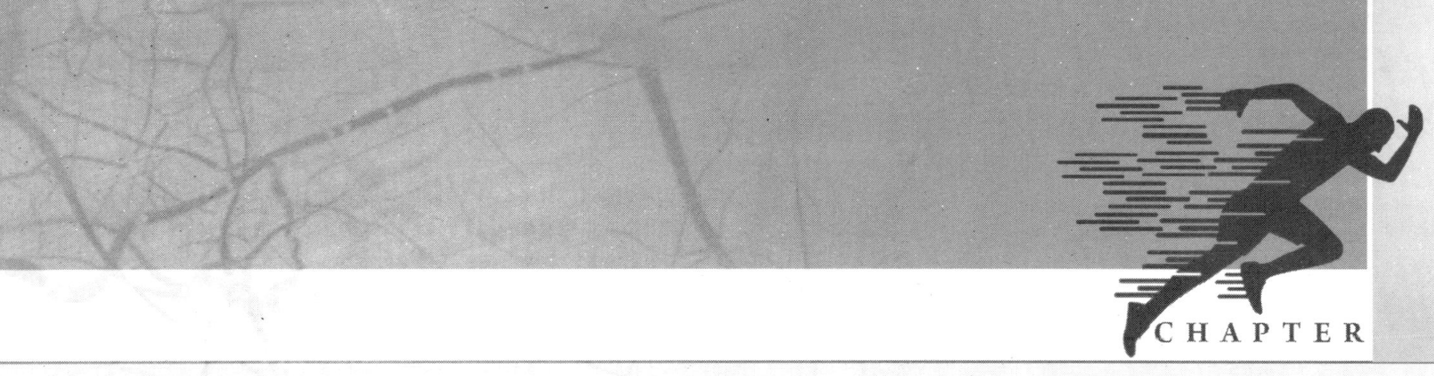

Nerve Conduction Studies

Learning Objectives

At the end of this practical, the students shall be able to:
- Describe the clinical significance of doing nerve conduction studies (NCS)
- Classify different types of nerve fibres with their functions
- Differentiate between sensory and motor nerve conduction
- Enumerate factors that affect nerve conduction
- Describe normal compound muscle action potential (CMAP)

■ INTRODUCTION

Nerve conduction studies are one of the important neuro-diagnostic tests. Sensory and motor nerve conduction helps to diagnose a variety of clinical conditions that affect functions of the nerve, neuromuscular junction, and muscle itself.

For most of the neuromuscular diseases, NCS helps to assess the peripheral nervous system. Responses can be recorded along peripheral sensory and motor axons. The response does show latency, amplitude, velocity, and duration of responses. With the help of the above parameters, one can identify abnormal conditions.

■ MOTOR NERVE CONDUCTION

Apparatus

Cathode ray oscilloscope, electronic stimulator, recording and stimulating electrodes, silver ring electrodes and spirit swab, electrode jelly.

Procedure

- Subject sits comfortably on a chair. The recording electrode, ground and surface electrodes are connected to the system.
- The site where the electrode is to be placed is cleaned and a jell is applied on the area where the electrode is to be placed to facilitate conduction.
- Motor nerve conduction requires stimulation of motor or mixed nerves. It is a record of motor action potentials from the muscle that is supplied by the nerve with help of surface electrodes.
- The active electrode is placed over abductor pollicis brevis, while the reference electrode is about 3 cm away from the active electrode and the ground electrode is placed between the two electrodes. The recording electrode is connected with CRO.
- Give supramaximal stimulus and obtain a response.

Observations

- With motor nerve conduction studies, there is stimulus artifact at the beginning, followed by latent period and biphasic muscle action potential (with initial negativity) or compound muscle action potential is recorded. Motor nerve responses range in millivolts.
- **Characteristics of CMAP**: It shows onset latency, duration, amplitude of biphasic AP.

Onset latency	It is the time from stimulus artifact to the first negative deflection. It indicates the time taken for NM transmission and excitation-contraction coupling
Amplitude of AP	It is measured from baseline to peak or between negative and positive peaks **(Fig. 36.1)**
Duration of AP	It is measured from onset to final return of wave to the baseline
Normal values	The median nerve (humans) normal velocity is 55 to 65 m/seconds

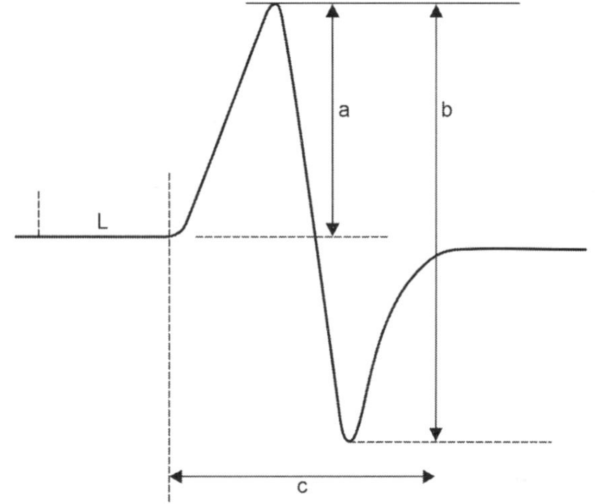

Fig. 36.1: Compound muscle action potential (L-latency, a and b - amplitudes, c-duration of CMAP)

■ SENSORY NERVE CONDUCTION

Apparatus

Cathode ray oscilloscope, electronic stimulator, recording and stimulating electrodes, silver ring electrodes and spirit swab, electrode jelly.

Procedure

- Subject sits comfortably on the chair. Recording electrode, ground and surface electrodes are connected to the system.
- The site where electrode is to be placed is cleaned and a jell is applied to the area where the electrode is to be placed to facilitate conduction.
- NCS can be done by electrically stimulating a pure sensory nerve percutaneously and recording sensory action potentials (SNAP) in specific nerve proximally or distally. The SNAP amplitude and conduction velocity are measured.
- Stimulation of the nerve at two different sites helps to find out conduction velocity between the two sites.
- The active electrode is placed on the middle phalanx and the other on the terminal phalanx, the recording electrode is placed about 3 cm apart (proximal to the wrist joint (near the skin crease and a ground electrode is placed between the two and all connected to CRO.
- Give supramaximal stimulus and obtain a response.

Observation

- With sensory nerve conduction studies sensory nerve action potential is recorded **(Fig. 36.2)**. Sensory nerve responses range in microvolts.
- SNAP has stimulus artefact, onset latency, amplitude, and duration as that of motor nerve conduction.
- Normal value – 50 to 65 m/seconds.

For most of motor conduction studies. Belly tendon montage is used where active electrode is placed on the belly of the muscle, the reference electrode on the tendon of the muscle and stimulator placed on nerve. Normal nerve requires current in range of 20–50 mA for supramaximal stimulation

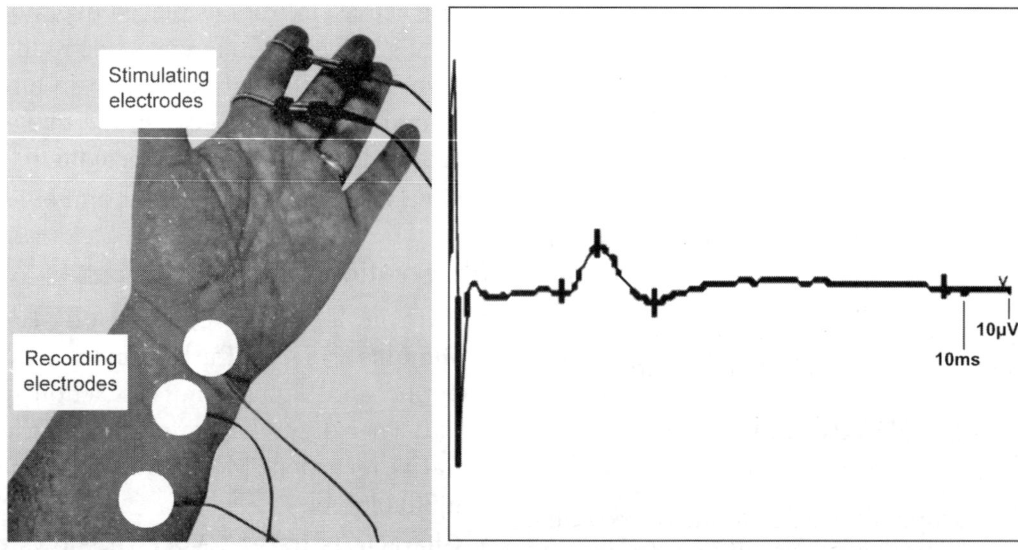

Fig. 36.2: Sensory nerve action potential (SNAP). Median orthodromic sensory study

■ IMPORTANT QUESTIONS AND ANSWERS

Q.1. Enumerate common indications for nerve conduction studies.

Common indications for NCS are:

- For diagnosis of dysfunction of the peripheral nervous system from peripheral nerve roots to NM junction to muscle.
- NCS also helps to understand if the disease is static or dynamic and the underlying pathophysiology of the same.
- NCS can also be advised to monitor the progress of diseases like multiple sclerosis.
- Any person in whom decompression of an entrapped nerve is suggested should get NCS done before surgery.

Q.2. What is the principle of NCS?

NCS involves activating the nerves electrically over a peripheral nerve and then producing:

- Propagation of nerve action potential (NAP) that is recorded at a distant point over the same nerve and compound muscle action potential (CMAP) that is obtained due to activation of muscle fibres supplied by the same nerve.
- Nerves can be stimulated by skin stimulators or by a needle placed close to the nerve root. The choice of stimulation is the area above and below the proposed area of focal lesion and the anatomical availability of appropriate structure for the same.
- PNS have different types of nerve fibers (afferents, efferents, myelination, diameters can be varied) NCS helps to document focal or continuous abnormality in the length of mixed, sensory or motor nerves. We try to asses, if conduction velocity, the gradient of conduction velocities and CMAP size and alterations if any.

Q.3. What are F waves?

- When motor nerve axon is stimulated, an action potential is propagated in both directions away from the site of stimulation.
- Distally propagated impulse gives rise to CMAP and impulse also conducts proximally to anterior horn cells causing depolarization of axon hillock and axon to backfire that leads to small additional muscle depolarization recorded as F wave. The latency and shape of F waves may vary depending on a number of neurons that backfire.
- Absence of F waves with nerve stimulation in response to normal evoked CMAP from same muscle indicates conduction block/recent axon loss proximal to point of stimulation of nerve.
- F waves are prolonged in demyelinating neuropathies.

Q.4. Which nerves are studied most in NCS?

NCS studies are commonly done in upper limbs for medial, ulnar and radial nerve and in lower limbs for femoral, peroneal, sciatic, tibial, and sural nerve.

Q.5. What factors can influence the recording of action potential?

Factors influencing the record of action potential are:

All the below factors can alter the shape, size, amplitude, and duration of the action potential.

General/Technical factors:

- Distance between active and reference recording electrodes
- Distance between the point of stimulation and to recording site
- Filter settings adjusted while recording
- Positioning of active or reference electrodes

Physiological factors:

- **Age**: Conduction velocity is low in infants and comes to adult level by about 5 years of age. Gradual loss of neurons with age (after 60 to 65 years) does cause decline in conduction velocity.
- **Gender**: Nerve conduction is more in males as compared to females.
- **Temperature**: As muscle temperature falls, SNAP, CMAP amplitude, duration, rise time, latency all increase (cooling is known to delay voltage-gated Na^+ channels inactivation and leading to excess depolarization).
- **Upper and lower limbs**: In upper limbs conduction velocity is higher than lower limbs. Length of nerves is more in upper limbs than lower limbs. The axonal diameter of nerves in lower limbs is lesser compared to upper limbs.

Q.6. What are the effects on motor NCS with axon loss?

- Most obvious abnormality with axon loss is reduced amplitude of CMAP (few functioning motor axons are connected to muscle fibres). As myelin is not affected, the remaining axons conduct normally which help to maintain latency and conduction velocities normal.
- With increasing axonal loss, some largest conducting fibres may be lost causing distal motor latency to get prolonged and even conduction velocity to reduce.
- However, if the axonal loss is very slow (as in generalized neuropathy) there can happen (collateral reinnervation via sprouting of unaffected axons) and CMAP may remain normal.

Q.7. What is the effect on motor NCS with demyelination?

With the loss of myelin nerve conduction slows down and if the loss is severe enough there is complete loss of salutatory conduction (conduction block). There is prolonged motor latencies observed. Changes do depend upon the site and extent of demyelination.

Q.8. What is the effect on sensory NCS with a generalized disorder of nerves?

In axonal as well as demyelinating pathologies, SNAP amplitude is reduced. Distribution of sensory NCS are helpful in determining etiology.

Neuropathies can involve only one nerve, i.e. mononeuropathy or many nerves, i.e. polyneuropathy.

Q.9. What are the features of the conduction block?

Conduction block is seen in demyelinating diseases. A drop in CMAP area is seen which is more than 50% and even noticeable reduced amplitudes are observed between proximal and distal stimulation sites.

Q.10. What are the symptoms of polyneuropathy?

- Axonal polyneuropathy usually starts with sensory symptoms like tingling and burning distally in feet. Symptoms gradually spread proximally to the calf and ankle leading to loss of ankle reflex. Once sensory loss reaches the knees, numbness of fingers is seen. This pattern results in a 'stocking-glove' distribution of sensory and motor findings.
- Demyelinating neuropathies do not show such a 'stocking-glove' type of loss but reflexes are lost and nerves often become abnormally palpable (as they enlarge).

Q.11. Define Carpal Tunnel syndrome and tarsal tunnel syndrome?

- **Carpal tunnel syndrome**: It is the most common **median entrapment neuropathy**. The median nerve is a mixed nerve and supplies flexors of the forearm (no innervation in the upper arm). After supplying muscles in the forearm, via the carpal tunnel, the nerve enters the hand to supply lumbricals I and II, flexor and abductor pollicis brevis and opponens pollicis. During the course of median nerve in carpal tunnel compression neuropathy occurs. This decreases the conduction velocity of median nerve (especially distal to site of compression). Carpal tunnel syndrome is common with hypothyroidism, acromegaly, more use of wrist (excess computer work).

- **Tarsal tunnel syndrome**: Similar to the median nerve, in lower limbs tibial nerve entrapment neuropathy via nerve passing via causes tarsal tunnel syndrome.

Q.12. What is sciatic neuropathy?

The sciatic nerve is the largest nerve in the body. Sciatic neuropathy is common in fracture/dislocation of hip joint or hip replacement surgery.

▮ COMMON STATIONS – SPOTS IN PRACTICAL EXAMINATION (2/3 MARKS)

Q.1. Diagram of SNAP or CMAP: To identify and label and any of the above questions can be asked.

Q.2. Electrodes can be kept: Identify and write about recording procedure and placements of electrodes.

Q.3. F waves: Identity in a given picture – Write its physiological significance.

▮ CASE-BASED SCENARIO/PROBLEM-BASED (2/3 MARKS)

1. A person with a known case of multiple sclerosis.
   - What are you likely to observe if NCS is done in him?
   - Give the physiological basis of your expected findings.
2. A 58-year-old diabetic patient complaining of numbness in the thigh, medial leg and foot. He was referred for NCS by a family physician.
   - Which nerves in the lower limbs you would like to test?
   - Femoral nerve conduction study showed small CMAP amplitude. What can be its physiological basis? (Clue-femoral neuropathy)
   - Describe normal characteristics of CMAP.
3. A 43-year-old female c/o bilateral hand numbness, and weakness for about one month. She works in an office with 7 to 8 hours of computer work. The doctor suggested her get NCS done.
   - What is your probable diagnosis? (Clue-carpal tunnel syndrome)
   - Which nerves in the upper limbs can be tested with NCS?

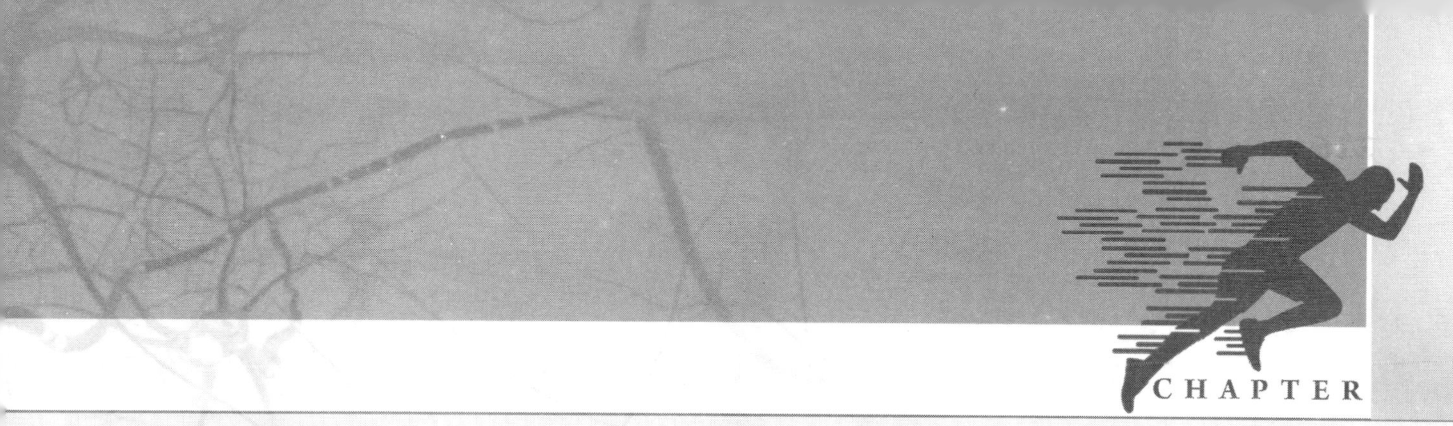

Electroencephalogram (EEG)

Competency:
PY 10.12: Identify normal EEG forms.

Learning Objectives

At the end of this practical, the students shal be able to:
- Define EEG and enumerate different waves of normal EEG
- Describe physiological basis of EEG
- Describe various normal waves in EEG
- Enumerate various clinical applications of EEG

■ INTRODUCTION

- EEG is a record of the brain's spontaneous electrical activity. This electrical activity is generated in the cerebral cortex and is picked up by electrodes that are placed on specific areas of the scalp and after amplification are recorded on paper or displayed on a monitor and recorded electronically. Electroencephalogram is the machine by which we record electroencephalogram. The records can be unipolar or bipolar.
- Potential changes recorded in EEG are due to the flow of current in fluctuating dipoles on cell bodies and dendrites of cortical cells.

Hans Berger in 1929 demonstrated electrical activities in the brain and labelled them as electroencephalogram.

Procedure

- Place a person in whom you are recording EEG in a recumbent position with neck support.
- Place electrodes with the international 10–20 system of electrode placement.
- Record EEG of the person with open eyes and then closed eyes (Even the effect of light and tactile stimuli can be recorded in EEG).
- In patients whose sleep study is done overnight, EEG is recorded as one of the important components of sleep study.
- In such subjects, EEG waves during different types of sleep can be recorded.
- Normal EEG records the alpha, beta, theta, and delta rhythm of waves. These waves are classified based on the amplitude and frequency of the waves. The normal range of frequency for EEG waves is 1 to 30 Hz and amplitude is about 20 to 100 microvolts.

Electrode Placement

- The standard set of electrodes used to record EEG are 22 in number. This included even ground electrodes. International 10–20 system of placement of electrodes uses the distance between body landmarks on the skull–nasion (bridge of the nose), inion (occipital protuberance at the back of the head) and pre-auricular points **(Fig. 37.1)**. Each site of electrode is labelled with a letter and number. Even numbers represent the right side and odd numbers represent the left side of the head.

Alphabetical Abbreviations

F= Frontal, C= Central, P= Parietal, Fp= Frontopolar, T= Temporal= Occipital, A= Auricular

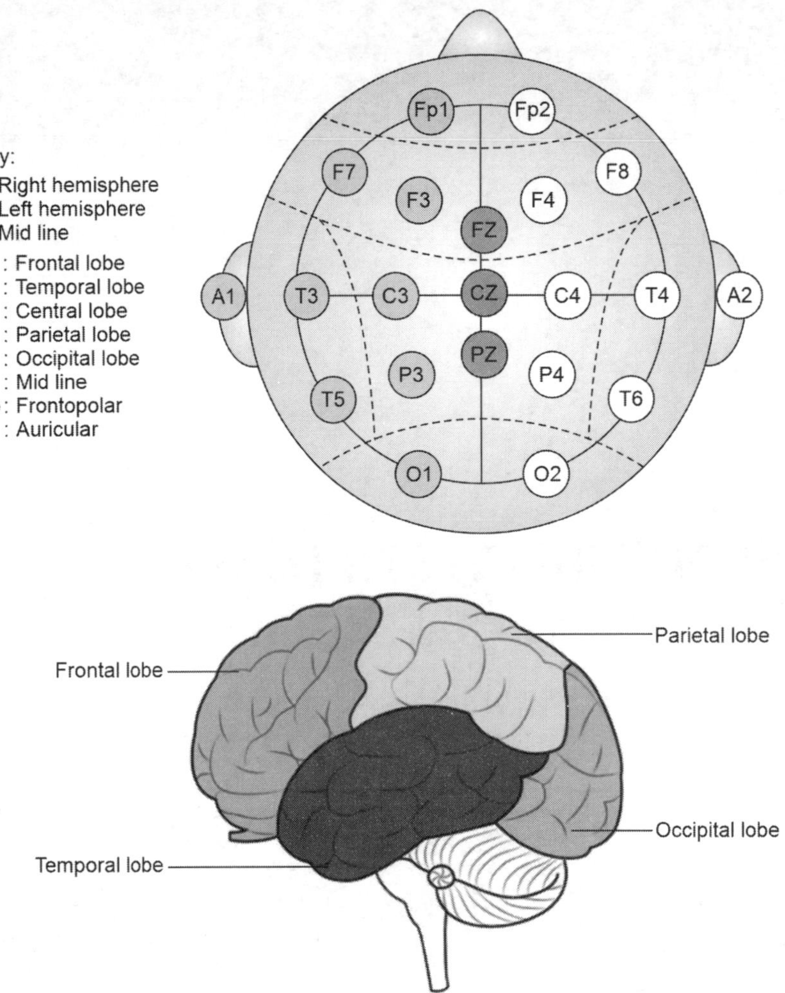

Fig. 37.1: International 10–20 system placement of electrodes

TABLE 37.1: Different types of EEG waves based on their frequency, amplitude, and the characteristics associated with their occurrence.

EEG wave	Frequency (Hz)	Amplitude (µV)	Characteristics
Alpha	8–13	50–100	Waves generated mainly in parieto-occipital region Recorded during rest or meditation Represents resting state of electrical activity EEG in this rhythm is said to be synchronized (due to synchronizing effect of densely packed dendrites in cortex
Beta	13–20	5–10	Waves generated mainly with eyes open Waves generated mainly in posterotemporal head regions
Delta	0.5–4	20–200	Waves are normally recorded during deep sleep Waves are not recorded in normal individual when awake (except infants) They are the slowest record of brain waves
Theta	4–8	Large	Waves are recorded mainly in the frontocentral region Waves are related to sleep or drowsiness

If electrical activity of active (exploring) electrode is positive as compared to activity of the reference electrode, downward deflection is recorded. A computerized EEG system with video recording is used to record EEG.

EEG waves are described with respect to their frequency and amplitude and depend on the consciousness state of a person **(Table 37.1)**. Awake state, waves are high frequency and low amplitude while waves recorded are low frequency and high amplitude **(Fig. 37.2)**.

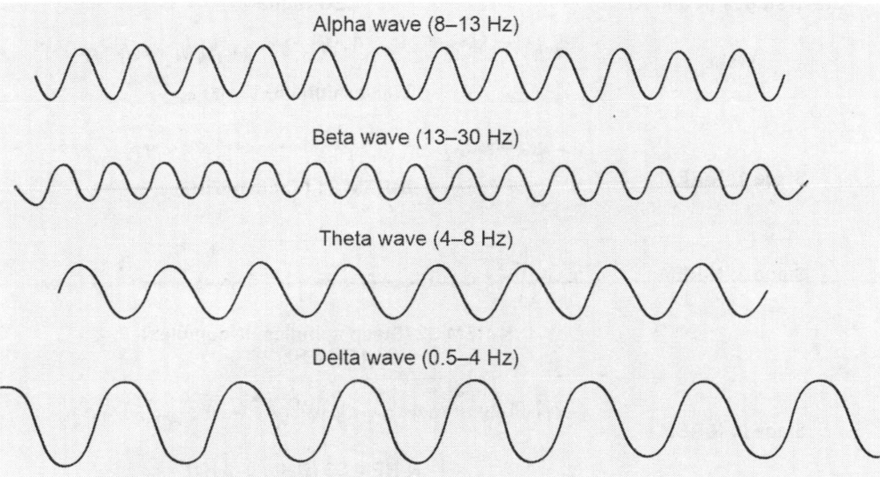

Fig. 37.2: EEG waves

■ IMPORTANT QUESTIONS AND ANSWERS

Q.1. Describe different EEG waves.
Refer to the table above (**Table 37.1, Fig. 37.2**).

Q.2. Enumerate physiological factors affecting EEG.
Physiological factors:
- Any type of sensory stimulus can give rise to high-frequency low voltage waves. This is called as desynchronization. Synchronized EEG (alpha rhythm) is recorded when a normal adult person is in a relaxed state.
- EEG waves are affected by different stages of sleep. Delta rhythm is observed during sleep.
- In awake infants, fast beta rhythm is recorded. This rhythm speeds up and theta rhythm s recorded in childhood. This rhythm is replaced by faster alpha rhythm as child matures.

Q.3. Enumerate pathological factors affecting EEG.
Pathological factors:
- Decreased alpha rhythm is observed with low blood glucose levels and low temperatures while hyperglycemia (high blood glucose levels) and rise in temperature increases alpha rhythm.
- With the tonic stage of epilepsy, high voltage and high-frequency synchronous waves are recorded and with the clonic stage of epilepsy slower and larger waves are recorded in EEG.
- With petit mal epilepsy typical spike and dome pattern is observed. In between the attack again normal waves are recorded.
- Brain tumours and subdural hematoma can give rise to the recording of delta waves in that specific area.

Q.4. What is alpha block?
With eyes closed and in a relaxed mental state alpha rhythm is recorded. As a person opens his/her eyes alpha rhythm disappears. This is called as alpha block This can be seen when you give any sensory stimulus to a person (tactile, auditory, visual, or cognitive stimuli).

Q.5. What is beta rhythm?
Predominant record of beta waves in EEG is called beta rhythm. These wave forms are especially recorded in awake state, or is focusing acutely on a particular thing or solving a mathematical problem.

Q.6. What is the clinical use of EEG?
- The main use of EEG is to help diagnose the type of epilepsy if it is focal or generalized. It has limitations to its use as it may not detect diagnostically useful abnormalities. MRI of head helps to diagnose the structural cause of epilepsy.
- It becomes difficult to diagnose with EEG if attack is epileptic or non-epileptic. But for it to be documented attack frequency has to be high so that it can be recorded.
- EEG may be useful in the diagnosis of brain tumours or encephalopathies, meningitis.
- Creutzfeldt-Jacob disease is a degenerative basic disorder that leads to dementia. In the early stages EEG shows frontal delta activity and in end stages of the disease typically shows periodic sharp wave complexes.
- EEG can help to diagnose non-convulsive status epilepticus in such situations show diffuse slowing patterns of waves in the background with generalized spikes with clinical myoclonus.

Q.7. How does EEG recording change with respect to sleep?
- Normally, sleep is divided into non-rapid eye movement sleep (NREM) and rapid eye movement (REM) sleep. NREM has four stages of sleep; N1, N2, N3, N4. Among these, N3 and N4 are also called as slow wave sleep (SWS) as shown in **Fig. 37.3**.
- Total NREM sleep is 75 to 80% and REM sleep is 25 to 30%.
- Any individual passes in deep sleep from N1 to N4 followed by Rem sleep to complete one sleep cycle. Like this, the cycle repeats every 70 to 90 minutes. Thus with 6 to 8 hrs. of sleep, there are 5 to 6 sleep cycles.

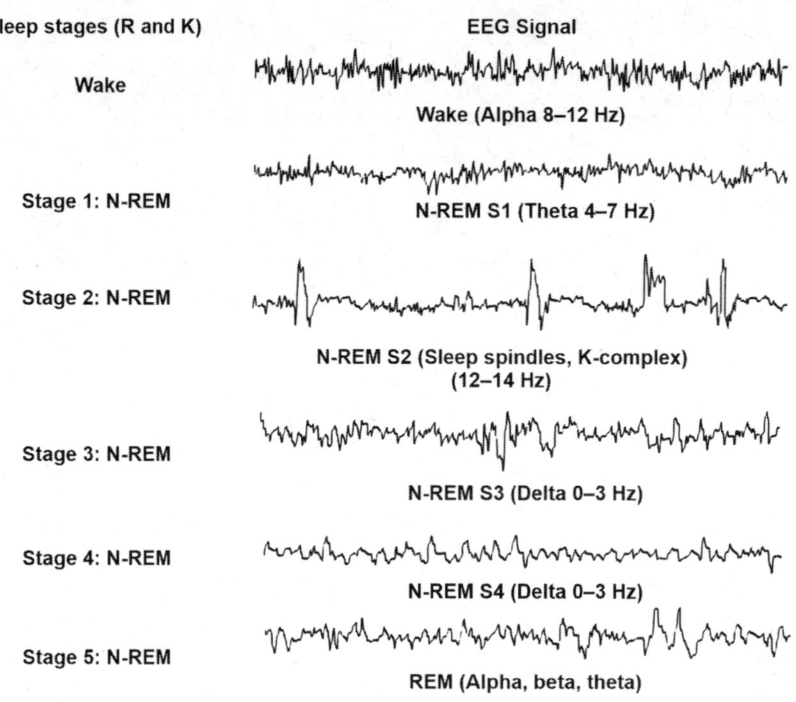

Fig. 37.3: EEG waves and stages of sleep

Normal sleep pattern:

Stages of sleep	EEG waves pattern
Stage I (N1): It is stage when body starts relaxing (3 to 8%)	EEG shows change from beta to alpha rhythm
Stage II (N2): Brain slows down and it is stable and light sleep (45–55%)	Wave amplitude increases. Sleep spindles (burst of alpha like waves with waxing and waning amplitude) K complex are characteristics of the stage
Stage III (N3 and N4): This is SWS (slow wave sleep). The body in this stage starts restoration, i.e. restorative sleep (15 to 20%)	Low-frequency high amplitude waves are recorded (delta waves)
REM sleep: It is stage associated with rapid eye movement. There are 4 to 5 cycles of REM sleep each night. In this stage learning and memory consolidation does happen and brain is quite active in this stage (so called as paradoxical sleep)	Slow waves are replaced by high frequency low voltage waves (like beta rhythm)

Q.8. What is the significance of EEG recording in a sleep study?

- Any complete sleep study (PSG) is incomplete without EEG recording in it.
- Person who undergoes a sleep study, has full night EEG recording which does make understand various details of sleep stages, duration, quality, sleep efficiency, number of arousals in between and so on.
- Various physiological parameters (especially related to cardiorespiratory and autonomic functions) do change when a person is awake, in REM sleep and NREM sleep. Thus, for diagnosis of various conditions sleep study with ECG becomes an important landmark.
- In the sleep study (PSG), we observe a hypnogram of sleep **(Fig. 37.4).**

■ COMMON STATIONS– SPOTS IN PRACTICAL EXAMINATION (2/3 MARKS)

Q.1. EEG recording: Identify and label any of the waves. Answer any one or two questions from the above **(Fig. 37.5).**

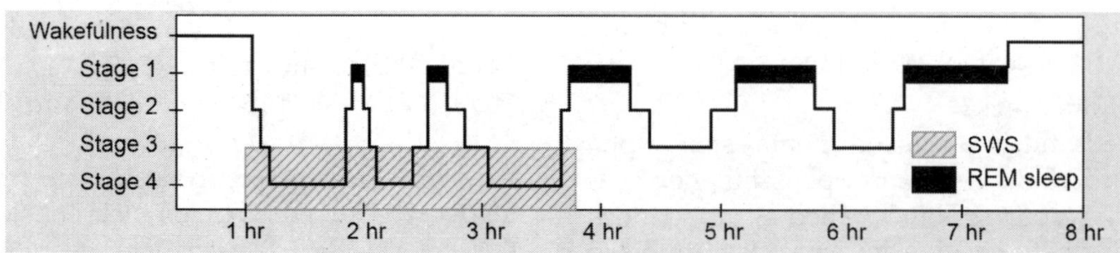

Fig. 37.4: Normal hypnogram in sleep study

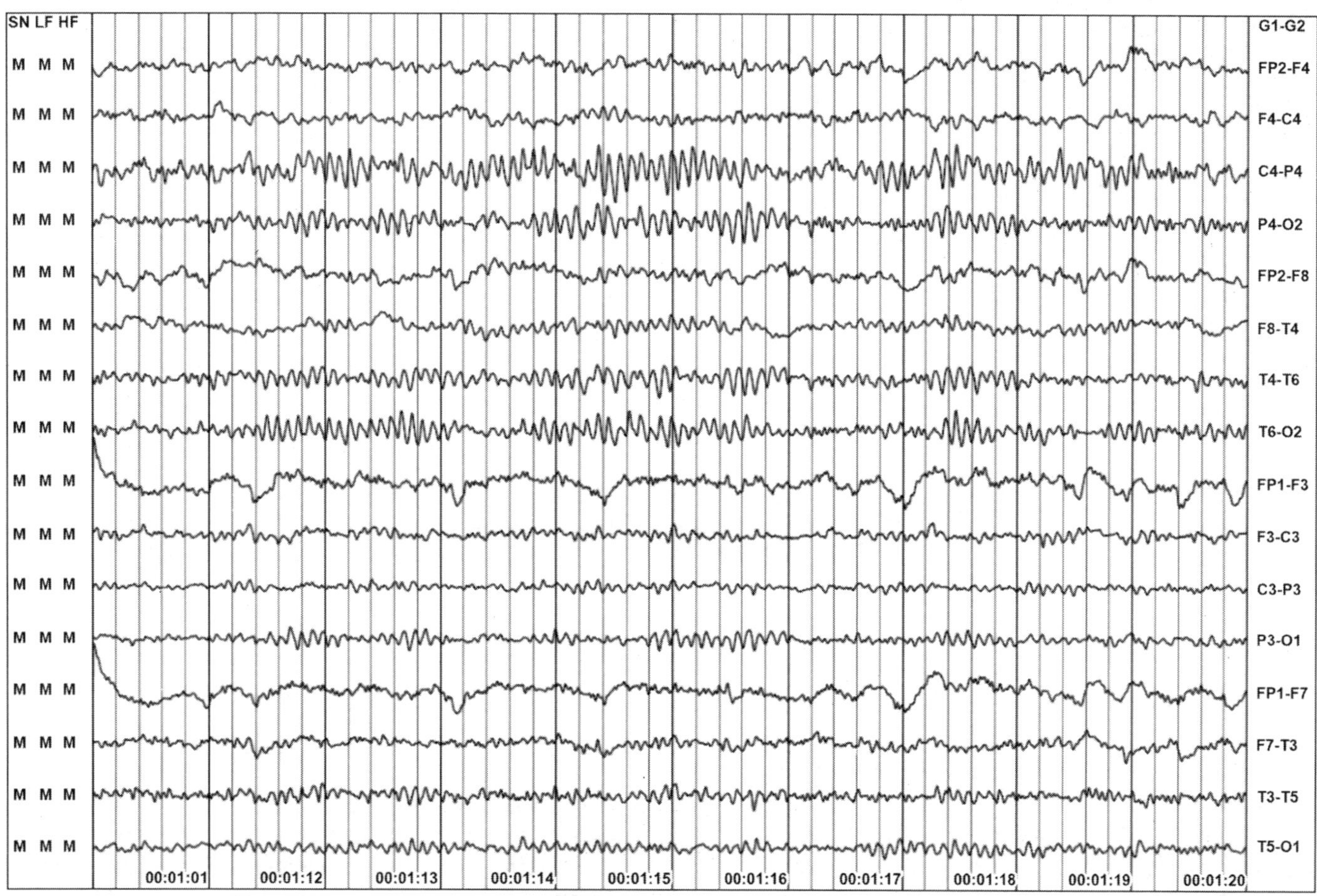

Fig. 37.5: Normal EEG recording

Q.2. EEG recording: Identify and write its physiological basis for recording **(Fig. 37.5)**.

Q.3. XYZ person is in deep sleep–What can be the stage of sleep and how will be EEG waves in that stage?

Give the physiological significance of this stage of sleep (Clue-restorative sleep).

Q.4. If an ABC person is solving some math puzzle and you record his EEG simultaneously-What waveform do you expect on the EEG?

Tests for Pregnancy Diagnosis

Competency:
PY 9.10: Discuss the physiological basis of various pregnancy tests.

Learning Objectives

At the end of the practical session, students should be able to:
- Describe the role of hormones in maintaining pregnancy
- Enlist various tests for diagnosis of pregnancy
- Discuss the physiological basis of pregnancy tests

■ INTRODUCTION

There are various biological immunological and radiographic tests available that help in detecting pregnancy. Some tests can be done within a few days of the conception. Biological tests are not done commonly as they are expensive and time-consuming. Immunological tests are preferred as they take less time and can detect pregnancy at a very early stage. However, ultrasonography techniques are used most commonly to diagnose pregnancy.

Tests for Pregnancy Diagnosis

Biological Tests

Various biological tests involve, injecting urine from pregnant women into female animals and its action on the morphology of ovaries is studied to detect pregnancy.

- **Friedman rabbit test:** Urine from pregnant women is injected in rabbits to see corpus luteum and corpus haemorahgia in the ovaries of rabbits in 2 to 3 days. Then the test is considered positive.
- **Aschheim–Zondek mouse test:** Urine from pregnant women is injected into female mice to check for ovarian changes in female mice. It may take 3 to 4 days. Then the test is considered positive.
- **Hogben test:** Urine from pregnant women is injected in female toads to check for ovulation that happens in toads in 18 hrs. Then the test is considered positive.
- **Galli-Mainini frog test:** Urine from pregnant women is injected in male toads. Positive test is indicated by release of sperms that get collected at cloaca of animal about 3 hrs after the injection.
- **Kupperman test:** Urine from pregnant women is injected in immature female rats subcutaneously to check for hyperemia of ovaries at a rate that occurs after 6 hrs of injection (then the test is considered positive).

Immunological Tests

These are the most commonly performed tests. They are reliable and give quick results. Human chrionic gonadotropin (hCG)-secreted syncytiotrophoblast (in pregnant women) has antigenic properties. By use of specific antibodies against hCG, their presence in serum or urine can be detected easily.

Procedure: Patient in whom a pregnancy test is to be done, a morning sample of urine is collected.

In pregnant women: When urine containing hCG is added to hCG antisera no agglutination will happen.

This means no agglutination is considered as positive for pregnancy.

In non-pregnant women: In contrast, if agglutination happens that means antibodies will remain available to agglutinate added hCG-coated particles and there will be agglutination. This means **agglutination present** is considered as **negative for pregnancy**.

- **Hemagglutination method**: In this to the urine sample of women, hCG antiserum and tagged sheep RBCs are added. If there is no agglutination, pregnancy is confirmed.
- **Latex agglutination inhibition test (Gravindex test)**: Small globules of latex (rubber) particles coated with hCG and antiserum to hCG are available in the market. A sample of urine is treated with antiserum. If there is no agglutination means test is positive and the woman is pregnant.
- **Enzyme-linked Immunosorbent assay (ELISA)**: In this test place of radioactive substance enzyme is used which is treated with a urine sample.
- **One-step immunoassay test**: A variety of kits are available to detect hCG in a urine sample.

Radioimmunoassay Test

Radiolabeled hCG with iodine is treated with a fixed amount of antibodies and urine sample. This is quite a sensitive method and can detect the presence of hCG even in the first week following fertilization.

Ultrasonography

This is the most reliable and commonly practised method to detect pregnancy. At the 5th week, approximately the gestational ring can be visible and cardiac pulsations also can be detected by the 8th to 10th week of gestation.

■ IMPORTANT QUESTION AND ANSWERS

Q.1. Enumerate different tests to detect pregnancy.
There are varieties of tests available to detect pregnancy as explained above.

Q.2. Enumerate various hormones released from the placenta during pregnancy.
Hormones released by the placenta are:
- **Human chorionic gonadotropin (hCG)**
- **Human chorionic somatotropin/human placental lactogen**
- **Progesterone:** Prepares endometrium during pregnancy and helps in the continuation of pregnancy and also prepares mammary glands for lactation.

- **Estrogen:** Prepares mammary glands for lactation. Estrogen secretion goes on increasing as pregnancy advances and helps in smooth parturition.
- **Corticotropic releasing hormone (CRH)**
- **Relaxin:** The initial stage relaxes the uterus and aids in the continuation of pregnancy, later stages help relax the pubic symphysis and dilate the cervix which aids in the parturition process.

Q.3. What is the function of hCG during pregnancy?
- hCG, i.e. human chorionic gonadotropin is secreted as early as even 6th day after fertilization.
- hCG does the function of luteinizing hormone (LH) and prevents degeneration of the corpus luteum
- hCG continues the production of estrogen and progesterone that helps the attachment of the embryo to the uterus. hCG secretion continues almost to about four to five months of pregnancy and later the level declines. The presence of hCG in urine is therefore used as the main principle to detect various pregnancy tests.

Q.4. What is the role of human chorionic somatotropin?
Human chorionic somatotropin (hCS) helps in the development of the fetus and prepares mammary glands for lactation. It is known to stimulate the synthesis of placental proteins. hCS is known to induce some maternal metabolic changes like increased mobilization of fat and decreased glucose utilization. It facilitates the supply of amino acids to the fetus by decreasing its maternal utilization. Levels of this hormone directly correlate with fetal and placental weight.

Q.5. What are the advantages of doing ultrasonography?
Ultrasonography is the most convenient and commonly practised test to detect pregnancy. Along with confirmation of pregnancy, it helps to understand the complete morphology of the fetus, any abnormalities can be detected. Ultrasonography is a noninvasive test and can be repeated if required.

■ COMMON STATIONS – SPOTS IN PRACTICAL EXAMINATION (2/3 MARKS)

Q.1. Enumerate any two pregnancy diagnostic tests.
Q.2. Answer any one or two questions from the above.

■ CASE-BASED SCENARIO/PROBLEM-BASED

Case 1: 25-year married female comes with c/o missed periods.
- Which pregnancy test you will advise her of?
- What is the physiological basis of the test?

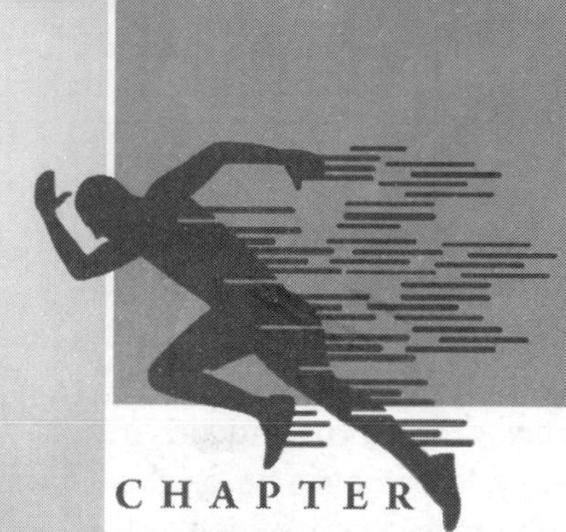

Cardiopulmonary Cerebral Resuscitation

Competency:

PY 11.14: Demonstrate basic life support in a simulated environment.

Learning Objectives

After completing this practical, students should be able to:
- Define CPCR
- Enlist indications for the same
- Understand the aim of CPCR
- Describe the procedure for mouth-to-mouth breathing
- Describe the procedure of external cardiac compression
- Describe the Holger Nielson method

■ INTRODUCTION

Cardiopulmonary/cerebral resuscitation (CPCR) is an emergency life-saving procedure that is performed to maintain oxygenation and blood circulation in a person in whom the heart suddenly stops working (cardiac arrest) and or even breathing stops (pulmonary arrest) or both things happens simultaneously (cardiopulmonary arrest). It becomes important that all health personnel are trained in this life-saving procedure. It involves repeated cycles of compression of the chest and artificial respiration in order to make oxygenated blood available to all vital organs in the body so that important cardiorespiratory function is restored immediately before one admits the patient.

■ PLAN OF CPCR

It is in two phases:
1. Basic life support (BLS)
2. Advanced cardiac life support

Phase 1: Basic Life Support

Basic life support (BLS): The sequence of BLS is CAB, i.e. circulation, airways and breathing. This procedure can be done anywhere in an emergency till medical help is reached.

Steps

1. Try to assess the responsiveness of the patient and call for emergency medical services (EMS).
2. Position a person on a flat surface.
3. Open mouth (remove vomitus, mucus, etc. if visible)
4. Place one hand on the victim's forehead and tilt the head backwards and the other hand under the chin to lift it (chin lift). This helps in neck extension and raises the tongue away to open airways.
5. Mouth-to-mouth respiration (as explained below).
6. External cardiac massage (as explained below)
   - **C-circulate:** Give an external cardiac massage, continuous compression at a rate of 100–120/minute
   - **A-airway:** Put the hand under the neck and tilt the head to maintain an open airway and prevent the fall of the tongue back into the pharynx (which can obstruct the airway)

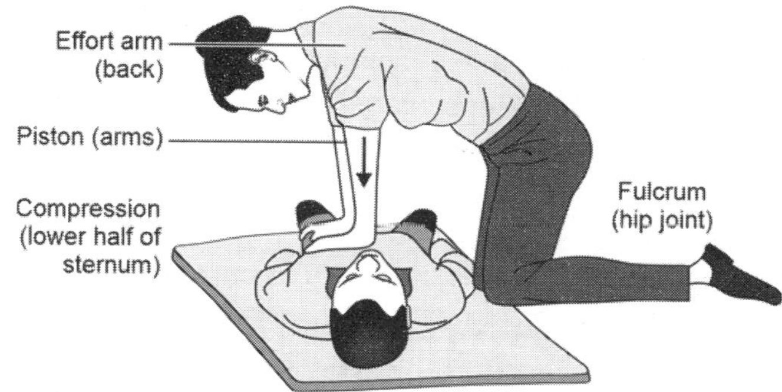

Fig. 39.1: Technique of chest compression

- **B-breathing:** Keeping the head tilted, give mouth-to-mouth respiration, and inflate lungs at least 14 to 16 times/min.

External Cardiac Compression

- Make the victim lie on a firm surface **(Fig. 39.1)**.
- Put the heel of one hand in the centre of the chest (approximately middle of the sternum) and then the heel of the other hand on it.
- Without touching the chest wall, keep the fingers of your hands interlaced.
- Keep elbows in complete extension, straight with shoulders in line with the heels of hands.
- Movement should be at the shoulders so that force is transmitted to the chest.
- Compression of the chest should be with a speed of about 100–120/minute.

- The chest has to be compressed approximately 5 cm and complete recoil of the chest is allowed after each compression.
- After every 30 compressions, 2 quick chest lung inflations are done.

Phase 2: Advanced Life Support

Advanced cardiac life support: The sequence of this phase is DEFGHI, i.e. drugs, ECG, and fibrillation, gauging and restoration of breathing, hypothermia, and management of patient in ICU. This procedure is done in a hospital setup only. The chain of survival inside hospital and outside hospital is shown in **Fig. 39.2**.

The basic steps of advanced life support include:

1. **Defibrillation:** As explained below.
2. **Airway management and O$_2$ therapy:** Endotracheal intubation has to be done by a physician (skilled person) at the earliest.
3. **Atropine sulphate:** Injectable atropine sulphate is given to restore normal heartbeat. It is known to inhibit parasympathetic influence (vagus). It's an anticholinergic drug.
4. **Sodium bicarbonate:** Cardiac arrest is known to cause acidosis, and hyperkalaemia (with low/absent circulation, metabolic end products do accumulate). To treat this sodium bicarbonate injection is given.
5. **Pacemakers:** If required
   - **D – Drugs:** Drugs like adrenaline, and sodium bicarbonate can be given to patient

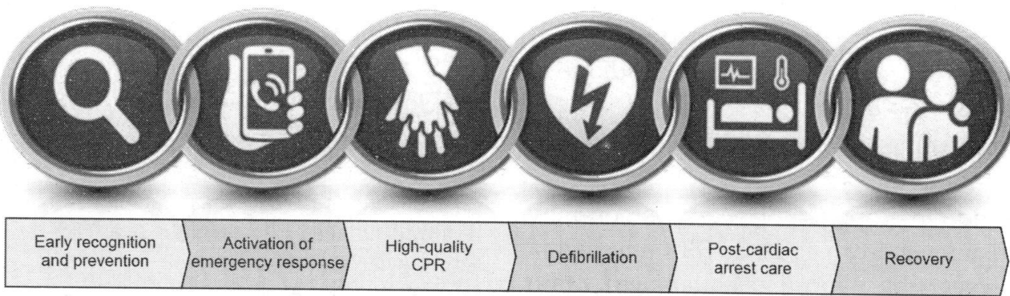

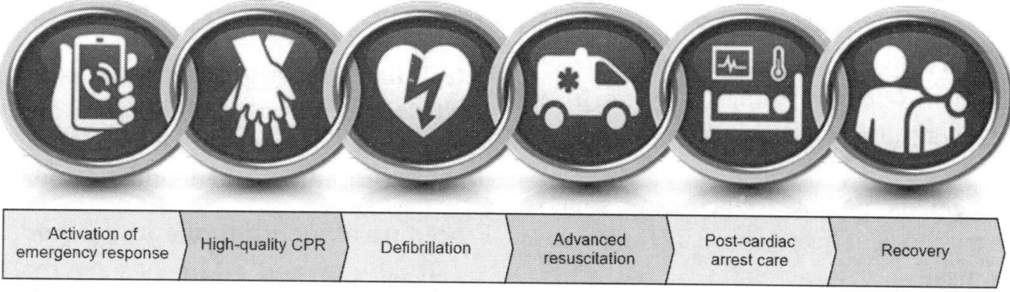

Fig. 39.2: Chain of survival inside hospital and outside hospital

- **E – ECG:** Start with continuous monitoring of ECG of the patient
- **F–** With the **defibrillator** start fibrillation treatment, procaine, lidocaine
- **G– Gauge** and try to restore normal breathing, and circulation.
- **H– Hypothermia**
- **I–** Management of patients in **ICU**.

■ IMPORTANT QUESTIONS AND ANSWERS

Q.1. What is the physiological basis of benefit of external chest compression?

Physiological basis of benefit of chest compression:

- When heart stops beating in an individual suddenly, it is understood that the left side of the heart and pulmonary veins do contain completely oxygenated blood.
- When on tries to compress the heart between the sternum and vertebral column, the heart gets squeezed and thus mechanical systole is produced which increases both ventricular pressures more than aortic and pulmonary pressures which help in forward movement (flow) of blood.

Importance of chest recoil: As one releases the pressure, diastolic filling of the ventricles happens (due to the pressure gradient between intrathoracic pressure and peripheral veins).

Q.2. What is cardiopulmonary arrest? What are the effects of cardiopulmonary arrest?

Cardiopulmonary arrest: It is an emergency medical condition when there is a sudden stoppage of heart/ respiration or both. There can be sudden loss of consciousness and vital organs can get damaged due to inadequate/Absent blood flow.

As heart stops beating suddenly, the effects are seen on various important vital organs.

- **Brain:** With sudden stoppage of heart, person may lose consciousness and can collapse (Brain ischemia can lead an irreversible neurological damage). Brain cannot withstand lack of O_2 for more than 20 seconds
- **Brain stem:** If brain ischemia continues for more than one minute, it can cause loss of brain stem functions.
- **Breathing:** Due to this (loss of brain stem functions) person can suddenly stop breathing. There can be no chest movement at all and no air coming out from nostrils.
- **Heart sounds:** One is not able to hear heart sounds when he/she tries to hear heart sound by putting ear over victim's chest.
- **Pupils:** Pupils may not respond to light and may become permanently dilated.

- **Heart:** With sudden stoppage of heart beating, there develops myocardial ischemia.
- **Pulse:** As heart stops beating, radial carotid or any other pulsations may not be palpable at all.
- **Blood pressure:** Blood pressure may not be recordable at all.
- **Skin:** Due to stoppage of circulation of blood, skin can be pale and cold.

Q.3. Enumerate common signs and symptoms/ Diagnosis of cardiopulmonary arrest.

Signs and symptoms of cardiopulmonary arrest:

- State of unconsciousness
- Dilated pupils (not responding to light)
- Cold, pale skin
- Absent/ feeble pulse
- BP not recordable
- Absent heart sounds
- Stoppage of breathing/gasping movements.

Q.4. What is basic purpose of CPR?

With sudden stoppage of heart beating, circulation of blood in the body comes to a holt. This leads to ischemia all over body including vital organs like brain.

By giving CPR one tries to:

- Restore blood flow and maintain circulation of the heart and brain.
- By restoring perfusion of vital organs try to prevent or postpone tissue death or permeant brain damage which might happen with lack of blood flow till cardiac activity is restored spontaneously or with help of an automated external defibrillator (AED).

Q.5. Enumerate common indications for CPCR.

CPCR is an emergency procedure which may be required in various acute conditions.

Acute conditions requiring CPCR are

- Acute and massive myocardial infarction leading to cardiac arrest (sudden stoppage of the heart)
- Cardiac arrhythmias
- Anaphylactic shock
- Head injuries
- Sudden obstruction of airways
- Hanging, drowning

Q.6. What is an artificial respiration?

Artificial respiration (pulmonary resuscitation) can be given by mouth to mouth method. This is one of the best first-aid procedure for adequate ventilation.

Procedure of mouth-to-mouth method

- Lift the chin and tilt the head so that patency of the airway can be maintained.
- With one hand close victim's nostrils

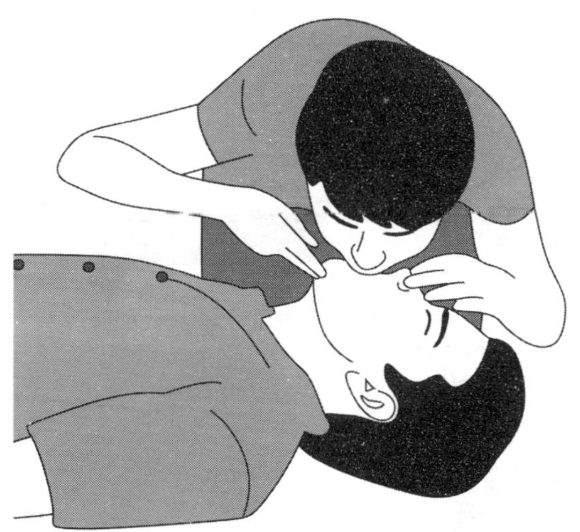

Fig. 39.3: Mouth-to-mouth respiration

- The resuscitator blows the expired air in the victim's mouth which will cause the victim's chest to rise
- A person who is trying to make the victim breathe, takes a deep breath and apply mouth close to the victim's mouth and exhales forcefully.
- Look for chest expansion in the victim.
- Repeat the procedure to maintain breathing at rate of 10 to 12 times/minute **(Fig. 39.3)**.

Advantages of mouth-to-mouth method
- It is a simple safe procedure
- It does not need any training and no apparatus is required
- Helps to cause adequate ventilation of lungs
- There is minimum handling of the victim
- This method can be used in newborns
- Expired air from the resuscitator does contain CO_2 which helps stimulate the respiratory centre of the victim
- While performing mouth-to-mouth breathing, simultaneous cardiac resuscitation is possible.

Care while performing mouth-to-mouth breathing: There is a chance of the tongue falling back and obstructing the victim's airway which can be prevented by tilting the head to one side and slight extension at the neck.

Q.7. Enumerate other manual methods for artificial respiration.

Other methods for artificial respiration
- Schafer's method
- Sylvester method
- Holger-Nielsen method **(Fig. 39.4)**
  The first two methods are not practiced as they allow compression of the chest for expiration and then allow the lungs to expand passively. However, Holger-Nielsen method is used when mouth-to-mouth respiration is not used.

Q.8. What are the contraindications for performing mouth-to-mouth method for pulmonary resuscitation?

Contraindications for the mouth-to-mouth method are:
- Drowning
- Fracture of jaw
- Severe face injuries

  In such situations where mouth-to-mouth method cannot be used, the Holger Nielsen method is used.

Q.9. What is Holger Nielsen method?

Procedure
- Victim is placed in prone position with both elbows flexed as seen in diagram
- Kneel on knee near the victim
- Grip the victim's arms above elbows and pull them backwards while raising the arms till resistance is felt at the victim's shoulder. This position should last for two and a half seconds, and return to the expansion phase. Repeat this procedure for 10 to 12 times/minute
- In this method compression and expansion both are actively done by the resuscitator **(Fig. 39.3)**.

Q.10. Enumerate instrumental methods used for an artificial respiration.

In various conditions where artificial respiration support is required for a long time then the following methods are used to maintain alternate positive and negative pressures to assist ventilation.

Various methods are:
- Drinkers method
- Continuous insufflation method
- Bragg-Paul method
- Eve's rocking method

Principle of these methods: Air tight plastic/metallic devices placed around chest. With the application of negative pressure at certain intervals draws, the air in the lungs (inspiration) and elastic recoil of the chest and lungs are responsible for expiration.

  Instrumental methods of an artificial respiration are no longer practised nowadays.

Q.11. What is physiological basis for providing an artificial respiration?

With sudden cardiac arrest, as blood circulation stops, oxygenation of various vital organs in the body suffers. By trying artificial respiration in a victim, oxygenation of the blood is achieved and the respiratory centre as well receive its proper blood and O_2 supply. This helps respiratory centre to regain its function as it gets stimulated by alternate inflation and deflation of lungs.

Q.12. Describe steps to handle a case of drowning.
- **Step 1:** First and foremost, check for breathing and pulse as victim is out of water

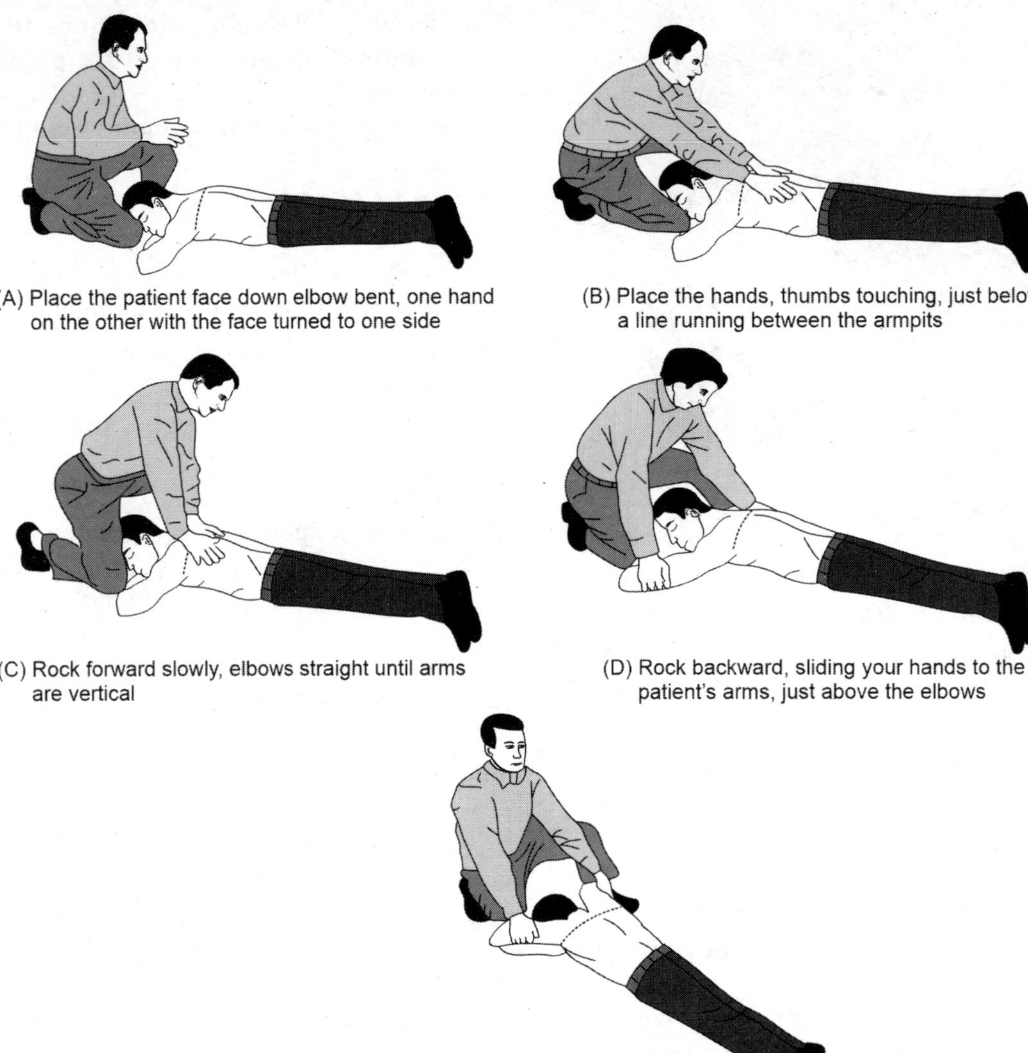

Fig. 39.4: Holger-Nielsen method.

- **Step 2**: If pulse is felt and breathing of victim is visible, then press lower abdomen to expel water
- **Step 3**: After this place a victim in recovery position It is a lateral position (right or left lateral) with head turned to one side, no pillow below head
- **Step 4**: Upper leg is folded at knee joint touching the ground/bed
- **Step 5**: Drain out all secretions from the pharynx so that the airway is kept patent
- **Step 6**: If the pulse of the victim is palpable but there is no breathing, immediately start with mouth-to-mouth breathing for artificial respiration
- **Step 7**: If pulse and breathing are absent, start with CPR till the victim is shifted to the hospital.

Q.13. Enumerate steps for external cardiac compression.
Please check above.

Q.14. What is open cardiac massage?

Open/ Internal cardiac massage: This procedure is done in a hospital setup only. The chest of a patient is opened, inserting hands in the thorax, heart is compressed against the chest wall rhythmically at a rate of 80/minute.

Q.15. What is an immediate treatment for ventricular fibrillation/cardioversion?

A strong high-voltage current is applied to the chest via electrodes to reset fibrillation. The procedure and physiological basis of this are explained below.

Q.16. What is the physiological basis of cardioversion/ defibrillation?

- With a cardiac arrhythmia, cardio-version is a common, effective technique. This is one of the most important treatments of CPR.

- When the heart is in defibrillation, it cannot pump blood, as there is no effective systole as well as diastolic filling of the heart.
- When the heart is in fibrillation when the heart is firing arrhythmically, (due to MI or some ectopic focus that sets up abnormal rhythms) a strong high-voltage current is applied to the chest with the help of electrodes to stop fibrillation.
- Shock causes a large portion of cardiomyocytes to depolarize simultaneously which helps in interrupting or terminating abnormal rhythms.
- Heart remains quiescent for a couple of seconds and starts taking its normal rhythm (shock can be repeated a couple of times).

Defibrillation tries to convert fibrillation into a normal rhythm so that effective contractions of the myocardium start and blood pumping and perfusion of the tissues start normally.

OBJECTIVE STRUCTURED PRACTICAL EXAMINATION (OSPE)

1. **Demonstrate CPR in a simulated environment/on a mannequin**

S. No.	Assessment criteria	Marks assigned	Marks given
1.	Verify the safety of the surroundings		
2.	Check the responsiveness of the patient/victim		
3.	Call for help/emergency medical service		
4.	Check for breathing and pulse if absent		
5.	Begin with external cardiac compression (as described above)		
6.	Report and answer the questions asked		
7.	Total		

COMMON STATIONS – SPOTS IN PRACTICAL EXAMINATION (2/3 MARKS)

Q.1. What is CPCR? Enumerate its common indications.

Q.2. Diagram of the person doing CPCR/mouth-to-mouth respiration–Answer any one or two questions from the above.

Q.3. Write basic life support steps.

40

Preparation of Diet Sheet

■ AIM OF NUTRITION

It is to supply energy for growth, repair, and enzymatic activity. Good nutrition is the basis of good health and plays an important role in the attainment of normal growth and development. Wrong and right food choices are one of the prime determinants of our long-term health.

■ BALANCED DIET

It is a diet which contains different types of food in such quantity and proportion that needs energy, essential amino acids, fatty acids, vitamins, and minerals to be adequately met for maintaining health, vitality and general well-being.

■ CALORIC VALUES

It is energy released when one gram of a particular type of food is metabolized.

Type of food	Caloric value (kcal)
Protein	4.1
Carbohydrate	4.1
Fat	9.3

For calculation purposes, caloric values of proteins, carbohydrates and fats can be taken as 4, 4, and 9 respectively. From these values, if one knows the quantities of protein, fat and carbohydrate taken in the diet, one can calculate the total calories taken in the food.

In planning a diet following requirements are taken into consideration:

- Total caloric requirement
- Proportion of different foods
- Giving enough minerals and vitamins in the diet

Calculation of total calorie requirement:

- From the age and sex of a person BMR is determined. BMR is determined from the chart given
- From height and weight of a person, the surface area is determined from the chart
- BMR = Number of calories expended/sq meter
- Calories/hour can be calculated by BMR surface area
- In a day subject is awake for 16 hrs
- So caloric requirement during waking hrs = 16 × BMR × surface area
- A person sleeps for 8 hrs during which caloric expenditure is equal to 90% of BMR
- Thus, calories consumed during sleep = 8 × surface area × 90/100
- Calories consumed during work are calculated depending upon the type of work as follows:

Type of work	Calories/hr/kg
Light	1.7
Moderate	2.5
Heavy	5.9

A person normally works for 8 hrs.

Work allowance:

Work allowance = 8 × 1.7 × weight of person in kg

- Non-working allowance for ordinary movements which a person does when awake (e.g. taking a bath, putting on clothes, talking, etc.) is taken as 400 kilocalories. The total calories required are total calories calculated in (6, 7, 8, 9 and 10) above.

  10% of the above total is added for specific dynamic action of food.
- **Climate:** After calculating the total calories required/day temperature correction is made. If the environmental temperature is 25°C no correction is required environmental temperature is 5°C to 10°C higher, then the calorie requirement is reduced by 5%. If environmental temperature is less by 5°C to 10°C, the caloric requirement is increased by 3%.
- Different physiological conditions:

  Pregnancy– 300 kcal/day should be given extra

  Lactation– 600 kcal/day should be given extra
- Age-wise caloric requirement should be calculated as shown in given below:

Age	Calorie requirement
1–3 months	120 cal/kg/day
4–9 months	110 cal/kg/day
10–12 months	100 cal/kg/day
1–3 years	90 cal/kg/day
4–6 years	90 cal/kg/day
7–15 years	60 cal/kg/day
16–25 years	46 cal/kg/day
25–30 years	Calories need to be decreased by 5 to 10% over 16–25 years
After 50 years	Calories need to be still decreased by 5% over 25–30 years
After 60 years	Calories need to be still decreased by 5% after 50 years

Proportion of Different Foodstuffs

- **Proteins**: For the adult diet should be 0.8 to 1g/kg/day. For growing children, the protein content of the diet should be 1.7 to 2 g/kg/day. Proteins in general should be given 15% of the total caloric requirement.
- **Fats**: Fats increase the palatability of the food. They act as a concentrated source of energy (9 kcal/g) They are also important for supplying fat-soluble vitamins and essential fatty acids in the diet. Fats therefore should supply about 15% of the total calories in the diet. A high-fat diet is responsible for causing atherosclerosis and therefore fat content of the diets should not extend beyond 25 to 30% of total calories.
- **Carbohydrates**: Carbohydrates are the main source of calories (70% of total calories in the diet). The carbohydrate requirement is about 4 to 6 g/kg/day. Carbohydrates are the cheapest and thus form a major source of calories in people with poor economic status (even 80 to 90% of calories may come from carbohydrates).
- **Requirement of minerals:** Important minerals and their daily requirement is given below:

Name of the mineral	Daily requirement
Sodium chloride	3 to 5 g
Calcium	0.9 to 1 g
Phosphorus	0.88 g
Iron	10 mg in males 20 mg in females (as only 10% is absorbed) The requirement is more in pregnancy and lactation (daily 2 mg extra iron should be absorbed, i.e. 10 to 15 mg extra iron should be taken in diet per day extra

Requirement of vitamins: Important vitamins and their daily requirement is given below:

Name of the vitamin	Daily requirement
Thiamine	0.5 to 1 mg in children 1 to 1.5 mg in adults
Nicotinic acid	10 to 15 mg
Riboflavin	2 mg
Vitamin A	4000 to 5000 IU
Vitamin D	400 to 500 IU
Vitamin C	75 mg
Vitamin B12	1 µg
Folic acid	100 µg

Approximate Measures

1 medium cup—150 ml

1 big cup—200 ml

1 medium glass—200 ml

1 teaspoon—5 ml or 4 grams

1 tablespoon—15 ml or 12 grams

1 medium wati—150 ml

1 small wati—80 ml

One serving—one exchange

This is the basic diet proforma one can plan for an individual. It has to be kept in mind that the diet requirement varies with different age groups and different physiological conditions like lactation and pregnancy, etc. Diet recommendations do vary in different clinical conditions. While prescribing a diet plan to any person it has to be individually tailored considering in detail his or her lifestyle.

41

Autonomic Function Tests

Competency:

PY 5.14: Observe cardiovascular autonomic function tests in a volunteer or simulated environment.

Learning Objectives

After completing this practical, the students shall be able to:

- Explain the physiological significance of testing autonomic functions in the body
- Enumerate and describe various autonomic function tests
- Enumerate the functions of autonomic nervous system (ANS)
- Perform non-invasive autonomic function tests and explain their principle
- Enumerate precautions taken during the tests
- Able to co-relate the physiological basis of various dysfunctions of ANS to various clinical conditions.

■ INTRODUCTION

The autonomic nervous system term was suggested by Langley for the part of the nervous system that controls all visceral activities of cardiac muscle, smooth muscles, and activities of all glands. ANS innervates the entire neuroaxis and permeates all organ systems. As it operates in the background, its importance is understood when any of ANS functions becomes compromised causing dysautonomia.

ANS has two components one that of visceral afferent (sensory) neurons and second that of visceral efferent (motor) neurons. Although ANS control is autonomic, it is controlled by various centres in the brain. ANS is known to excite or inhibit visceral structures in response to continuous sensory input.

ANS does control blood pressure, heart rate, sleep, bowel, and bladder functions. ANS is divided into the sympathetic nervous system and the parasympathetic nervous system. Activation of both often has opposite effects that allow simultaneous integration of multiple body functions.

Functional Anatomy of ANS

- ANS has two important components – sympathetic and parasympathetic.
- Both have their respective preganglionic (myelinated) neurons and postganglionic neurons (unmyelinated) as shown in **Fig. 41.1**.
- Preganglionic sympathetic, preganglionic para-sympathetic and postganglionic parasympathetic secrete acetylcholine at their nerve endings.
- Postganglionic sympathetic nerve endings secrete adrenaline (except fibres that innervate blood vessels in skeletal muscle and sweat glands).
- The sympathetic nervous system has thoracolumbar outflow and the parasympathetic has craniosacral outflow.
- Sympathetic preganglionic neurons synapse with postganglionic sympathetic neurons in the para-vertebral sympathetic chain of ganglia.

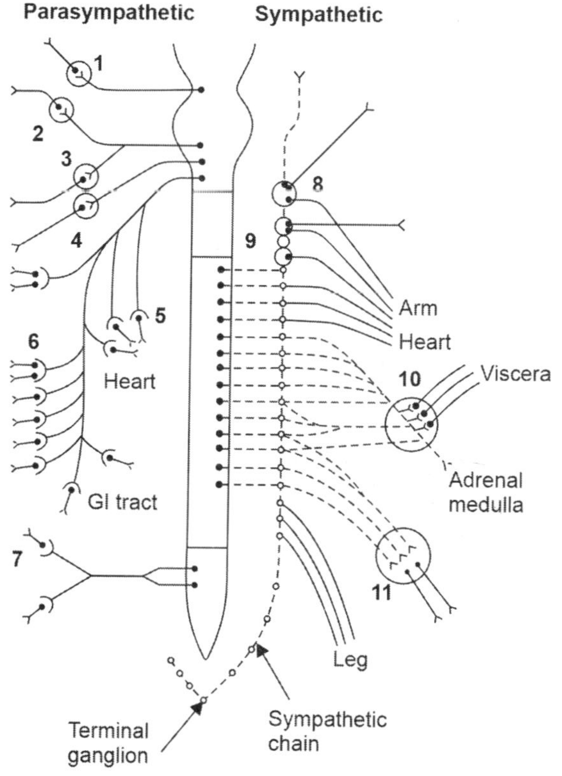

Parasympathetic—Craniosacral outflow
Sympathetic—Thoracolumbar outflow
1   Ciliary ganglion
2   Pterygopalatine ganglion
3   Submandibular ganglion
4   Otic ganglion
5   Vagal to heart
6   Vagal to GI tract (wall)
7   Pelvic ganglia
8   Superior cervical
9   Middle cervical and stellate ganglion
10 Coeliac
11 Lower abdo—sympathetic ganglion

Fig. 41.1: ANS organization

- Parasympathetic preganglionic neurons synapse with postganglionic parasympathetic neurons which are very close to the viscera they serve.

Effects of Stimulation of ANS

- Normally, activation of sympathetic and parasympathetic systems shows opposite effects **(Table 41.1)**.
- The effect of parasympathetic stimulation is usually short-lived and that of sympathetic stimulation effect lasts longer.
- Sympathetic stimulation is important when the body responds to acute stress (fight or flight response). In acute stress, it tries to maintain homeostasis.
- Parasympathetic stimulation helps to conserve and restore body energy.
- A fine balance is maintained between the two systems to maintain homeostasis.

TABLE 41.1: Activation of sympathetic and parasympathetic systems

Functional consequences of normal ANS activation		
	Sympathetic	**Parasympathetic**
Heart rate	Increased	Decreased
Blood pressure	Increased	Mildly decreased
Bladder	Increased sphincter tone	Voiding (decreased tone)
Bowel motility	Decreased motility	Increased
Lung	Bronchodilation	Bronchoconstriction
Sweat glands	Sweating	–
Pupils	Dilation	Constriction
Adrenal glands	Catecholamine release	–
Sexual function	Ejaculation, orgasm	Erection
Lacrimal glands	–	Tearing
Parotid glands	–	Salivation

- Various autonomic reflexes regulate various functions in the body. For these reflexes ANS is the integrating center and visceral organs are the effectors.

Classification of ANF Tests

- Autonomic function tests are broadly classified as activity tests (subject does some activity) and reactivity tests.
- When we ask the patient/subject to change position, take deep breaths, immerse the hand in cold water, Valsalva maneuver, etc. we are performing activity tests.
- Various tests that we perform without disturbing subjects, it is called as reactivity tests (discussed later).

Reactivity Tests

- Resting heart rate
- Resting blood pressure
- Heart rate variability

Activity Tests

For sympathetic functions	*For parasympathetic functions*
• Cold pressor response • Hand grip strength • Sympathetic skin response	• Standing test • Heart rate and BP response to passive tilting • Deep breathing test • Valsalva ratio • Standing to lying ratio

■ SYMPATHETIC NERVOUS SYSTEM TESTS

Sympathetic Skin Response/Galvanic Skin Response

Apparatus

Electrodes, EMG equipment.

Principle

It is studying functions of peripheral sympathetic cholinergic fibres. This is tested by evaluating changes in skin resistance with respect to electrical stimuli.

Procedure

- Give proper instructions to the subject for the test.
- Do appropriate low-frequency filter settings (0.1 to 0.5 Hz) and high-frequency (500–1000 Hz) filter settings.
- Connect electrodes from hands/feet to EMG machine (proper placement of active and reference electrodes).
- After providing a stimulus (usually a startling sound–handclap near the subject's head), record SSR potential and note its amplitude and latency.

Result

- SSR in hands and feet are noted with their amplitude and latencies. Normally, amplitude of SSR amplitude ranges from 1.6 mV to 2.1 mV.
- Various physiological as well as pathological factors can alter SSR.

Cold Pressor Response/Test

This test is preferred to be done at the end of other ANS tests.

Apparatus

Sphygmomanometer, cold water.

Principle

Any physical or mental stress is known to stimulate or activate the sympathetic nervous system. Putting a hand in cold water (acts as a stress-like painful stimulus) increases blood pressure.

Procedure

- Proper instructions are given to the subject about the test
- Record the blood pressure
- In a container take cold water (at or below 4°C) and ask the subject to put his/her hand in it for about one minute
- Record BP after 30 seconds and 60 seconds when the hand is submerged in water.

Result

When a person submerges their hand in cold water there is a rise in his/her systolic as well as diastolic BP (systolic BP can increase in the range of 10 to 20 mm of Hg) and diastolic BP increase in the range of 5 to 10 mm of Hg). There can be variations with respect to age and gender. Very small or no rise in BP indicates reduced sympathetic activity **(Fig. 41.2)**.

Hand Grip Strength

Apparatus

Electrodes, sphygmomanometer, ECG machine, hand grip dynamometer.

Principle

A sustained handgrip against the resistance is known to increase the activity of the sympathetic nervous system and increase heart rate and BP.

Procedure

- Proper instructions are given to the subject about the test

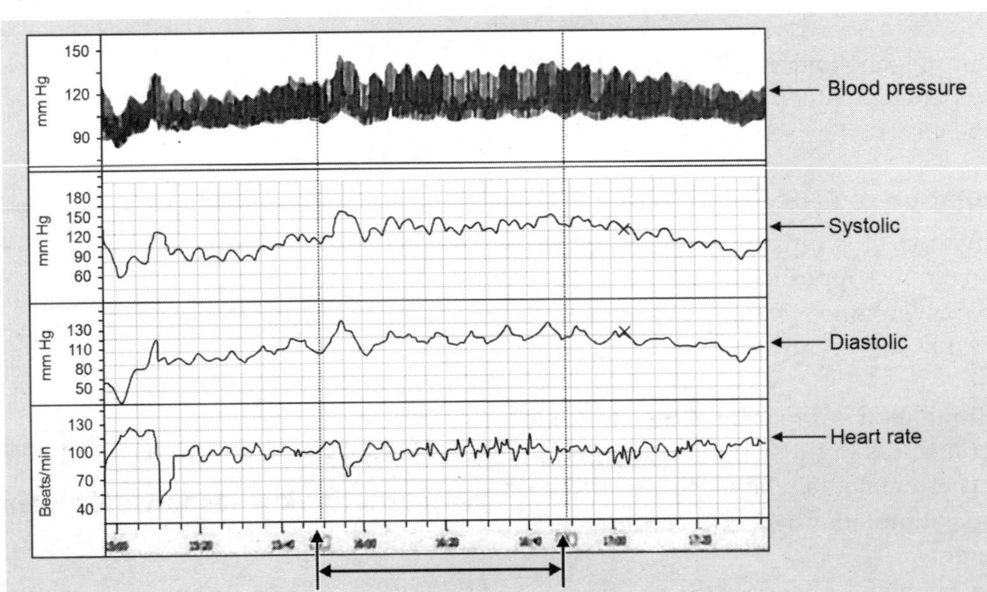

Fig. 41.2: Cold pressor test

- Proper electrodes are placed on the body surface area connected to the ECG machine
- Connect simultaneously sphygmomanometer (to the non-exercising hand)/NIBP monitor (continuous record of BP)
- Ask the subject to hold the dynamometer in the other hand (exercising one) and to take a full grip on it
- Ask the subject to exert maximum force and note the maximum tension (T_{max}) developed
- Repeat the procedure three times (at intervals of 2 minutes) record the highest tension and note that as maximum isometric tension
- Ask the subject to maintain a 30% maximum pressure for about 5 minutes
- Record heart rate and blood pressure.

T_{max} can be affected by age, gender, nutritional state of muscle, pain, fatigue, and mental state of person

Precautions

- Proper instructions and practising the hand grip is a must before the test
- Basal BP (systolic/diastolic) must be noted down
- Before the release of the grip, BP is recorded

Result

In a normal subject, a rise in diastolic BP to about 10 to 15 mm of Hg is noted and even a rise in heart rate (about 20 to 30%) is noted.

■ PARASYMPATHETIC SYSTEM TESTS

Standing Test (Effect on BP and Heart Rate on Standing)

Apparatus

Multichannel polygraph, non-invasive blood pressure (NIBP) monitor.

Principle

When a person stands suddenly from a supine position, there is a reflex fall in BP and an increase in heart rate is observed. This occurs between 3 to 12 seconds from immediate standing.

Procedure

- Explain the complete procedure to the subject.
- Ask him to lie in the supine position and connect him to the polygraph machine and apply ECG electrodes, tie the cuff of NIBP around his arm.
- Let him relax in the same position for about 10 to 15 minutes and note down his basal heart rate and BP.
- Ask the subject to stand up and immediately note changes in BP and heart rate, on NIBP.
- Record BP and heart rate serially for about 3 minutes. Record BP and BP at the end of 3 minutes (the point of standing is marked on ECG paper).
- Calculate heart rate from R-R interval at 15th beat (fastest HR and shortest R-R interval) and 30th beat (slowest HR and longest R-R interval) after standing.
- Determine a 30:15 ratio. It is calculated as the ratio between the longest R-R interval (at the 30th beat)/shortest R-R interval (at the 15th beat) as shown in **Fig. 41.3**.

Result

Normally, there is an increase in heart rate followed by a decrease in heart rate and a fall in BP. In a normal person fall in systolic BP ranges from 7 to 10 mm of Hg. If the fall is more than 30 mm of Hg it is considered abnormal. A normal 30:15 ratio is more than 1.04, if it is less than 1.0 it is abnormal.

Effect on Heart Rate and BP to Passive Tilt/Tilting Test

Apparatus

Multichannel polygraph, tilt table, ECG electrodes, and NIBP.

Principle

This test tries to assess cardiovascular response on passive tilt to a person from supine to inclination about 80%.

Procedure

- Explain the complete procedure to the subject and ask him to lie down on the tilt table.

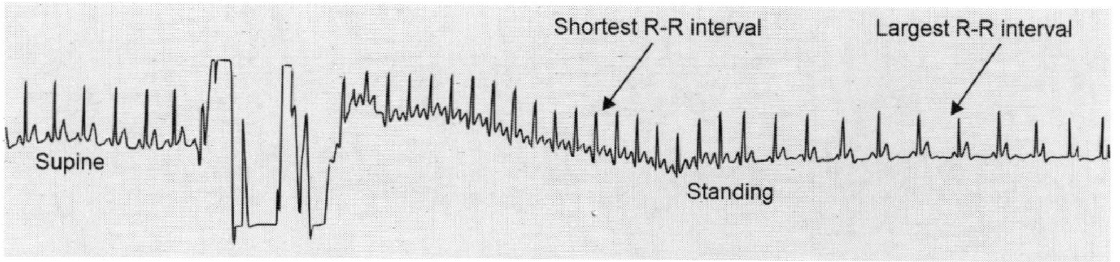

Fig. 41.3: Standing test (30:15 R-R ratio)

- Connect ECG, polygraph, and NIBP.
- Let him lie down for 10 minutes. Note his heart rate and BP.
- Put a 80° head-up tilt from a supine position.
- Record/note BP and heart rate immediately and then at one-minute intervals for about 3 minutes.

Result

On changing to head up position from supine, there is the pooling of venous blood to the periphery. This decreases cardiac filling pressure and even the stroke volume. This is corrected within a few minutes due to a decrease in parasympathetic and an increase in sympathetic activity.

Deep Breathing Test

Apparatus

ECG machine, electrodes, and jelly.

Principle

There is a change in heart rate with respect to phases of respiration, i.e. inspiration (heart rate increases) and expiration (heart rate decreases). This normal phenomenon is called as sinus arrhythmia.

Two Ways for Deep Breath

1. Using a single deep breath to see the effect on heart rate with respect to respiration.
2. Ask the subject to take deep breaths at a rate of 6 breaths/min and note variations in heart rate with respiration.

Procedure

- Explain complete procedure to the subject
- Ask him to lie in supine position with head tilted at about 30°

- Six breaths/min method of deep breathing is usually preferred over a single deep breath
- Note heart rate with respect to inspiration and expiration.

Result

An increase in heart rate with inspiration and a decrease in heart rate with expiration is observed.

Valsalva Ratio

Apparatus

ECG machine, electrodes, jelly, nose clip, mouthpiece, a mercury manometer.

Principle

When one tries to do forced expiration against a closed glottis, it is called as Valsalva maneuver, (effort) and is associated with changes in heart rate and blood pressure. For the response to occur afferents are sympathetic and parasympathetic and efferents are sympathetic pathways. This effort mainly assesses the baroreceptor activity.

Phase I and II are phases of strain.

Phase III and IV are phases of release of strain **(Fig. 41.4)**.

Procedure

- Explain the complete procedure to the subject (he/she has to be explained how to exhale forcefully in a manometer and maintain pressure at 40 mm of Hg)
- Connect ECG machine to subject (with proper placement of electrodes)
- Close nostrils using nose clip
- Put mouthpiece in the mouth of subject, and connect it with a mercury manometer

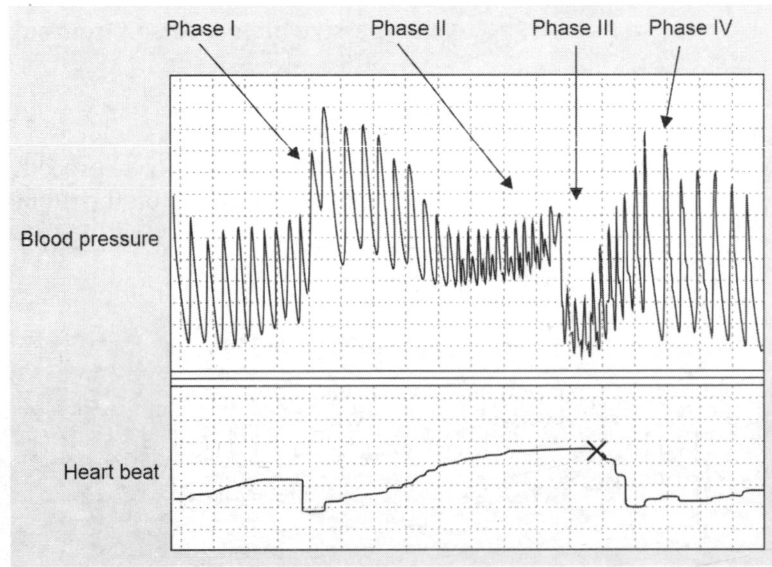

Fig. 41.4: Phases of Valsalva maneuver

Phases of Valsalva Maneuver (Phase I and II) Phases of Strain		
Phase	*Changes observed in heart rate and blood pressure*	*Cause*
Phase I (onset of strain)	Transient increase in BP for few seconds but no change in heart rate	On the onset of straining activity, there is rise in intrathoracic pressure which compresses large veins in the thorax
Phase II (two parts)	Part one- Fall in BP (for about 4 seconds)	*Part one:* Due to compression of large veins, (as explained above) there is a decrease in venous return that in turn decreases cardiac output and hence BP (lasts for 4 seconds only)
	Part two- BP comes to normal and heart rate increases.	*Part two:* Due to the effect written above (fall in BP), there is strong sympathetic vasoconstriction and increase in peripheral resistance-BP comes to normal Increase in heart rate that is observed in this phase is due to simultaneous sympathetic stimulation and vagal (parasympathetic) stimulation

Phases of Valsalva maneuver (Phase III and IV) phases of release strain		
Phase	*Changes observed in heart rate and blood pressure*	*Cause*
Phase III (release of strain)	Decrease in BP (for few seconds) and no change in heart rate	With the release of strain, there is sudden displacement of blood in the pulmonary vascular bed (as intrathoracic pressure is lessened now) that decreases BP but no change in heart rate
Phase IV (further release of strain)	BP steadily increases and heart rate decreases (occurs about 15 to 20 seconds after release of strain and lasts for few minutes)	With the release of strain in next 15 to 20 seconds after phase III, there is an increase in venous return, stroke volume and cardiac output, which increases BP with a simultaneous fall in heart rate.

- Ask the subject to blow forcefully in manometer and then to maintain pressure at 40 mm of Hg for 10 to 15 seconds
- Repeat the same procedure with a gap of 5 minutes between for three times
- Calculate the valsalva ratio and note down the largest ratio of the three.

Result

Valsalva ratio is the ratio of the longest R-R interval during phase IV to the shortest R-R interval during phase II. The normal ratio is 1.45 and above. Below that is abnormal and indicates autonomic dysfunction.

$$VR = \frac{\text{Longest R-R interval during phase IV}}{\text{Shortest R-R interval during phase II}}$$

Standing-to-lying Ratio

Principle

Heart rate does change when person lies down from standing position and it helps us to assess vagal tone (parasympathetic system) which is done with the help of continuous ECG monitoring of the patient.

Procedure

- Explain the complete procedure to the subject.
- Connect ECG leads for recording ECG (all precautions that are taken while recording ECG).
- Instruct the subject to stand quietly for about 2 minutes and then lie down in a supine position (without any support).
- Record ECG for 20 beats before and 60 beats after the subject lies in the supine position.
- Do mark the point of change of position of the subject (from standing to supine) on ECG paper.
- Repeat the same procedure thrice with an interval of 5 minutes each.

Result

Standing lying ratio (SLR) is calculated by measuring the ratio of R-R intervals from ECG. For these first five R-R intervals average is taken (before lying down position) and the shortest R-R interval during 10 beats (after lying down) is taken and a maximum ratio of three trials is reported.

Another way to calculate SLR is the longest R-R interval in standing/shortest R-R interval in lying down is noted.

Activity Tests

Resting heart rate and resting blood pressure assessment of a patient indicates parasympathetic and sympathetic activity respectively.

Heart rate variability is one of the important reactivity tests to assess autonomic functions.

Heart Rate Variability

Introduction

HRV is one of the non-invasive autonomic function test that is highly sensitive. Variation in cardiac activity with respect to respiratory cycle is called as Sinus arrhythmia and is completely a physiological phenomenon.

Beat-to-beat variations in the heart are directly co-related to discharge from SA node (pacemaker of the heart) and SA node is influenced mainly by vagal (parasympathetic) activity analysis thus helps us understand the balance between sympathetic and parasympathetic systems and thus one of the important autonomic function tests used to assess cardiovascular risk and cardiovascular health in an individual **(Fig. 41.5)**.

Apparatus

ECG machine, electrodes, jelly, software for HRV analysis.

Principle

Heart rate variability does happen with respect to variation in the length of cardiac cycle that is correlated with respiratory cycle.

Methods to Determine HRV

HRV can be measured by two methods.
1. **Short-term method:** In this method HRV is recorded for 5 minutes. The short-term method is mainly used for clinical investigations or in research.
2. Time and frequency domain analysis.

Procedure

- Before the recording, person is made to be in supine position for 15 minutes and rest.

- Person is instructed not to sleep/talk/move any body parts and close his/her eyes.
- ECG electrodes are placed on limbs and connected to ECG machine.
- ECG signal is amplified, digitized and stored in a computer for analysis and is further processed with software to get HRV analysis.
- Remove artefacts, if present.
- Using an R wave detector software, an R-R tachogram is taken out which should have at least 288 R-R intervals, and HRV analysis is done using HRV analysis software.

Analysis of HRV

Analysis of HRV: Variations in heart rate can be analysed by either time domain analysis or frequency domain analysis.

Time domain analysis: From a continuous ECG record, each QRS complex is detected and all intervals between adjacent QRS complexes are determined. They are termed as N-N intervals (instead of R-R intervals) as they denote normal beats. Time domain analysis is one of the simplest methods to determine HR. All the variables mentioned below indicate parasympathetic activity.

Time domain variables that are counted are:
- SDNN: Standard deviation of R-R interval
- RMSSD: Root square of mean of sum of all squares or difference between adjacent R-R intervals.
- NN50: Number of pairs of successive R-R (N-N) intervals that differ by more than 50 m seconds
- pNN50: It is percentage of NN50.

Frequency domain analysis: HRV is recorded in various frequencies **(Fig. 41.6)**. Frequency components that are analysed which indicate autonomic activity. Three main frequency bands includes:
1. High frequency (HF) – 0.15 to 0.4 Hz
2. Low frequency (LF)– 0.04 to 0.15 Hz
3. Very low frequency (VLF)– 0.0 to 0.04 Hz

Both LF and HF components are expressed as normalizing units (nu), i.e. (HF nu and LF nu). LF

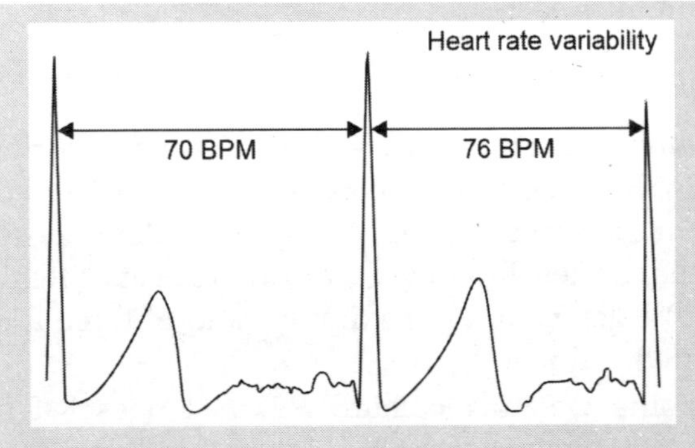

Fig. 41.5: Variation in cardiac cycle with respect to heart rate

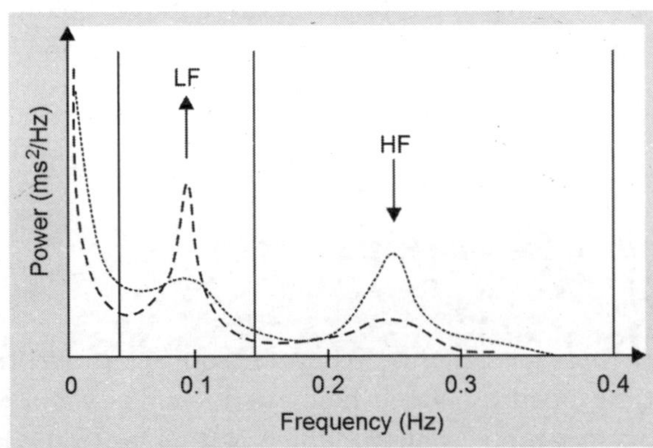

Fig. 41.6: Short-term power spectral density

component reflects sympathetic and HF component reflects vagal (parasympathetic activity). Normally, HF constitutes 60% and LF constitutes 40% thus LF-HF ratio of less than one indicates a good cardiovascular health. Total LF and HF together is called as total power of HRV.

■ IMPORTANT QUESTION AND ANSWERS

Q.1. Enumerate factors that alter SSR.
- **Physiological factors:** Age, skin temperature, and mental state of a person can affect SSR.
- **Pathological conditions:** Progressive autonomic failure, multisystem atrophy, diabetes, or alcoholic neuropathies can alter SSR.

Q.2. Trace the pathway involved in the cold pressor response test.
- **Stimulus:** Cold water (at or below 4°C)
- **Afferents:** Nociceptors
- **Efferent:** Sympathetic (adrenergic)
- **Response:** Rise in BP

Q.3. What is the physiological basis of the handgrip strength test?
- When a person holds a strong grip on the dynamometer, it is the response of the cardiovascular system mainly that is mediated due to the contraction of skeletal muscle due to hand grip. It becomes an isometric type of exercise (where length remains constant, and tension in the muscle changes).
- With a hand grip, there is stimulation of the sympathetic nervous system and its effects are recorded on heart rate and BP. Change in heart rate can also be noticed on ECG (about 30% rise of heart rate from its basal level) and diastolic BP does increase by 10 to 15 mm of Hg.
- It is one of the significant tests to study the sympathetic system function.

Q.4. Trace the pathway involved in the handgrip test.
- **Stimulus:** Isometric exercise
- **Afferents:** Mechanosensitive receptors from skeletal muscle
- **Efferent:** Sympathetic nerve endings
- **Response:** Increased heart rate and rise in diastolic BP.

Q.5. Trace the pathway involved in the standing test.
- **Stimulus:** Standing position from supine (Baro-receptors get stretched)
- **Afferents:** IXth and Xth cranial nerve
- **Efferent:** Sympathetic and parasympathetic
- **Response:** Initial increase in heart rate, followed by a decrease in heart rate and fall in BP.

Q.6. What is the physiological basis of the response obtained when a person suddenly stands from a supine position? How is it corrected immediately?

- As a person stands from a supine position, there is a pooling of blood in the lower parts of the body that causes a fall in venous return.
- When venous return falls, there is a decrease in cardiac output and BP.
- This decreased BP is sensed by baroreceptors which decreases the rate of firing of baroreceptors and is responsible for a fall in BP and heart rate (for a few seconds after standing).
- **Correction:** A fall in BP that happened immediately on standing, decreases inhibition of the vasomotor centre which increases sympathetic activity causing vasoconstriction, increased heart rate and increased force of contraction and simultaneous inhibition of the cardio-inhibitory centre causes decreased vagal activity which also helps to increase the heart rate.

Q.7. What is the clinical significance of studying the standing test?
This test helps to assess the integrity of the sympathetic nervous system and the sensitivity of baroreceptors. If systolic BP falls to 20 mm of Hg and diastolic falls to 10 mm of Hg or more, it is labelled as orthostatic hypotension.

Q.8. How can one calculate deep breathing difference?
- Normal sinus arrhythmia is heart rate rise with inspiration and heart rate falling with expiration. This is a normal observation in each person. This is mediated by pulmonary stretch receptors, cardiac mechanoreceptors, and parasympathetic innervation to the heart.
- The difference between maximum heart rate and minimum heart rate during deep breathing is called as deep breathing difference. For a normal person, this difference is about 15 beats. The test helps to assess parasympathetic activity. This difference with deep breathing can vary with age.
- Altered deep breathing difference–Seen with autonomic neuropathy, diabetes, and pulmonary diseases.

Q.9. What is the expiration to inspiration ratio (E:I ratio)?
E:I ratio: It is mean of maximum R-R intervals during deep expiration to the mean of minimum R-R intervals during deep inspiration. The normal ratio varies from 1:23 to 1:11. It does decrease with age.

Q.10. What is the physiological basis of alteration in heart rate observed with respect to standing and lying down?
When a person goes into a lying position from a standing position, there is an increase in the venous return which causes reflex bradycardia, due to a rise in vagal tone (Bainbridge reflex).

When we monitor ECG continuously in a person, this change is recorded and can be calculated by measuring the R-R interval (as it helps to calculate heart rate) called SLR as explained above. A value of SLR below 1 is considered as abnormal. It indicates parasympathetic insufficiency.

Q.11. What is the Valsalva maneuver?

It is forced expiration against a closed glottis. It has four phases I to IV. Phase I and II are phases of strain and phase III and IV are phases of release of strain. Various cardiovascular changes that do happen in various phases of the maneuver (as explained above) and they help to assess the baroreceptor activity and parasympathetic efficiency of a person.

Q.12. Enumerate factors that affect the Valsalva maneuver.

Factors affecting the Valsalva maneuver are age, sex, duration of strain, expiratory pressure and position of the patient.

Q.13. Trace pathway for Valsalva maneuver.

- **Stimulus**: Forced expiration with closed glottis
- **Afferents:** Baroreceptors, IXth and Xth cranial nerve
- **Efferent:** Sympathetic and parasympathetic

Q.14. Give the clinical application of the Valsalva maneuver.

- The cardiovascular changes observed in the Valsalva maneuver, are due to changes in intrathoracic pressure that do change sympathetic vasomotor activity and vagal activity which cause changes in BP and heart rate.
- During strain, there is an increase in sympathetic activity that increases heart rate, if there is no increase in heart rate, it suggests sympathetic dysfunction or insufficiency and in contrast, failure of heart rate to slow down or decrease (on release of strain) indicates parasympathetic dysfunction/ insufficiency.
- Such abnormalities are common with autonomic failure, diabetes, and various neuropathies.

Physiological basis of the Valsalva ratio: When we find out longest R-R interval in phase IV, we are assessing the parasympathetic sufficiency (vagus).
When we assess the shortest R-R interval in phase II, we are assessing the sympathetic sufficiency.
Note: Long R-R interval indicates a decrease in heart rate (which should happen with proper parasympathetic stimulation). The shortest R-R interval indicates an increase in heart rate (which should happen with proper sympathetic stimulation).

Q.15. What is the physiological significance of heart rate variability?

Assessment of heart rate variability is one of the most used autonomic function assessment tests. It reflects a sympathovagal balance of a person which indicates the risk of a person to cardiovascular diseases. When a person breathes in (inspiration) there is inhibition of vagal tone, which increases the heart rate with inspiration and decreases heart rate with expiration. SA nodal activity is best assessed by balance between sympathetic and vagal activity which is reflected in heart rate variability in a person. This HRV can be altered in various clinical conditions.

Q.16. What is the clinical application of the HRV test?

HRV is used as a very common effective tool for assessment of the sympathovagal activity of a person and is one of the important tests that help to determine cardiovascular health and risk of an individual. More LF activity indicates more sympathetic activity less LF activity indicates less sympathetic activity. In contrast, more HF activity indicates increased vagal drive (parasympathetic) and less HF activity indicates decreased vagal drive. LF and HF together are called as total power of HRV.

Increased LF-HF ratio indicates increased sympathetic activity and decreased LF-HF ratio indicates increased parasympathetic activity.

Alterations in HRV (decreased total power of HRV) can be picked up before any clinical symptom manifestation in the patient and thus become an effective tool to assess cardiovascular health. HRV is also used as a prognostic tool after myocardial infarction.

With interventions like yoga, exercise, and meditation, there can be an improvement in HRV and the overall cardiovascular health of a person.

Q.17. Enumerate common indications for ANS testing.
Common indications of ANS testing:

- Long-standing diabetes
- Long-standing hypertension
- Spinal cord injury
- Chronic fatigue syndrome
- Allergic conditions
- To analyze the effect of intervention with drugs, yoga, exercise, etc.

■ COMMON STATIONS – SPOTS IN PRACTICAL EXAMINATION (2/3 MARKS)

Q.1. Any of the above questions or sub-questions can be asked at practical exam stations.

Q.2. Enumerate indications for ANS testing.

Q.3. Write clinical applications of HRV testing.

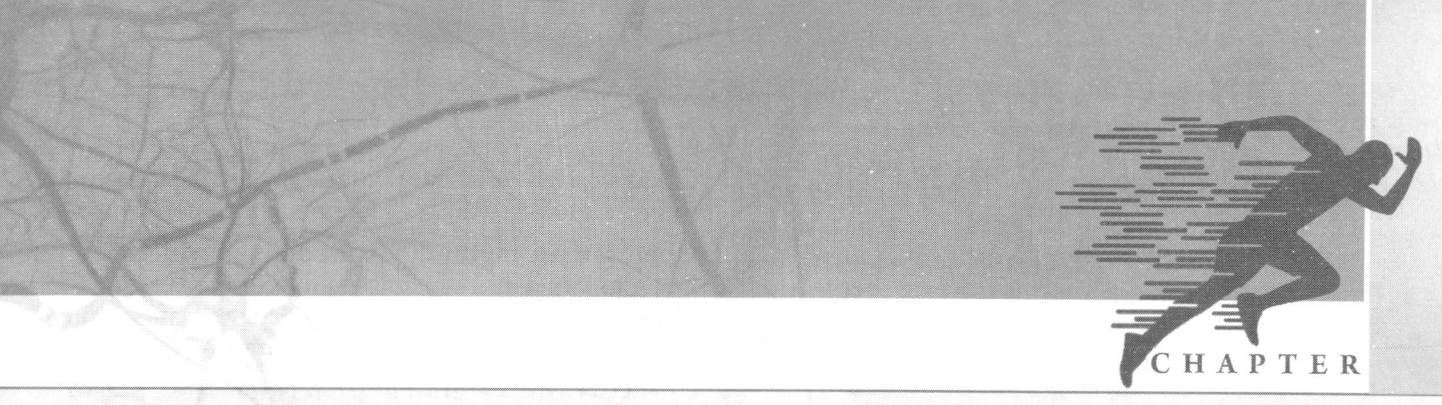

Body Composition Analysis and Calculation of BMR

Learning Objectives

At the end of this session, students should be able to:

- Understand the importance of assessment of body composition in health and disease
- Enumerate common methods to assess body composition
- Enumerate factors influencing body composition
- Understand the importance of measurement of BMR in health and disease
- Enumerate factors affecting BMR

■ INTRODUCTION

Body composition can be affected by a variety of clinical conditions like obesity, metabolic syndrome, insulin resistance and so on. Adipose tissue is an important factor in regulating lipid flux and modulating lipid and glucose homeostasis. Body composition can be assessed by various direct as well as indirect methods.

Methods of Measurement of Body Composition

The human body can be quantified at several levels. It includes atomic level (assessment of basic elements like carbon, calcium, hydrogen, potassium, etc.) to molecular (amount of protein, water and fat) and cellular level (like ECF, body mass and body cell mass, distribution of skeletal, adipose and muscle tissue). Methods for assessment include **direct methods** like densitometry, CT, MRI and DXA. **Indirect methods** include anthropometry and bioelectrical impedance analysis (BIA).

Indirect Methods

Anthropometry: These are the basic methods of assessing body composition. They include measurement of body mass, size, shape and level of fatness. Anthropometry gives an idea about the adiposity of an individual.

Body mass index (BMI), waist circumference (WC), waist-to-hip ratio (WHR), waist-to-height ratio (WHtR) and skin fold thickness are important predictors of cardiovascular risk of a person. BMI levels of about 25 are associated with an increased risk of morbidity and mortality.

Bioelectric impedance analysis (BIA): This method involves the measurement of bioelectrical resistive impedance (R). It is based on the principle that the electrical conductivity of fat-free tissue mass is greater than that of fat.

BIA include body fat, lean body mass, body cell mass (BCM) total and intracellular body water (TBW and ICW) and extracellular body water (ECW). BIA device determine body composition by measuring the electrical impedance of an imperceptible electric current passing through the body.

Impedance has two parameters – resistance and reactance. **Resistance** reflects total body water and **reactance** measures body cell mass. BIA assessment is a simple, non-invasive technique that is used commonly to measure various body composition parameters.

Apparatus

Body stat Quad Scan 4000 with accessories.

Preparation of Patient

The following instructions are given to the patient:

- No eating and drinking at least 4 hrs before the test
- No exercise for 12 hrs before the test
- No alcohol, tea, or coffee consumption 24 hrs before the test.

Procedure

- Written consent of the patient must be taken.
- After recording the name, age, and other basic information of the patient, note his/her height, weight, and waist-to-hip ratio and feed it into the machine.
- The physical activity of the patient is assessed with the help of the International Physical Activity Questionnaire (IPAQ).
- Ask the patient to lie down for 10 minutes and electrodes are placed (after aseptic precautions) on the dorsum of the hand (right hand) and metacarpophalangeal and right foot and metatarsophalangeal joints.
- Usually current of 50 kHz frequency and 500–800 microamperes current is applied via BIA equipment.
- Body composition results are displayed on the screen.
- Various body composition parameters are recorded with the help of the BIA equipment.

Basal Metabolic Rate

With the help of BIA, one can measure a patient's BMR. The BIA equipment helps to measure the body's basal and active metabolism.

BMR: It is the sum of energy required to carry out various body activities. It is measured as $kcal/h/m^2$ of body surface area.

Normal values of BMR in adults – 40 $kcal/h/m^2$ BSA (males) and 37 $kcal/h/m^2$ BSA in females (±10% is considered in the normal range).

Preparation of Patient

- Patient should be a minimum of 12 hrs fasting.
- Temperature should be comfortable (approx. 25°C)
- The patient should be in complete physical and mental relaxed state

O_2 consumption at basal rate is measured. There are three methods for the measurement of O_2 consumption:

Open circuit method: Expired air is collected in a Douglas bag. Air in the bag is analysed for O_2 and CO_2 content. The composition of atmospheric and expired air is analysed to find out O_2 consumption.

Closed circuit breathing: This is the most practised method for the measurement of BMR.

O_2 consumption = Initial level of O_2-final level of O_2 (after 6 minutes)/6

BIA method: BMR is assessed by the BIA method as discussed above.

■ IMPORTANT QUESTIONS AND ANSWERS

Q.1. What are the various body composition parameters that can be assessed with the help of BIA?

With the help of BIA, we can assess various body parameters like body weight, body cell mass, body mass index, extracellular mass, fat-free mass (%), body fat (%), total body water (TBW), basal and active metabolism.

Q.2. What is the clinical significance of doing body composition analysis?

Body composition helps one to diagnose various dysregulations in body composition by which one can also assess the cardiovascular or metabolic risk of the patient. One can also access and help understand the effects of various interventions on body composition that help us to monitor the health of our patients. We can give an individually tailored diet plan to each of our patients depending on his/her body needs.

Q.3. Enumerate factors that can affect BIA parameters.
Common factors that can affect BIA parameters:

- Position of body limbs
- Environmental conditions
- Medical conditions/drugs that can affect body compositions
- Level of physical activity before body composition analysis

Q.4. Enumerate factors that increase and decrease BMR.

Factors that increase BMR	Factors that decrease BMR
Males, pregnancy, more muscle mass, hyperthyroidism	Females, hypothyroidism, old age, fasting, starvation

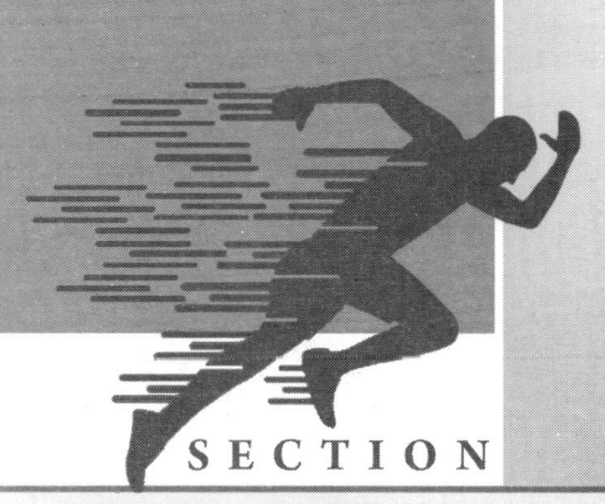

Charts, Calculations, and Endocrine Disorders

Chapter Outline

PART A: Charts

- Action Potential in Nerve Fibres
- Action Potential in Purkinje Fibres
- Compound Action Potential
- Arterial Pulse Tracing
- Cystometrogram
- Gastric Analysis
- Glucose Tolerance Test
- Ishihara's Chart
- Jaeger's Test
- Jugular Venous Pulse Tracing

- Snellen's Chart
- Strength Duration Curve
- Volume and Pressure Changes in Different Chambers of the Heart
- Oxygen Dissociation Curve
- Semen Analysis
- TPR Chart
- Growth Charts and Anthropometric Assessment of Infants

PART B: Calculations

PART C: Endocrine Disorders

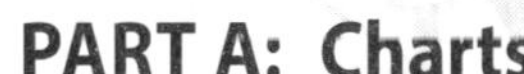

Action Potential in Nerve Fibres

■ INTRODUCTION

Nerves and muscles are excitable tissues in the body. There exists resting membrane potential across the membrane of all excitable tissues due to differences in the ionic concentration of different ions. Different muscles, nerve fibres and neurons respond by firing an action potential when a threshold stimulus is applied.

■ IMPORTANT QUESTIONS AND ANSWERS

Q.1. Define action potential. Name various components of action potential in nerve fibre.

Action potential (AP)

It is a rapid change in the membrane potential of any excitable tissue due to the application of a threshold stimulus. This change in the potential is self-propagatory and non-decremental **(Fig. 43.1)**.

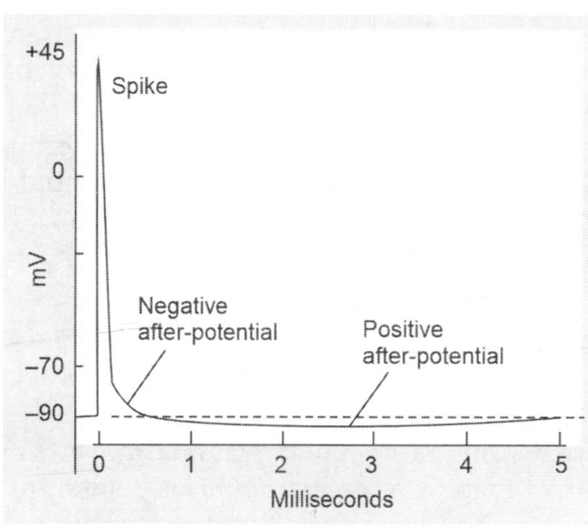

Fig. 43.1: Action potential in nerve fibre

Components of action potential
- Spike potential
- Negative after-potential
- Positive after-potential

Q.2. What is spike potential? What is its cause?
- When nerve fibre is stimulated with threshold stimulus, there is a rapid rise in membrane potential from −90 mV to +35 mV which is followed by rapid repolarization to −70 mV. This is called as spike potential.
- The reason for the rapid rise in potential from −90 mV to +35 mV is the diffusion of Na$^+$ ions in the nerve membrane (due to 5000-fold increased permeability

of the membrane for Na^+ ions with simultaneously no change in permeability for K^+ ions). This makes the inside of the membrane more positive leading to depolarization.

- The rapid repolarization from +35 mV to –70 mV occurs due to increased permeability of the membrane for K^+ ions than for Na^+ ions (decreased permeability of Na^+ ions happens due to closure of voltage-gated Na^+ channels). This causes diffusion of more number of K^+ ions out of the membrane than a number of Na^+ ions moving in. This leads to the return of inside negativity. This is called as repolarization.

Q.3. What is depolarization?

- **Depolarization**: Loss of inside negativity is depolarization. When an excitable tissue is stimulated with threshold stimulus, there is a rapid rise in potential from –90 mV to +35 mV, which happens due to Na^+ ions entry into the nerve fibre (due to increased permeability of the membrane to Na^+ ions).
- Simultaneously there is no change in the permeability of the membrane for K^+ ions, thus changing potential to a positive value (depolarization).

Q.4. What is repolarization?

- **Repolarization:** The returning of inside negativity is repolarization. Following depolarization at around +35mV, there is increased permeability of the membrane for K^+ ions.
- Simultaneously permeability of the membrane for Na^+ ions decreases, thus changing potential back to the negative value that is repolarization (from +35 mV to –70 mV).

Q.5. What is negative after potential?

- **Negative after potential:** The slow phase of repolarization from –70 mV to –90 mV is called as negative after potential.
- **Cause**: During rapid repolarization (from +35 mV to –70 mV) there is a large amount of potassium ions accumulation outside the membrane. This reduces the concentration gradient for potassium ions across the membrane, reducing the rate of diffusion of potassium ions from inside to outside, causing slow repolarization from –70 mV to –90 mV.

Q.6. What is positive after potential?

- **Positive after potential**: Even after resting membrane potential is reached (–90 mV) potassium ions efflux (movement outwards) continues which makes the membrane still more negative than RMP this causes the development of the first part of positive after potential (hyperpolarization).
- The later part of positive after potential is due to the activation of the $Na^+ K^+$ pump. When many impulses pass through a nerve fibre, with each impulse transmission there is depolarization due to Na^+ influx (moving in) and repolarization due to K^+

efflux (moving out). When this happens many times then the concentration of Na^+ inside and K^+ outside the fibre rises which acts as a stimulus for activation of $Na^+ K^+$ pump.

- $Na^+ K^+$ pump with each cycle pumps two potassium ions in and throws three sodium ions in, thus accepting one positive charge less with each cycle, creating inside negativity. This is responsible for the second half of positive after potential.

Q.7. What is recharging?

When several impulses pass through the nerve fibre, there is a change in ionic concentration of Na^+ and K^+ (as explained above) this stimulates $Na^+ K^+$ pump activity that brings the Na^+ ions and K^+ ions concentration back to normal inside and outside of the nerve fibre. This is called as **recharging.**

Q.8. What is the absolute refractory period?

- **Absolute refractory period**: It is the period following action potential during which there is a complete loss of excitability of the excitable tissue. It corresponds with spike potential.
- Even if the second subsequent stimulus is given to the excitable tissue in that period, there is no response at all from excitable tissue.
- **Cause of absolute refractory period**: Loss of excitability is due to the closure of inactivation gates of Na^+ channels (which do not open unless membrane potential reaches to RMP). During depolarization activation gates of Na^+ channels open to cause Na^+ influx inside the membrane.

Q.9. What is the relative refractory period?

Relative refractory period: It is a period following an absolute refractory period during which there is a partial loss of excitability of excitable tissue.

Q.10. How is action potential recorded?

- Action potential is recorded with the help of a cathode ray oscilloscope (CRO). It can be recorded monophasically or biphasically.
- It is obtained by placing one microelectrode (tip less than one micron) into the nerve fibre and one electrode placed outside the surface of the nerve fibre and then connecting the two to a cathode-ray oscilloscope.

We do record the electrical activity of excitable tissues like the heart, brain and muscle when we record ECG, EEG, and EMG respectively.

COMMON STATIONS – SPOTS IN PRACTICAL EXAMINATION (2/3 MARKS)

Q.1. Diagram of action potential in nerve fibre– Identify and label phases of AP, and answer any one or two questions.

Q.2. Diagram of AP in nerve fibre– Label absolute and relative refractory period.

Q.3. Draw a neatly labelled diagram of AP in nerve fibre.

▌CASE-BASED SCENARIO/PROBLEM-BASED/ CLINICAL APPLICATIONS (2/3 MARKS)

Case 1: A 45-year-old patient diagnosed with multiple sclerosis for a couple of years complains of muscle fatigue.

- What is the physiological basis of his fatigue?
- What is the pathophysiology of multiple sclerosis (clue-autoimmune disorder due to demyelination of nerve fibre, causing depression or no AP generations)?

Case 2: A 12-year-old boy comes with an injury to his right leg while playing. On examination, it is found that the wound will require suturing. To reduce pain doctor injected local anaesthetic near the injured area.

- What is the physiological basis of the mechanism of action of the local anaesthetic? (clue- anaesthetic drugs block AP conduction by acting on various ion channels).

■ KEY POINTS TO REMEMBER

- Action potential can be generated when any excitable tissue is stimulated with a threshold stimulus.
- Depolarization, repolarization, negative and positive after potential are various phases of action potential.

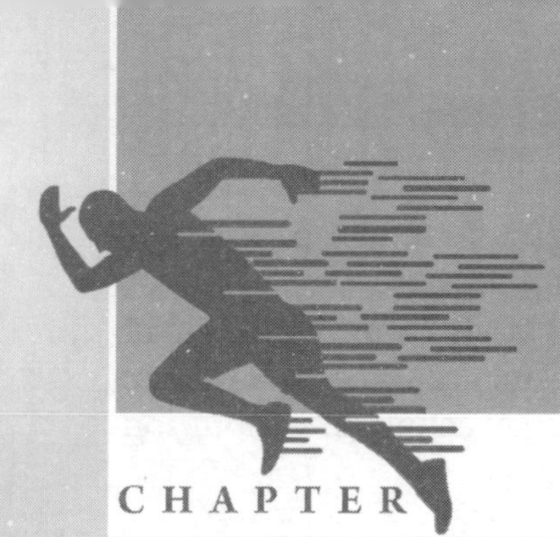

44

Action Potential in Purkinje Fibres

Learning Objectives

At the end of this practical, the student shall be able to:
- Define action potential and identify the chart of action potential in Purkinje fibre
- Enumerate various phases and describe the causes of all phases of action potential in a Purkinje fibre
- Describe the significance of the plateau
- Describe the significance of the long refractory period of the heart

■ INTRODUCTION

Purkinje fibres are one of the important structures in the specialized conductive system of the heart that is responsible for the excitation of the innermost layer of the myocardium when the impulse is generated at the SA node (pacemaker of the heart). Like all other cardiac tissues, Purkinje fibres also display a plateau phase in their action potential as atria and ventricular muscle fibres **(Fig. 44.1)**.

Purkinje fibres conduct impulses more efficiently and quickly than other tissues in the conduction system of the heart.

■ IMPORTANT QUESTIONS AND ANSWERS

Q.1. Describe action potential in Purkinje fibres of the heart.

- Action potential in cardiac muscle (Purkinje, atrial or ventricular muscle fibres) is unique from skeletal and smooth muscle fibres action potential. The duration

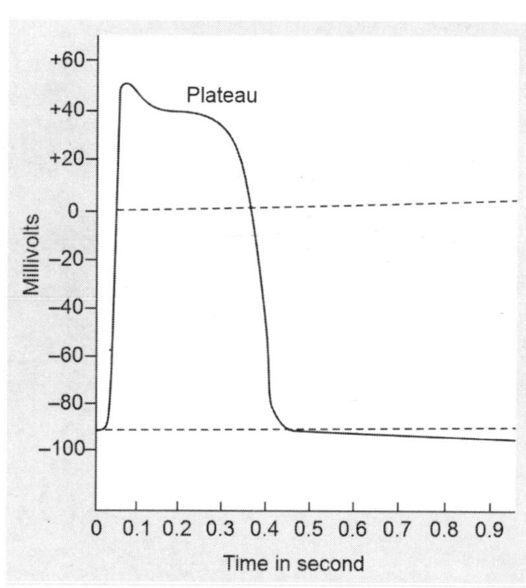

Fig. 44.1: Action potential in Purkinje fibre of the heart

of AP in Purkinje fibres is 300 to 350 ms. The action potential is characterized by the plateau phase.

- As seen in **Fig. 44.1**, it has following phases (1) **0 phase-** acute depolarization, (2) **1 phase-** a short phase of depolarization, (3) **2 phase** is plateau phase, (4) **3 phase** of repolarization, (5) **4 phase** is resting membrane potential.

- **Phase 0**: This is a rapid phase of depolarization that changes potential from −90 mV to +35 mV. This is due to the opening of fast voltage-gated Na^+ channels (upstroke).

- **Phase 1**: This is a short phase of repolarization
- **Phase 2**: Plateau
- **Phase 3**: Repolarization
- **Phase 4**: RMP

Q.2. What is plateau potential? Enumerate causes of plateau/phase 2.

A sustained state of depolarization that you see in AP in cardiac muscle (Purkinje, atrial, ventricular muscle fibres) is known as a plateau.

Causes of plateau

- Opening of slow Na^+ Ca^{++} channels causing Na^+ and Ca^{++} influx, trying to maintain inside positivity.
- Throughout the plateau phase, there is decreased permeability of membrane for K^+ ions thus hardly K^+ ions movement is allowed outwards, trying to maintain inside positivity.

  Thus, by maintaining inside positivity, depolarization is maintained. Thus, the plateau is a sustained state of depolarization that is unique in cardiac muscle action potential.

Q.3. What is the significance of the plateau phase?

Significance of plateau: Ca^{++} ions do enter the cardiac membrane during this phase (via Na^+ Ca^{++} channels) that add to the Ca^{++} released from terminal cisternae of muscle. This availability of Ca^{++} ions makes the contractile process of the myocardium more strong.

Q.4. What is the difference between the AP of the SA node and Purkinje fibres?

SA node fibre AP	Purkinje fibre AP
RMP is –55 to –60 mV	RMP is –85 to –90mV
Membrane at resting stage is leaky to Na^+ ions	The membrane is not leaky to Na^+ ions
Depolarization is due to Na^+ and Ca^{++} ions influx due to the opening of Na^+ Ca^{++} channels	Depolarization is due to Na^+ influx (from fast voltage-gated Na^+ channels)
Plateau is not seen	Plateau is seen
Duration of AP 200 to 250 msec	Duration of AP 300 to 350 msec

Q.5. How much is the absolute refractory period of the heart? Give its advantage.

- The absolute refractory period for Purkinje fibres or atrial or ventricular muscle fibres is 0.3 seconds (throughout the plateau phase) which means the whole of the contraction phase.
- Due to this long refractory period, the second subsequent stimulus is not effective and thus heart shows properties of non-tetanizability and non-fatigability and thus heart acts as an effective pump.

Q.6. What is the physiological basis of the fast conduction of impulses via Purkinje fibres of the heart?

- Purkinje fibre cells are larger than other myocardial cells and have fewer myofibrils.
- As compared to other cells and glycogen content of Purkinje fibre cells is high as compared to other cells and thus are capable of withstanding hypoxia than other cardiac cells.
- Special connexin protein in the cells in Purkinje fibres make them efficient in the conduction of impulses faster (2–4 m/s) than other cardiac tissue. Purkinje fibres are responsible for controlling the time of ventricular conduction of impulses.

▮ COMMON STATIONS – SPOTS IN PRACTICAL EXAMINATION (2/3 MARKS)

Q.1. Diagram of action potential in Purkinje fibre: Identify and label phases of AP in Purkinje fibre of the heart and answer any one or two questions on it.

Q.2. Diagram of AP in Purkinje fibre: Label the plateau phase and enumerate its causes.

Q.3. Enumerate points that differentiate AP in Purkinje and AP in SA nodal fibre of the heart.

▮ CASE-BASED SCENARIO/ PROBLEM-BASED/ CLINICAL APPLICATIONS

- Dysfunction in conduction via Purkinje fibres can be one of the most common causes
- Re-entry or abnormal impulse conduction leading to ventricular arrhythmias, ventricular tachycardias and ventricular fibrillation.
- Purkinje fibre dysfunction is one of the common causes of arrhythmia post-heart failure as well.
- Various antiarrhythmic drugs are acting on the various ion channels to slow excitability (mainly by blocking Na^+ and Ca^{++} channels), especially in Purkinje fibres, or SA or AV nodes that can help slow down electrical impulses in the heart.
- Cardiac pacing or Purkinje system pacing has been found to improve cardiac function.

▮ KEY POINTS TO REMEMBER

- Action potential can be generated when any excitable tissue is stimulated with a threshold stimulus.
- Depolarization, plateau, and repolarization are unique features of cardiac muscle.
- Purkinje fibres are responsible for impulse conduction through ventricles (to the innermost layer of the myocardium).

45

Compound Action Potential

■ INTRODUCTION

Compound action potential is a record of action potential from a nerve trunk. A nerve trunk contains different types of nerve fibres **(Fig. 45.1)**.

It is the result of the summation of many action potentials from different nerve axons in a nerve trunk. The compound action potential is used to assess peripheral nerve functioning.

■ IMPORTANT QUESTIONS AND ANSWERS

Q.1. What is a compound action potential?
Compound action potential: It is an algebraic summation of all action potential recorded from a nerve trunk containing many types of nerve fibres.

Q.2. How is compound action potential recorded?
- One part of the nerve trunk is injured and one electrode is kept on it. The injured area is permanently depolarized. Let that electrode be 'B'. Another

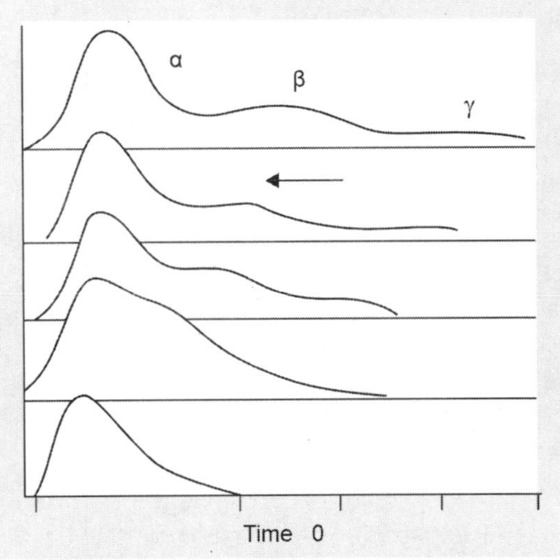

Fig. 45.1: Compound action potential

electrode is placed on an uninjured area let that electrode be 'A'. These two electrodes are connected to CRO.

- As the membrane under B is depolarized permanently (injured) and the membrane under A is positive, A and B are not equipotential. Thus, the current of injury is recorded on CRO.

- Now, nerve trunk is stimulated with the help of stimulating electrodes at some distance from electrodes A and B. Due to this stimulating electrode action potential is initiated in the nerve trunk.

- Action potential initiated by fast-conducting fibres first reaches electrode A, making the area under electrodes A and B equipotential thus no current flows between them. This causes loss of current of injury and the graph comes to baseline (which is an alpha wave). When the membrane under A gets repolarized again, A and B electrodes are no longer equipotential as B records the current of injury (upstroke).

- Now medium conducting fibres conduct impulses under the membrane of electrode A, making it depolarized, which again makes the A and B electrodes equipotential and the current of injury disappears recorded as a beta wave. When again membrane under A is repolarized again, makes A and B electrodes again no longer equipotential and the current of injury is recorded from the membrane under electrode B as an upstroke.
- In a similar way gamma wave is recorded due to impulse transmitted by slow conducting fibers **(Fig. 45.1)**.

Q.3. What can be done for better separation of waves while recording compound action potential?

For better separation of waves, stimulating electrodes should be away from recording electrodes.

Q.4. What do numbers written on the graph indicate?

Numbers written on the graph indicate the distance between stimulating and recording electrodes in millimetres.

Q.5. How nerve fibres are classified?

Nerve fibres are classified according to diameter and conduction velocity:

- *A group:* 1 to 20 microns in diameter. Conduction velocity 5 to 120 m/s. They are myelinated and are sensory as well as motor in function

- *B group:* 1to 3 microns in diameter. Conduction velocity 3 to 14 m/s. They are myelinated. They are found in preganglionic autonomic nerves.
- *C group:* Less than 1micron diameter conduction velocity 2 m/s or less. Mostly these fibers are unmyelinated and found in visceral and cutaneous nerves.

■ COMMON STATIONS – SPOTS IN PRACTICAL EXAMINATION (2/3 MARKS)

Q.1. Diagram of compound action potential: Identify, label and answer any one or two questions (check above).

Q.2. In a nerve trunk which nerve fibres will get stimulated first, explain.

Q.3. What is the physiological basis of the current of injury?

■ CASE-BASED SCENARIO/PROBLEM-BASED/ CLINICAL APPLICATIONS

Compound nerve or muscle action potential is studied as a part of a complete neurophysiological examination and is done with the help of an electromyogram (EMG). (Please refer to Human Experiments).

■ KEY POINTS TO REMEMBER

Compound action potential is the algebraic summation of all action potentials generated in different axons in the nerve trunk.

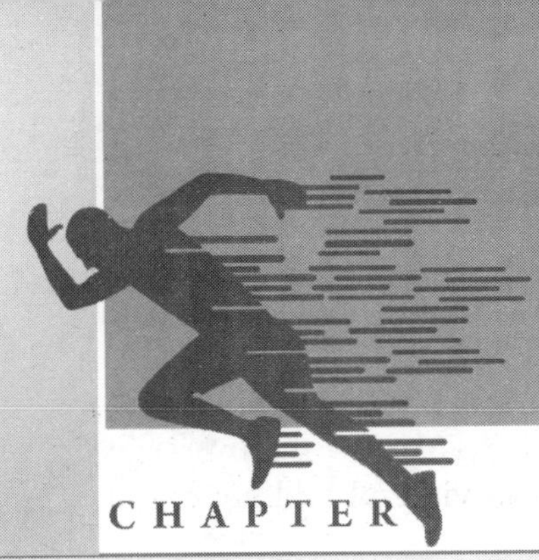

Arterial Pulse Tracing

Learning Objectives

At the end of this practical, students shall be able to:
- Describe different waves in normal arterial pulse tracing
- Understand the significance of arterial pulse tracing
- Explain the significance of the dicrotic notch followed by the dicrotic wave
- Understand different variations in pulse with respect to various conditions and their physiological basis

■ INTRODUCTION

Arterial pulse tracing can be recorded with the help of Dudgeon's sphygmograph **(Fig. 46.1)**. During ventricular systole when blood is suddenly ejected in the aorta and is then transmitted throughout the arterial system is the record of the same.

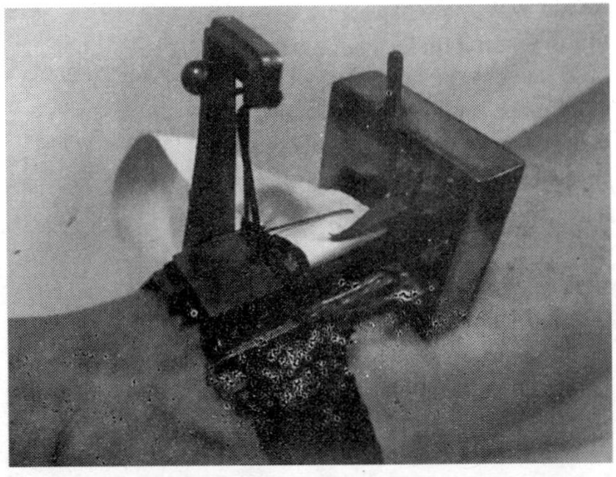

Fig. 46.1: Dudgeon's sphygmograph

■ IMPORTANT QUESTIONS AND ANSWERS

Q.1. How is arterial pulse tracing recorded and what are the important waves recorded in it?

Arterial pulse is recorded with the help of a sphygmograph. This has to be placed on the radial artery to record arterial pulse tracing. The wave recorded in pulse tracing is an anacrotic limb that records upstroke (also called as percussion wave). This occurs due to ventricular systole and the catacrotic limb that records a downstroke. Radial pulse recording is shown in **Fig. 46.3**.

Q.2. Write the cause of the dicrotic notch followed by the dicrotic wave. What is its significance?

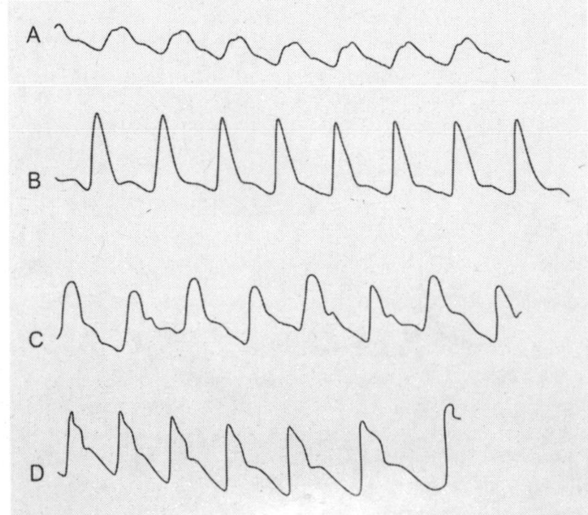

Figs. 46.2A to D: (A) Aortic stenosis; (B) Aortic regurgitation; (C) Pulsus alternans; (D) Normal arterial pulse tracing

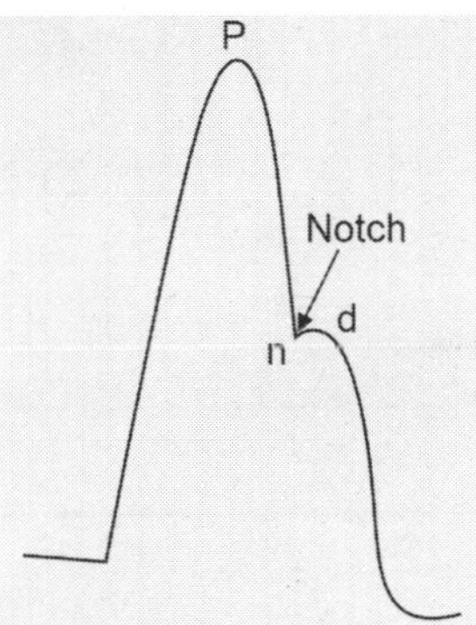

Fig. 46.3: Radial pulse recording p- Percussion wave, d- Dicrotic wave, n- Dicrotic notch

- Dicrotic notch (it's a sharp depression near the middle of downstroke) followed by the dicrotic wave is recorded on a catacrotic limb.
- Dicrotic notch is a small downward deflection found in arterial pulse tracing following the closure of semilunar valves.
- It is caused due to backflow of blood from the aorta to the ventricle (it indicates the end of ventricular systole). This slightly increases the pressure in the aorta causing a dicrotic wave in pulse tracing.

Q.3. What is a primary wave? What is its significance?
- The wave from the beginning of the tracing up to the dicrotic notch is called a primary wave.
- Large primary wave is due to larger stroke volume, bradycardia or due to low peripheral resistance.
- Wide and small primary wave is due to tachycardia, increased stiffness (less compliance) of blood vessels, and increased peripheral resistance.

Q.4. What is anacrotic pulse/ slow rising pulse?
- It is a small volume pulse with a late systolic peak (i.e. pulse is slow to rise). It occurs in aortic stenosis.
- Obstruction at the level of the aorta restricts the rate at which blood can be ejected from the left ventricle **(Fig. 46.2A)**.

Q.5. What is a water hammer pulse or collapsing pulse?
- Collapsing pulse is characterized by rapid ascent and descent of the pulse wave. This type of pulse is seen with aortic regurgitation.
- In aortic regurgitation, during diastole, the left ventricle receives blood not only from normal pulmonary venous return but also some amount of blood ejected in the aorta during previous systole as it flows from the aorta due to an incompetent valve **(Fig. 46.2 B)**.
- Resultant large stroke volume that is rapidly ejected produces a rapidly rising carotid pulse that collapses in early diastole (due to backflow from aortic valve).
- This collapsing pulse can be exaggerated at the radial artery by lifting the arm.

Q.6. What is pulsus parvus?
- Parvis means small. When the amplitude of the pulse wave is small, it is known as pulsus parvus. It indicates low cardiac output.

- It is seen with coarctation of the aorta, myocardial infarction, and severe hypotension.

Q.7. What is a dicrotic pulse?
- When there is a small second wave (dicrotic wave) following the peak of the main wave, it is called as dicrotic wave.
- This makes the dicrotic wave prominent than normal therefore two pulse waves are felt during one heartbeat. It is seen in heart failure.

Q.8. What is plateau pulse?
If a delayed systolic peak in aortic stenosis is sustained, it is labelled as a plateau pulse.

Q.9. What is pulsus alternans?
There is a regular alteration in the size of the beats. The beats are regularly placed but are alternately large and small. It is seen in left ventricular failure or severe ventricular dysfunction **(Fig. 46.2C)**.

Q.10. What is pulsus bisferiens?
It shows two peaks in systole. It is observed in combination with aortic regurgitation and aortic stenosis.

Q.11. What is pulsus paradoxus?
- It is an exaggerated decrease in the strength of arterial pulse during inspiration, with more than 10 mm Hg fall in systolic BP.
- It can be seen with cardiac tamponade, constrictive pericarditis, and acute asthma.

▌COMMON STATIONS– SPOTS IN PRACTICAL EXAMINATION (2/3 MARKS)

Q.1. Diagram of arterial pulse tracing: Identify and label anacrotic and dicrotic wave and dicrotic notch, and answer any one or two questions (check above).

Q.2. Diagram showing pulsus alternans, collapsing pulse, etc.: Identify and answer questions (check above).

Q.3. Describe normal arterial pulse tracing.

▌CASE-BASED SCENARIO/ PROBLEM-BASED/ CLINICAL APPLICATIONS

- Arterial pulse wave analysis helps to understand the complex interplay of left ventricular stroke volume, vascular compliance, systemic resistance, and other physiological factors.
- Wave analysis helps us give clues to estimate the cardiac output of a person and helps to assess cardiovascular elasticity.
- The contour of pulse waves varies in different parts of circulation and depending on which artery, one is recording pulse waves.

OSCE– For Clinical Examination of Pulse – Refer to Clinical Physiology (Chapter on Examination of Arterial Pulse)

Cystometrogram

■ INTRODUCTION

- Cystometrogram is a part of urodynamic testing. One can assess the bladder functions with this.
- It helps understand pressure changes in the bladder when it gets filled. It tries to assess detrusor function and bladder sensation.
- Record is monitored via intravesical catheters and signal is transmitted and recorded on a recorder.

■ IMPORTANT QUESTIONS AND ANSWERS

Q.1. What is cystometrogram? Explain the normal graph of cystometrogram.

- Cystometrogram is a graph indicating a relationship between intravesical volume and intravesical pressure.
- As the volume of urine in the bladder rises there is only a slight rise in pressure. If volume rises beyond that, pressure in the bladder remains constant (between the volume of 50 ml to 400 ml). This is shown as a plateau again, an increase in volume increases the pressure and thus causes the stretch of the bladder muscle and initiation of the micturition reflex **(Fig. 47.1)**.
- Plateau indicates that a large volume of urine can be stored in the bladder without a rise in pressure. This

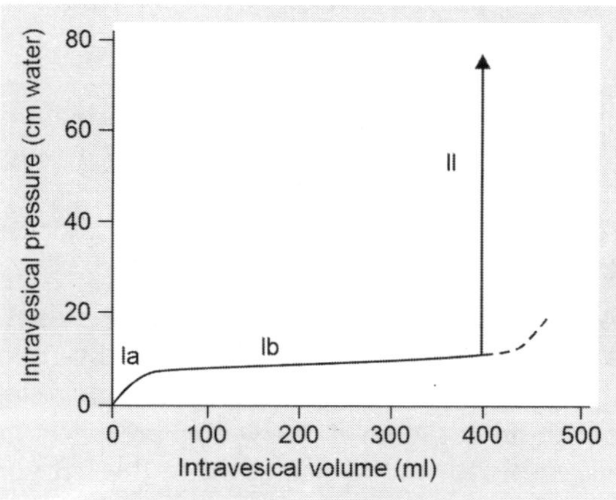

Fig. 47.1: Cystometrogram

is possible because of the property of plasticity of the bladder muscle. Tension in the wall varies according to Laplace's law as given below:

$$\text{Collapsing pressure} = 2T/r$$

Where,

T = tension in the wall

r = radius of the bladder

Q.2. How much is the normal capacity of the bladder?
The physiological capacity of the bladder is 400 to 500 ml. The anatomical capacity of the bladder is 700 to 800 ml.

Q.3. What is the use of cytometry?
Uses:
- To measure bladder capacity and pressure.

- To assess the integrity of sphincters when urine is stored and passed.

COMMON STATIONS – SPOTS IN PRACTICAL EXAMINATION (2/3 MARKS)

Q.1. Cystometrogram graph: Identify and answer any one or two questions as given above.

KEY POINTS TO REMEMBER

- The physiological capacity of the bladder is 400 to 500 ml. The anatomical capacity of the bladder is 700 to 800 ml.
- Due to the plasticity of the bladder muscle, a large amount of urine can be stored in the bladder without much rise in pressure.

Gastric Analysis

Learning Objectives

At the end of this practical, students shall be able to:
- Enumerate indications for gastric analysis
- Describe the procedure of gastric analysis
- Describe free, total and combined acidity
- Define achlorhydria, hypochlorhydria and hyperchlorhydria
- Describe insulin test and its significance

■ INTRODUCTION

Measurement of gastric acid secretion was done previously to assess and diagnose peptic ulcer diseases. In a normal person, basic acid output is not more than a few millimetres per hour containing up to 10 mmol/L of hydrogen ions. In patients with **Zollinger-Ellison syndrome (ZES),** the ratio of basal and maximum acid secretion is increased more than six-fold **(Fig. 48.1).**

■ IMPORTANT QUESTIONS AND ANSWERS

Q.1. Describe the procedure of gastric analysis.

The gastric analysis is done to study the secretory function of the stomach. The patient is asked to take a light diet, the previous night and has to come fasting in the morning. Ryle's tube is introduced (up to the second mark) till it enters the stomach. Fasting juice is collected and analyzed.

Test meals:
- 7% 50 ml alcohol
- 300 ml oatmeal gruel
- Dry toast with a cup of tea

Any one of the above test meals is given. After giving the test meal, gastric samples are collected every 15 minutes for 3 hrs. Each time 10 ml of contents are aspirated. Each sample is placed in different tubes for analysis.

S. No.	Test	Procedure
1.	Free acid	Is titrated with standard alkali (0.1NaOH) till pH 3.5 is obtained. Topfer's reagent is used as an indicator. Acidity is expressed in clinical units as the number of millilitres of standard alkali required to titrate 100 ml of gastric sample to a pH of 3.5
2.	Total acid	The sample is titrated further with alkali till a pH of 8.5. Phenolphthalein is used as an indicator. Acidity is expressed in clinical units as explained above
3.	Combined acid	It is obtained by subtracting free acid from total acid. It includes HCl combined with proteins, mucus and organic acids
4.	Total chloride	Total chloride content is determined. It includes chloride of HCl, combined HCl, inorganic chloride, etc. It is not affected by the entry of bile. Free acidity and estimation of chloride further give better information about the secretory ability of the stomach
5.	Starch and sugar	When starch and sugar are present in the stomach, it indicates that stomach emptying is not complete. The emptying time of the stomach can be analyzed when starch and sugar are absent in the sample
6.	Bile	Bile regurgitates from the duodenum thus; its presence indicates that stomach emptying has started and the pyloric sphincter is open
7.	Lactic acid	It is a product of fermentation and thus lactic acid secretion is high when acid secretion is less
8.	Blood	The presence of blood first one or two samples can be due to injury caused while passing Ryle's tube. Its presence in other samples may indicate gastric ulcer or cancer
9.	Mucus	Normally, some amount of mucus is present in the sample. Excess of it may indicate irritation of gastric mucosa
10.	Pepsin	The presence of pepsin in a sample indicates that peptic cells are functional

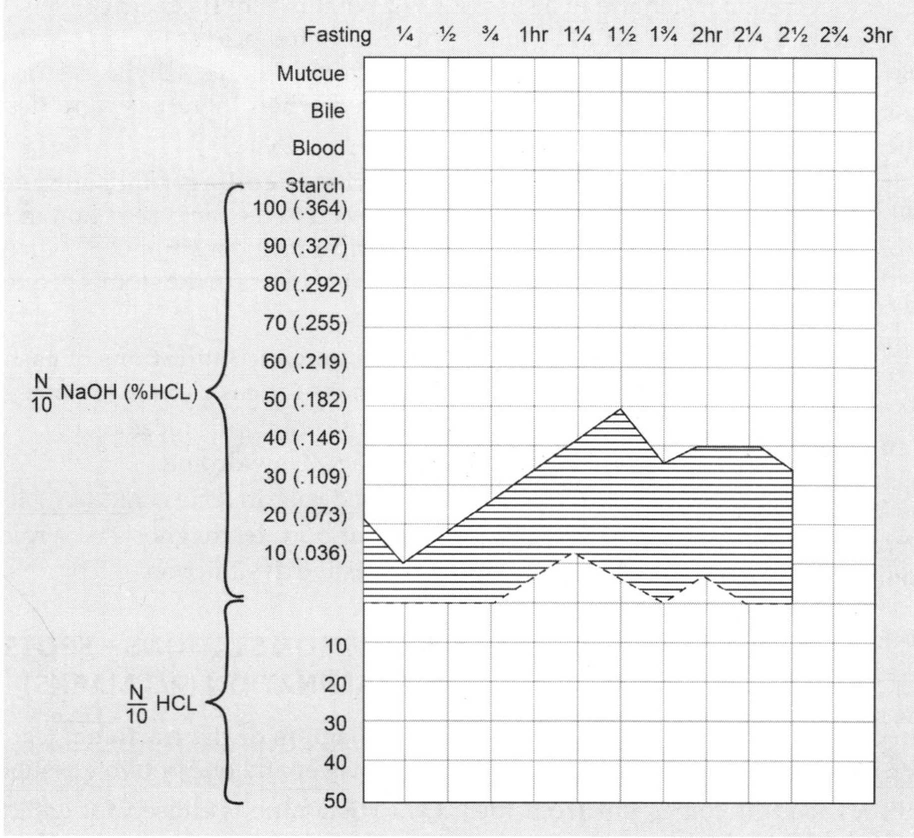

Fig. 48.1: Gastric analysis

Q.2. Describe curves of free acidity and total acidity.

- **Free acidity**: As we find out levels of free acid from each sample, the curve of free acidity is obtained against time. Usually in fasting samples level is less than 20 clinical units.
- **Normal pattern of the curve**: Immediately after giving the test meal, free acid level drops due to the dilution of acid with a meal. Then gradually it starts rising and reaches a peak at the end of one hour (40 to 70 ml units), remains high for about 1 to one and a half hr. and then declines within 3 hrs.
- **Total acidity**: As a free acidity curve, the total acidity curve is plotted. Maximum level of total acidity is about 80 to 120 clinical units.

Q.3. What is combined acidity?

Portion between free and total acidity curves denotes combined acidity. It is the amount of HCl in a combined form with protein, mucus, and organic acids.

Q.4. What is hypochlorhydria and hyperchlorhydria?

- **Hypochlorhydria:** When there is decreased secretion of acid and on analysis, it is found that free acid levels are below normal, this is known as hypochlorhydria.
- **Hyperchlorhydria:** When free acid levels on gastric analysis are higher and the dose does not come to normal in 3 hours, it is known as hyperchlorhydria.

Q.5. What is achlorhydria? What is true and false achlorhydria?

- **Achlorhydria**: It is a condition where there is a complete absence of acid secretion in all gastric samples.
- **False achlorhydria**: It is a condition where acid secretion does happen from the stomach but is not detected in any gastric samples as acid gets neutralized.
- **True achlorhydria**: It is a condition where there is no secretion of acid from the stomach at all.

Q.6. How to differentiate between true and false achlorhydria? Histamine is used to detect true chlorhydria. Justify.

- A histamine test is done to differentiate between true and false achlorhydria. This test is the same as a test meal but instead of a test meal, a histamine injection is given (40 micrograms/kg of body weight).
- After histamine injection if acid is not secreted then it is a true achlorhydria or histamine-fast achlorhydria. It is observed with chronic gastritis, stomach cancer or any other condition where there is destruction of gastric mucosa.

Cause of choosing histamine:

- Histamine is a potent stimulator of the gastric mucosa to stimulate acid secretion if the test meal has failed to do it.

- Histamine causes acid secretion faster and in a short time so that there is no time available for neutralization so can be detected as free-acid.

Q.7. What is an insulin test?

- Insulin test is the same as fractional test meal but insulin injection is given instead of test meal. About 7 units of insulin are injected subcutaneously. This causes hypoglycemia which in turn stimulates the vagal nerve which stimulates the secretion of gastric juice with acid secretion.
- As test indicates the integrity of the vagus nerve. Thus, this test is used to assess if a vagotomy operation done in patients is successful or not.

Q.8. Can there be any other condition coexisting with achlorhydria?

Oxyntic cells in the stomach that secrete acid, are also responsible for secretion of intrinsic factor (Castle's intrinsic factor) required for vitamin B12 absorption. If for any reason if oxyntic cells are damaged, then along with achlorhydria there can be associated pernicious anaemia (B12 deficiency anaemia).

Q.9. How is gastric secretion studied in animals?

- **Sham feeding:** The oesophagus is cut in the neck region and cut ends are brought to the exterior. As the animal swallows food, it comes out from the proximal opening. Gastric juice is collected by passing a tube from the distal opening. An important point to understand here is juice uncontaminated with food is collected. This test usually tests the cephalic phase of gastric secretion.
- Gastric acid secretion can also be studied by creating various pouches of the stomach like Pavlov's pouch, Heidenhain's pouch, and Bickel's pouch and collecting and analyzing gastric secretions collected from the pouch.

Q.10. What is gastroscopy?

The interior of the stomach can be studied with the help of a long tubular instrument. With gastroscopy, one can take a biopsy from the stomach region for study.

Q.11. What is tubeless gastric analysis?

For doing tubeless gastric analysis, cation resin exchange is given by mouth. This gets dissociated in the stomach by HCl. Liberated cations are absorbed and excreted in urine. The amount of cations excreted in urine indicates the amount of acid secreted.

Q.12. What is achylia gastrica?

Absence of free acid as well as pepsin collected in gastric samples is called as achylia gastrica. This condition is observed when there is severe destruction of gastric mucosa.

Q.13. What is Zollinger-Ellison syndrome (ZES)?

There is an excess acid secretion in the stomach due to a gastrin-producing tumour which causes the development of ulcers in the stomach, duodenum, and upper jejunum.

Q.14. Enumerate indications of gastric analysis.

Indications for gastric analysis are:

- To rule out peptic ulcers
- Detect ZE syndrome
- Raised gastrin levels
- To support the diagnosis of pernicious anaemia
- Digestive dysfunction.

▌ COMMON STATIONS – SPOTS IN PRACTICAL EXAMINATION (2/3 MARKS)

Q.1. Diagram of the fractional test meal. Identify and answer any one or two questions.

Q.2. Histamine is chosen for detection of true achlorhydria. Give physiological basis.

▌ CASE-BASED SCENARIO/PROBLEM-BASED/ CLINICAL APPLICATIONS

Nowadays gastric analysis is done rarely. A variety of other investigations are available by which gastric functions; and ulcers can be diagnosed. If required endoscopic gastric analysis can be done for diagnosis of ulcers or ZE syndrome. It takes less time and is easy compared to conventional gastric analysis.

▌ KEY POINTS TO REMEMBER

- Gastric function studies are done to assess the secretory capacity of the stomach.
- It includes a variety of tests like fractional test meal, insulin test meal, and histamine test meal.
- Patient comes after 12 hrs. of fasting. Tests are time-consuming and better tests via endoscopy can help access gastric secretory functions better.

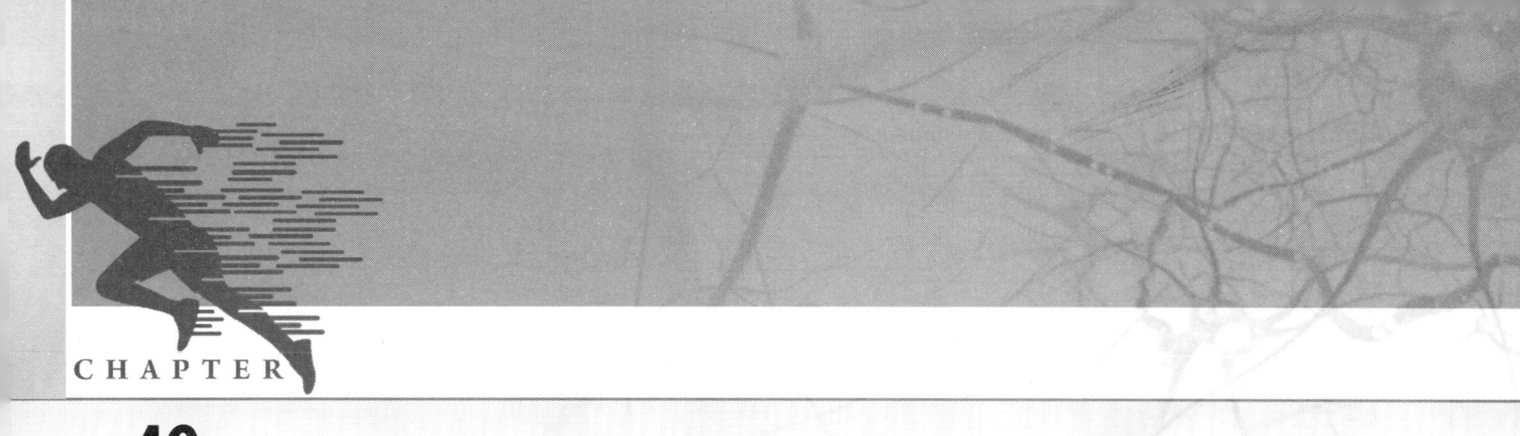

Glucose Tolerance Test

■ INTRODUCTION

A glucose tolerance test is done to assess the body's response to glucose, that is how glucose is utilized in your body. It is one of the important methods for screening diabetes.

■ IMPORTANT QUESTIONS AND ANSWERS

Q.1. How is the glucose tolerance curve obtained?
- Before this test, it is ensured that 8 days before the person takes a minimum of 100 grams of carbo-hydrate/day in his/her diet. Starvation can give rise to a diabetic type of curve.
- A person is called fasting in the morning. Blood and urine sample is collected to test the presence of sugar in them. After this person is given glucose as 1 g/kg of body weight or 50 g. After giving glucose, every half an hour urine and blood samples are collected for two and a half to three hrs.
- Glucose levels are plotted against the time to obtain the glucose tolerance curve. None of the urine samples show the presence of glucose.
- Instead of oral glucose as mentioned above, one can give intravenous glucose and can plot a glucose tolerance curve.

Q.2. Describe the normal glucose tolerance curve.
- Fasting level of glucose in a normal person varies from 80 to 120 mg/100 ml.
- After administration of glucose, the blood glucose level rises to a peak level up to 140–150 mg/100 ml in one or one and a half hour. It does not cross the renal threshold.
- After that blood glucose level falls and reaches to fasting level within two and half to three hours **(Fig. 49.1)**.
- A curve is plotted with blood glucose levels on the vertical axis and time on the horizontal axis.

Q.3. What is the tubular load of glucose?
The amount of glucose which is filtered by renal tubules every minute is known as the tubular load for glucose, e.g. when blood glucose is 180 mg/100 ml, the tubular load is 220 mg as each minute 125 ml of plasma is filtered through glomeruli.

Q.4. What is the renal threshold for glucose?
- Renal threshold for glucose is 180 mg%. This means that as long as the blood glucose level is below 180 mg% glucose is not excreted in urine.

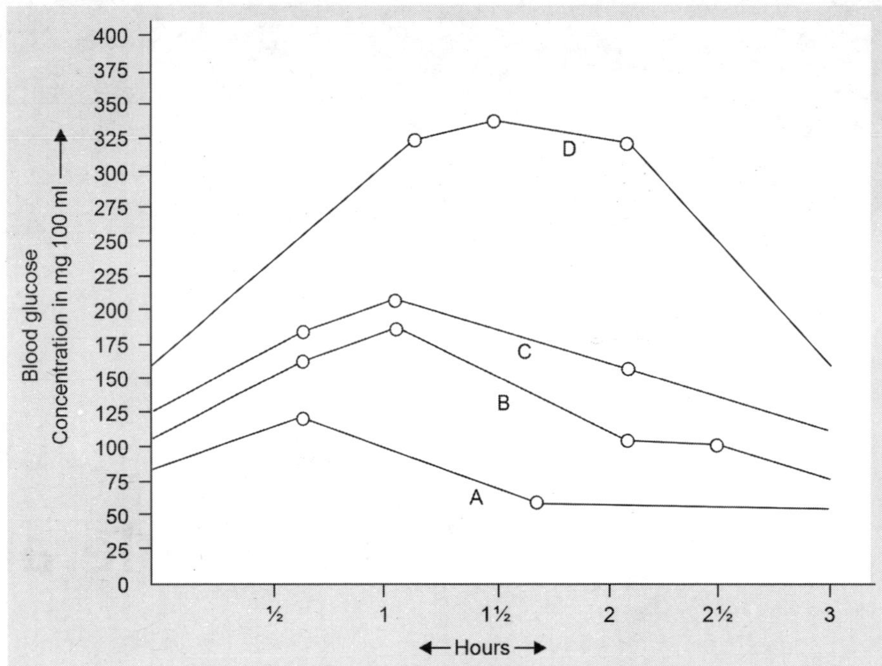

Fig. 49.1: Glucose tolerance test (GTT): A. Normal, B. Pre-diabetic, C. Borderline (mild) diabetic, D. Severe diabetic

- When blood glucose level rises above 180 mg% all excess glucose is excreted in urine.

Q.5. What is the transport maximum? How much is it for glucose?

Transport maximum is the maximum rate at which renal tubules can absorb a particular substance. It is different for different substances, for glucose TmG (tubular maximum for glucose) is 320 mg/minute.

Q.6. Describe the glucose tolerance curve obtained in a diabetic person.

- In a diabetic person, the fasting blood glucose level is more than 120 mg%. This level varies with respect to the severity of diabetes. After giving glucose, the peaked level reached is more than 180 mg% (i.e. above renal threshold). The peak value of glucose depends on the severity of the diabetes. At this time, glucose is excreted from urine and can be detected in urine samples.
- The raised blood glucose level does not come to a fasting level in two and a half to three hours.

Q.7. Even though the tubular maximum for glucose (TmG) is 320 mg/min, why does glucose appear in the urine when blood glucose levels are just above 180 mg% (resulting in a tubular load of 220 mg/min)?

Though the tubular maximum for glucose is 320 mg/min, glucose appears in urine with tubular load of 220 mg/minute. This is called as splay.

Causes of splay:

- Although the affinity of the transport system for glucose is high, the finite concentration of glucose must remain in tubular fluid to saturate the transport system. Some amount of glucose is thus excreted prior to saturation.
- There is considerable variability in filtration capacity of glomeruli as well variable reabsorptive capacity of renal tubules. Few nephrons may have subnormal reabsorptive capacity and thus would excrete glucose at lower glucose levels than other nephrons.

Q.8. What is hypoglycemia? Why it is dangerous?

- Decrease in blood glucose level below 50 to 70 mg/100 ml is termed hypoglycemia. Brain tissue cannot tolerate hypoglycemia for more than a few seconds.
- Hypoglycemia can be fasting or post-prandial.
- Symptoms of hypoglycemia-sweating, dryness of mouth, anxiety, tremors, etc.

Q.9. Define glycosuria.

The presence of glucose in the urine is known as glycosuria. It is seen when the blood glucose level rises above the renal threshold, i.e. 180 mg/100 ml.

Q.10. What is renal glycosuria?

Presence of glucose in urine even if the renal threshold of 180 mg/100 ml is not exceeded in blood, is known as renal glycosuria. This is because there is a lowering of the renal threshold for glucose (normally, it is congenital).

Q.11. What is a prediabetic state?

- **Prediabetic state:** It is a condition where a person has not developed or been diagnosed as diabetic, but is at increased risk of getting diabetes in the near future. There can be many risk factors that he/she may be associated with, some of which may include, obesity, a sedentary lifestyle, less vegetables and fruits in diet, high cholesterol levels, family h/o diabetes, hypertension, etc.

- If timely intervention is done, the condition can be completely reversed if appropriate lifestyle changes are made.
- In prediabetic people it may take more time for glucose levels to return to normal after glucose ingestion than a normal person (as the body's capacity to handle carbohydrates is altered).
- If glucose level remains above 130 after 2 hrs of glucose ingestion, it is said to be impaired tolerance to glucose.

Q.12. Enumerate conditions that can decrease or increase glucose tolerance.

Decrease glucose tolerance:

Whenever the body is not able to utilize carbohydrates properly, it is said that glucose tolerance has decreased. It is seen in all situations when there is hyperglycemia (increased blood sugar levels). Such conditions include:

- Diabetes mellitus
- Hyperthyroidism
- Excess cortisol secretion in the body (stress)
- Excess activity of the anterior pituitary or adrenal cortex

Increase glucose tolerance:

It is seen in all situations when there is hypoglycemia (decreased blood sugar levels). Such conditions include:

- Decreased GI absorption (e.g. celiac disease)
- Hyperinsulinism
- Hypothyroidism
- Adrenocortical hypofunction

■ COMMON STATIONS – SPOTS IN PRACTICAL EXAMINATION (2/3 MARKS)

Q.1. Normal glucose tolerance curve: Identify and explain and answer any one or two questions.

Q.2. Glucose tolerance test in prediabetic, severe diabetic: Identify and comment.

■ CASE-BASED SCENARIO/PROBLEM-BASED/ CLINICAL APPLICATIONS

Case 1: A 35-year-old person comes for a glucose tolerance curve for screening for diabetes. His GTT was done as explained above (by giving oral glucose) and the findings are as shown below (clue- as glucose is well tolerated in this person, it is a normal glucose tolerance curve).

	Fasting	30 minutes	60 minutes	90 minutes	120 minutes	180 minutes
Blood glucose	80	100	150	120	110	80
Urine glucose	Nil	Nil	Nil	Nil	Nil	Nil

Case 2: A 34-year-old obese male comes with a history of diabetes in his family. The doctor advises him to get GTT done. His report on GTT is as shown below.

- Comment on the findings.
- Describe normal glucose tolerance curve response.

	Fasting	30 minutes	60 minutes	90 minutes	120 minutes	180 minutes
Blood glucose	190	225	350	300	275	225
Urine glucose	+	++	+++	++	++	++

Case 3: A 10-year-old boy comes to the clinic to get a glucose tolerance test as advised by his family doctor. His GTT is normal. Blood glucose levels are also normal. However, it was observed that glucose is being present in urine samples despite normal blood sugar levels.

	Fasting	30 minutes	60 minutes	90 minutes	120 minutes	180 minutes
Blood glucose	90	128	150	120	100	90
Urine glucose	-	+	++	+	+	Nil

Based on your physiology knowledge answer the following:

- Comment on findings.
- What is the probable diagnosis? (Renal glycosuria check answers above).

■ KEY POINTS TO REMEMBER

- The glucose tolerance test is one of the important tests for screening for diabetes.
- Good glycemic control (maintaining normal blood sugar levels) is very important for health and hyperglycemia and hypoglycemia, both have different ill effects on the body.

50

Ishihara's Chart

■ INTRODUCTION

- The human eye is sensitive to wavelengths of light from 400 nm to 700 nm. Cones are responsible for colour vision. Colour vision can be assessed by various methods. Ishihara 's chart was initially used to assess or test congenital colour blindness, but now it is also used to assess acquired visual disorders.
- Most inherited colour blindness occurs in males. It is sex-linked recessive inheritance **(Fig. 50.1)**.

■ IMPORTANT QUESTIONS AND ANSWERS

Q.1. What is Ishihara's chart used for?

Ishihara's chart is used for testing the colour vision of the subject.

Q.2. Describe Ishihara's chart. Explain how colour vision can be tested with it.

Ishihara's chart: It consists of a series of pages on which either letters or numbers are written in different colours on a background of coloured dots. If the person is

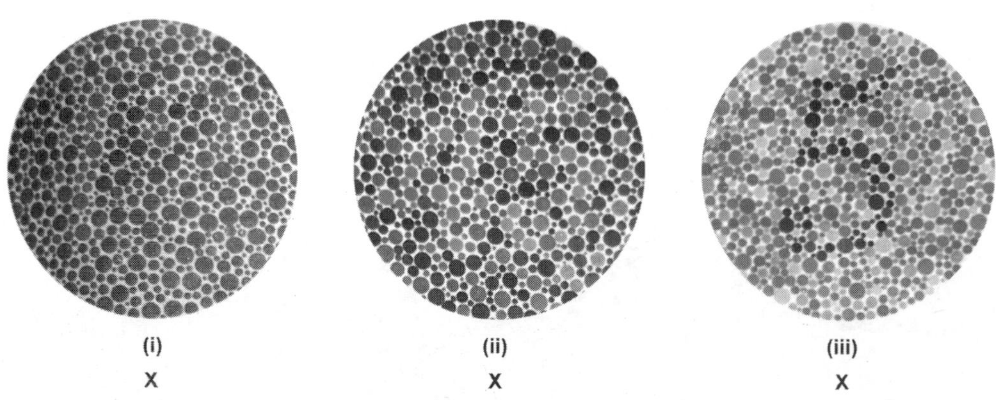

Fig. 50.1: Ishihara's chart *(For colour version, See plate 2)*

colour-blind he/she is not able to read letters or numbers or may be read wrongly.

The answers are given at the end of the chart thus even if one who is examining a patient is himself/herself colour-blind, he/she can carry out the test for the patient.

Q.3. What is deuteranopia?
It is the condition in which a person is blind to green colour due to the absence of green-sensitive cones.

Q.4. What is protanopia?
It is red blindness, i.e. person is blind to red colour due to absent red-sensitive cones.

Q.5. What is red-green blindness?
It is blindness in which a person is not able to differentiate between red and green colour as he/she is either deuteranope or protanope.

Q.6. What is tritanopia?
It is blue blindness and is a rare condition.

Q.7. What is deuteranomaly, protanomaly and tritanomaly?
The suffix anomaly is for colour weakness (the suffix anopia is for colour blindness). Thus deuteranomaly is green colour weakness, protanomaly is red colour weakness and tritanomaly is blue colour weakness.

Q.8. In which person colour perception is of vital importance?
Colour perception is of vital importance in:
- Air, sea, and road drivers
- Paints and printing industries
- Textile industries

Q.9. Enumerate methods to test colour vision.
- **Ishihara chart**: (as explained above)
- **Holmgren's wools**: Small pieces of different colours of woolen threads are used here. The subject is asked to match the colours.
- **Edridge–Green lantern**: Different coloured glass pieces of different sizes are fitted in a rotating disc. The subject is made to sit about 6 feet distance from the lantern and is asked to name the colours that are shown to him in front of the aperture.

There are about 38 plates in Ishihara's chart. Different numbers, letters, and designs that can be read by normal people and that can be read or perceived by a colour-blind person are given at the end of the book.

▌COMMON STATIONS – SPOTS IN PRACTICAL EXAMINATION (2/3 MARKS)

Q.1. **Ishihara's chart:** Identify and answer any one or two questions as given above.

▌KEY POINTS TO REMEMBER
- Ishihara's chart is used to assess the colour vision of an individual.
- Different numbered plates or designs are shown to the patient and the patient is asked to identify them. Scores are given according to the results obtained.

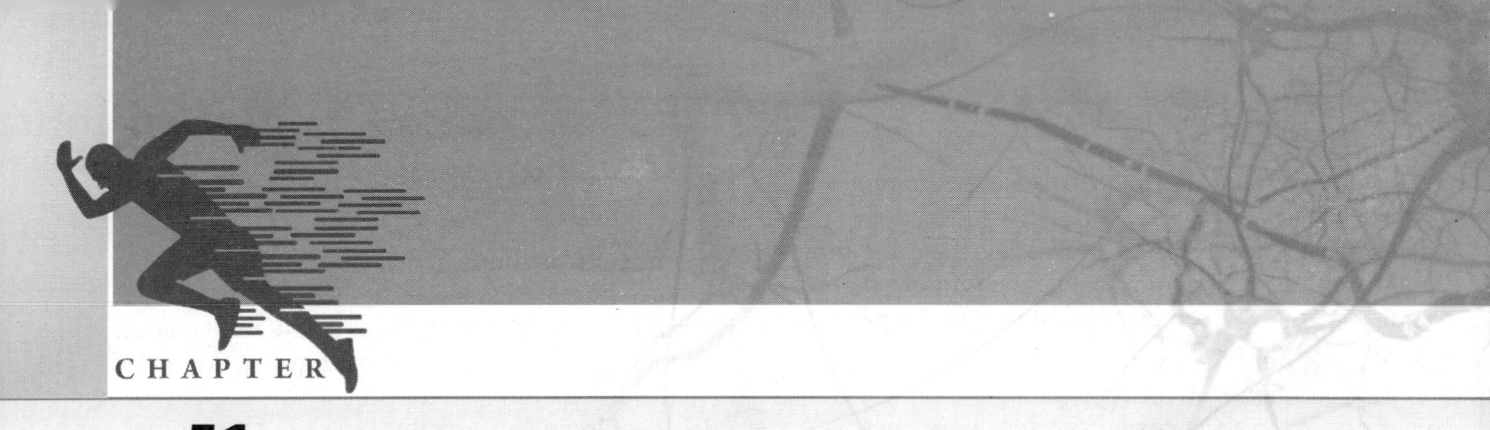

51

Jaeger's Chart

Learning Objectives

At the end of this practical, students shall be able to:
- Define visual acuity
- Enumerate factors affecting visual acuity
- Identify and describe Jaeger's chart
- Demonstrate test for near vision

■ INTRODUCTION

- Visual acuity is the ability of the eye to recognize two-point sources of light or two parallel lines as separate rather than one.
- It has to be tested for near vision and far vision.
- Jaeger's chart is used to assess the near vision of a person.

■ IMPORTANT QUESTIONS AND ANSWERS

Q.1. Describe Jaeger's chart with its use.

- The Jaeger's chart is used for testing visual acuity (for near vision). Acuity for near vision depends on the power of accommodation for near vision in addition to all factors on which distant vision depends.
- **Jaeger's chart:** It consists of various test types printed in different letter sizes with the smallest size at the bottom (J1, J2, J3, etc.). J1 is the smallest type indicating normal vision.
- Near vision is tested by noting the smallest type which the subject can read comfortably at a distance of the eye from the chart at which the test type is used. For children near-vision charts with pictures are available.

Modified Jaeger's chart: This chart is used nowadays where visual acuity is expressed in terms of printer's point system as N36, N18, N8, N6, N5 instead of J1, J2, etc. N5 is considered the smallest type instead of J1.

Q.2. How is the eye accommodated for near vision?

- The eye is accommodated for near vision by increasing the power of the lens of the eye. The power of the lens of the eye can vary from +15D to +29D.
- The power of lens is increased due to the contraction of ciliary muscles with various degrees.
- Contraction of ciliary muscles makes the suspensory ligament lax and reduces the tension of the capsule of a lens. Lens due to its elastic nature, assumes a globular shape when tension on the capsule is reduced.

Q.3. What is the amplitude of accommodation?

- The difference in refractory powers of the lens with ciliary muscles maximally contracted and with ciliary muscles completely relaxed is called as the amplitude of accommodation.
- In a young adult person, it is 14 diopters because the minimum lens power with ciliary muscles completely relaxed) is +15D and the maximum lens power (with ciliary muscles maximally contracted) is +29D.

Q.4. What is the range of accommodation?

- The distance between the far point and the near point is known as the range of accommodation.
- Far point is the farthest distance from the eye at which an object can be seen clearly.
- Near point is the nearest distance from the eye at which an object can be seen clearly.

Q.5. What is presbyopia?
It is a condition where the amplitude of accommodation is reduced. It is seen in old age due to loss of elasticity of the lens (due to denaturation of lens proteins). Correction is done by convex lenses.

Q.6. What are errors of refraction?
- **Myopia:** It is also called as short-sightedness. Parallel rays coming from distant objects are focused in front of the retina. Thus, distant objects cannot be seen clearly. It is corrected by using concave lenses.
- **Hypermetropia:** It is also called long-sightedness. Parallel rays coming from distant objects are focused behind the retina. Thus, near objects are not seen clearly. It is corrected by using a convex lens.
- **Presbyopia:** As explained above.

▌COMMON STATIONS – SPOTS IN PRACTICAL EXAMINATION (2/3 MARKS)

Q.1. Jaeger's chart: Identify and write one or two questions from the above.

Q.2. Enumerate errors of refraction/draw any error of refraction with its correction.

■ KEY POINTS TO REMEMBER
- Jaeger's chart is used to test near-vision
- Normally, near vision N5 or J1 is considered normal.
- Various factors do affect visual acuity.

Jugular Venous Pulse Tracing

Learning Objectives

At the end of this practical, students shall be able to:
- Define jugular venous pulse and describe the normal recording of waveform
- Describe the cause of the upstroke and downstroke of each wave with respect to phases of the cardiac cycle.
- Give a physiological basis for some abnormal pulse waves in different clinical conditions

■ INTRODUCTION

Jugular venous pulses (JVP) are the pulsations that are recorded in the neck. These pulsations are due to pressure changes in the right atrium which are reflected in large veins and can be recorded by placing a transducer on the vein and connecting it to the recording system **(Fig. 52.1)**. There can be physiological variations in JVP waves with respect to respiration (it normally decreases with inspiration) and posture.

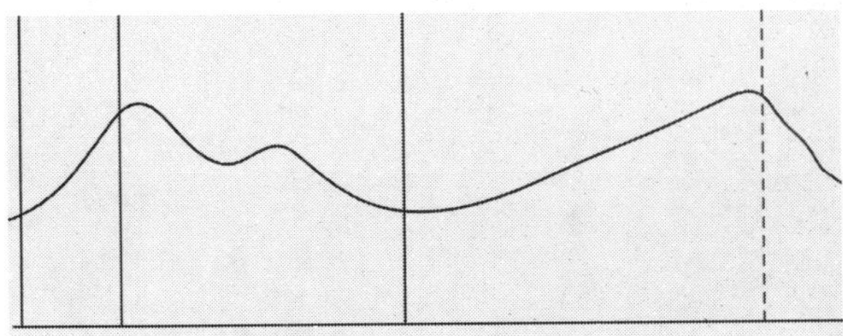

Fig. 52.1: Jugular venous pulse tracing

■ IMPORTANT QUESTIONS AND ANSWERS

Q.1. What is the jugular venous pulse? Name various waves in it. How is it recorded?
- Fluctuations in right atrial pressure during the cardiac cycle generate a pulse which is transmitted backwards into jugular veins.
- Basic waves in jugular pulse tracing are 'a', 'c', 'v' waves. A jugular venous pulse is recorded with the help of Mackenzi's polygraph.

Q.2. What is the cause of upstroke and downstroke for a wave?
Atrial systole is responsible for wave generation. The upstroke of a wave is due to the dynamic phase and the downstroke of a wave is due to the dynamic phase of atrial systole.

Q.3. What is the cause of the upstroke and downstroke of the c wave?
- In jugular venous pulse tracing c wave is recorded during the isovolumic contraction phase of ventricular systole.
- Upstroke of c wave—at the end of atrial systole, when AV valves close and semilunar valves are also closed and the isovolumic contraction phase starts, there is increased pressure in the ventricles which causes bulging of AV valves towards the atrial cavity-causing rise in atrial pressure recorded as upstroke of c wave.
- **Downstroke of c wave:** As the isovolumic contraction phase gets over and the ejection phase starts due

to which the AV valves come back to their normal position (no more bulging in the atrial cavity) this causes a drop in atrial pressure recorded as a downstroke of c wave.

Q.4. What is the cause of the upstroke and downstroke of v wave?

In jugular venous pulse tracing, the cause of the v wave is atrial diastole (filling phase).

- **Upstroke of v wave:** When atrial diastole is going on, atria get filled with blood which causes a rise in atrial pressure recorded as upstroke of v wave.
- **Downstroke of v wave:** At the beginning of the isovolumic relaxation phase of ventricles, AV valves open and the first rapid passive filling phase starts during which blood flows from the atria to ventricles, this causes a drop in the atrial pressure is recorded as downstroke of v wave.

Q.5. Enumerate common conditions causing prominent a wave and canon a wave.

Prominent a wave is seen in:
- Pulmonary stenosis (as the forceful right atrial contraction is required)
- Pulmonary hypertension
- Cardiomyopathy
- While a wave is absent in atrial fibrillation.
- Cannon a wave—This is high amplitude a wave. This is caused due to atrial systole against a closed tricuspid valve. It is seen with ventricular tachycardia, a complete heart block.

Q.6. When is giant v wave obtained?
- **Giant v wave:** It is obtained during tricuspid regurgitation. Due to the regurgitation of blood, there is a fusion of the downstroke of the c wave with the v wave upstroke giving the appearance of a giant v wave.
- Regurgitant jet leads to pulsatile systolic waves in JVP.

Q.7. What is the relationship between ECG and jugular pulse waves?

All electrical events precede mechanical events, thus P wave and QRS complex (atrial and ventricular depolarization) precede a wave and c wave respectively.

■ COMMON STATIONS – SPOTS IN PRACTICAL EXAMINATION (2/3 MARKS)

Q.1. Jugular venous pulse: Identify the chart and answer any one or two questions as given above.

■ CASE-BASED SCENARIO/PROBLEM-BASED/ CLINICAL APPLICATIONS

Kussmaul's sign: It is a paradoxical increase in JVP that occurs during inspiration. Kussmaul's sign along with pulsus paradoxus (drop in systolic BP more than 10 mm Hg with inspiration are important in the assessment of pericardial disease).

■ KEY POINTS TO REMEMBER

- Jugular venous pulse is a record obtained from jugular veins in the neck.
- They reflect right atrial pressure changes during the cardiac cycle.
- A variety of clinical conditions can alter normal waveforms of JVP.

53

Snellen's Chart

Learning Objectives
At the end of this practical, the students shall be able to:
- Define visual acuity
- Enumerate factors affecting visual acuity
- Demonstrate, how the distant vision is tested
- Describe Snellen's chart

■ INTRODUCTION

- Visual acuity is the ability of the eye to recognize two-point sources of light or two parallel lines as separate rather than one.
- It has to be tested for near vision and far vision.
- Snellen's chart is used to test acuity for distant vision.

■ IMPORTANT QUESTION AND ANSWERS

Q.1. Describe Snellen's chart. What is it used for?
- **Snellen's chart**: It consists of letters written in different lines. The letters in each line vary in size. Against each line, a number is written as 60, 36, 24, etc. This number indicates the distance in meters from which letters in that line can be read by the normal eye.
- At this distance each letter in that line makes an angle of five minutes to the nodal point of the eye whereas the gap between two lines or two curves in the letter subtends an angle of one minute at the nodal point of the eye.
- The total number of lines from above downwards is eight in number and they are read from distances of 60, 36, 24, 18, 12, 9, 6 and 5 meters respectively by the normal eye **(Fig. 53.1)**.

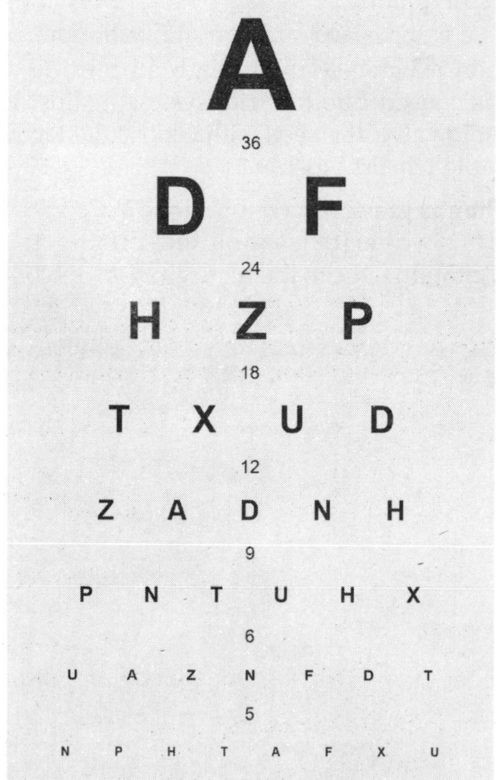

Fig. 53.1: Snellen's chart

Q.2. How visual acuity is tested with the help of Snellen's chart?
- Snellen's chart is placed at a distance of 6 meters from the subject in a well-lighted room. The person is asked to read the chart with each eye separately.

- Visual acuity in each eye is expressed as a fraction, the numerator corresponding to the distance from the patient to the chart (6 meters) and the denominator indicating the distance at which the smallest row of letters read by the patient should be read by the normal eye.
- Normally from a distance of 6 meters the subject should be able to read up to last but one line against which '6' is written. Then acuity of that eye is expressed as 6/6.

Q.3. What do you mean by visual acuity 6/36 for a left eye?

- If the subject can read only the first two lines with his/ her left eye, the visual acuity of his/ her left eye is 6/36. This means that a normal person can read that particular line of letters from a distance of 36 meters, he/she can read that line from 6 meters of distance only, and that much is the defect.
- If a person is not able to read even the first line from a distance of 6 meters then, the chart can be brought nearer and then visual acuity is expressed accordingly.

Q.4. Define visual acuity. Enumerate factors affecting it.

- **Visual acuity:** It is the resolving power of the eye and is expressed as minimum separable, i.e. minimum distance at which two-point sources of light (or two-point objects) can be recognized as separate.
- The point objects can be recognized as separate when they make an angle of 'one minute' at the nodal point of the eye (at fovea even if the angle is subtended by two-point objects in 26 seconds they can be recognized as separate objects. But the fovea is very small and therefore the gaze cannot be fixed for a long to keep the images of two objects required to recognize them separately is considered as one minute).

Factors affecting visual acuity:
- Illumination
- Wavelength of light
- Brightness contrast
- Errors of refraction
- Exposure time

Q.5. What can be done if a person is not able to read the largest letter at 60?

- Get the Snellen's chart still closer to the subject (from 6 meters of distance.) and try to assess if he/she can read. Go on reducing the distance between the chart and the subject.
- If at one meter of distance also, the letter at the 60 cannot be read, then try to assess
  - Counting fingers (at 1 m distance)
  - Hand movements
  - Perception of light

▮ COMMON STATIONS – SPOTS IN PRACTICAL EXAMINATION (2/3 MARKS)

Q.1. Snellen's chart: Identify and write any one or two questions as given above.

▮ KEY POINTS TO REMEMBER

- Snellen's chart is used to test distant vision.
- Normally distant vision is 6/6. Where numerator 6 is fixed (distance between Snellen's chart and subject). The denominator can vary depending on which particular line the subject can read.
- Various factors do affect visual acuity.

Strength Duration Curve

Competency:
PY 3.17: Strength duration curve.

Learning Objectives

At the end of this practical, the students shall be able to:
- Define chronaxie and rheobase
- Enumerate factors affecting chronaxie

■ INTRODUCTION

- The strength-duration curve is a graphical represen-tation of the relationship between the intensity of the stimulus and the time taken for the muscle to respond.
- Strength refers to the intensity of stimulus represented on the vertical axis and duration (time) on the horizontal axis.

■ IMPORTANT QUESTIONS AND ANSWERS

Q.1. What is chronaxie? What is its significance?
- **Chronaxie**: Is the minimum time required to excite the excitable tissue when the strength of the current used is double the rheobase. Chronaxie helps us measure the excitability of excitable tissues. Lesser is the chronaxie greater the excitability of tissues.
- Large myelinated nerve fibres are the most exci-table tissues with a chronaxie of 0.0001 seconds followed by small myelinated (0.0003 seconds) and unmyelinated nerve fibres (0.0005 seconds). Thus most excitable tissue will have the least chronaxie **(Fig. 54.1)**.

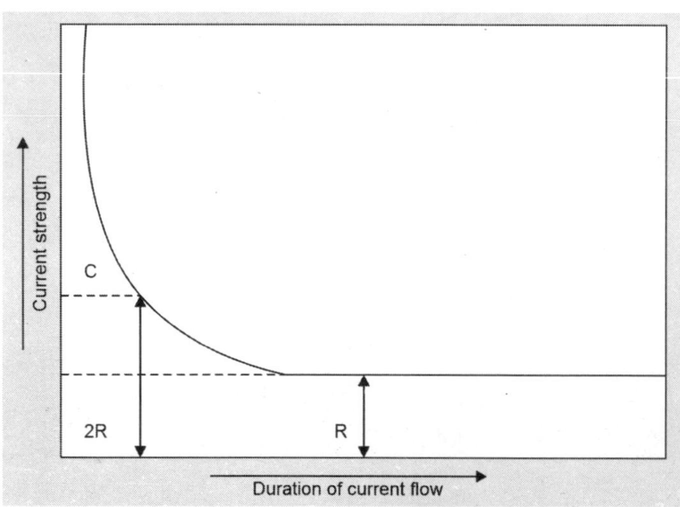

Fig. 54.1: Strength duration curve

Q.2. What is Rheobase?

It is the minimum strength of current that is allowed to pass through a tissue for an infinite length of time which elicits a response from the excitable tissue.

Q.3. What is utilization time?

It is the minimum time required to excite the tissue when rheobase strength is used.

Q.4. Enumerate factors affecting chronaxie.

As chronaxie is a measure of the excitability of the tissue, any condition that affects the excitability of tissue will also affect chronaxie.

Factors affecting chronaxie:

- **Temperature**: Rise in temperature will decrease while cold temperature will increase chronaxie.

- **Injury**: Any injury or degeneration of tissue will decrease its excitability and thus increase chronaxie.

- **Agents acting at NM junction**: Any agent that stimulates neuromuscular junction will decrease and any agent inhibiting neuromuscular junction will increase chronaxie.

COMMON STATIONS – SPOTS IN PRACTICAL EXAMINATION (2/3 MARKS)

Q.1. Strength duration curve: Identify the graph and answer any one or two questions from above.

KEY POINTS TO REMEMBER

- Chronaxie determines the excitability of tissue.
- Large myelinated nerve fibres are the most excitable tissues in the body.

Volume and Pressure Changes in Different Chambers of the Heart

Competency:

PY 5.3: Discuss events occurring during the cardiac cycle.

Learning Objectives

At the end of this practical, students shall be able to:

- Describe left ventricular pressure changes during the cardiac cycle
- Describe right atrial pressure changes during the cardiac cycle
- Describe ventricular volume changes with the cardiac cycle
- Correlate ECG waves with cardiac cycle
- Correlate heart sounds with cardiac cycle

■ INTRODUCTION

- In between two consecutive heartbeats, various electrical and mechanical events happen in the heart in a sequential manner which is called as cardiac cycle.
- It becomes important to understand the detailed pressure-volume changes and their correlation with heart sounds in order to understand and diagnose various types of murmurs heard in various clinical conditions **(Fig. 55.1)**.

■ IMPORTANT QUESTIONS AND ANSWERS

Q.1. Define cardiac cycle. Enumerate various phases with respect to the time duration of each

Cardiac cycle: Various sequential electrical and mechanical events that occur in between two consecutive heartbeats. The normal duration of the cardiac cycle is 0.8 seconds.

Phases of cardiac cycle

Atrial systole (0.1 s)

Ventricular systole (0.3 s)

- Isovolumic contraction (0.05 s)
- Rapid ejection (0.11 s)
- Reduced ejection (0.14 s)

Ventricular diastole (0.5 s)

- Protodiastole (0.04 s)
- Isovolumic relaxation (0.06 s)
- First rapid passive filling phase (0.11s)
- Reduced filling phase (diastasis 0.19s)
- Second rapid filling phase (atrial systole 0.1s)

Q.2. How much is pressure variation (max and minimum pressure) in the left ventricle?

- Maximum pressure in the left ventricle is 120 mm Hg and it occurs during the rapid ejection phase
- Minimum pressure in the left ventricle is almost 0 mm Hg. It occurs during the first two third phases of ventricular diastole **(Fig. 55.1)**.

Q.3. Define end diastolic and end-systolic volume and stroke volume.

- **End-diastolic volume**: It is the volume of blood present in the ventricle at the end of ventricular diastole. It is about 120 to 130 ml.
- **End-systolic volume**: It is the volume of blood present in the ventricle at the end of ventricular systole. It is about 40 to 50 ml.

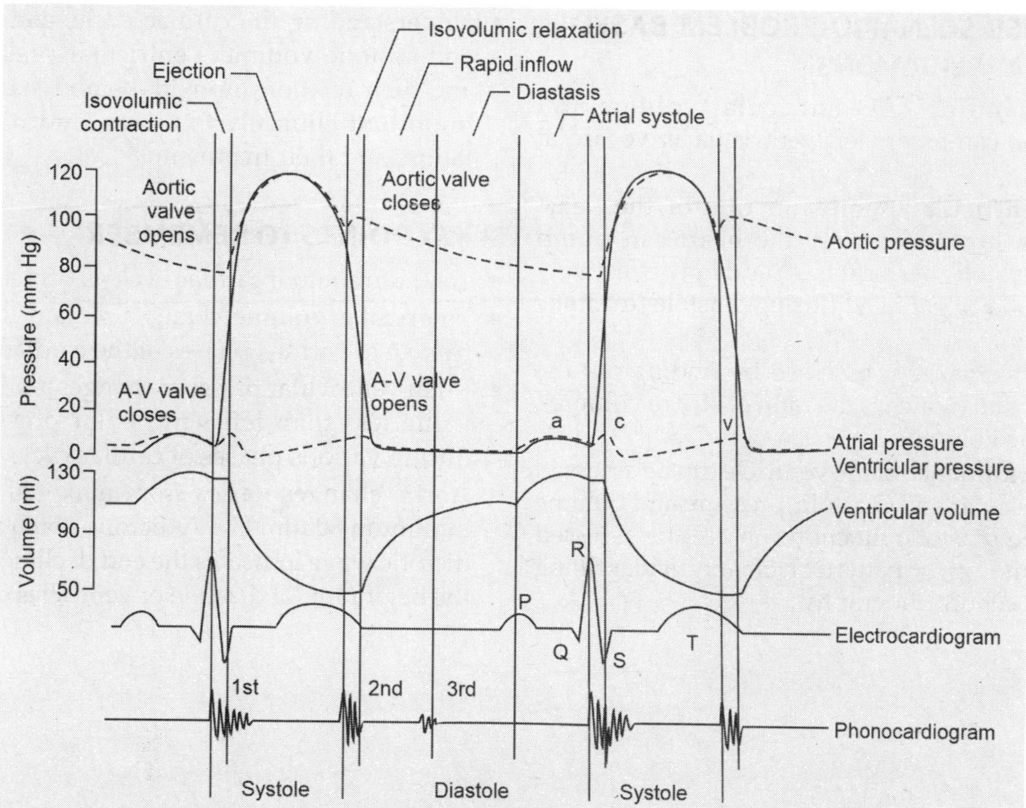

Fig. 55.1: Pressure and volume changes, aortic pressure changes, and atrial pressure changes during various phases of the cardiac cycle, correlating heart sounds and ECG with events in the cardiac cycle

- **Stroke volume**: The volume of blood ejected by each ventricle per beat is known as stroke volume. It is about 70 to 75 ml.

Q.4. Describe right atrial pressure changes during the cardiac cycle.
Please refer to Chapter – Jugular Venous Pulse Tracing

Q.5. What is a dicrotic notch and wave? Give its clinical significance. Where is it seen in this chart?
Please refer to Chapter – Arterial Pulse Tracing

Q.6. What is pressure variation in the aorta with systole and diastole?
- Pressure wave of the aorta during the cardiac cycle varies from a maximum of 120 mm Hg to a minimum of 80 mm Hg
- At the end of protodiastole, when semilunar valves close, there is a small drop in aortic pressure (due to the tendency of blood to flow back to the left ventricle) which is prevented by sudden closure of semilunar valves and as they close, they snap back the blood again in aorta (which causes a small rise in aortic pressure), then pressure falls to about 80 mm Hg (as oxygenated blood flows to all body through aorta)
- This dicrotic notch is followed by a dicrotic wave.

Q.7. Explain the physiological significance of the isovolumic contraction phase of the ventricle.

- The isovolumic contraction phase of the ventricle occurs at the beginning of ventricular systole. At this time A-V valves are closed, but semilunar valves are not yet open. Ventricles therefore contract isometrically as a closed chamber.
- This increases pressure inside the ventricle greatly and when the pressure becomes higher than that of the corresponding artery (aorta, pulmonary artery) semilunar valves open.

Q.8. What is protodiastole?
- Protodiastole is a period occurring at the beginning of ventricular diastole. In this period ventricular muscle relaxes allowing rapid fall in intraventricular pressure.
- At the end of protodiastole, there is closure of semilunar valves.

■ COMMON STATIONS – SPOTS IN PRACTICAL EXAMINATION (2/3 MARKS)

Q.1. Diagram of pressure changes, volume changes in ventricles, ventricular volume changes, right atrial pressure changes, and aortic pressure changes can be shown separately or together– to identify explain, and answer any one or two questions from the above.

Q.2. Corelate heart sounds with phases of the cardiac cycle.

CASE-BASED SCENARIO/PROBLEM-BASED/ CLINICAL APPLICATIONS

- By understanding left ventricular volume and pressure one can assess left ventricular myocardial function.
- The left ventricular pump function of the heart depends on how effectively the heart can pump blood out (systolic performance) and how effectively it allows blood to get filled during diastole (diastolic performance).
- Systolic performance is assessed by finding out the ejection fraction (which is the ratio of stroke volume/ end-diastolic volume).
- Diastole performance of the ventricle can be assessed by left ventricular end-diastolic pressure and volume relation. The diastolic function can also be assessed by understanding the pattern of left ventricular filling by Doppler echocardiography.
- Understanding the cardiac cycle, end-diastolic and end-systolic volume, ventricular pressure changes and their relationship with hemodynamics becomes important clinically to assess, and diagnose heart failure and their treatment.

■ KEY POINTS TO REMEMBER

- Total duration of cardiac cycle is 0.8 seconds.
- Ventricular volume changes remain the same with respect to various phases of the cardiac cycle.
- Right ventricular pressure changes are 1/6th to 1/8th value less than left ventricular pressure changes during various phases of cardiac cycle.
- Aortic changes varies from max 120 mm Hg to a minimum 80 mm Hg. A dicrotic notch followed by a dicrotic wave indicates the end of clinical systole and the beginning of diastole of ventricles.

Oxygen Dissociation Curve

Learning Objectives

At the end of this practical, students shall be able to:
- Describe O$_2$ dissociation curve
- Explain and enumerate various factors that cause right and left shift of the curve
- Explain the significance of the steep and plateau parts of the curve

◼ INTRODUCTION

The O$_2$ dissociation curve explains the binding ability of O$_2$ with Hb at different partial pressures of O$_2$. The curve is normally sigmoid in shape. It is also referred to as the oxyhaemoglobin dissociation curve **(Fig. 56.1)**.

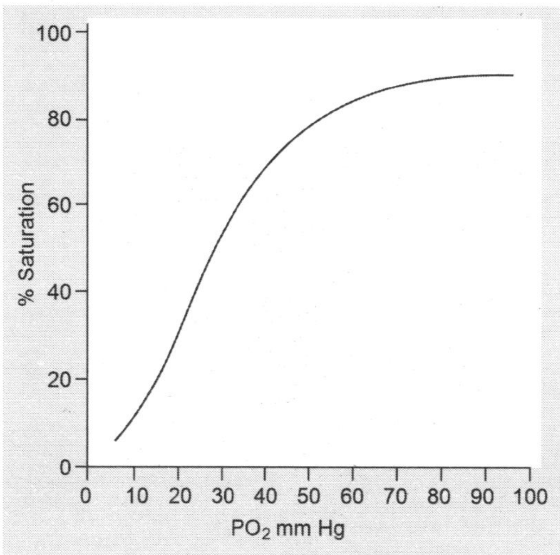

Fig. 56.1: O$_2$ dissociation curve

◼ IMPORTANT QUESTION AND ANSWERS

Q.1. Describe O$_2$ dissociation curve.

The O$_2$ dissociation curve is a sigmoid-shaped curve that is plotted by keeping pO$_2$ (mm Hg) on the X-axis and % saturation of Hb with O$_2$ on the Y-axis.

O$_2$ dissociation curve:

- **Flat upper part of O$_2$ dissociation curve**: The O$_2$ dissociation curve is flat in the upper portion, i.e. if pO$_2$ varies from 100 to 60 mm Hg, the percent saturation of Hb does not vary much (it only varies from 97% to 90%).
- If pO$_2$ increases from 100 to 300 mm Hg still percent saturation can increase from 97 to 100%. This means that with great atmospheric variation in pO$_2$ from 60 to 300 mm Hg percent saturation of Hb with O$_2$ varies only from 90% to 100%.
- In other words, it means that even if there is great atmospheric variation in pO$_2$, the amount of O$_2$ supplied to tissues does not vary much (large safety factor).
- **Lower steep part of the curve**: Lower part, of the curve is steep, that is between 60 to 20 mm Hg pO$_2$. It is beneficial at the tissue level. A slight fall in tissue pressure would allow a larger amount of O$_2$ to be given out from Hb. If tissue O$_2$ rises above 60 mm Hg then a very small amount of O$_2$ is released from Hb. These steep curve characteristics help to maintain a constant supply of O$_2$ to tissues (normal tissue pO$_2$ is 40 mm Hg). Thus due to this peculiar shape of the

curve, Hb acts as a buffer to maintain tissue pO_2 at 40 mm Hg.

Q.2. Enumerate various conditions that cause a shift of the curve to right and left.

Factors causing a right shift of the curve	Factors causing a left shift of the curve
• Increase pCO_2 of blood • Increase H^+ ion concentration in blood • Increase in temperature • Increase in 2,3-diphosphoglycerate level of blood	• Decrease in pCO_2 of blood • Decrease in H^+ ion concentration of blood • Decrease in temperature • Fetal haemoglobin

Q.3. What is p_{50}?

The partial pressure of O_2 at which haemoglobin (Hb) is 50% saturated with O_2 is known as p_{50}, and it is normally 26 mm Hg. This value indicates the affinity of Hb for O_2. A decrease in p_{50} signifies an increased affinity of Hb for O_2, corresponding to a leftward shift of the O_2 dissociation curve. Conversely, an increase in p_{50} signifies a decreased affinity of Hb for O_2, corresponding to a rightward shift of the O_2 dissociation curve.

Q.4. What is Bohr's effect?

- Shift of the O_2 dissociation curve that occurs due to changes in pCO_2 of blood is termed Bohr's effect.
- Shifts in the O_2 dissociation curve due to changes in blood pCO_2 is termed the Bohr effect.
- At the tissue level, an increase in pCO_2 causes the O_2 dissociation curve to shift to the right, leading to more O_2 dissociating from Hb and being released to the tissues. In the lungs, a decrease in pCO_2 causes the O_2 dissociation curve to shift to the left, increasing the affinity of Hb for O_2, thus promoting O_2 binding to Hb.

Q.5. What is Haldane's effect?

- The increased capacity of deoxygenated Hb to carry more CO_2 is called Haldane's effect.
- CO_2 uptake is thus facilitated at tissues and CO_2 release is facilitated at lungs.

■ COMMON STATIONS – SPOTS IN PRACTICAL EXAMINATION (2/3 MARKS)

Q.1. O_2 dissociation curve: Identify and label different parts. Answer any one or two questions from the above.

■ KEY POINTS TO REMEMBER

- Various physiological factors can cause the O_2 dissociation curve to shift either to the right or left. A leftward shift favours O_2 loading, while a rightward shift favours O_2 unloading.
- Fetal haemoglobin (Hb) causes a leftward shift, which is beneficial in utero as it helps draw O_2 from maternal blood to support the growing fetus.
- An increase in temperature, pCO_2, and 2,3-diphosphoglycerate, along with a decrease in pH, shifts the curve to the right, which is particularly useful for oxygen delivery to mechanically active tissues.

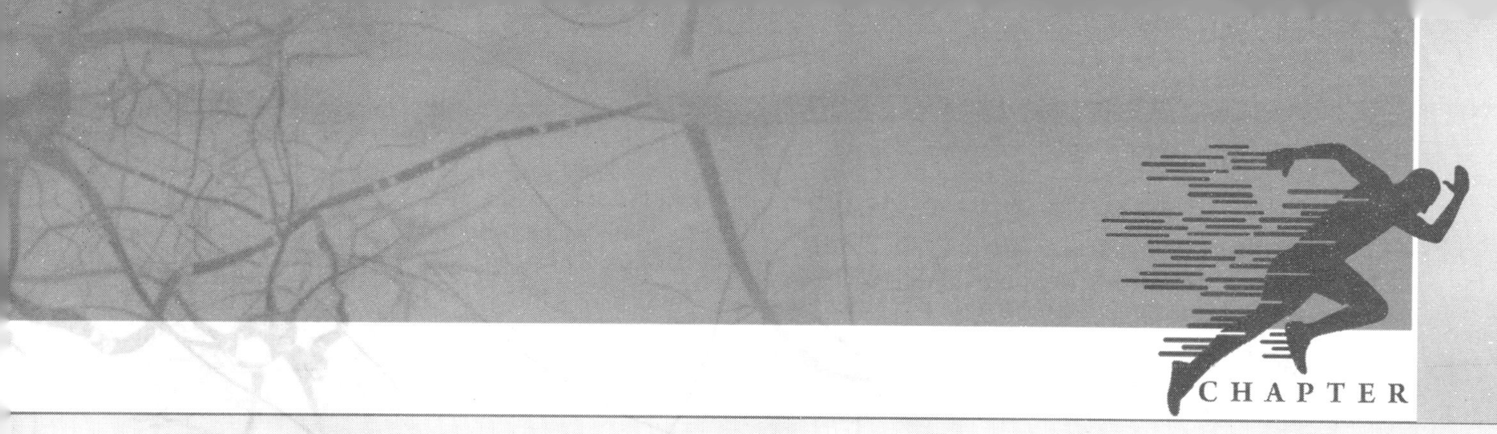

Semen Analysis

Competency:

PY 9.9: Interpret normal semen analysis reports including sperm count, sperm morphology, and sperm motility as per WHO guidelines and discuss the results.

Learning Objectives

After completing this practical, students should be able to:

- Enumerate indications for semen analysis
- Describe the importance of semen analysis in clinical practice
- Enumerate precautions while doing semen analysis
- State the composition of normal sperm and correlate any abnormal findings with their physiological basis

■ INTRODUCTION

Semen analysis is one of the basic investigations that is asked while investigating infertility cases. Normal semen analysis helps us to understand not only sperm count but even its morphology and motility which can be altered in various clinical conditions.

Principle

Semen that is collected from a patient must be analyzed within half an hour after collection. The semen is diluted 20 times using a WBC pipette and examined under the microscope for sperm morphology and motility under high and low power.

Apparatus

Freshly collected semen, Neubauer's chamber, WBC pipette.

Procedure

- Collect semen from a patient after at least 2 days of sexual abstinence.
- Semen analysis is performed 30 minutes after collection of the sample (as after collection, semen coagulates and then liquefies in 15 to 20 minutes).
- After confirming that the sample is liquified completely.
- Assess all physical characteristics of semen.
- Assess sperm motility and morphology under low and high power under a microscope.
- *For sperm count:* Fill semen in WBC pipettes up to 0.5 mark and then dilute it up to 11-mark (using 4% sodium bicarbonate in 1% phenol). Mix contents for 2 to 2 minutes.
- Discard the first few drops and charge Neubauer's chamber and sperm count is done in WBC squares ($N \times 50,000$ gives sperm count per ml of fluid). For details check the calculation of total WBC count.

Observations/Results

Observe for physical characteristics and sperm count, sperm motility and any abnormal findings (details see below).

■ IMPORTANT QUESTIONS AND ANSWERS

Q.1. What does normal semen analysis include?

It includes macro and microscopic analysis of semen samples.

Normal semen analysis		
Macroscopic examination		*Microscopic examination*
Appearance	Whitish, opaque and sticky	Sperm count
Volume	2–5 ml	Total sperm motility
pH	7.2–7.7	Progressive motility and non-progressive motility
Self-liquefaction	30 minutes	Immobile
Fructose content	Present	Agglutination (negative)
Count	60–120 million/ml	Pus cells/macrophages/RBCs/epithelial cells–Nil
Motility	More than 80%	Abnormal forms (abnormalities more than 30 % indicates pathology) Head defects Neck and midpiece defects Tail defects Excess residual cytoplasm

Q.2. What is the significance of knowing sperm count?

The normal sperm count is between 60 to 120 million/ml. A sperm count between 20 to 40 million/ml is seen with borderline cases of infertility and a count below 20 million/ml indicates sterility.

Q.3. Enumerate indications for sperm/semen analysis.

Indications for sperm analysis:
- Investigate cases of infertility
- To confirm if vasectomy is successful
- To diagnose any disease of the genital tract
- To investigate for any genetic disorders (e.g. Klinefelter's syndrome)

Q.4. What is the reason for abstinence that is advised to a patient before semen collection?

Frequent ejaculations are considered to affect volume and sperm count and may give a false low count. To avoid this usually, abstinence is suggested for about 2 to 4 days before semen collection.

Q.5. What is the significance of clotting and liquefaction of semen?

Initial coagulation that happens is said to be due to fibrinogen present in semen and after about 1 to 20 minutes, there is self-liquefaction of semen. This is due to the presence of plasmin in prostatic fluid. Delayed liquefaction of more than 2 hrs. indicates enzyme defects in secretory products of the glands or inflammation of accessory glands.

Q.6. What is vasectomy? When semen analysis is done post vasectomy and why?

- Vasectomy is the main method for sterilization in males. It is the procedure by which new blocks entry of sperm in the semen when a person ejaculates.
- Semen analysis is advised to confirm the success of the vasectomy procedure (this is advised after about 2 months of surgery). Immediately after bilateral vasectomy, sperm can be visible in semen analysis as they may be released from storage in the ampullae of seminal vesicles.

Q.7. Define the following terms

- **Normozoospermia:** Normal sperm (volume of semen is over 2 ml, more than 20 million sperm with at least 25% of good motility and at least 4% look normal)
- **Azoospermia:** Total absence of sperms in semen
- **Oligospermia:** Total sperm count less than 20 million/ml of semen
- **Aspermia:** It is a complete lack of semen with ejaculation
- **Asthenozoospermia:** It is a decrease in sperm motility. According to WHO progressive motility of more than 32% is considered normal while total motility is 40% (progressive plus non-progressive)
- **Leukospermia:** It is an abnormally high concentration of WBCs in semen. It can be due to infection or inflammation of the genitourinary tracts.
- **Haemospermia/Haematospermia:** It is blood in the ejaculate.
- **Oligoasthenozoospermia:** It is a decrease in concentration and percentage of motile spermatozoa in the given sample.
- **Teratozoospermia:** It is abnormal sperm morphology caused due to defects in the sperm head, mid-piece or tail.
- **Oligoasthenoteratozoospermia:** It is a condition where a semen sample has oligozoospermia (i.e low sperm count), asthenozoospermia (that is poor motility of sperms) and teratozoospermia (i.e. abnormal morphology of sperm).

Q.8. How normal semen reporting is done?

Semen analysis–seminogram		
Name of the patient	*Age–years*	*Method of collection*
Specimen produced at 10:30 am Specimen examined at 11:10 am	Duration of abstinence-	Reg. no
Macroscopic examination		*Reference value*
Appearance	Opaque	
colour	Whitish	

Contd...

Contd...

Name of the patient	Age–years	Method of collection
Self-liquefaction	— minutes	30 to 60 minutes
volume	5 ml	2 to 7 ml
Viscosity	Normal	
Microscopic examination		
Sperm count	80 million/ml	>20 millions/ml
Total sperm motility	70%	>50%
Progressive motility	40%	>32%
Non-progressive motility	75%	
Immotile	5%	
Agglutination	Negative	
Pus cells	Negative / (1-2 hpf)	Nil
Macrophages	Negative / (1-2 hpf)	Nil
RBCs	Nil/HPF	Nil
Epithelial cells	Nil/HPF	Nil
Abnormal forms	20%	
Head defects	10%	
Neck and midpiece defects	5%	
Tail defects	0%	
Excess residual cytoplasm	0%	
Chemical examination		
pH	7.5	
Fructose	Present	

COMMON STATIONS– SPOTS IN PRACTICAL EXAMINATION (2/3 MARKS)

Q.1. Enumerate indications of semen analysis.

Q.2. Answer the questions below looking at the semen report.

Name–ABC	Age–35 years	Duration of abstinence–4 days
Method of collection— Masturbation	Specimen produced at 10:30 am Specimen examined at 11:10 am	Sperm count– 80 million/ml pH– 7.5

- Is the sperm count in the normal range?
- Why does one have to wait for 30 minutes to do a test after sample collection?

Q.3. Answer the questions below by looking at the semen report.

Name–ABC	Age–32 years	Duration of abstinence–2 days
Method of collection— Masturbation	Specimen produced at 10:30 am Specimen examined at 11:10 am	Sperm count – 15 million/ml pH 7.5 Progressive motility – 25%

- Comment on sperm count and progressive motility of sperms.
- Define asthenozoospermia.

CASE-BASED SCENARIO/PROBLEM-BASED/ CLINICAL APPLICATIONS

Case 1: A couple visited a gynecologist for infertility. The doctor had advised semen analysis and ovulation studies. He did his semen analysis. His sperm count is 10 million/ml and sperm abnormalities were detected in about 40%.

- How much is the normal sperm count?
- What can be different abnormalities with respect to the morphology of sperms?

TPR Chart

Competency:

PY 11.13: Perform general examination in the volunteer/ simulated environment.

PE 23.9: Record pulse, blood pressure, temperature, and respiratory rate, and interpret as per age.

Learning Objectives

At the end of this practical, the students shall be able to:
- Record the body temperature of the given subject
- Enumerate various sites at which body temperature is recorded
- Enumerate clinical significance of hyperthermia and hypothermia
- Enumerate various types of fever
- Understand the significance of recording of temperature, pulse and respiration in health and disease

■ INTRODUCTION

Recording of vital signs like pulse, temperature and blood pressure plays a very important role in understanding the patient's course of disease as well as prognosis and patient's response to treatment especially when the patient is admitted to hospital. It therefore becomes very important for a medical student to understand how and when to record these vital signs and to correlate the same with the clinical findings of the patient in order to go correctly on the path of treating the disease of the patient.

Procedure

- TPR chart helps combinedly to record the pulse, temperature and blood pressure of a patient **(Fig. 58.1)**.
- One should correctly record the pulse (as discussed in the (as discussed in Chapter on examination of pulse and Examination of blood pressure).
- With the help of a clinical thermometer, body temperature is recorded from the mouth/axilla.

■ IMPORTANT QUESTIONS AND ANSWERS

Q.1. What is the significance of the TPR chart?
Significance of TPR chart:
- To diagnose various types of fever
- To detect the time of ovulation
- To judge the prognosis of the patient

Q.2. Enumerate physiological and pathological variations in body temperature.

Physiological variations	Pathological variations
Diurnal variation: Temperature is maximum in the late afternoon and minimum at 3 to 5 am	*Infections:* In all types of body infections, there is a rise in body temperature
Exercise: Temperature rises after exercise. It depends on the severity of the exercise (up to 104.6°F)	*Sunstroke:* During extreme heat, body temperature can rise to a high degree causing heat stroke

Contd...

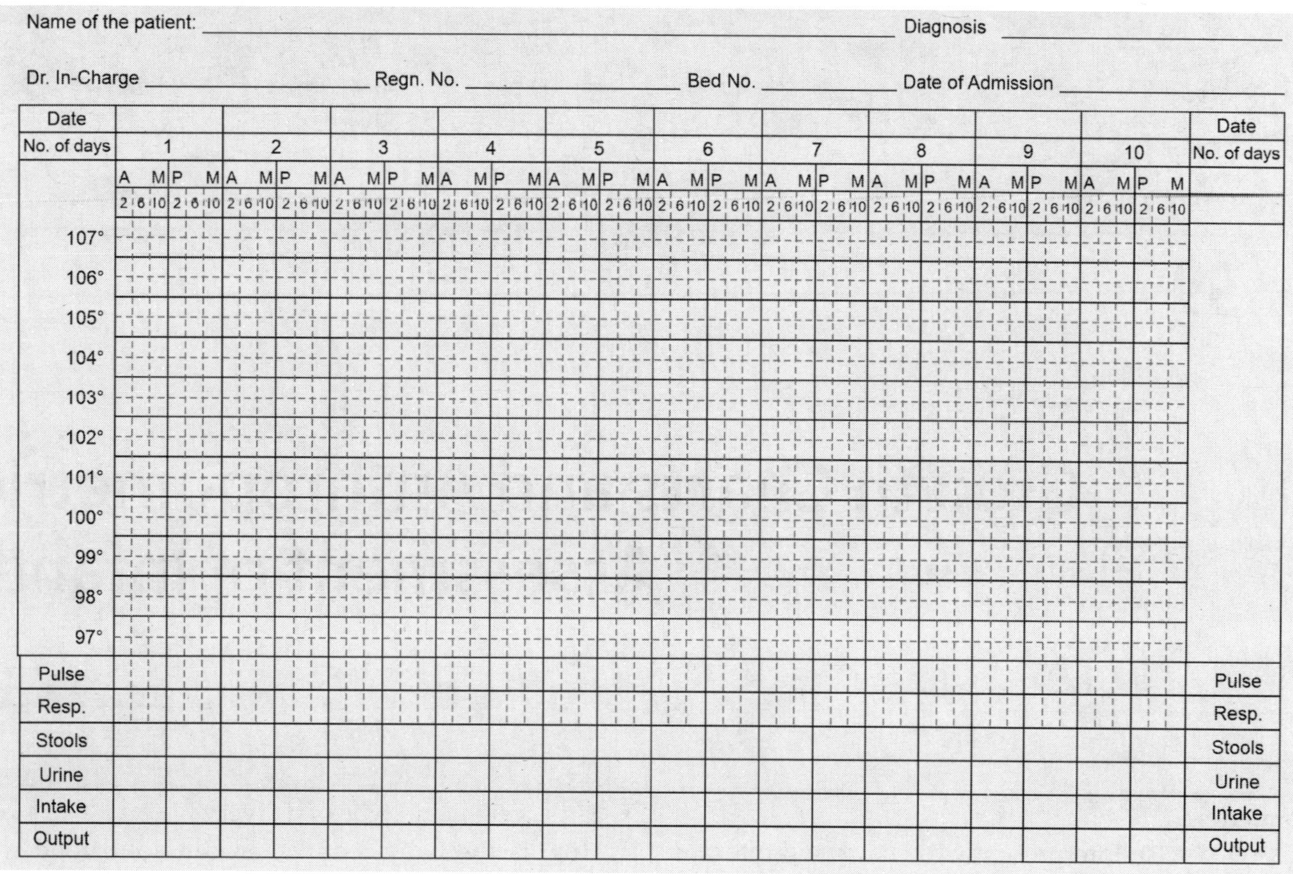

Fig. 58.1: TPR chart

Contd...

Physiological variations	Pathological variations
Age: In babies body temperature might vary with surrounding temperature as the temperature regulating centre is not well developed	*Hyperthyroidism:* Due to an increase in BMR body temperature is greater than normal
Sex: In females variation with phases of the menstrual cycle is noted, ovulation is associated with a 0.5°C rise in temperature	*Circulatory shock:* Body temperature decreases in shock *Frostbite:* Occurs due to very low surrounding temperature *Myxedema:* Low thyroid hormone level, decreases BMR and one can have body temperature less than normal

Q.3. What is fever? What are the different types of fever?

An increase in body temperature above normal (more than 37 °C) is termed as fever.

The following are common types of fever:

- **Remittent fever**: When daily temperature fluctuations exceed two degrees centigrade, it is termed as remittent fever, e.g. tuberculosis, infective endocarditis, various bacterial and viral infections.
- **Relapsing fever**: Fever is present only for certain hours during the day, i.e. febrile episodes are separated by intervals of normal temperature, e.g. malaria, tuberculosis

If this happens daily, it is called as quotidian fever, e.g. *P. falciparum*

If it occurs every 48 hrs it is called as tertian fever, e.g. *P. falciparum, P. vivax,* etc.

If it occurs every 72 hrs it is called quartan fever.

- **Continuous/sustained fever**: Fever does not fluctuate more than 1 to 1.5°F during 24 hours but at no time touches normal, e.g. pneumonia, meningitis, etc.
- **Step ladder fever**: A type of sustained fever where temperature rises gradually to a higher level with every spike, e.g. typhoid.
- **Intermittent fever**: There is an exaggeration of circadian rhythm. The variation between high and low temperatures is very high, e.g. deep-seated infection, kala-azar, drug fever.
- **Inverse fever**: Temperature rises in the early hours of the morning rather than in the evening, e.g. some type of miliary tuberculosis.

COMMON STATIONS – SPOTS IN PRACTICAL EXAMINATION (2/3 MARKS)

- *TPR chart:* Identify the chart and write its uses.
- Enumerate different types of fever.
- *Anyone diagram of types of fever:* Define and identify.

Growth Charts and Anthropometric Assessment of Infants

Competency:

PY 11.9, 11.10: Interpret growth charts and interpret anthropometric assessments of infants

Learning Objectives

After completing this practical, the students shall be able to:
- Understand the importance of assessing growth in infants and children
- Enumerate important parameters that need to be assessed especially in children
- Interpret weight, height, and length in children below two years
- Understand and interpret the importance of measurement of head circumference and chest circumference
- Understand and interpret the target height and weight of children with respect to their age

■ INTRODUCTION

Even though the basic structure of taking history remains the same as that in adults, in children, more emphasis needs to be given to developmental history. Various things like maternal illness during pregnancy, type of delivery, full-term or premature delivery, immunization of child, etc. can help us give clues towards the diagnosis.

Some important questions that are to be addressed while assessing children:

- Any illness of the mother during pregnancy
- Full-term or premature delivery
- Birth-weight and type of delivery
- How is the baby fed? When did solid food was introduced?
- Immunization status of child
- If satisfactory weight gain?

General Questions

- Child's present diet, bowel, and micturition habits, behaviour of child with siblings, classmates, etc. Child's academic performance, missing school, etc.
- Any behaviour of child, parents worried about should be enquired. Normal developmental milestones must be enquired.

Scheme of Examination in Children

General examination: Besides normal general examination, try to assess the nutrition of the child and observe if speech and behaviour are appropriate with age and if growth and milestones are appropriate with age.

Examination of head, face, and neck: Observe the child's face properly and note if any unusual features are noted as many syndromes are diagnosable just by looking at the face. Look for the shape of the head (look for micro and macrocephaly) and feel for fontanelles and sutures. Normally, anterior fontanelle closure happens by 18 months. Delayed closure is common with rickets hypothyroidism, etc. Sunken fontanelle indicates a state of dehydration. Sutures and normally closed and ossified by the age of six months. Measurement of head circumference is very crucial in children. The neck should be examined for lymph nodes, tonsils, etc.

Limbs: Limbs should be examined for any obvious abnormality or painful or swollen joints etc. Similarly, hands should be examined for any obvious abnormality, extra or missing digits.

Abdomen: Abdomen must inspected and palpated carefully. It should be remembered that up to 3 years of age abdomen may appear protuberant (due to laxity of the rectus muscle). Look for any obvious distensions and pulsations. Liver edge can be felt in kids up to the age of 4 years (2 cm below the costal margin).

Chest: Chest examination becomes important for cardiovascular or respiratory systems. Look for any obvious deformity, movement, obvious abnormal pulsations, etc. Palpate for cardiac impulse and thrills, and palpate for the position of the trachea, suprasternal notch and intercostal spaces. Normal percussion and auscultation of the chest is significant. Appreciate splitting of heart sounds (it is more obvious in children). Observe for any murmurs or arrhythmias.

Neurological examination: Extensive neurological examination in children will depend upon the child's age.

In a walking child, gait has to be observed. Note for coordination, and tone of the muscles. Look for any obvious spine abnormalities and abnormal movements. Checking for neck stiffness is important in children. Careful examination of eyes, nose and genitalia for any obvious abnormality has to be checked.

Routine Measurement in Children

Height and weight: Childhood is a period of growth, the pattern of which may be adversely affected by many disturbances of health. Measurements of height and weight are therefore essential in the examination of children. In children able to stand, height can be measured against a wall-mounted who gauge. Younger children can be measured lying down on special measuring height boards. Height and weight should be compared with those of healthy children of similar sex, age and built on percentile charts. The different types of growth charts are shown below **(Figs. 59.1 to 59.8)**. There are special growth charts for children with Down's syndrome and Turner's syndrome.

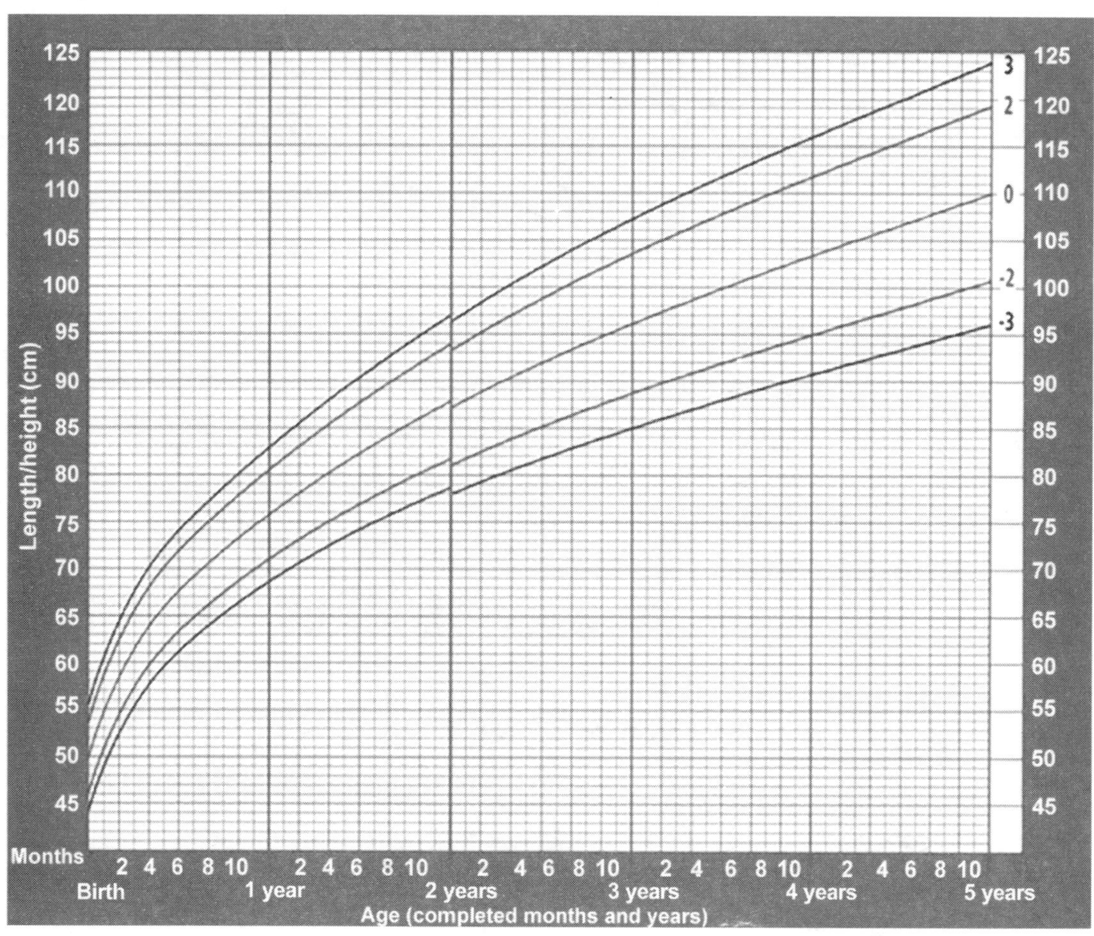

Fig. 59.1: Growth chart for boys, birth to 5 years: Length/height for age.

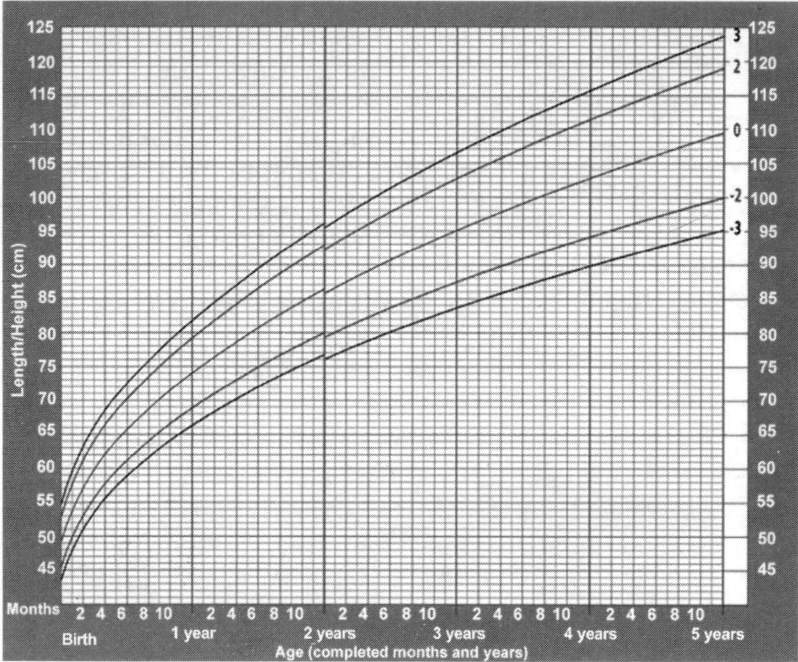

Fig. 59.2: Growth chart for girls, birth to 5 years: Length/height for age

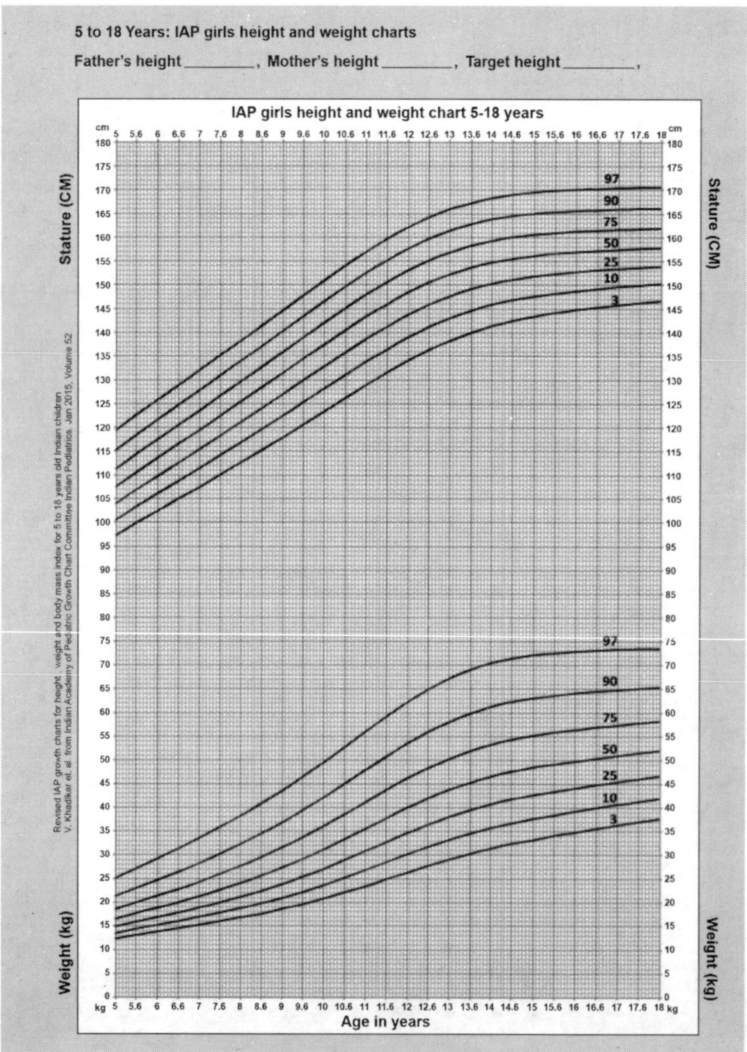

Fig. 59.3: Growth chart for girls, 5 to 15 years: Height and weight charts for age

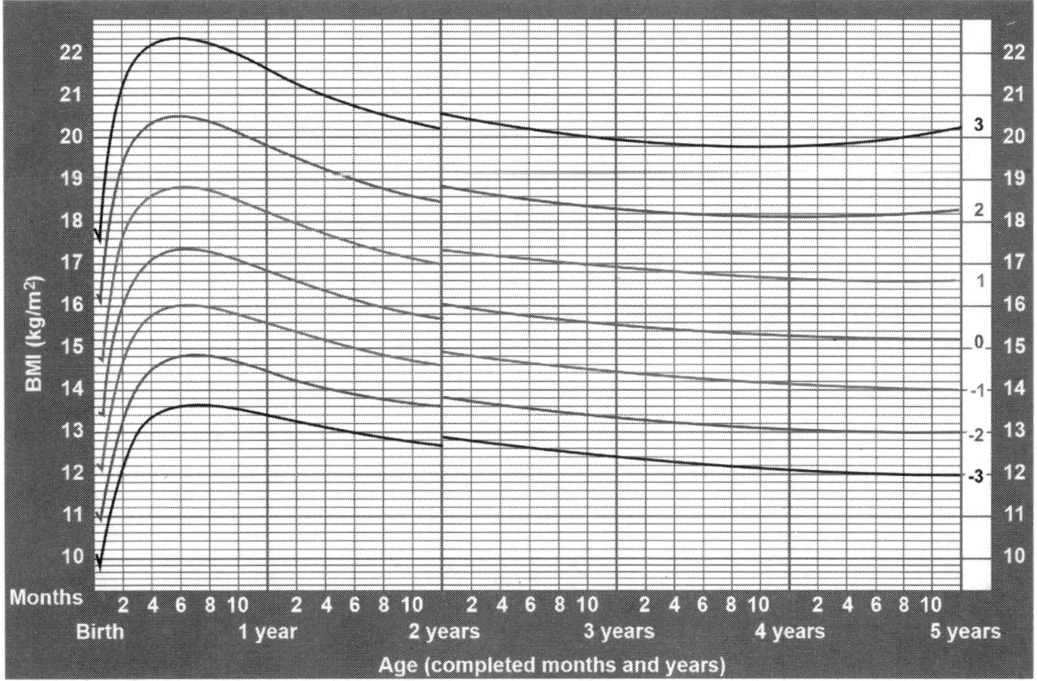

Fig. 59.4: Birth to 5 years boys: BMI for age

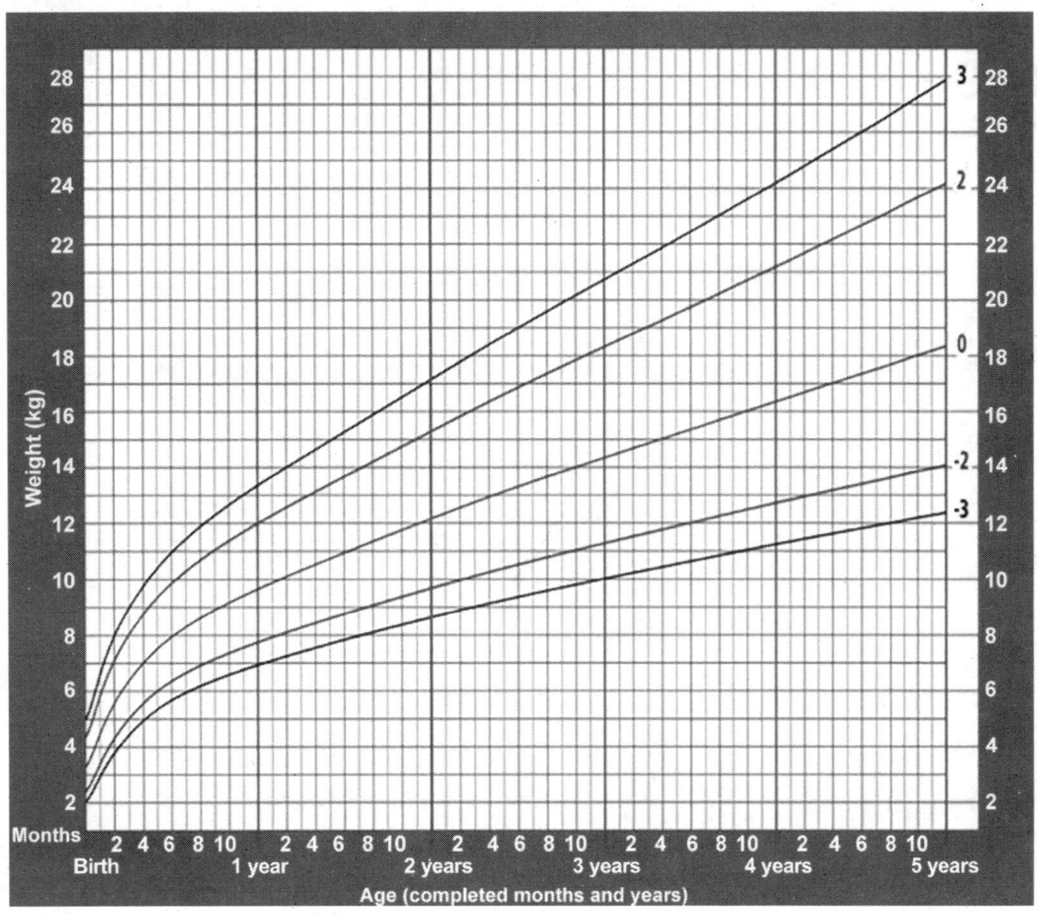

Fig. 59.5: Birth to 5 years boys: Weight for age

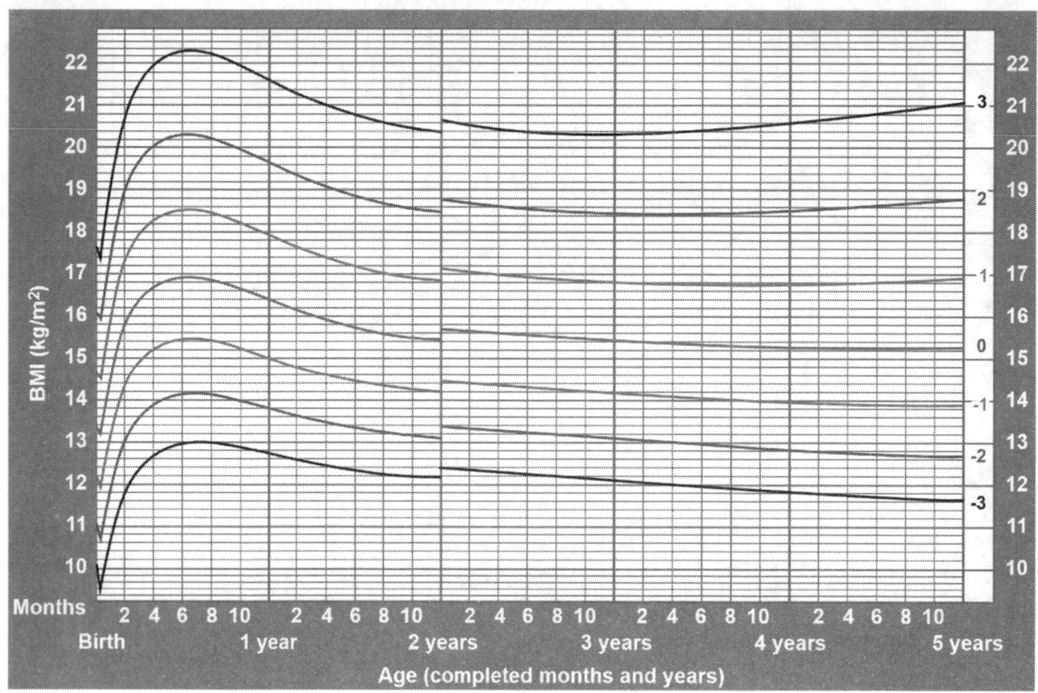

Fig. 59.6: Birth to 5 years girls: BMI for age

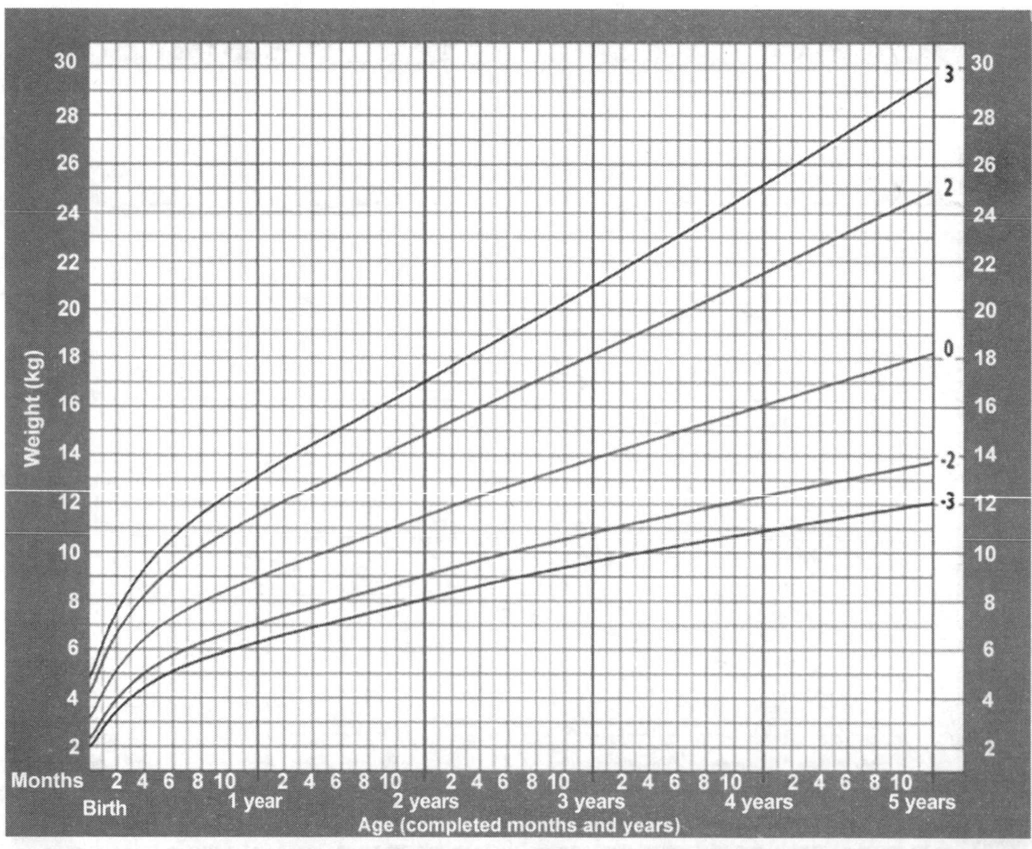

Fig. 59.7: Birth to 5 years girls: Weight for age

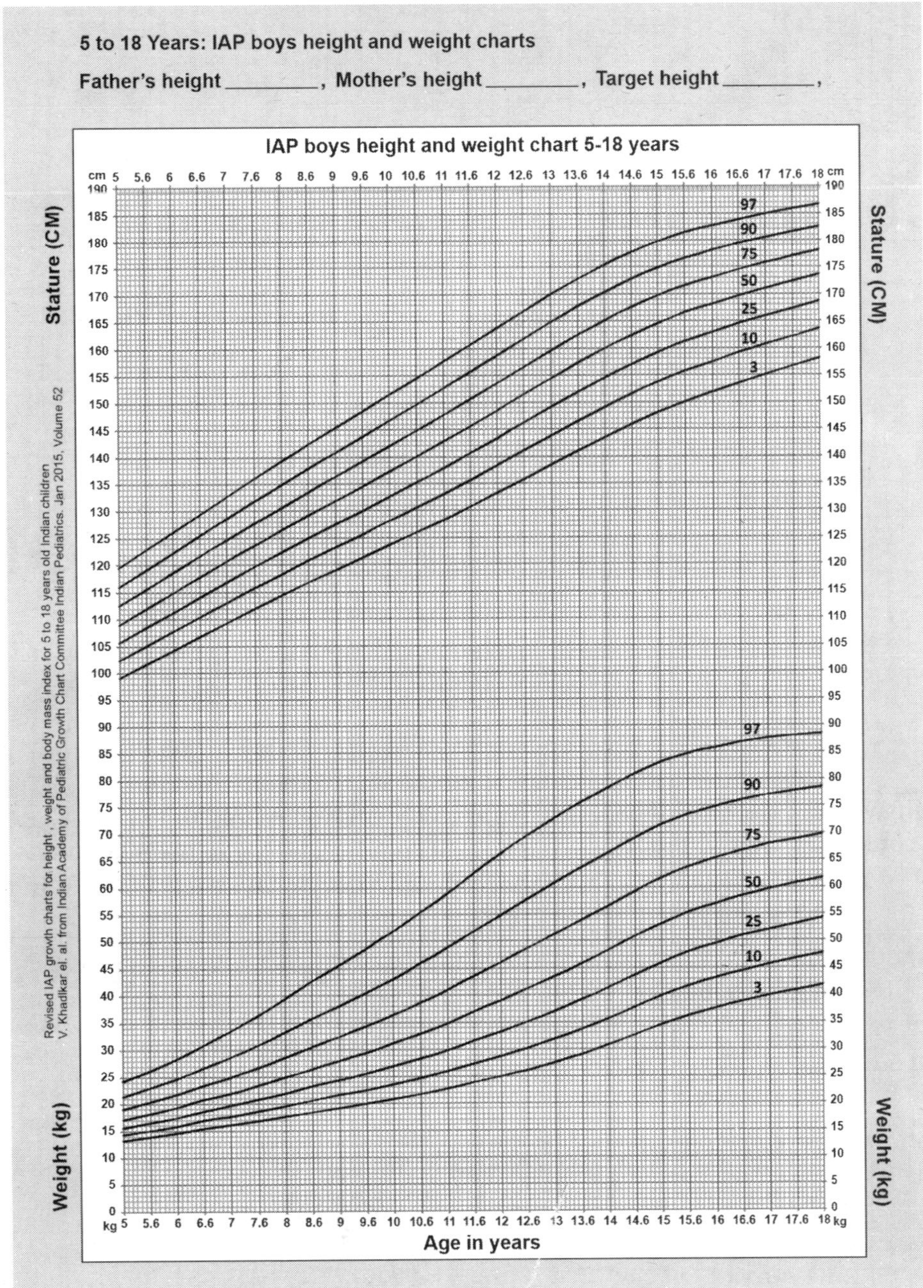

Fig. 59.8: 5 to 15 years girls: Height and weight charts for age

Preterm infants graph should be plotted according to their corrected age (chronological age minus the number of weeks born early) up until the age of 2 years.

Head circumference: In children below 2 years, head circumference is a better parameter to estimate linear growth than height and weight. The standard measurement is the largest occipitofrontal circumference.

Microcephaly: Baby's head is smaller than expected when compared to babies of the same age and sex. Common causes of microcephaly–Perinatal insult, fetal alcohol syndrome, genetic mutations.

Macrocephaly: Baby's head is about 2 standard deviations above that of 97 percentile. Common causes of macrocephaly–Hydrocephalus, excess brain growth.

Blood pressure: A variety of cuff sizes are available for children of different ages for recording blood pressure. The blood pressure should be checked in all four limbs to exclude coarctation of the aorta when congenital heart disease is suspected.

Temperature: Fever is one of the very common findings in children. Axillary or rectal measurement of temperature is a common site for temperature recording. Febrile convulsions can occur in children between 6 months and 6 years of age when the temperature rises rapidly to 39.5°C or above.

Examination of stools and urine: Examination of urine and stool plays a very important role in children.

CHAPTER

60

Calculations

1. From the following values determine the O_2 carrying capacity and O_2 content in arterial blood.

Data:

Hb – 15 g%

Arterial O_2 saturation– 80%

O_2 carrying capacity of blood = Hb in g% × 1.34

$$\text{Formula for } O_2 \text{ content} = \frac{\% \text{ saturation} \times O_2 \text{ carrying capacity}}{100}$$

From the given data oxygen carrying capacity of the blood can be found.

$$O_2 \text{ carrying capacity} = 15 \times 1.34$$
$$= 20.10/100 \text{ ml}$$

$$O_2 \text{ content of blood} = \frac{(O_2 \text{ carrying capacity})}{100}$$

$$= \frac{80 \times 20.10}{100}$$

$$= \frac{1608}{100}$$

$$= 16.08/100 \text{ ml}$$

Ans: O_2 content in the arterial blood of the given sample is 16.08/100 ml of blood.

2. Find out the dyspneic index and breathing reserve from the given data.

Data:

Maximum ventilatory volume (MVV) = 100 L/min

Tidal volume = 500 ml

Respiratory rate = 10 breaths/min

To find out the dyspneic index from the above data.

Step 1:

Respiratory minute volume (RMV)
$$= TV \times \text{Respiratory rate}$$
$$= 500 \times 10$$
$$= 5000 \text{ ml}/5L$$

Step 2:

Breathing reserve
$$= MVV\text{-}RMV$$
$$= 100\text{-}5$$
$$= 95 \text{ L}$$

Step 3:

$$\text{Dyspneic index} = \frac{MVV\text{-}RMV}{MVV} \times 100$$

$$= \frac{100\text{–}5}{100} \times 100$$

$$= 95\%$$

Ans: Dyspneic index is 95%.

3. The cardiac output of the subject is 5 L/min and his body surface area is 1.6 sq. metre. Calculate cardiac index.

The cardiac index is cardiac output per minute per square meter of body surface area.

Data:

Cardiac output	= 5 L/min
Body surface area	= 1.6 sq m

$$\text{Cardiac index} = \frac{\text{Cardiac output/min}}{\text{Surface area}}$$

$$= 5/1.6$$

$$= 3.125$$

Ans: Cardiac index is 3.125 L/min/m^2 of body surface area.

4. Calculate heart rate from the given ECG.

To find out heart rate from ECG, count the number of smallest squares in between two successive R waves.

- Two ways by which heart rate can be found out are:

$$\text{Heart rate} = \frac{1500}{\text{Number of smallest squares between two successive R waves}}$$

OR

- Find out the time interval in seconds between two successive R waves

$$\text{Heart rate} = \frac{60}{\text{Time interval in seconds between two successive R waves}}$$

5. Calculate work done in gm cm in isotonically contracting skeletal muscle.

Data:

Load attached = 20 g

Height of contraction = 3 cm

Length of the lever from the fulcrum to the point of attachment of load = 3 cm

Length of the lever from the fulcrum to the writing point = 12 cm

To find out the work done by the muscle,

Step 1:

$$\text{Magnification factor} = \frac{\text{Length of the lever from the fulcrum to the writing point}}{\text{Length of the lever from the fulcrum to the point of attachment}}$$

$$= 12/3 \text{ cm}$$

$$= 4 \text{ cm}$$

Step 2:

$$\text{True height (h)} = \frac{\text{Height of contraction (H)}}{\text{Magnification factor}}$$

$$= 3/4 \text{ cm}$$

$$= 0.75 \text{ cm}$$

Step 3:

Work done	= Load × true height (h)
	= 20 × 0.75
	= 15.00 g cm

6. From the given data find out the absolute counts of eosinophils and neutrophils.

Data:

Total WBC count = 8000/cu mm of blood

Eosinophil = 4%

Neutrophil = 60%

- Absolute eosinophil count:
  100 WBCs contain 4 eosinophils
  8000 WBCs contain 8000/100 × 4 = 320 eosinophils
  Thus, the absolute count of eosinophils is 320 cu mm of blood

- Absolute neutrophil count
  100 WBCs contain 60 neutrophils
  8000 WBCs contain 8000/100 × 60 = 4800 neutrophils
  Thus, the absolute neutrophil count is 4800 cu mm of blood.

7. Find out the expiratory reserve volume and inspiratory reserve volume.

Data:

Total lung capacity = 5800 ml

Inspiratory capacity = 3500 ml

Tidal volume = 500 ml

Vital capacity = 4600 ml

- Residual volume
  = Total lung capacity–Vital capacity
  = 5800–4600
  = 1200 ml

- Inspiratory reserve volume (IRV)
  = Inspiratory capacity–Tidal volume
  = 3500–500
  = 3000 ml

- Expiratory reserve volume (ERV)
  = Vital capacity–Inspiratory capacity
  = 4600–3500
  = 1100 ml

8. From the given data find out the physiological dead space.

Data:

Tidal volume = 500 ml

Alveolar pCO$_2$ = 40 mm Hg

Expired air pCO$_2$ = 28 mm Hg

Formula for physiological dead space

$$\text{Physiological dead space air} = \frac{\text{Alveolar air pCO}_2 - \text{Expired air pCO}_2 \times \text{Tidal volume}}{\text{Alveolar air pCO}_2}$$

Thus substituting it from the provided data,

$$\text{Physiological dead space} = \frac{40-28 \times 500}{40}$$

$$= 12 \times 500/40$$

$$= 150 \text{ ml}$$

Ans: Physiological dead space air is 150 ml.

9. Determine mean corpuscular volume (MCV) from given data.

Data:

RBC count = 4 million/cu mm of blood

PCV= 40%

ESR = 30 mm at the end of one hour

Formula for MCV

$$MCV = \frac{PCV}{RBC\ count\ in\ million/cu\ mm\ of\ blood} \times 10$$

Substituting it from the provided data,

MCV = 40/4 × 10

       = 100 cubic microns.

Ans: MCV is 100 cubic microns.

10. Calculate reticulocytes (%) in peripheral blood from given data.

- In 5 high power fields number of RBCs = 100,000
  In 10 high power fields number of RBCs = 8000

In 5 high power fields if number of RBCs are 100,000

Then, in 10 high power fields number of RBCs = 200,000

In 10 high power fields number of reticulocytes = 8000

(given)

Therefore,

Per 200,000 RBCs there are 5000 reticulocytes

Therefore,

Per 100 RBCs there are 8000 × 100/200,000

     = 4 Reticulocytes

Ans: Reticulocytes % in peripheral blood is 4%.

11. Determine respiratory quotient from given data.

Data:

Total expired air volume in 6 minutes = 30 L

% of CO_2 in expired air = 4%

O_2 consumption = 250 ml/min

100 ml of expired air contains 4 ml of CO_2

Therefore,

5000 ml of expired air contains 200 ml of CO_2 (CO_2 output/min)

$$RQ = \frac{CO_2\ output/min}{O_2\ consumption/min}$$

     = 200/250

     = 0.8

Ans: Respiratory Quotient (RQ) is 0.8.

12. Calculate MCHC from the given data.

Data:

PCV = 32%

Hb = 8 g%

RBC count–4 million/cu mm of blood

Formula for MCHC, i.e. mean corpuscular haemoglobin concentration

$$MCHC = \frac{Haemoglobin\ in\ g\% \times 100}{PCV}$$

By substituting the data

MCHC = 8 × 100/32

       = 25%

Ans: MCHC is 25%.

13. Calculate the velocity of the nerve impulse from the given data.

When the stimulus is applied to the spinal end of the nerve in an experimental animal, the latent period is 0.01 second.

When the stimulus is applied at the muscle end of the nerve, the latent period is 0.006 second.

The length of the nerve between these two points is 7 cm

In one second, the distance travelled is 7 × 1000/4.

     = 1750 cm

     = 17.5 metre/second

Ans: The velocity of nerve impulse from given data is 17.5 m/sec.

14. Calculate urea clearance from the given data.

Data:

Concentration of urea in the urine = 21 mg/ml

Concentration of urea in the blood = 30 mg/100 ml

Flow of urine/min = 1 ml/min

Formula for finding out urea clearance is

$$Urea\ clearance = \frac{Conc.\ of\ urea\ in\ urine \times \sqrt{volume\ of\ urine/min} \times 100}{Conc.\ of\ urea\ in\ blood}$$

Substituting these values from given data,

$$Urea\ clearance = \frac{21 \times 1 \times 100}{30}$$

     = 70 ml

Ans: Urea clearance is 70 ml.

15. Find out the platelet count from the given data.

Data:

1/250 cu mm of blood contains 6 platelets (Dilution = 1:200)

Calculation:

1/250 cu mm of blood contains 6 platelets

Then, 1 cu mm of blood contains 1500 platelets (Dilution = 1: 200)

Therefore,

Platelets/cu mm = 1500 × 200

       = 3 lack per cu mm of blood

Ans: Total platelet count is 3 lakh per cu mm of blood.

16. Find out GFR from given data.

Data:

Concentration of inulin in plasma = 0.25 mg/ml
Concentration of inulin in urine= 30 mg/ml
Urinary output = 1.0 ml/min

Formula for finding out plasma clearance is:

$$\text{Plasma clearance} = \frac{\text{Conc. of substance in urine} \times \text{Volume of urine per minute}}{\text{Concentration of inulin in plasma}}$$

Substituting with given values

$$\text{Plasma clearance} = \frac{30 \times 1}{0.25}$$
$$= 120 \text{ ml/min}$$

Ans: GFR is 120 ml/min.

17. Determine renal blood flow from the given data.

Data:

Concentration of PAH in urine = 7.2 mg/ml
Concentration of PAH in plasma = 0.02 mg/ml
Urinary output = 2 ml/min
Haematocrit = 45%

Formula

$$\text{Plasma clearance of PAH} = \frac{\text{Conc. of PAH in urine} \times \text{Urine volume/min}}{\text{Concentration of PAH in plasma}}$$

$$= \frac{7.2 \times 2}{0.2}$$
$$= 720 \text{ ml/min}$$

Actual plasma flow = PAH clearance/0.9
$$= 720/0.9$$
$$= 800 \text{ ml/min}$$

$$\text{Renal blood flow} = \frac{100}{100\text{-Haematocrit}} \times \text{Renal plasma flow}$$

$$= 100/100\text{-}45 \times 800$$
$$= 80000/55$$
$$= 1454.5 \text{ ml/min}$$

Ans: Renal blood flow is 1454.5 ml/min.

18. Calculate creatinine clearance from the given data.

Data:

Creatinine concentration in urine (Uc) = 2 mg/ml
Creatinine concentration in plasma (Pc) = 1.5 mg%
Urine volume for 24 hrs = 1440 ml
Therefore, urine volume/min (Uv) = 1 ml

Formula

$$\text{Creatinine clearance} = \frac{Uc \times Uv}{Pc} \times 100$$
$$= 2 \times 1/1.5 \times 100$$
$$= 133 \text{ ml/min}$$

Ans: Creatinine clearance is 133 ml/min.

19. Calculate basal metabolic rate (BMR) from the given data.

Data:

O_2 consumption = 250 ml/min
Surface area = 1.5 m^2
Standard BMR for the person = 45 cal/hr/m^2
O_2 consumption per min = 250 ml
Thus O_2 consumption/hour = 15 litres.

When one litre of O_2 is consumed, 4.8 calories are released per hour.

Therefore, for 15 liters of O_2 consumed 4.8 × 15 = 72.0 cal/hour will be released.

BMR = Calories consumed/hour/surface area
$$= 72/1.5$$
$$= 48 \text{ cal/hr/m}^2$$

The standard BMR for a person is 45 cal/hr/m^2
Calculated BMR is in excess by 3 cal/hr/m^2
% excess = 3/45 100
$$= 6.6\%$$
BMR $= 6.6\%$

20. Calculate effective filtration pressure for GFR.

Data:

Hydrostatic pressure in glomerular capillaries = 60 mm Hg
Bowman's capsular fluid pressure = 10 mm Hg

Formula

Effective filtration pressure = Hydrostatic pressure of blood- (Colloid osmotic pressure of blood + Bowman's capsular pressure)
$$= 60\text{-}(28\text{+}10)$$
$$= 60\text{-}38$$
$$= 22 \text{ mm Hg}$$

Ans: Effective filtration pressure for GFR is 22 mm Hg.

21. Calculate the O_2 carrying capacity of blood.

Hb = 14.5 g/dl
O_2 carrying capacity of blood = Hb × 1.34
$$= 14.5 \times 1.34$$
$$= 19.43 \text{ ml/dl}$$

Ans: O_2 carrying capacity of blood is 19.43 ml/dl of blood.

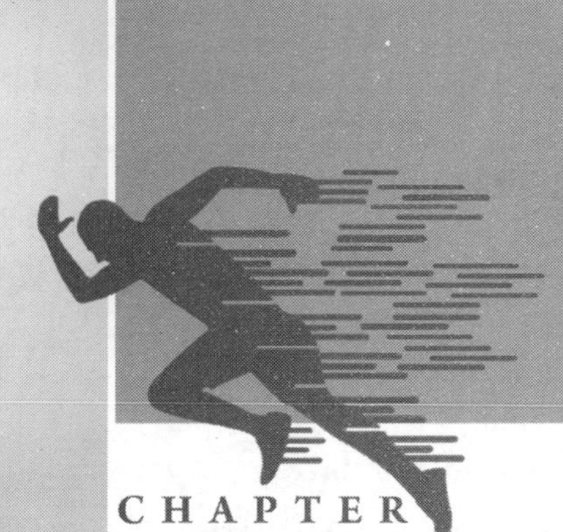

Endocrine Disorders

Learning Objectives

At the end of this practical, the students shall be able to:

- Describe various common endocrine disorders due to growth hormones and understand the physiological basis of gigantism, acromegaly, and dwarfism, identify their main features, findings on clinical examination and physiological basis for their treatment.
- Describe various common endocrine disorders due to thyroid hormone and understand the physiological basis of cretinism, Grave's disease and myxedema identify their main features, findings on clinical examination and the physiological basis for their treatment.
- Describe various common endocrine disorders due to parathyroid hormone and understand the physiological basis of tetany and its various forms, identify their main features, findings on clinical examination and the physiological basis for its treatment.
- Describe various adrenocortical disorders and understand the physiological basis of Cushing's syndrome and identify their main features, findings on clinical examination and physiological basis for its treatment.

■ INTRODUCTION

The endocrine system consists of the pituitary, thyroid, parathyroid, adrenal, and islets cells of the pancreas and gonads. Symptoms of any endocrine disorder may not be specific to a particular system and can be presented as some non-specific symptoms.

Common symptoms include weight gain/loss, peculiar deposition of fat, heat or cold intolerance, thirst, polyuria, sweating, amenorrhea, muscle weakness, etc.

Approach to a Patient with Endocrine Disorder

General Assessment of Patient

- It includes height, weight BMI, state of nutrition, and peculiar fat deposition in body parts.
- **Examination of skin**: For pigmentation, striae, abnormal dryness or coarseness of skin, etc.
- **Examination of hair**: For texture, less or more hair growth, hair loss, localized thickening of dermis, etc.
- **Examination of thyroid**: Palpation of thyroid should be carried out standing posterior to the patient with the neck slightly extended, try to inspect below cricoid cartilage and palpate for isthmus. Try to palpate lobes of the thyroid, and enlargement of thyroid (if any) and nodule/nodules palpable.
- **Examination of cardiovascular system**: In particular try to look for, tachycardia, postural hypotension, sinus tachycardia or atrial fibrillation on ECG, any autonomic dysfunctions like heart rate variability, etc.
- **Breast and genitalia**: Examination of breasts and genitalia should be examined thoroughly when relevant.
- **Examination of the nervous system**: Especially look for any tremors, hyperreflexia, etc.

Gigantism and Acromegaly

Gigantism

It is due to hypersecretion of growth hormone in childhood (before fusion of epiphyses with shafts of bones).

Cause
Acidophilic tumour.

Characteristic features
- *Skeleton:* The person is tall (6 to 8 feet)
- Muscles and viscera are proportionately large
- Hyperglycemia and reduced sugar tolerance
- Fat is used as fuel than carbohydrates (fat catabolic effect).

Treatment
Microsurgical removal of tumour or irradiation of gland.

Acromegaly

It is due to hypersecretion of growth hormone after adolescence (i.e. after fusion of epiphyses with shafts of the bones).

Cause
Acidophilic tumour.

Characteristic features
- *Skeleton:* The person is not tall as seen in gigantism but bones do grow in thickness
- There is an overgrowth of the jaw, slanting forehead, prominent supraorbital ridges, and kyphosis (all due to enlargement of membranous bones) as shown in **Fig. 61.1**.
- With excess soft tissue growth, the tongue, liver, spleen, and kidneys get enlarged
- Hyperglycemia and reduced sugar tolerance

Treatment
Microsurgical removal of tumour.

Dwarfism

It is stunted growth with respect to the age of a person.

Causes

- Hyposecretion of growth hormone
- Hyposecretion of all anterior pituitary hormones (Panhypopituitarism)

Characteristic Features

- *Skeleton:* There is a stunted physical growth but no deformity proportions of different body parts are normal **(Fig. 61.2)**.
- Intelligence is normal.
- Reproductive function is affected if dwarfism is due to panhypopituitarism.

Treatment

- If dwarfism is due to growth hormone deficiency, then it is treated by supplementing with human growth hormone.
- If dwarfism is due to panhypopituitarism, along with growth hormone, adrenocortical and thyroid hormones are administered.

Cretinism

It is a state of thyroid deficiency that is mainly seen in fetal life, infancy or childhood.

Causes

It develops due to less or no availability of thyroid hormone in fetal life due to the hyposecretion of thyroid hormone by the mother or congenital hypothyroidism in newborn

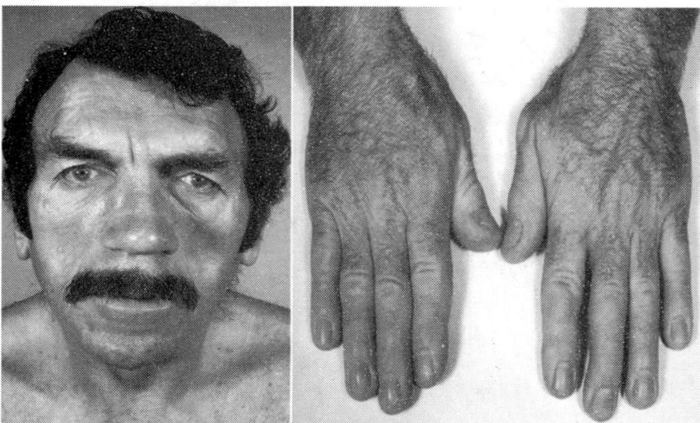

Fig. 61.1: Hand appearance in acromegaly
Source: Hutchison Clinical Methods, 24th edition

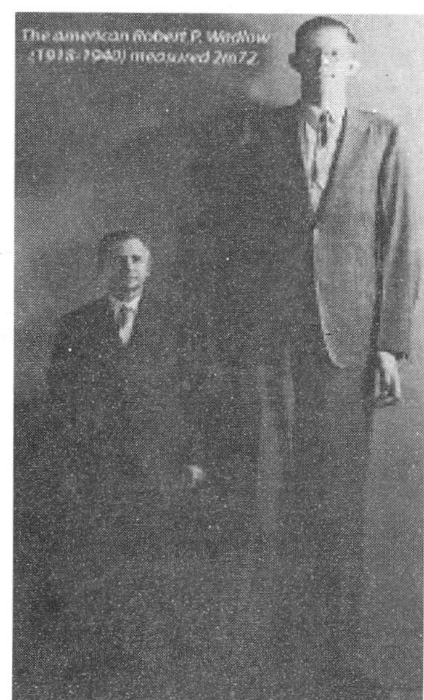

Fig. 61.2: Comparison of a patient with dwarfism and a normal individual

Characteristic Features

- Milestones in child are delayed
- *Skeleton:* Stunted growth is observed. Skeleton growth is more affected than soft tissue growth, this leads to a disproportionate rate of growth
- Skin is dry, rough, wrinkled. Scanty hair growth
- *Face:* The child has an idiotic expression (retarded mental growth), thick parted lips, a large protruding tongue with dribbling saliva, broad nose with a depressed bridge **(Fig. 61.3)**
- *Abdomen:* Pot belly appearance with protruding umbilicus
- Sex organs and all secondary sexual characters are retarded.

Treatment

Neonate with cretinism is treated with adequate iodine or thyroxine. This causes the normal return of physical growth but unless cretinism is treated within a few weeks after birth, mental growth remains permanently retarded.

Hyperthyroidism/Grave's Disease

It is a state of excess secretion of thyroid hormone.

Cause

It develops due to excess secretion of thyroid hormone.

Characteristic Features

- Raised BMR, body temperature (heat intolerance)
- Increased sweating
- Resting tachycardia, atrial fibrillation, heart failure
- Excess hyperactivity of neurons- causing fine tremors, difficulty in sleeping
- *Exophthalmos:* Protrusion of the eyeballs (due to edematous swelling of retro-orbital tissue and degenerative changes in extraocular muscles) shown in **Fig. 61.4**.
- Increased appetite with loss of weight
- Muscle weakness
- Thyroid enlargement may or may not be there.

Treatment

- Most direct treatment is the surgical removal of the gland (total/partial thyroidectomy)
- Anti-thyroid drugs (different types of drugs that affect/block steps in the synthesis of thyroid hormones)
- Treatment with radioactive iodine.

Hypothyroidism/Myxedema

It is a state of less secretion of thyroid hormone.

Causes

It develops due to less secretion of thyroid hormone by the thyroid gland in adults. It can be due to thyroiditis, endemic colloid goitre, idiopathic colloid goitre, irradiation of the thyroid gland or surgical removal of the thyroid gland.

Characteristic Features

- Reduced BMR, body temperature (cold intolerance)
- Excess sleep and muscle sluggishness
- Resting bradycardia, heart blocks
- Decreased appetite with weight gain
- Depressed hair growth and scaliness of skin
- Swelling of tongue and larynx causing hoarseness of voice and slow slurred speech
- Swollen, puffy and edematous look on face, bagginess under eyes as shown in **Fig. 61.5**
- Thyroid enlargement may or may not be there.

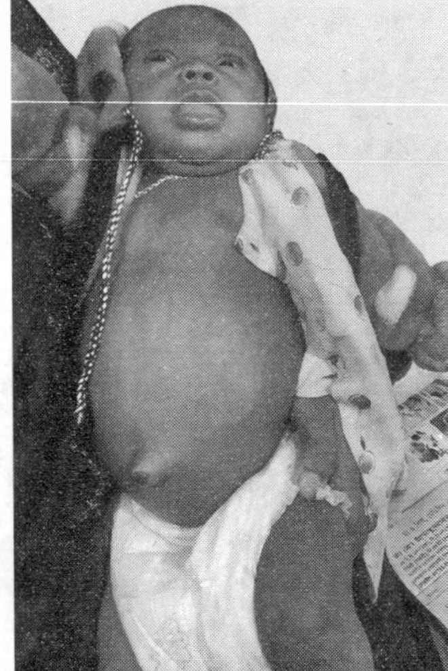

Fig. 61.3: Cretinism

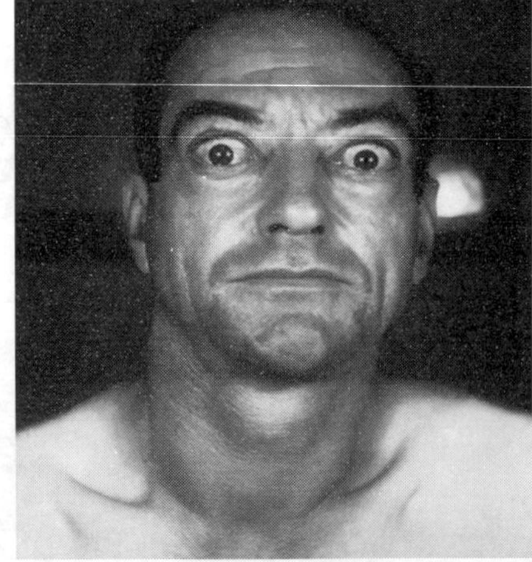

Fig. 61.4: Grave's disease (Thyrotoxicosis)
Source: Hutchison Clinical Methods, 24th edition

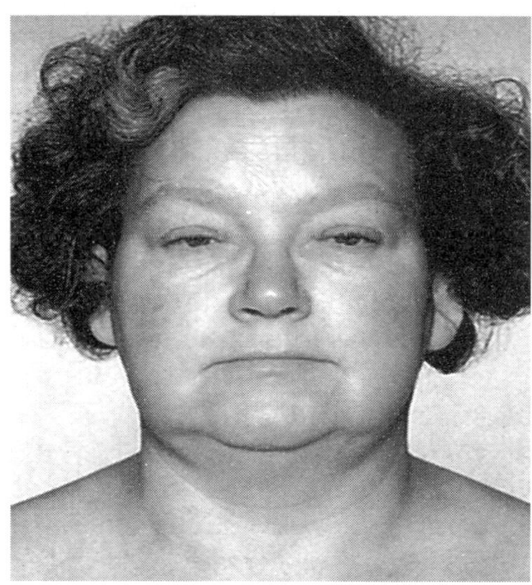

Fig. 61.5: Myxedema (Hypothyroidism)
Source: Hutchison Clinical Methods, 24th edition

Treatment

Thyroxine tablets.

Hypocalcemia – Tetany/Carpopedal Spasm

Tetany

It is a state that can be developed with low serum levels of calcium.

Causes

Low serum calcium levels (hypocalcemia) can happen due to a deficiency of parathyroid hormone, or surgical removal of the parathyroid gland. When calcium levels go below 6 to 7 mg/dl (normal level 9 to 11 mg/dl) nerves become hyperexcitable leading to spasms of muscles.

Carpopedal spasm

- This characteristic sign is seen with hypocalcemia. The elbow and wrist are flexed. Fingers are flexed at metacarpophalangeal joints but extended at interphalangeal joints. The thumb is in the palm and the fingertips are drawn together **(Fig. 61.6)**.
- In addition to the generalized convulsions, and spasms in the larynx and face (Chvostek's sign) are seen.

Other forms of tetany: Besides parathyroid deficiency, tetany can be observed in rickets, renal failure, and impaired absorption of calcium.

Treatment

Parathyroid hormone is occasionally used for treating hypoparathyroidism as the hormone is expensive and the body does have a tendency to develop antibodies against it. Usually, administration of a high dose of vitamin D–1000,000 units/day along with 1 to 2 g calcium helps in keeping calcium levels normal.

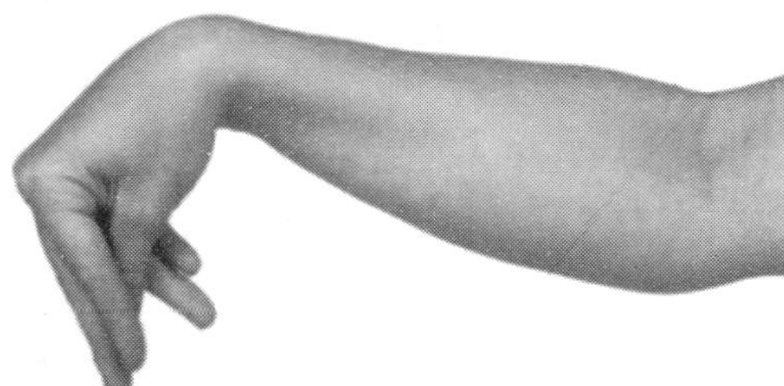

Fig. 61.6: Carpopedal spasm

Cushing's Syndrome

Excess secretion of adrenocortical hormone (mainly cortisol) due to excess secretion of ACTH by the anterior pituitary.

Causes

- Adenomas of the anterior pituitary that secretes a large amount of ACTH
- Excess CRH (corticotropic releasing hormone)
- Ectopic secretion of ACTH (by tumour elsewhere in the body).

Characteristic Features

- Increased deposition of fat peculiarly on the trunk, face, back and not on limbs.
- Rounded/moon face appearance.
- Pad of fat on the neck giving buffalo hump appearance **(Fig. 61.7)**.
- Excess cortisol causes protein catabolic effect, leading to muscle weakness, asthenia and muscle wasting.
- The protein catabolic effect also suppresses immunity, making a person susceptible to infections.
- Diminished protein collagen fibers in subcutaneous tissues so that they tear easily causing large purplish striae on skin.
- Cortisol prevents carbohydrate utilization causes hyperglycemia and can lead to insulin-resistant DM.

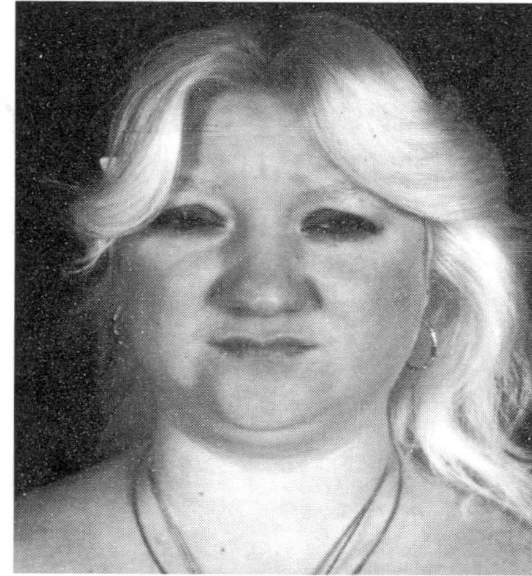

Fig. 61.7: Facial appearance Cushing's syndrome
Source: Hutchison Clinical Methods, 24th edition

- Due to loss of protein matrix and decalcification, osteoporosis is observed.
- Excess excretion of 17-keto steroids and 17-hydroxy corticosteroids.

Treatment

Removal of adrenocortical tumours can be done. Drugs blocking steroid synthesis, or removal of pituitary tumour, if it is due to excess secretion of ACTH.

Addison's Disease

Decreased secretion of adrenocortical hormone (mainly cortisol).

Causes

- Damage to adrenal glands, tuberculosis of adrenal glands
- Primary adrenal insufficiency (outer layer of adrenal gland damaged)
- Secondary adrenal insufficiency (less ACTH secretion due to some pituitary condition).

Characteristic Features

- Fatigue, weight loss, loss of appetite
- Hyperpigmentation, muscle weakness
- Low BP, fainting
- Salt craving, hypoglycemia.

Treatment

Supplementing cortisol orally or injectable.

- **Addisonian crisis:** It is a medical emergency developed during stress/infection/injury where adrenal glands normally can double or triple the cortisol production, which is not possible in a person with Addison's disease ending in Addisonian crisis.
- Addisonian crisis can cause low BP, high levels of potassium and low levels of blood sugar. It requires immediate treatment.

■ COMMON STATIONS – SPOTS IN PRACTICAL EXAMINATION (2/3 MARKS)

Q.1. Photographs of any of the above-mentioned disorders: Identify, and write any two features, and the physiological basis of treatment (refer above).

Q.2. A baby developed carpopedal spasm and came with c/o twitching of muscles after thyroidectomy. What is it? (clue-tetany; probably acci- dental removal of parathyroid glands with thyroidectomy).

Q.3. A 16-month-old baby was brought to OPD by the mother, c/o delayed milestones. The child had a pot belly and poor muscle strength. What is it? (Cretinism– refer above).

Q.4. A 45-year-old lady came with c/o fatigue and weight gain. She also, c/o loss of appetite and sleepiness. On examination, generalized non-pitting oedema was observed. What is the probable diagnosis? (Myxedema – refer above).

Q.5. A 50-year-old man came with pigmentation on his extremities and showed his blood reports blood glucose–60 mg/dl, serum K$^+$ 5.2 mEq/L, serum Na$^+$ 128 mEq/L. What is the probable diagnosis? (clue- Addison's disease – refer above).

■ CASE-BASED SCENARIO/ PROBLEM-BASED/ CLINICAL APPLICATIONS

Case 1: A photograph of myxedema– Identify the disorder. What you expect for this patient's TSH level (clue- It should be raised in hypothyroidism patients with negative feedback regulation).

Case 2: A photograph of Cushing's syndrome– Identify the disorder. Write the cause of suppressed immunity in the patients.

Case 3: A patient comes with h/o palpitations and weight loss. His TSH level is below normal and T3 and T4 levels are high. Give the physiological basis of the findings (clue- TSH low and T3, T4 high negative feedback).

Case 4: A photograph of acromegaly– Identity the disorder. On examination, there is a huge splenomegaly. Blood sugar levels are high. Give a physiological basis for both.

Case 5: A picture of Grave's disease, this person has a resting pulse rate of 110 beats/min. Give the physiological basis of tachycardia.

Case 6: Addison's disease – Identify the condition. What do you expect from his serum K$^+$ levels? Why?

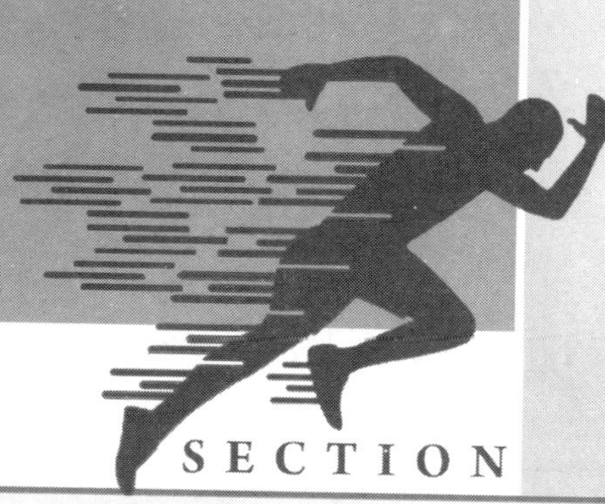

Experimental Physiology

Introduction to Experimental Physiology (Amphibian Experiments)

Competency:
PY 3.18: Observe with computer-assisted learning, amphibian nerve muscle experiments.

Learning Objectives

After completing this practical, the students shall be able to:
- Name and describe different apparatus used in experimental physiology
- Define stimulus and enumerate a different variety of stimuli and describe why electrical stimulus is preferred over the other types of stimuli
- Enumerate the advantages of using frogs in the experiments

■ INTRODUCTION

- Different instruments are used in experimental physiology
- One must know the use and principle on which different instruments work
- In experimental physiology, we study the response of tissues to various stimuli.

Stimulus

- It is defined as any change in the external environment that elicits a response from excitable tissue
- Stimulus can be mechanical, electrical, chemical, thermal, etc.
- In experiments, an electrical stimulus is used.

Advantages of Electrical Stimulus

- Electrical stimulus causes the least damage to the tissues
- It can be easily quantified thus its duration and strength can be exactly known
- Stimulus can be easily controlled
- Excitation and conduction of impulses in tissue are electrical in nature
- Electrical stimulation can be localized to a tissue.

Tissue Preparation

- For amphibian nerve–muscle experiments, the sciatic nerve and gastrocnemius muscle of a frog are used
- Frogs are preferred because:
  - Frogs are easily available and can be handled easily
  - Maintenance of tissue preparation is easy and can be kept for a long time (as no extra O_2 is required for frog muscles as they imbibe O_2 from the environment directly).

Source of Current

- Faradic current is preferred over galvanic current
- Faradic current is short-lived and causes the least damage to the tissues
- Faradic current is obtained from an induction coil or a stimulator
- Strength of current depends on the strength of the current in the primary circuit and the distance between the primary and secondary coil.

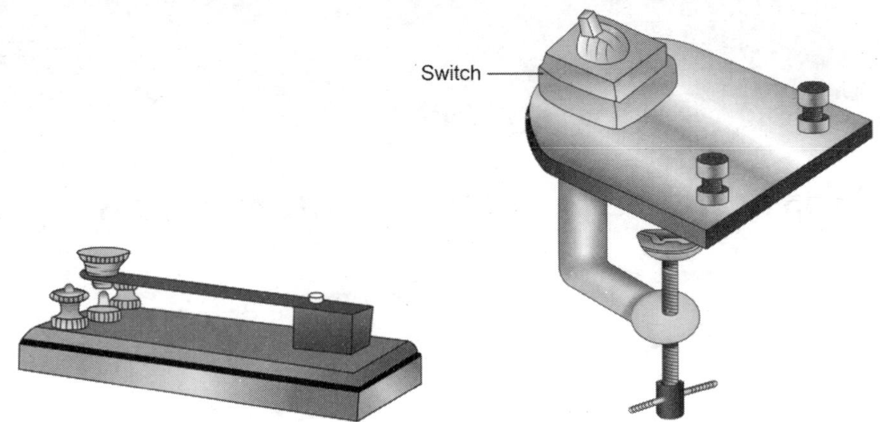

Fig. 62.1: Simple (primary) key

Common Appliances

Wires

- Copper or aluminium wires are used in laboratories to carry current
- There should not be any damage or cracks in wires. If there is a break in insulation, such wires should not be used.

Keys

- This is a device used to complete or interrupt the circuit.

  Two types of keys:
  1. **Tap key**: It is used to make or break the circuit. The key is connected to a primary circuit **(Fig. 62.1)**.
  2. **Dubois Raymond key (short-circuiting key)**: Connected in a secondary circuit usually in parallel (to prevent leakage of current into tissues). The key is usually kept closed and is left open when stimulation is desired **(Fig. 62.2)**.
- Key convert continuous current into induced current.
- **Reversing key:** It is used when two electrodes are required and current from one electrode has to be shunted.
- **Tapping key:** It is used to make or break a circuit for a short period. It is connected in series with low-voltage mains in the primary circuit.

Stimulating Electrodes

- They are used for delivering electrical stimulus to the tissues.
- It consists of two copper wires.

Induction Coil (Dubois Raymond Induction Coil)

It consists of primary and secondary coils.
- **Primary coil** has 300 turns of insulated thick copper wire wound around the soft iron core.

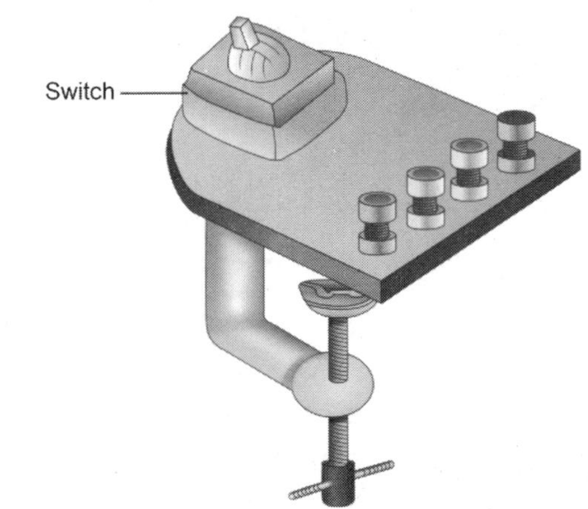

Fig. 62.2: Secondary key (short-circuiting key)

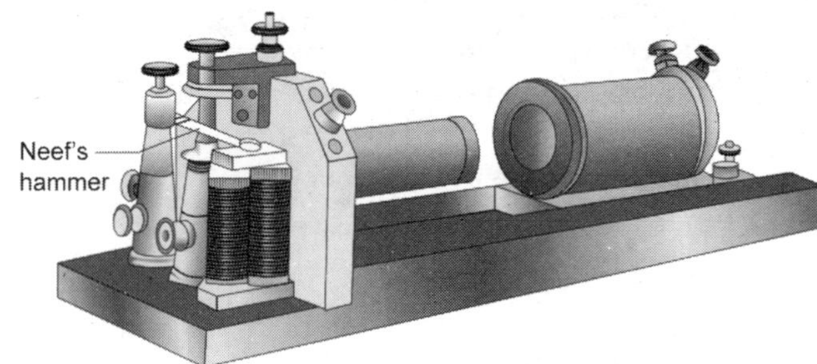

Fig. 62.3: Dubois Raymond induction coil.

- **Secondary coil** is made up of 5,000 turns of fine copper wire. There is a scale marked by which the distance between the primary and secondary coil can be measured.
- A current is induced in the secondary coil only when there is a change in the strength of the magnetic field of the primary coil.
- Thus, starting, stopping, and altering the strength of the current in the primary circuit induces a current of momentary duration is the secondary coil **(Fig. 62.3)**.
- In induced or faradic current, break shock is stronger than make shock.

- The strength of the stimulating current can be increased or decreased by changing the distance between the primary and secondary coil.

Factors affecting the strength of induced current are:

- **Distance between two coils:** Less the distance between two coils, the more the strength of the stimulus and vice versa
- **Strength of direct current fed in the primary coil**
- **Angle between two coils:** Maximum strength of current when coils are laced straight.

> **Break stronger than make:** A change in the magnetic field caused by current flowing in the primary coil produces a momentary current of opposite direction not only in the secondary coil but also in the primary coil. This self-induced current impeds the development of the original current in the primary coil.
>
> During break, the circuit is broken and self-induced current cannot develop and flow. The change in the magnetic field occurring during the break is thus greater as compared to make a circuit.
>
> As the induced current developed in the secondary coil is proportional to the change in the magnetic field, the induced current developed during break is stronger than developed during make.

Kymograph (Sherrington–Starling Drum)

- It records movements on a moving surface.
- It has a metal gearbox to which a vertical rotating shaft is connected.
- Shaft can be stationary or can be rotated with a suitable pulley connection.
- A cylinder or drum is fixed to the shaft. The drum rotates with the shaft.
- Gear switch present on the left side of the kymograph.
- In each gear, different speeds of the drum can be obtained.
- At the base of the shaft, there is a projecting striker that has two parts that can be separated by drawing them apart (for giving two successive stimuli).
- There are two electrical terminals for electrical connection.
- Circuit can be made or broken when the tip of the contact arms makes and breaks contact with the insulated spring **(Fig. 62.4)**.

Keith Luca's Moist Chamber

- It is an aplastic chamber used to keep muscle moist in Ringer solution.
- At the bottom, it has two holes with corks.
- One end of the muscle is fixed to one of these holes. The other end of the muscle is tied to the hook firmly **(Fig. 62.5)**.
- A block carrying stimulating electrodes is fixed on the side walls of the chamber.

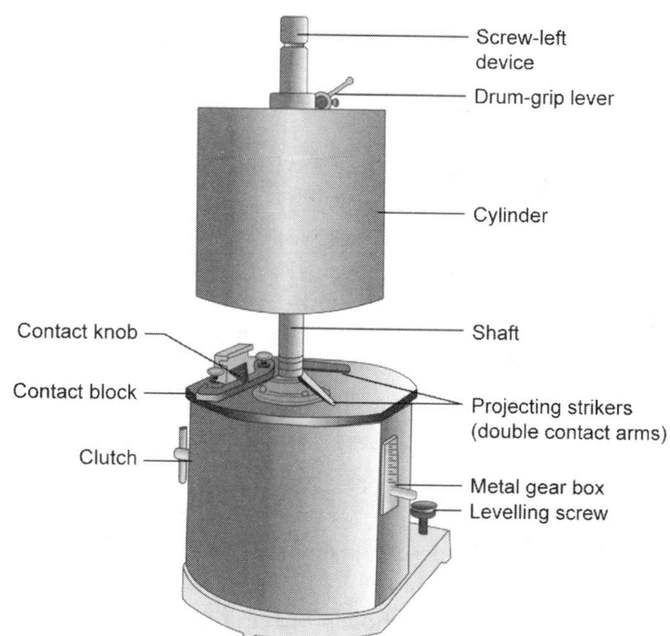

Fig. 62.4: Sherrington-Starling drum

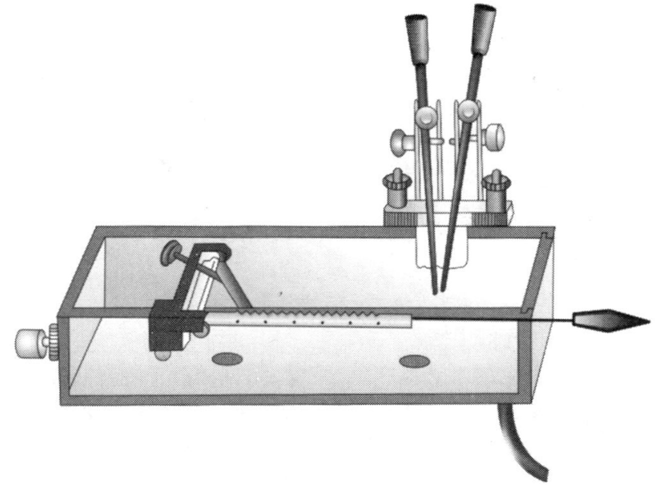

Fig. 62.5: Luca's moist chamber

- The writing lever is fixed to the other side of the chamber, it is so adjusted that it remains tangential to the surface of the cylinder on which the record is obtained.
- At one end of the lever, there is an afterload screw to prop up the lever. When in use, it does not allow the load to stretch the muscle at rest.
- When the screw is removed, load acts on the muscle at rest and hence, it becomes freeloaded state of muscle.
- At the base of the chamber, a drainage pipe is provided, that helps to drain Ringer solution from the chamber when required.
- Chamber is completely filled with 0.65% NaCl (it is normal saline for frogs) so that muscle can be completely immersed in the solution.

Vibrating Reed

- It is a long and thin metal strip fixed at one end.
- To the other end, there is a pin, which acts as a contact point.
- When the pin makes contact with mercury present in the cup, the circuit is completed.
- Vibrating reed is used for the experiment of the genesis of tetanus.
- We can give the desired number of stimuli per second with the help of a vibrating reed (5 to 30 stimuli/ second).

Writing Lever (Simple Lever)

- This is used to magnify and record muscle contraction on the drum.
- The writing point of the lever is made up of a triangular piece of photographic film.
- There are notches or holes for hanging the weights.

Starling's Heart Lever

- It consists of two bars that are placed at right angles to each other.
- The horizontal bar has got a socket for bearing the liver and a vertical bar for holding the spring.
- One end of the spring is attached to the writing lever. There is an arrangement to vary the tension of the spring on the lever.
- It is used to measure the contraction of a frog's heart.

Isometric Lever

It has a holder which carries a spring and flat writing lever. It is used to record isometric muscle contractions.

Myograph Stand

- This is a vertical rod fixed to a heavy and triangular base.
- Luca's moist chamber can be fitted to this rod **(Fig. 62.6)**.

Tuning Fork

- A tuning fork with a frequency of 100 vibrations per second (100 Hz) is used for measuring different time intervals.
- The tuning fork is set to vibrate and then made to write on a rotating drum.
- Each wave of tracing measures 0.01 seconds **(Fig. 62.7)**.

Electromagnetic Time Marker

- It consists of two coils around two soft iron bars, as electric current is made to flow they get magnetized.

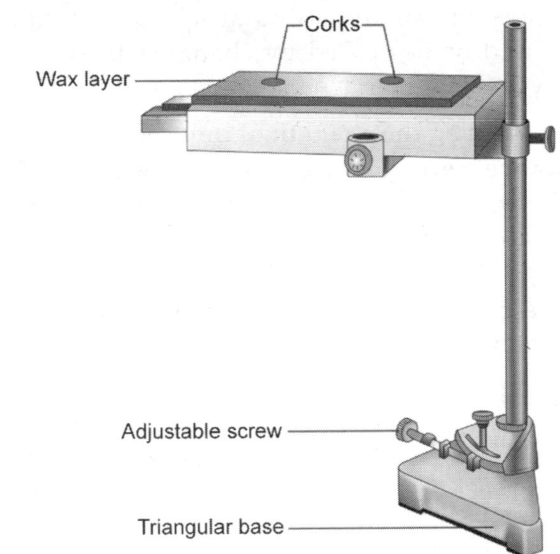

Fig. 62.6: Myograph stand

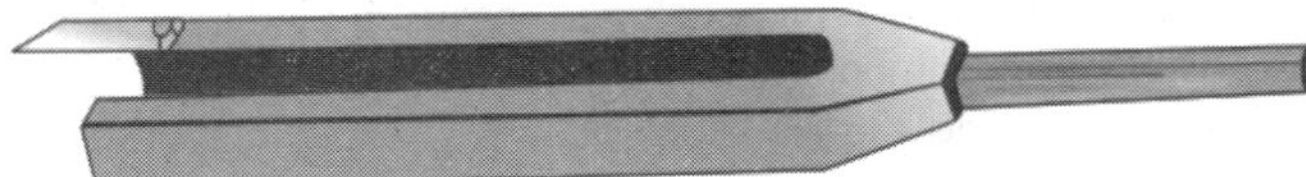

Fig. 62.7: Tuning fork

- A soft iron plate placed over them is attracted towards them.
- The writing lever is attached to the iron plate and records the movement of the iron plate on the recording drum.
- Electromagnetic marker is used to mark the point of stimulus in the primary circuit.

Primary and Secondary Circuits

Primary Circuit

- Battery, key and induction coil are arranged in the circuit to form the primary circuit.
- This is a continuous current circuit.
- A constant strength low voltage current flows through this circuit **(Fig. 62.8)**.

Secondary Circuit

- A constant strength of high voltage current flows through this circuit.
- Secondary induction coil and electrodes are connected through the short-circuiting key to form a secondary circuit **(Fig. 62.9)**.

▌COMMON STATIONS– SPOTS IN PRACTICAL EXAMINATION (2/3 MARKS)

Q.1. Any of the instruments can be kept – Identify the instrument and write its use. Additionally, answer one or two questions about the instrument from the options provided above.

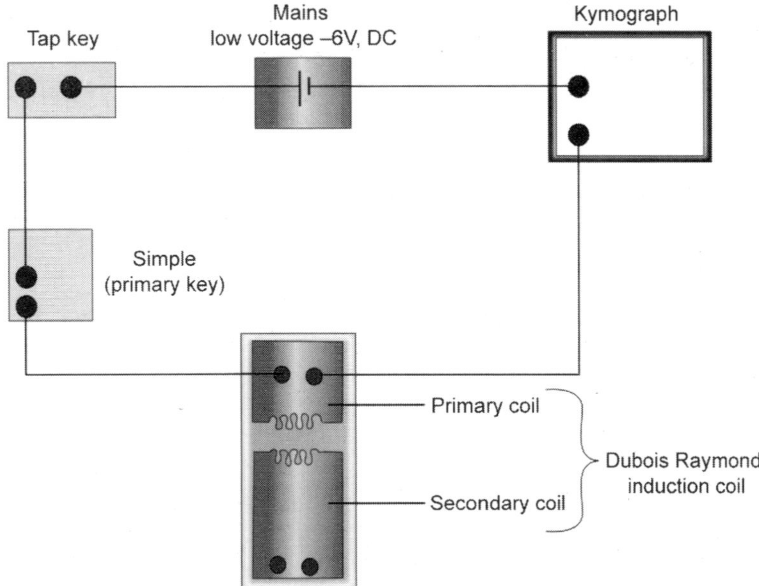

Fig. 62.8: Primary circuit

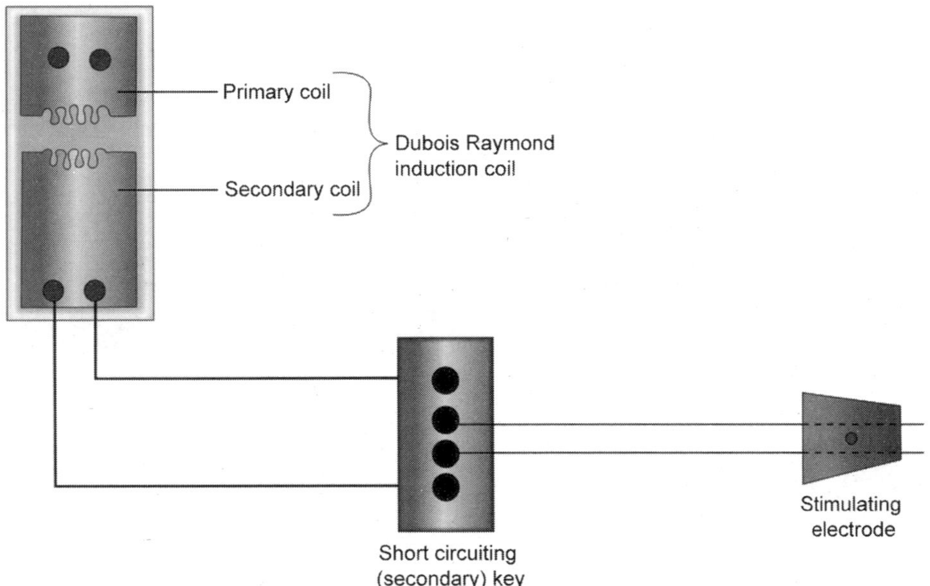

Fig. 62.9: Secondary circuit

Q.2. Draw a diagram of the primary and secondary circuits.

Q.3. Define stimulus and write preferring electrical stimulus over others (check above).

Q.4. The break circuit is stronger than the make. Justify.

■ KEY POINTS TO REMEMBER

- Electrical stimulus is preferred over all other types of stimulus and faradic current is used than galvanic.

- The strength of the stimulus can be increased by decreasing the distance between the primary and secondary coil.

- Luca's moist chamber is used to mount the sciatic nerve and gastrocnemius muscle of the frog (nerve-muscle preparation).

- Vibrating reed is used when one demonstrates the genesis of tetanus in skeletal muscle.

- Starling's heart lever is used to record contraction from a frog's heart.

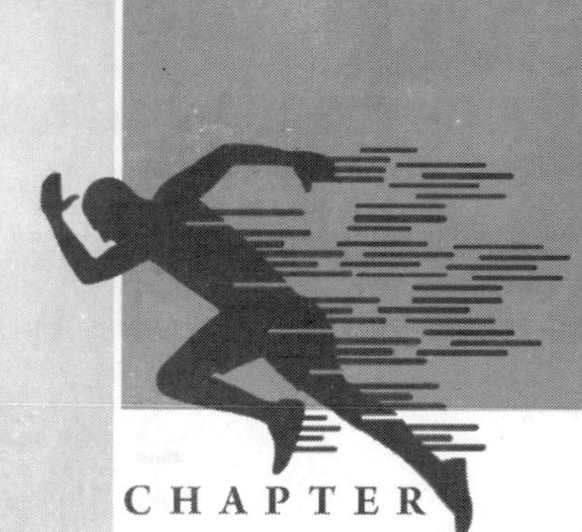

Nerve Muscle Preparation in Frog

Competency:
PY 3.18: Observe with computer-assisted learning, amphibian nerve muscle experiments.

Learning Objectives

After completion of this practical, the students shall be able to:
- Give the composition of Ringer's solution
- Give reasons as to why the sciatic nerve and gastro-cnemius muscle are selected for nerve-muscle experiments
- Explain what is pithing

■ INTRODUCTION

- In the amphibian experiment, the frog's sciatic nerve and gastrocnemius muscle are used.
- As the sciatic nerve is long, it can be mounted easily. Electrode placement also becomes easy on the sciatic nerve.
- Gastrocnemius muscle being bulky gives good amplitude of contraction **(Fig. 63.1)**.
- For nerve-muscle preparation, the frog is pithed by destroying the brain and spinal cord.

■ PRINCIPLE

The pithed frog is dissected and intact nerve–muscle preparation is mounted on Luca's moist chamber.

■ APPARATUS

Frog, pithing needle. Ringer solution, forceps, glass rod, scissors.

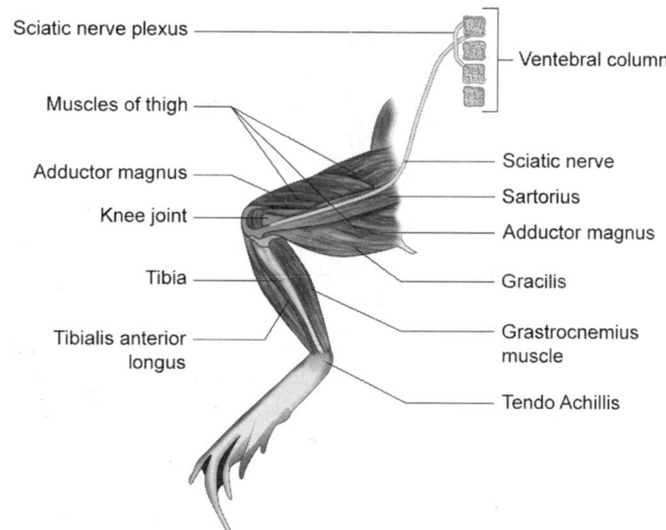

Fig. 63.1: Origin and course of sciatic nerve through the muscles of the thigh in a frog

■ PROCEDURE

Pithing of a Frog

- Animal must be held with dry cotton.
- Blow is given on the head (the animal becomes unconscious) this is stunning.
- Frog's head is ventroflexed. Depression at the junction of the skull and vertebral column is felt.
- Pithing needle is inserted firmly through skin, muscle, and bone tissue into the spinal cord.
- The needle is manipulated anteriorly to destroy the brain.

- The needle is withdrawn and is directed to the spinal cord and rotated to destroy the spinal cord.
- After pithing, the animal loses its voluntary and reflex movements. However, heart muscles are alive and used in experiments to study the properties of muscles.

Dissection

- The skin of the frog is cut along the midline of the trunk.
- Skin from the trunk and hind limb is striped off.
- The frog is placed on its abdomen.
- Pelvic girdle is cut and sciatic plexus is identified.
- About a 2 cm long piece of the vertebral column is isolated by cutting the vertebral column above and below the exit of the sciatic nerve.
- With the help of bone-cutting scissors, the vertebral column is bisected vertically in two halves.
- The sciatic nerve in the thigh is exposed lying between the muscle masses.
- Nerve is cleaned and handled only with a glass rod.
- Identify and cut the gastrocnemius tendon from its attachment. Free muscle from tibia and cut it close to the knee joint.
- Nerve muscle preparation is kept in Ringer's solution to avoid drying.
- Preparation is mounted on Luca's moist chamber.
- Different properties of skeletal muscle are studied using this nerve-muscle preparation.

■ COMPOSITION OF RINGER SOLUTION

- Sodium chloride (NaCl)– 0.6% (isotonic to frog)
- Potassium chloride (KCl)– 0.014 % (maintains membrane potential)
- Calcium chloride ($CaCl_2$)– 0.012% (maintains muscle excitability)
- Sodium bicarbonate ($NaHCO_3$), disodium phosphate ($Na_2H_2PO_4$)– maintains pH
- Dextrose– 0.1% (nutrition).

■ PRECAUTIONS

- Nerve muscle preparation should be handled with care to cause minimum/no injury to it.
- Nerve is not to be stretched or handled with metal objects.
- Care is taken not to allow NM preparation to dry (use an adequate amount of Ringer solution).

■ IMPORTANT QUESTIONS AND ANSWERS

Q.1. What is the pithing of a frog?
Pithing is destroying the spinal cord and brain of frogs.

Q.2. What is the composition of the Ringer solution?
The composition of the Ringer solution is explained above.

Q.3. Why frog is not anaesthesized?
If we anaesthesize the frog, then due anaesthetic drug, the excitability of nerves and muscles will be suppressed and thus we will not be able to study the properties of the same.

Q.4. Why is a frog used as an experimental animal?
Frog is used in experimental physiology because:
- It is cheap and easily available.
- As a frog is a cold-blooded animal, it can withstand changes in temperature, pH and O_2 content of the blood.

Q.5. Why gastrocnemius muscle and sciatic nerve preparation is used for experimental purposes?
- The gastrocnemius muscle and the sciatic nerve are ideal nerve-muscle preparations as the gastrocnemius muscle is bulky, it gives good amplitude of contraction on stimulation. Thus, it becomes easy to study the properties of skeletal muscle.
- The sciatic nerve is along the nerve that makes its mounting easy.

■ COMMON STATIONS – SPOTS IN PRACTICAL EXAMINATION (2/3 MARKS)

Q.1. Ringer solution bottle: Identify, enumerate its contents and write the use of each content.

Q.2. The frog to be studied for nerve-muscle properties is not anaesthetized. Justify.

■ KEY POINTS TO REMEMBER

- Frog's sciatic nerve and gastrocnemius muscle are used, as the sciatic nerve is long and can be mounted easily.
- Luca's moist chamber is used for it and one hole is used to fix one end of muscle.
- Chamber is filled with 0.65% saline and muscle is completely immersed in saline.
- Different properties of skeletal muscle are studied.

Effect of Gradation of Stimuli

Competency:
PY 3.18: Observe with computer-assisted learning, amphibian nerve muscle experiments.

Learning Objectives

After this practical, the students shall be able to:
- Identify the graph of the effect of increasing strength of stimuli on skeletal muscle contraction
- Define a motor unit
- Define subminimal, minimal, maximal, submaximal, and supramaximal stimuli
- Define all-or-none law
- Explain why the response with supramaximal stimulus is the same as that for maximal stimulus

■ INTRODUCTION

- The magnitude of contraction increases with an increase in the strength of stimuli.
- As muscle is stimulated with increasing strength, more motor units get recruited (quantal summation).
- A motor unit is defined as a single alpha motor neuron along with its axon and the number of muscle fibres it innervates.

■ PRINCIPLE

- Amplitude of muscle contraction increases with an increase in the strength of stimuli.
- Increasing strengths of single make and break stimuli are applied to muscle by stimulating the nerve (from subminimal to suprathreshold strength).

Apparatus

Kymograph, muscle trough, lever, and nerve-muscle preparation.

Procedure

- Simple make and break circuit is used.
- Nerve–muscle preparation is mounted in Luca's moist chamber.
- Nerve–muscle preparation is stimulated with different intensities of stimuli.
- First secondary coil is kept far away from the primary (to give minimal strength of stimulus).
- Distance between primary and secondary coil is noted.
- Stimulation is given at make-and-break shock separately. After every stimulus, the drum is moved by hand with 2 cm.
- The strength of the stimulus is increased by decreasing the distance between the secondary and primary coil by 2 cm at each step pressing the tap key and releasing it (every time, the distance between the primary and secondary coil is noted).
- Procedure is repeated till a further increase in strength of the stimulus does not alter the height of contraction. Label response as M for make stimulus and B for break stimulus **(Fig. 64.1)**.

Observations/Results

- There is no contraction at subminimal stimuli.
- First contraction recorded at break stimulus at minimal strength.

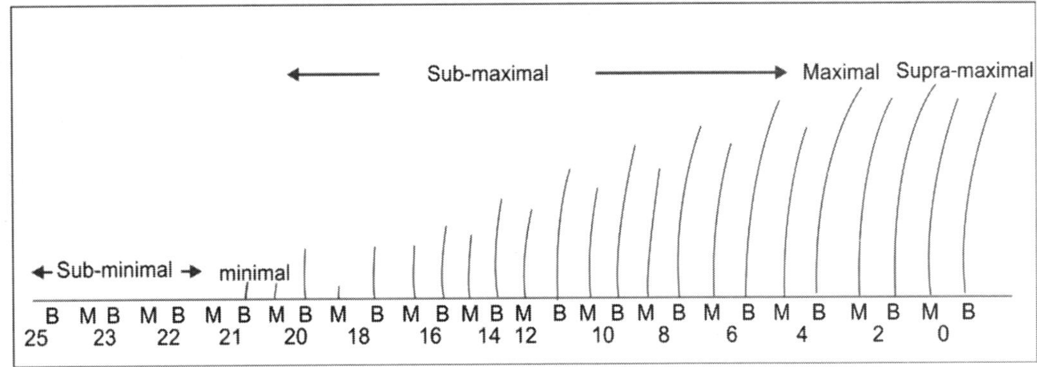

Fig. 64.1: Gradation of stimuli (M: Make shock; B: Break shock)

- With further increase in strength of stimuli, contractions are recorded at make as well as at break.
- Heights of contractions are more during break than make.
- At maximal stimulus, the height of contraction is maximum.
- Beyond that with supramaximal stimulation, the height of contraction remains the same.

Precautions

- Contraction of both make and break is to be recorded.
- Drum is not taken in the primary circuit.
- Minimum of 15 seconds of gap between make and break stimuli in order to avoid beneficial effect on muscle contraction.

■ IMPORTANT QUESTIONS AND ANSWERS

Q.1. Define subminimal stimulus.

It is defined as a stimulus, which fails to elicit a visible response from excitable tissue.

Q.2. Define minimal stimulus.

- It is defined as the weakest strength of stimulus that elicits a visible response from excitable tissue.
- Break is stronger than the make, so the first response is obtained at the break.

Q.3. Define submaximal stimuli.

It is a range of stimuli that are between minimal and maximal. During this, the effect of break is more than the make stimulus.

Q.4. Define maximal stimulus.

- It is defined as the strength of stimulus producing maximum response from excitable tissue. Further, an increase in the strength of stimulus does not increase the response.
- The strength of stimulus above the maximal is known as supramaximal.
- The height of contraction with supramaximal stimulus is the same as that for maximal stimulus.

Q.5. Why response obtained increase during the submaximal range?

With increasing strength of stimulus during the submaximal range of stimuli, more and more motor units get recruited (quantal summation). Therefore, the response obtained also goes on increasing, with the response at break more than that at make.

Q.6. What is the response with maximal strength of stimulus?

- With maximal stimulus, all motor units in the muscle are recruited.
- Thus maximum response is obtained with maximal strength of stimulus.

Q.7. What is the effect of supramaximal stimulus?

At the maximum strength of the stimulus, all motor units in the muscle contract to its maximum. Therefore, even if the strength of stimulus increases further, there is no further increase in response.

Q.8. What is an all-or-none law?

All-or-none law: It states that under the same physiological conditions, the excitable tissue when stimulated with threshold stimulus responds to its maximum or does not respond at all. In skeletal muscle, each motor unit obeys the all-or-none law.

Q.9. What is quantal summation?

- With increasing stimulus strength, a greater response is obtained due to the increased number of motor units participating in the contraction process.
- This greater recruitment of motor units with an increase in stimulus intensity is known as quantal summation.

Q.10. Define motor unit.

- **Motor unit:** It is defined as an alpha motor neuron along with its axon and the number of muscle fibres it innervates. The motor unit is a functional unit of skeletal muscle.
- In the case of skeletal muscle each individual motor unit obeys all or none law.
- In the case of cardiac muscle whole of myocardium obeys all or none law.

■ COMMON STATIONS – SPOTS IN PRACTICAL EXAMINATION (2/3 MARKS)

Q.1. Graph of gradation of stimuli: Identify and answer any one or two questions from the above.

Q.2. What do you mean by M and B in the graph/what do those numbers down in the graph indicate? (clue- M- make, B- break, numbers- indicate the distance between the primary and secondary coil, as distance reduces, the strength of stimulus increases).

■ KEY POINTS TO REMEMBER

- Motor unit is defined as an alpha motor neuron, along with its axon and the number of muscle fibres it innervates.
- **All-or-none law:** Within physiological limits, any excitable tissue when stimulated with an adequate stimulus will either respond to its maximum or will not respond at all.
- Each motor unit obeys the all-or-none law.
- As the gradation of stimulus strength increases, more and more motor units are recruited (quantal summation).

Simple Muscle Curve

Competency:
PY 3.18: Observe with computer-assisted learning, amphibian nerve muscle experiments.

Learning Objectives

At the end of this practical, students shall be able to:
- Identify a graph of a simple muscle curve
- Define and identify the latent period, contraction period, and relaxation period
- List causes of the latent period
- Calculate contraction period, latent period and relaxation period

■ INTRODUCTION

- When a muscle is stimulated with a single adequate stimulus, it exhibits twitch-like contraction.
- Thus, it is defined as the response of a muscle to a single adequate stimulus.
- Contraction recorded on a moving kymograph is called a simple muscle curve **(Fig. 65.1)**.
- By recording simple muscle curve excitability, and contractility of the muscle is studied.

■ PRINCIPLE

- When a muscle is stimulated with a single adequate stimulus, it contracts.
- This lifts the lever to record a curve on the revolving smoked drum.

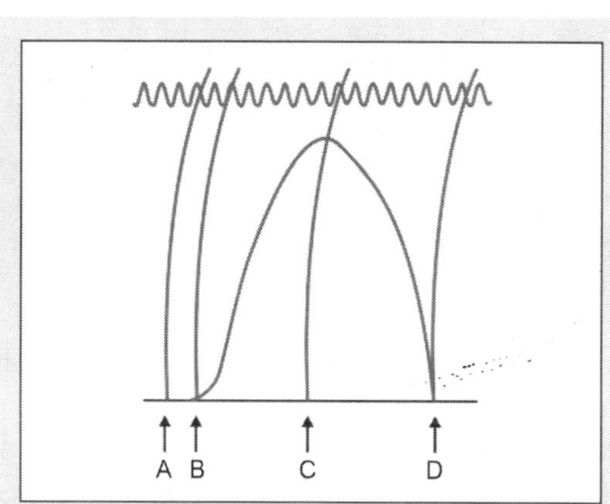

Fig. 65.1: Simple muscle curve or twitch (A. Point of stimulus, B. Start of contraction, AB. Latent period, C. Point of maximum contraction, D. End of relaxation, BC. Contraction period, CD. Relaxation period)

Apparatus

Dissection instruments, Ringer solution, Luca's moist chamber, tuning fork (100 Hz), induction coil, smoked drum.

■ PROCEDURE

- Arrange primary and secondary circuits.
- Take drum in circuit.
- Fix nerve-muscle preparation in Luca's moist chamber.
- Adjust the secondary coil to obtain contraction at break only.

- Rotate the drum at a fast speed and record the baseline.
- Close the key to complete the circuit and obtain a simple muscle curve.
- Stop the drum and open the key and mark the point of stimulus.
- Time tracing is recorded with the help of a tuning fork.
- Mark the beginning of contraction, peak of contraction, and end of relaxation.
- Find out the latent period, contraction period, and relaxation period.

Observations/Results

Rewrite the following data in proper format

- **Latent period** (AB): 0.01s
- **Contraction period** (time interval between initiation of contraction and maximum contraction; BC): 0.04s
- **Relaxation period** (time interval between the point of maximum contraction and point of complete relaxation; CD): 0.05s.

Precautions

- Mark accurately the point of stimulus
- Take time tracing below the recording of SMC.

■ IMPORTANT QUESTIONS AND ANSWERS

Q.1. What is the latent period?

The latent period is the time interval between the application of stimulus and the start of response.

Q.2. What are the causes of the latent period? What are the factors affecting the latent period?

Causes of latent period:

- Time taken for the impulse to travel along the nerve to the neuromuscular junction.
- Time taken for impulse to travel through the neuromuscular junction.
- Time required for spread of impulse and various changes to occur in muscle for initiation of contraction.
- Time taken by lever to overcome inertia at rest.
- Time taken to overcome viscous resistance of muscle.
- **Latent period increases with**—cold saline, attaching more loads, and repetitive stimulation.
- **Latent period decreases with**—direct stimulation of muscle, short length of nerve, and warm saline.

Q.3. What is an isotonic and isometric contraction?

- **Isotonic contraction**: Tension of muscle remains the same, and the muscle shortens.
- **Isometric contraction**: Tension of muscle changes without change in muscle length.

Q.4. What is excitation-contraction coupling?

The mechanism by which the action potential of nerve fibres leads to the contraction of muscle fibres is called as excitation-contraction coupling. It occurs as follows:

- When the excitatory impulse reaches the sarcoplasmic triad via T tubules, it causes the release of calcium into the sarcoplasm. This calcium binds with troponin that moves the tropomyosin molecule away from the active sites of actin filaments (normally tropomyosin covers the active site of actin filament).
- Cross bridges of myosin molecule get attached to these sites, initiating muscle contraction.

Q.5. Enlist the factors responsible for the relaxation of muscles.

Factors responsible for relaxation are:

- Load acting on the muscle.
- Removal of calcium ions from sarcoplasm to sarcoplasmic reticulum (active process, requires energy).
- Once the concentration of calcium in the sarcoplasmic reticulum lowers, calcium is removed from troponin and there is no more interaction between actin and myosin and muscle relaxes.

Q.6. Define the load and tension of the muscle.

- **Load**: It is the force exerted by the weight of the object on a contracting muscle.
- **Tension**: It is the force exerted by contracting muscle on the object.
- Load and tension are opposite to each other.
- In order to lift the load, tension developed in the muscle should be more than the load or else the load will not be lifted by the muscle.

Q.7. Why is the drum taken in the circuit?

A drum is taken in the circuit to mark the point of stimulus.

Q.8. What is freeloaded and after-loaded muscle?

- When load acts on the muscle only during contraction and not at rest is called as after loaded condition.
- When load acts on the muscle during contraction as well as when the muscle is at rest in freeloaded condition.

Q.9. How can one identify that the SMC obtained is in the freeloaded state or after-loaded state?

- After recording a simple muscle curve, small curves are recorded. These curves are not a part of muscle contraction, but they are recorded as a result of the elasticity of the muscle and the inertia of the instrument (momentum of the lever). These are termed shatter curves/physiological curves.
- When the SMC is recorded in a freeloaded state, shatter curves below the baseline are recorded.

- If SMC is recorded in after loaded state, shatter curves are not recorded below the baseline.

Q.10. Enumerate the factors affecting the height of contraction of a simple muscle curve.

Factors affecting the height of contraction of SMC are:

- **Strength of stimulus:** The greater the strength of the stimulus, the higher the contraction height, as more motor units contract with increasing stimulus strength.
- **Temperature:** Warmer saline results in a greater height of contraction.
- **Type of load:** Up to an optimum load, if the muscle is freeloaded, the height of contraction will be greater compared to when the muscle is in an after-loaded state.
- **Instrumental inertia:** The greater the inertia, the lesser the height of contraction.
- **Type of muscle fibres:** Whether the fibres are fast-twitch or slow-twitch affects contraction.

COMMON STATIONS – SPOTS IN PRACTICAL EXAMINATION (2/3 MARKS)

Q.1. Graph of SMC: Identify and label various periods. Write the cause and duration of any period and answer any one or two questions from the above.

Q.2. Graph of SMC: Identify, whether it is in the freeload state or after loaded state (clue- Q no. 9).

Q.3. If time tracking is not recorded can we get the duration of different phases of SMC? (clue- yes if we know the speed of the drum).

KEY POINTS TO REMEMBER

- Simple muscle twitch is the response of skeletal muscle to a single adequate stimulus.
- Relaxation is longer (passive + active process) than contraction (active process).
- **Contraction period:** Time interval between initiation of contraction and point of maximum contraction.
- **Relaxation period:** Time interval between the point of maximum contraction and the point of complete relaxation.

Effect of Two Successive Stimuli on Skeletal Muscle of Frog

Competency:

PY 3.18: Observe with computer-assisted learning, amphibian nerve muscle experiments.

Learning Objectives

After this practical, students shall be able to:

- Identify a graph of the effect of two successive stimuli on the skeletal muscle of a frog
- Define the absolute and relative refractory period
- Explain the effect of the second stimulus falling in the first half of the latent period
- Explain the effect of the second stimulus falling in the second half of the latent period
- Explain the effect of the second stimulus falling in the contraction period
- Explain the effect of the second stimulus falling in the relaxation period
- Give physiological basis of beneficial effect

■ INTRODUCTION

- When two successive stimuli are paired, the response of the muscle to a paired stimulus depends upon the timing of the second stimulus.
- Second stimulus is applied in different phases and the effect is seen.

Principle

When two successive stimuli are paired and applied to the muscle, the magnitude of contraction depends on the timing of the second stimulus.

Apparatus

Kymograph, muscle trough, Ringer solution, dissection instruments, induction coil, tuning fork, tap and short-circuiting key.

■ PROCEDURE

- Take the drum in the primary circuit.
- Set up nerve-muscle preparation for recording simple muscle curves. Record simple muscle curves.
- Arrange an induction coil to get the maximal stimulus.
- Separate two arms attached to the spindle of the drum to make two points of stimulation.
- Every time the distance between two arms is adjusted, so that the second stimulus will fall in:
  - First half of latent period
  - Second half of latent period
  - During contraction
  - During relaxation
  - After relaxation
- Both points of stimuli are recorded every time. Each time, the cylinder is rotated to obtain separate graphs.

All stimuli given in the experiment are maximal/supramaximal so that all motor units in the muscle are recruited.

Precautions

- Decrease the distance gradually between contact arms so that the second stimulus can be applied to different phases of contraction due to the first stimulus.

- The point of stimulus for both contractions should be marked.
- Maximal strength of stimulus is to be given every time (as it recruits all motor units in the muscle).

■ OBSERVATION/RESULTS

When the second stimulus falls in:

1. **First half of the latent period (Fig. 66.1):**
   - There is no effect of the second stimulus on muscle contraction if the impulse falls in the first half of the latent period.
   - As this second stimulus falls in the absolute refractory period of the muscle, the second stimulus does not show any response.
2. **Second half of latent period (Fig. 66.2):**
   - If the second stimulus falls in the second half of the latent period, the magnitude of contraction increases. As this second stimulus falls in the relative refractory period of the muscle.
   - Second stimulus causes summation of stimuli and thus simple muscle curve obtained is of higher magnitude.

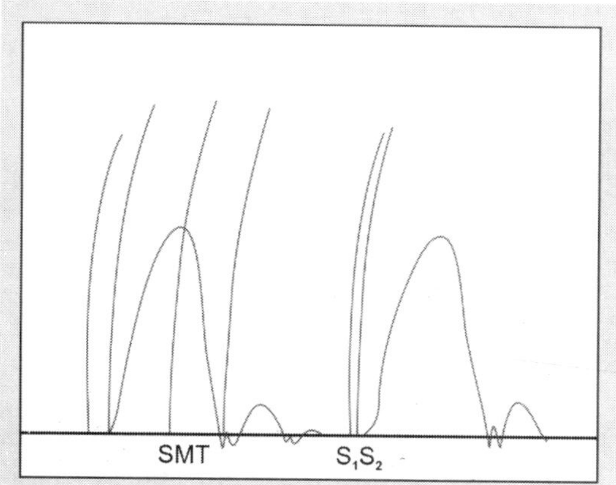

Fig. 66.1: S₁ is the first stimulus and S₂ is the stimulus in the first half of the latent period

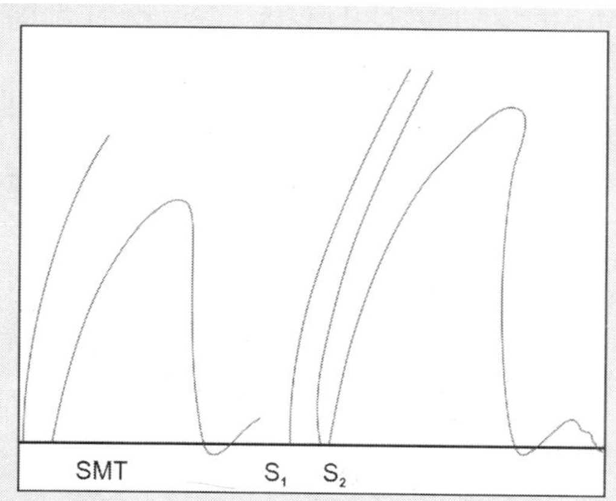

Fig. 66.2: Second stimulus falls in the second half of the latent period

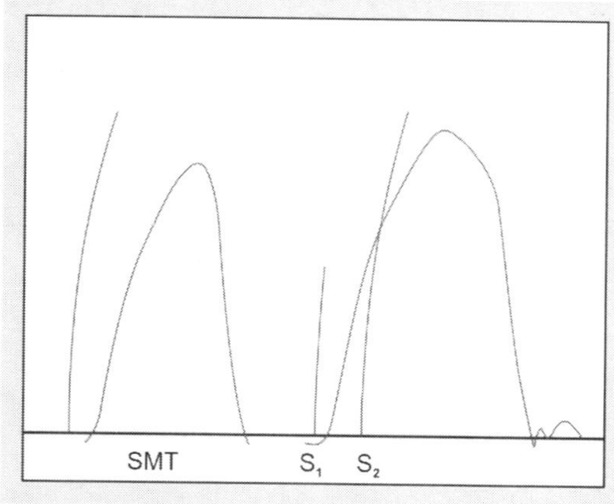

Fig. 66.3: Second stimulus falls in contraction period (SMT: simple muscle twitch)

3. **Contraction period (Fig. 66.3):**
   - When a second stimulus is applied during the contraction phase, the magnitude of contraction increases. This is due to wave summation.
   - When a second stimulus is applied during contraction, muscle contracts vigorously with high speed.
4. **Relaxation period (Fig. 66.4):**
   - When the second stimulus is applied during the relaxation period, the second contraction starts before the completion of relaxation. This is called as imposition of waves.
   - The height of the second contraction is higher than the first due to the beneficial effect.

Reasons for beneficial effect:
   - Release of more calcium from sarcoplasmic reticulum.
   - Increase in temperature of muscle.
   - Decrease in viscosity and resistance of the muscle.
   - Decrease in the inertia of the recording system.
5. **After relaxation period (Fig. 66.5):**
   - When a second stimulus is applied after the relaxation period, two separate simple muscle curves are obtained.

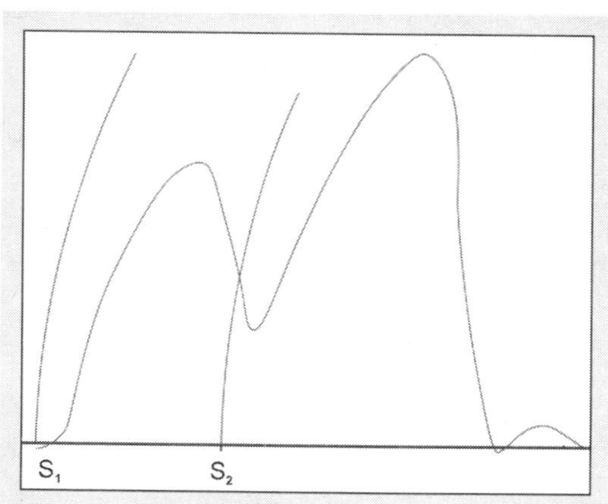

Fig. 66.4: Second stimulus falls in the relaxation period

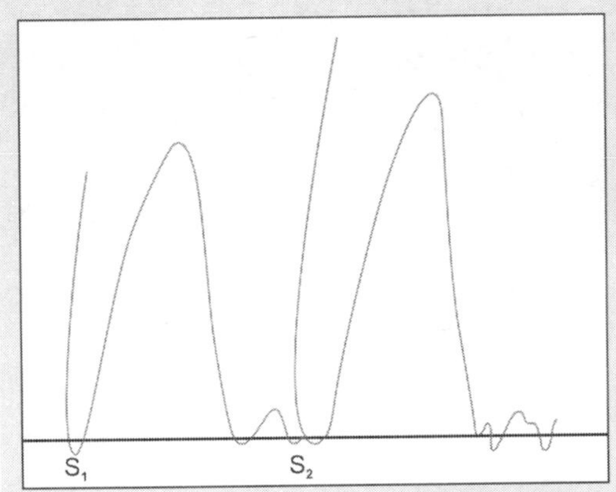

Fig. 66.5: Second stimulus is applied after the relaxation period

- The second curve is of higher magnitude as compared to the first curve.
- The increase in height of the second curve is due to a beneficial effect.

■ IMPORTANT QUESTIONS AND ANSWERS

Q.1. What is the absolute refractory period?
- Absolute refractory period is defined as a short period following the stimulus during which there is a complete loss of excitability of excitable tissue.
- In a simple muscle curve, the first half of the latent period acts as the absolute refractory period.

Q.2. What is the relative refractory period?
- Relative refractory period is defined as small period following absolute refractory period during which the excitability of tissue is lesser than normal.
- In a simple muscle curve, the second half of the latent period acts as a relative refractory period.

Q.3. What is the beneficial effect?
When the muscle is stimulated with two successive stimuli, the magnitude of contraction of the second stimulus is greater. The first stimulus becomes beneficial for the second one. This is called a beneficial effect. This is due to changes in viscosity, change in temperature and pH due to previous contraction.

Q.4. What is summation?
- When two stimuli do reach a neuron from two different afferent neurons, the effect is added up which is called as summation. It is the summation of response.
- **Spatial summation:** An increase in response when two or more nerve fibres are stimulated is termed as spatial summation.
- **Temporal summation:** An increase in response when a single nerve fibre is stimulated repeatedly is termed as temporal summation.

Q.5. Describe the graph obtained when the second stimulus is applied during the first half of the latent period.
Explained above.

Q.6. Describe the graph obtained when the second stimulus is applied in the later half of the latent period
Explained above.

Q.7. Describe the graph obtained when the second stimulus is applied during the contraction phase
Explained above.

Q.8. Describe the graph obtained when a second stimulus is applied during the relaxation phase.
Explained above.

Q.9. Describe the graph when the second stimulus is applied after the relaxation period.
Explained above.

■ COMMON STATIONS – SPOTS IN PRACTICAL EXAMINATION (2/3 MARKS)

Q.1. Graph with the second stimulus in different phases: Identify and answer any one or two questions as explained above.

Q.2. State the physiological significance of the beneficial effect.

Q.3. Summation effect: Identify and write it as the summation of stimuli or responses (clue- it is the summation of response).

■ KEY POINTS TO REMEMBER

- When the second stimulus is applied during the first half of the latent period, it is ineffective as it falls in an absolute refractory phase of the first stimulus.
- When the second stimulus (stronger one) is applied during the second half of the latent period, i.e. in the relative refractory phase due to the first stimulus, a greater magnitude of response is obtained (summation of stimuli).
- When the second stimulus is applied during the contraction phase, increased contraction is seen due to wave summation.
- When the second stimulus is applied during the relaxation phase, a better response is obtained due to the beneficial effect.

Genesis of Tetanus

Competency:
PY 3.18: Observe with computer-assisted learning, amphibian nerve muscle experiments.

Learning Objectives

After completion of this practical, the student shall be able to:
- Identify the graph of the genesis of tetanus
- Define staircase, trappe, clonus, and tetanus
- Define critical fusion frequency
- Explain the mechanism of tetanus

■ INTRODUCTION

- Tetanus refers to a sustained state of contraction of the muscle due to rapid and repeated stimulation.
- When the muscle is stimulated below the tetanizing frequency, incomplete tetanus (clonus) is obtained.

Principle

- If muscle is stimulated at higher frequencies tetanus develops in the muscle.
- Nerve–muscle preparation is stimulated at different frequencies till tetanus is obtained.

Apparatus

All apparatus same as that required for simple muscle curves, vibrating reed (which is calibrated to vibrate at a particular frequency).

Procedure

- For giving multiple stimuli, a vibrating reed is taken in the circuit.
- Nerve–muscle preparation is mounted as for a simple muscle curve.
- With the help of a vibrating reed, 5 stimuli/second are given.
- With an increasing number of stimulations/seconds as 10, 20, 30, 40, and so on the record is obtained.
- Frequency of stimulation that produces complete tetanus is noted.

Precautions

- Muscle has to be stimulated from low to high frequencies
- If tetanus is not obtained then Kneef's hammer can be taken in circuit.

■ OBSERVATIONS/RESULTS

- With 5 stimuli/second, staircase is obtained **(Fig. 67.1)**
- With 10 stimuli/second, trappe is obtained **(Fig. 67.2)**
- With 15–20 stimuli/second, incomplete tetanus is obtained **(Fig. 67.3)**
- With more than 30 stimuli/second, tetanus is obtained **(Fig. 67.4)**.

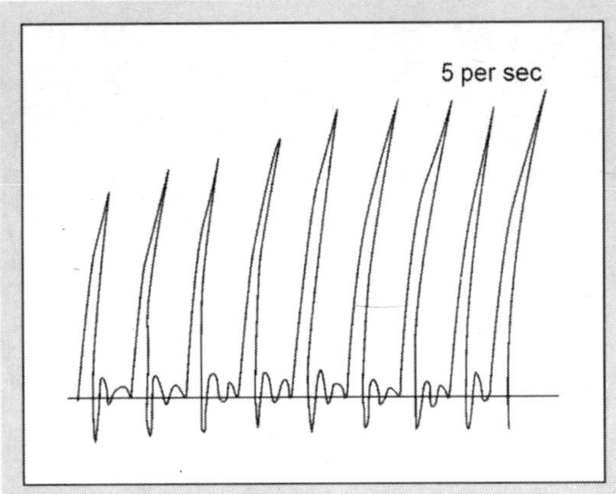

Fig. 67.1: Staircase

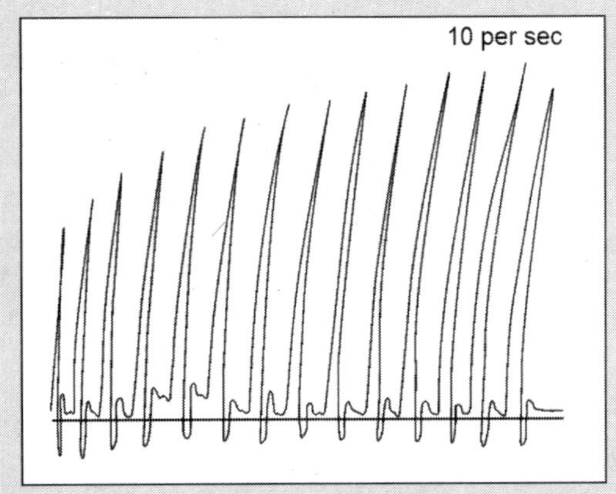

Fig. 67.2: Trappe

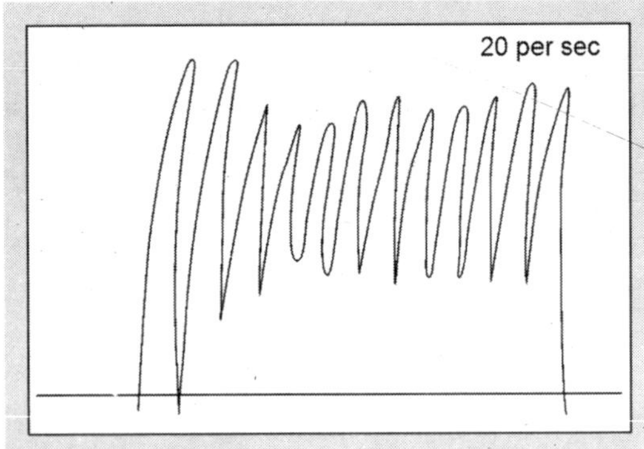

Fig. 67.3: Clonus

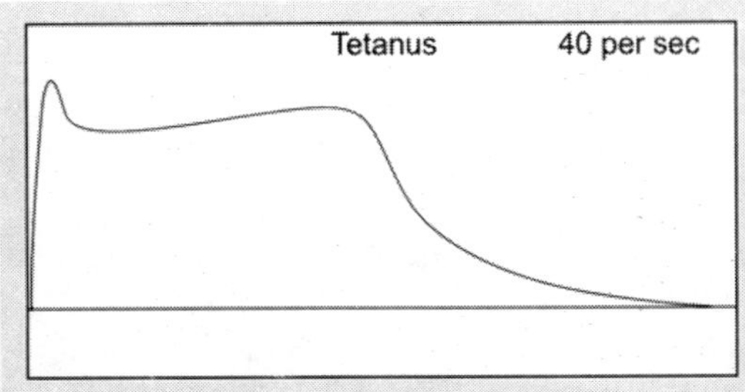

Fig. 67.4: Genesis of tetanus

■ IMPORTANT QUESTIONS AND ANSWERS

Q.1. What is a staircase? What is the effect of skeletal muscle response with 5 stimuli/sec?

When one stimulates muscle with 5 stimuli/second, the staircase is obtained. Each contraction starts after the complete relaxation of the previous one. Each successive contraction is higher than the previous due to beneficial effect.

Q.2. What is a trappe? What is the effect of skeletal muscle response with 10 stimuli/sec?

- When a muscle is stimulated with 10 stimuli/sec, trappe is obtained.
- Each successive contraction starts immediately after the lever touches the baseline during relaxation. Each successive contraction is higher than the previous due to beneficial effects.

Q.3. What is clonus? What is the effect of skeletal muscle response with 15–20 stimuli/sec?

- When the muscle is stimulated with 15–20 stimuli/sec, clonus is obtained.
- Each successive contraction starts before the previous relaxation is complete. Lever does not touch the baseline during relaxation.

Q.4. What is tetanus? What is the effect of skeletal muscle response with more than 30 stimuli/sec?

When a muscle is stimulated with more than 30 stimuli/sec, tetanus is obtained. The muscle remains in a sustained state of contraction.

Q.5. What is genesis of tetanus?

It is obtaining tetanus by gradually increasing the number of stimuli/second.

Q.6. What is mechanism of tetanus?

- When a muscle is stimulated repeatedly, successive action potential causes the release of calcium from the sarcoplasmic reticulum before all the calcium from the previous action potential is pumped back. This maintains a high concentration of calcium in the sarcoplasm.
- This prevents a decline in available binding sites for cross-bridges, which maintains the sustained state of contraction.

Q.7. What are the factors affecting tetanus?

Factors affecting tetanus are:

- Type of muscle fibre
- Load
- Strength of stimulus
- Refractory period
- Temperature
- Fatigue

Q.8. What is critical fusion frequency/minimal tetani sable frequency (MTF)?

Critical fusion frequency: It is the frequency of stimulation at which tetanus is generated. In the case of amphibian muscle, critical fusion frequency is about 30 stimuli/seconds and is almost double for mammalian muscle. Critical fusion frequency or MTF is 1/contraction period. It is written in Hz.

Q.9. Skeletal muscle can be completely tetanized. Justify.

- The refractory period of skeletal muscle is short (compared to cardiac muscle), due to this skeletal muscle does respond to second subsequent stimuli.
- As we increase the number of stimuli/sec, it can be completely tetanized (sustained state of contraction).

When a person is infected with *Clostridium tetani*, (that usually follows after a cut or injury). Tetanus toxin released by the bacteria does affect motor neurons and can lead to tetanus. Prevention is immunization with tetanus toxide injection.

◼ COMMON STATIONS – SPOTS IN PRACTICAL EXAMINATION (2/3 MARKS)

Q.1. Any of the graphs (with different frequencies of stimulations): Identify and answer one or two questions from the above.

Q.2. If the contraction period of muscle is 0.04 seconds find out its critical fusion frequency. (*See* above).

◼ KEY POINTS TO REMEMBER

- Sustained state of contraction of a muscle due to its repeated stimulation at high frequency.
- Repeated stimulation of muscle causes Ca^{++} ion concentration to build up as calcium ions are not allowed to move back to the sarcoplasmic reticulum causing a sustained state of contraction.

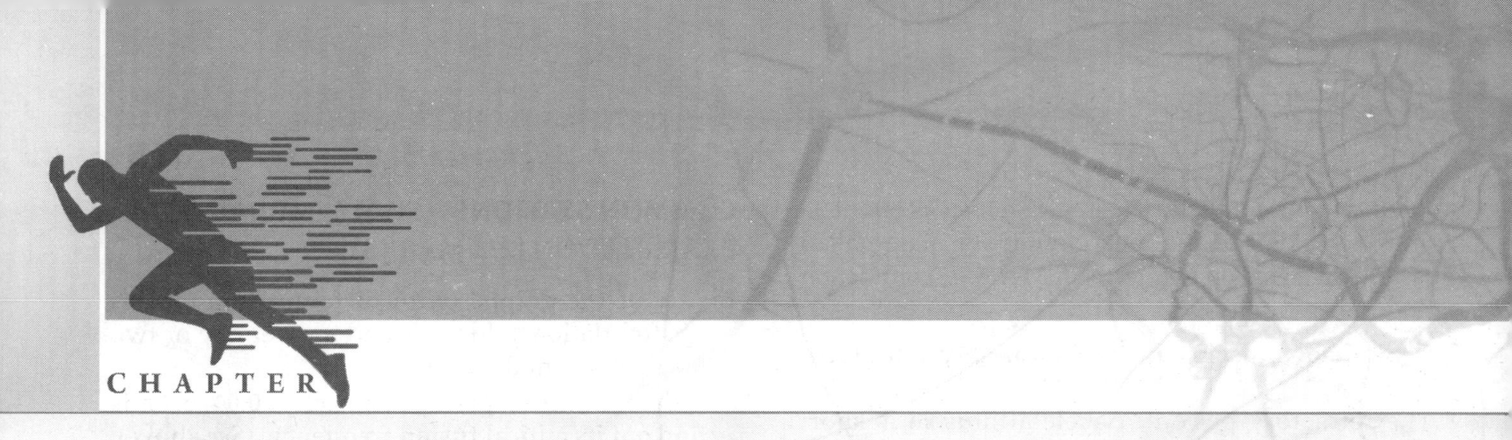

Genesis of Fatigue

Competency:

PY 3.18: Observe with computer-assisted learning, amphibian nerve muscle experiments.

Learning Objectives

After completion of this practical, the students shall be able to:

- Identify a graph of fatigue
- Define fatigue
- Give the cause and site of fatigue in nerve-muscle preparation
- List factors affecting fatigue

■ INTRODUCTION

- Failure of a muscle fibre to maintain tension as a result of previous contractile activity.
- It can occur in an intact body or nerve-muscle preparation.
- In fatigue, there is no structural or functional damage to the tissues.
- Fatigue is completely reversible.
- In human beings, fatigue resides in the central nervous system (CNS synapse); and in nerve-muscle preparation, it resides in the neuromuscular (NM) junction.

Principle

- A muscle is fatigued when it is stimulated repeatedly and continuously.
- Fatigue is recorded by stimulating with the same strength of stimulus.

Apparatus

Kymograph, muscle trough, dissection instruments, induction coil. Ringer solution, tap key.

Procedure

- Nerve–muscle preparation is fixed in Luca's moist chamber.
- Drum is taken in the circuit.
- First simple muscle curve is recorded.
- Repeatedly, muscle is stimulated and contractions are recorded on the fast-moving drum, till fatigue sets in.
- After some time, the muscle stops responding. However, if the muscle is stimulated directly, the response is obtained.
- Observe for height of contraction, and relaxation period **(Fig. 68.1)**.
- A similar graph can also be obtained on stationary drums **(Fig. 68.2)**.

Observations/Results

- There is a progressive increase in the relaxation period.
- There is a decrease in the height of contraction.
- Contracture remainder is observed (as relaxation becomes incomplete).

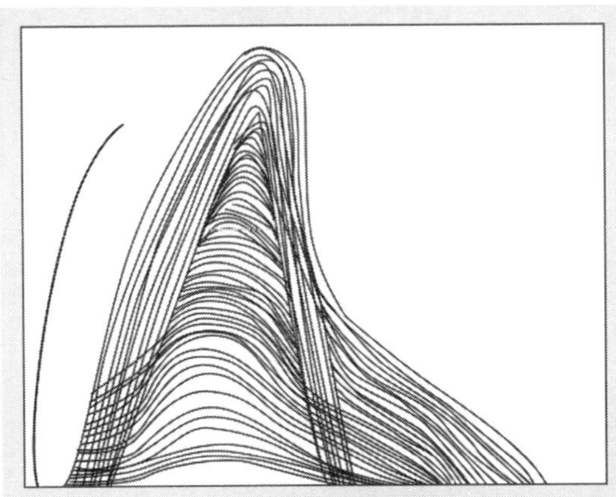

Fig. 68.1: Muscle fatigue (recorded on moving drum)

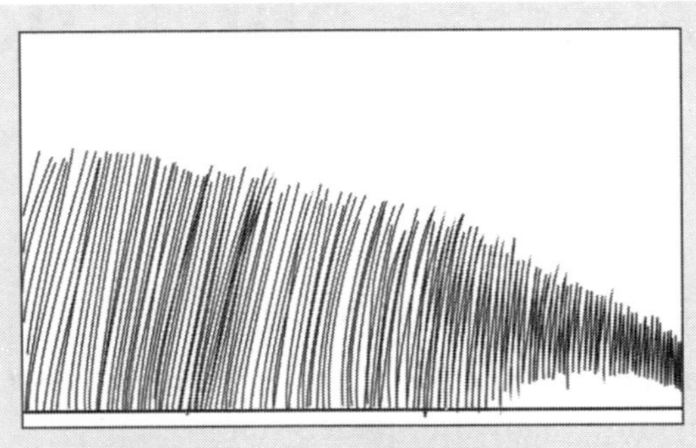

Fig. 68.2: Fatigue (recorded on stationary drum)

■ IMPORTANT QUESTIONS AND ANSWERS

Q.1. What is the seat of fatigue in isolated nerve-muscle preparation?
- The seat of fatigue is in the NM junction in a nerve-muscle preparation.
- If the nerve is stimulated directly, it responds (a nerve is not fatigable).
- Muscle, if stimulated directly, also responds. This shows that fatigue lies at the level of the neuromuscular junction.

Q.2. What is the cause of fatigue?
- Cause of fatigue is depletion (exhaustion) of acetylcholine at the NM junction.
- If rest is given for some time (resynthesis of acetylcholine occurs at the NM junction) it again starts responding.
- So, fatigue is a completely reversible phenomenon.

Q.3. How to study fatigue in human beings?
- Fatigue in human beings is studied with the help of the ergo graph (Mosso's ergograph or bicycle ergograph).
- The seat of fatigue lies at the level of synapse.

Q.4. What is contraction remainder?
- When a muscle is fatigued, it cannot completely relax and remains slightly contracted. This is known as contraction remainder.
- It occurs due to a decrease in adenosine triphosphate (ATP) content and accumulation of metabolites in the muscle. ATP is required for the pumping of calcium ions back into the sarcoplasmic reticulum.
- Lack of ATP inhibits ca^{++} pump and thus prevents entry of calcium ions in SR from sarcoplasm. Sarcoplasmic calcium level thus remains high which is responsible for maintaining muscle in a contracted state.

Q.5. What are the factors affecting fatigue?
Various factors affecting fatigue are:

	Local factors	
General factors	**In intact muscle**	**In intact body**
• Motivation and training • Efficiency of the cardiovascular system and respiratory system • Nutrition • pH–Acidosis sets early fatigue • Hormones–Thyroxine, adrenaline, steroids	• Type of muscle fibre- fast-twitch glycolytic fibres fatigue early than slow-twitch oxidative fibres • Speed of movement–Faster movement, earlier is fatigue • Collection of waste products-fatigue sets early	• Strength of stimulation • Load- greater load early fatigue • Duration and frequency of stimulation • State of muscle before fatigue

Q.6. Why is fatigue reversible?
Fatigue is a completely reversible phenomenon. There is no structural damage to skeletal muscle. Taking rest thus can completely reverse fatigue.

■ COMMON STATIONS – SPOTS IN PRACTICAL EXAMINATION (2/3 MARKS)

Q.1. Graph of fatigue (stationary/slow-moving drum): Identify and answer any one or two questions from the above.

Q.2. Graph of fatigue: Identify and label the contracture remainder and write its cause.

■ KEY POINTS TO REMEMBER

- Inability of the muscle to maintain muscle twitch tension due to repeated stimulation of muscle is fatigue.
- In the intact body, the seat of fatigue is at the level of the synapse; and in nerve-muscle preparation, it is at the level of NM junction.

Effect of Freeload and Afterload on Skeletal Muscle Contraction

Competency:

PY 3.18: Observe with computer-assisted learning, amphibian nerve muscle experiments.

Learning Objectives

After completion of this practical, the students shall be able to:

- Identify the graph of the effect of freeload and afterload on the frog's muscle
- Define freeload and afterload
- Give the effect of the afterloaded state of muscle on— the latent period, contraction period, and relaxation period
- Give the effect of the freeloaded state of muscle on— the latent period, contraction period, and relaxation period
- Define Starling's law
- Give the physiological basis for why freeloaded muscle works better
- Calculate work done by muscle in freeload and afterload states

■ INTRODUCTION

- Load is defined as the force exerted by the weight of an object on the muscle.
- Tension is the force exerted by contracting muscle on an object.
- When the load is applied on the muscle before the muscle starts contracting, it is a freeloaded state.
- When the load is applied to muscle only when it starts contracting in an afterloaded state.
- Freeloaded state muscle works better than afterloaded state.

Principle

The efficiency of muscle to do the work is different in the freeloaded state and afterloaded state.

Apparatus

Muscle trough, kymograph, dissection instruments, weights, Ringer solution, drum, Starling's lever.

Procedure

- Drum is taken in the circuit.
- Nerve–muscle preparation is mounted in Luca's moist chamber.
- Simple muscle curves are obtained with 10, 20, 30, 40, and 50 g of weight (afterloaded state) as shown in **Fig. 69.1**.
- Each time, the point of stimulus and strength of stimulus are kept the same.
- Muscle is freeloaded and simple muscle curves are recorded by adding weights as mentioned above **(Fig. 69.2)**.
- Similarly, the record is also obtained on a stationary drum in afterloaded **(Fig. 69.3)** and freeloaded state of muscle **(Fig. 69.4)**.

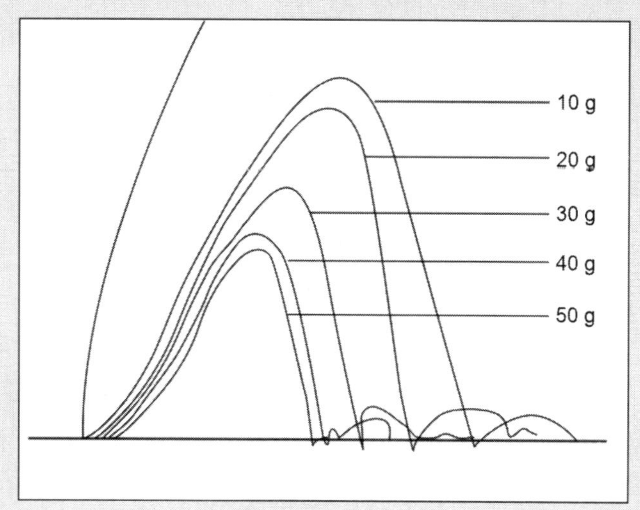

Fig. 69.1: Effect of afterloading (on moving drum)

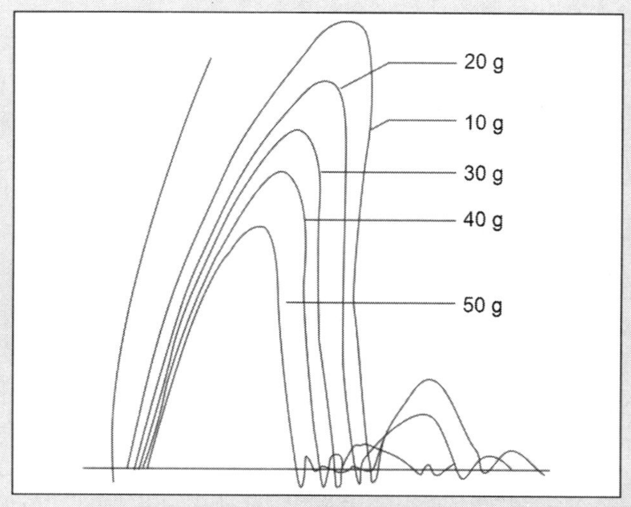

Fig. 69.2: Effect of freeloading (on moving drum)

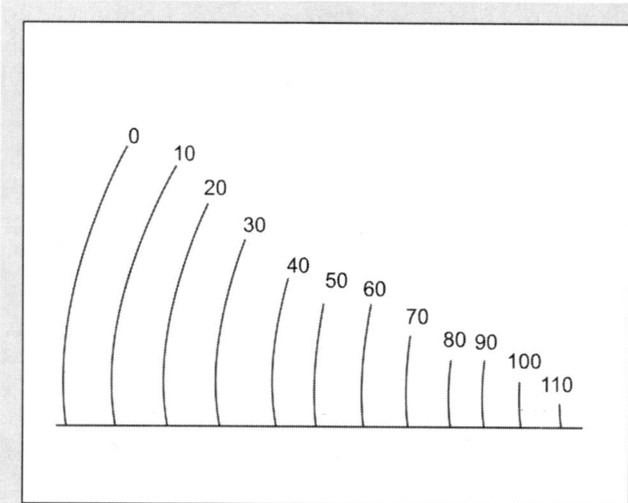

Fig. 69.3: Effect of afterloading (stationary drum)

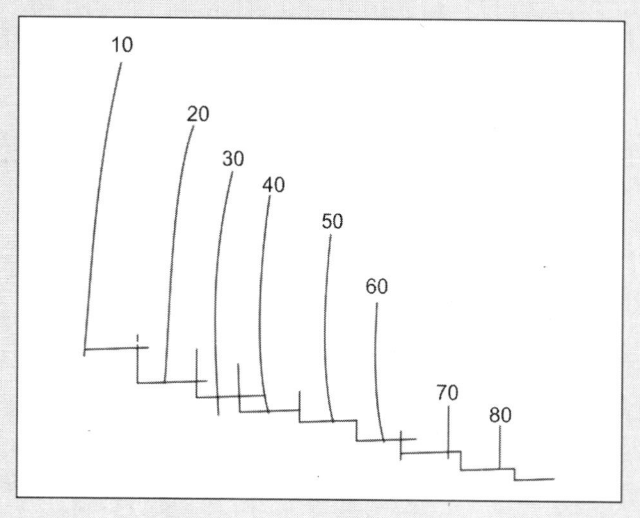

Fig. 69.4: Effect of freeloading (stationary drum)

Observations/Results

In Afterloaded State

With the increase in load:

Latent period: Latent period increases.
Cause: By the addition of load inertia of the lever increases.

Contraction period: Contraction period decreases.
Cause: Due to a decrease in the active state of muscle.

Relaxation period: Relaxation period decreases.
Cause: As load facilitates bringing down of lever.

Height of contraction: Height of contraction decreases.
Cause: As muscle has to lift the larger load.

In Freeloaded State

With the increase in load:

* *Latent period:* With load, the latent period decreases for the first few contractions and then it increases.
* *Contraction period:* Contraction period remains the same.
* *Relaxation period:* The relaxation period decreases, as load facilitates the bringing down movement of the lever.
* *Height of contraction:* The height of contraction increases for the first few contractions but later it decreases.

In Freeloaded State of a Muscle

* Load acts on a muscle even at rest, i.e. before it starts contracting.
* According to Starling's law, within physiological limits muscle works better for the first few contractions **(Fig. 69.5)**.
* Once the limit is reached, the muscle works as in an afterloaded state.

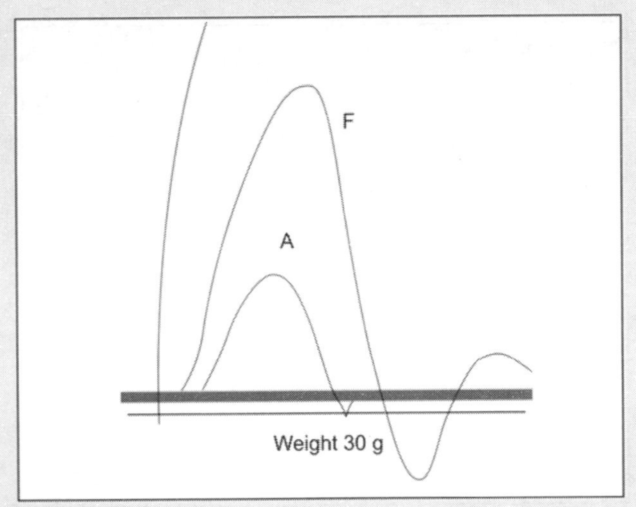

Fig. 69.5: Starling's law; A. Afterloaded state, F. Freeloaded state

Calculation of Work Done

- For comparing the work done, heights of contractions at different loads in freeloaded and after loaded are measured.
- The observed height of contraction in each case is denoted as H (it is magnified height).
- True height through which load is lifted is h.
- To find out the magnification factor, the total length of the lever (L) is divided by the length of the lever from the fulcrum to the point of attachment of load (l).
- This L/l gives the magnification factor.
- True height is calculated as, h = H/magnification factor

$$h = H/L/l$$
$$\text{Work done} = \text{Weight} \times h$$

Work done can be calculated for each weight in the freeloaded and afterloaded state. The unit for work done is g/cm.

■ IMPORTANT QUESTIONS AND ANSWERS

Q.1. What is Frank Starling's law? What is its significance?
- **Frank Starling's law**: It states that within physiological limits, the height of contraction is directly proportional to the initial length of muscle fibre.
- This can be proved by recording muscle contraction in the freeloaded state and afterloaded state.
- The length of muscle fibre decides the amount of overlap between actin and myosin filaments.

- At optimal sarcomere length (2.2 micrometres) every myosin head is opposite to the active site of the actin filament and maximum force is generated.
- At shorter and longer lengths (less than or more than 2.2 micrometres) there is decreased overlap and the force obtained is less.

Q.2. What is the mechanical efficiency of muscle?
It is the amount of energy converted into work during muscle contraction.

Q.3. What is optimum load?
It is defined as the load at which maximum work is done by the muscle.

Q.4. Define the freeloaded and afterloaded state of the muscle. How latent period, contraction and relaxation period is affected by free and afterload states?
- **Freeloaded state**: Muscle is said to be freeloaded when the load acts on the muscle even in a resting state.
- **Afterloaded state**: Muscle is said to be afterloaded when the load acts on muscle only when it starts contracting. Effects on latent period, contraction, relaxation period and height of contraction are explained above.

Q.5. Give examples of the freeloaded and after-loaded state of muscle.
- Afterloaded: Lifting a bag from the ground
- Freeloaded: Carrying a bucket full of water.

■ COMMON STATIONS–SPOTS IN PRACTICAL EXAMINATION (2/3 MARKS)

Q.1. Graph of freeloaded and after loaded (moving/stationary drum): Identify and answer any one or two questions from the above.

Q.2. State Frank Starling's law and its significance.

Q.3. Pictures of the person throwing a stone, carrying a bucket full of water: Identify the freeloaded/afterloaded state of muscle (clue- It is freeloaded).

Q.4. Pictures of a person lifting a bag, lifting a load: Identify free-loaded/afterloaded?

Q.5. In Fig. 8.5 identify which is freeloaded and which is afterloaded state of muscle.

■ KEY POINTS TO REMEMBER

- Load is the force exerted by the weight of an object on a muscle.
- Tension is the force exerted by contracting muscle on an object.
- Freeloaded state muscle works better than afterloaded state.

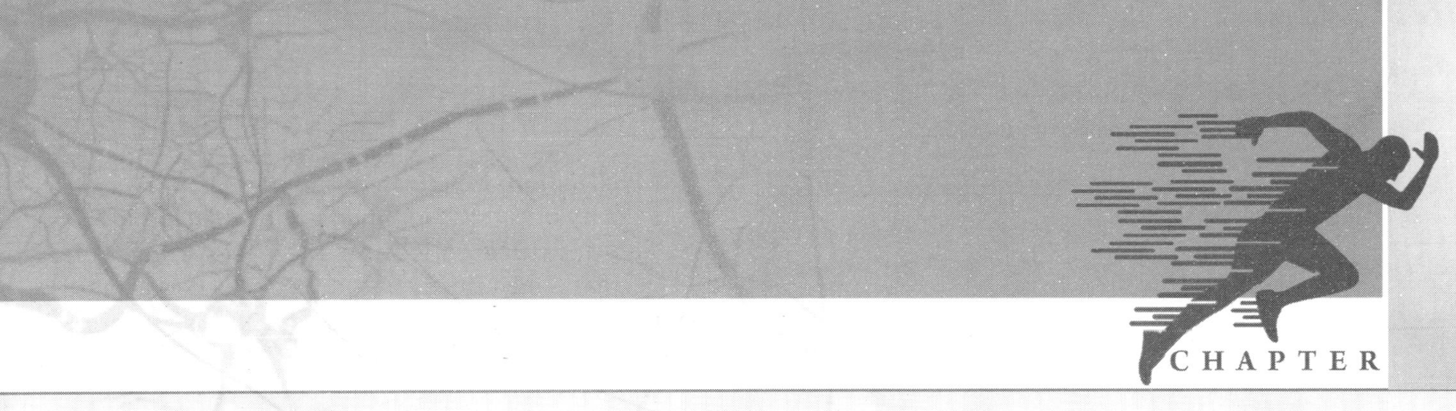

Conduction Velocity of Nerve Impulse

Competency:
PY 3.18: Observe with computer-assisted learning, amphibian nerve muscle experiments.

Learning Objectives
After completion of this practical, students shall be able to:
- Demonstrate velocity of nerve impulse in frog
- Enumerate factors affecting the velocity of nerve impulses.

■ INTRODUCTION
- Nerves carry impulses at different rates. In this experiment velocity of nerve impulse in the sciatic nerve is determined.
- Nerve conduction velocity largely depends on the myelination of nerves and the diameter of nerve fibres.

Principle
The velocity of conduction of an impulse can be found by dividing the distance between the point of stimuli (proximal and distal). It is in cm and different in the latent period of both recordings. It is in milliseconds.

Apparatus
Dissection instruments, kymograph, ringer solution, pin, cotton, thread, and stimulator.

Procedure
- Mount a nerve-muscle preparation in Luca's moist chamber.

- Distance between the primary and secondary coil is adjusted to obtain maximal stimulus.
- Take the drum in the circuit with the fastest speed (pulley 1:4, fast gear).
- With a tuning fork of 100/second frequency, record time tracing.
- Put electrodes towards the muscle end of the nerve to record simple muscle curve.
- Mark point of stimulus, as well as latent period (AB), is noted with the help of time tracing.
- Shift electrodes towards the vertebral end of the nerve and record another simple muscle curve without changing the point of stimulus. The latent period (AC) is noted with the help of time tracing **(Fig. 70.1)**.

Precautions
- Distance between the point of stimuli and two latent periods should be accurately measured.
- The point of stimulus should be properly marked.

Observations
- Velocity of nerve impulse is determined as follows:

$$\text{Velocity of nerve impulse} = \frac{\text{Length of the nerve (cm)}}{\text{Difference between two latent periods (AC-AB) in seconds}}$$

(1 second = 1000 milliseconds, 100 cm = 1 metre)
Convert velocity in metres/second

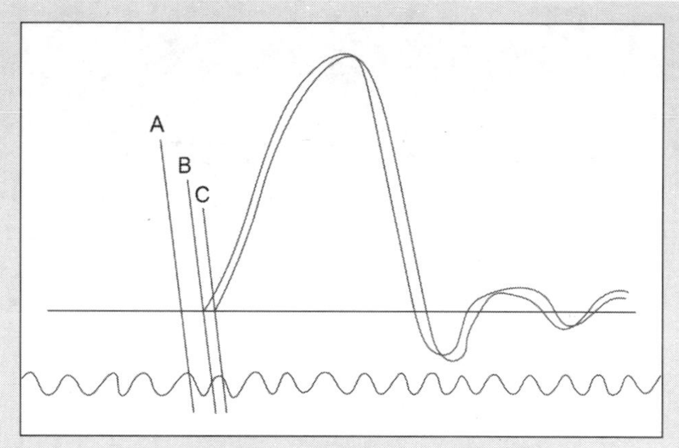

Fig. 70.1: Velocity of nerve impulse

■ IMPORTANT QUESTIONS AND ANSWERS

Q.1. Enumerate different factors affecting the velocity of nerve impulses.

Factors affecting the velocity of nerve impulses are:

- **Diameter of nerve fibre:** The larger the diameter, the faster is conduction velocity.
- **Myelination:** Myelinated nerve fibres have a faster velocity of conduction than unmyelinated ones.
- **Temperature:** Warming increases and cooling decreases the velocity of conduction of nerve impulse.
- **pH:** Acidosis decreases and alkalosis increases conduction velocity.
- **Hypoxia:** It decreases conduction velocity.
- **Drugs and chemicals:** Narcotics, ether, alcohol, and chloroform do decrease conduction velocity.
- **Mechanical pressure:** It decreases conduction velocity.

■ COMMON STATIONS – SPOTS IN PRACTICAL EXAMINATION (2/3 MARKS)

Q.1. Velocity of nerve conduction graph: Identify and enumerate factors affecting the velocity of nerve impulses.

Q.2. If the length of the nerve is 7 cm, calculate the conduction velocity if the tuning fork frequency is 100 Hz.

Ans. 7 m/s.

Effect of Temperature on Simple Muscle Curve

Competency:
PY 3.18: Observe with computer-assisted learning, amphibian nerve muscle experiments.

Learning Objectives

After completion of this practical, the students shall be able to:
- Identify the graph showing the effect of temperature on a simple muscle curve
- Explain the effect of temperature on muscle contraction

■ INTRODUCTION

- A change in the temperature of the Ringer solution can cause a change in muscle contraction.
- With temperature change, there are changes in the latent period, contraction period, and relaxation period of muscle.
- With temperature change, there is a change in the conduction velocity of the nerve, muscle viscosity, and enzymatic and chemical activities of the muscle.

Principle

The effect of change in muscle activity is studied by changing the temperature of the Ringer solution. Effects are studied on the same point of stimulus and same baseline. Changes in the latent period, contraction period, and relaxation period are noted.

Apparatus

Kymograph, Ringer solution (cold and warm), drum, thermometer.

Procedure

- With Ringer solution at room temperature, record a simple muscle curve.
- Replace that with warm Ringer solution (wait for 2–3 minutes, so that the muscle warms up). The temperature should not exceed beyond 42°C.
- Record simple muscle curve now at the same baseline, the same strength of stimulus, and the same point of stimulus.
- Repeat the same to see the effect of cold Ringer solution.
- Record time tracings below the recordings with the help of a tuning fork **(Fig. 71.1)**.

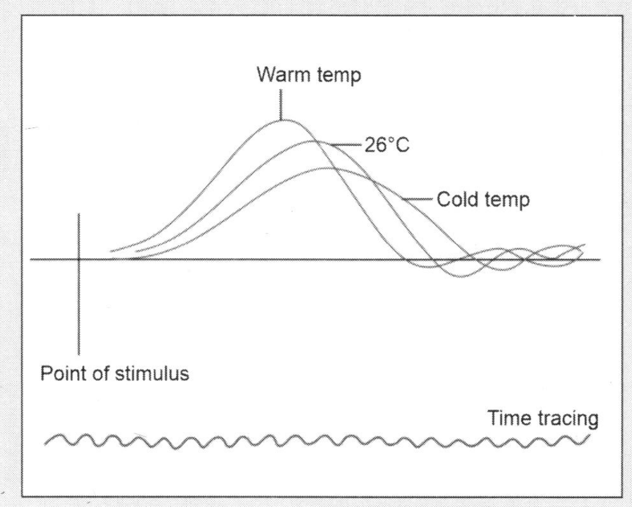

Fig. 71.1: Effect of temperature on the simple muscle twitch

Precautions

- Temperature of warm saline should not exceed 42°C.
- The temperature of the solution (warm or cold) should be checked just before muscle contraction.
- The warm saline effect is recorded first and then the effect of cold saline is recorded.

Observations/Result (Table 71.1)

TABLE 71.1: Observation of the effect of temperature on a simple muscle curve

Temperature of Ringer solution	LP	CP	RP	Height of contraction
Normal				
Warm				
Cold				

■ IMPORTANT QUESTIONS AND ANSWER

Q.1. What are the effects of different temperatures on muscle?

Effect of warm temperature

- Latent period, contraction period, and relaxation period decrease.
- There is an increase in the height of contraction.

Decrease in the latent period is due to:

- Increase in conduction velocity of the nerve.
- Increase in rate of neuromuscular transmission.

Decrease in contraction and relaxation period is due to:

- Activation of myosin adenosine triphosphatase (ATPase) activity and decreased viscosity of muscle.
- Amplitude of contraction increases due to increased enzymatic and chemical activities of the muscle.
- These effects cause faster contraction and relaxation and therefore decrease contraction and relaxation period.

Effect of Cold Temperature

All the effects are opposite to that seen with the effect of warm saline.

Q.2. Enumerate precautions taken while performing this experiment.

Precautions:

- Temperature of warm saline should not exceed 42°C. More temperature than this can cause denaturation of proteins in muscle.
- Temperature less than 4°C should not be used.
- Initially effect of warm and then the effect of cold saline is tested (as cold saline inactivates the muscle).

Q.3. What is heat rigour?

Heat rigour: This is observed due to the use of saline which is more than 42°C. High temperature causes denaturation of muscle proteins. Myosin filaments are not able to carry their functions which causes muscles to remain in permanent contraction, this is known as heat rigour.

■ COMMON STATIONS – SPOTS IN PRACTICAL EXAMINATION (2/3 MARKS)

Q.1. Effect of temperature on simple muscle curve: Identify the graph and answer any one or two questions from the above.

■ KEY POINTS TO REMEMBER

- With warm temperatures, the latent period, contraction, and relaxation period decrease, however amplitude of contraction increases.
- Thus, we can say that the efficiency of skeletal muscle contraction increases with an increase in temperature (in physiological limits).

CHAPTER

72

Recording of Normal Cardiogram in Frog's Heart

Competency:

PY 3.18: With computer-assisted learning, observe amphibian cardiac experiments.

Learning Objectives

After completion of this practical, the students shall be able to:

- Identify the graph of the normal cardiogram of the frog
- Enlist various waves in the cardiogram
- Enlist the differences between a frog's heart and a human heart
- Enumerate properties of the heart

■ INTRODUCTION

A normal cardiogram is recorded of a frog's heart. In contrast to the human heart, a frog's heart has three chambers and sinus venosus acts as a pacemaker of the heart.

Apparatus

Dissection apparatus, kymograph with drum, Luca's chamber, Starling's heart lever, myograph board.

Principle

We try to understand the initiation of impulses in a frog's myocardium and its conduction via different chambers of the heart. Thus, we do study the properties of excitability, contractility, and conductivity of the heart. Cardiac activities are recorded on a moving drum.

Procedure

- The heart of the frog is exposed and pericardium is removed.
- Bent pin (attached to Starling's heart lever) is passed via the apex of the heart. Care is taken not to puncture the ventricle.
- Cardiogram is recorded on the drum with different speeds.
- Contraction and relaxation of the heart is recorded. Downstroke is recorded as systole and upstroke is recorded as diastole of the heart.

Observation

- Normal cardiogram shows impulse generated from sinus venosus and then impulse going to atria and ventricle of frog's heart **(Fig. 72.1)**.

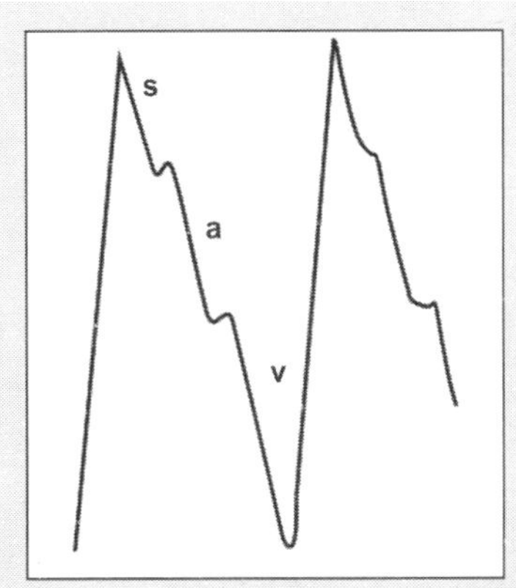

Fig. 72.1: Normal cardiogram of frog's heart

- Sinus venosus is a pacemaker of a frog's heart from where the impulse is conducted in the heart further. A normal frog's heart rate varies from 30 to 50 beats/minute.

Precautions

- Handle the heart carefully to prevent it from damaging.
- Remove the pericardium after the heart is fixed on the myograph board.

■ IMPORTANT QUESTIONS AND ANSWERS

Q.1. What are the components of a normal cardiogram in a frog?

Normal cardiogram shows contraction and relaxation of sinus venosus, followed by atrial contraction and relaxation and lastly ventricular contraction and relaxation.

> A cardiogram represents the mechanical activity of the heart and an electrocardiogram represents the electrical activity of the heart

Q.2. What is the pacemaker of the heart in frogs?

The pacemaker of a frog's heart is sinus venosus. In human beings, the SA node is the pacemaker of the heart.

Q.3. Why pericardium must be removed?

The pericardium must be removed in order to support the heart from the apex.

Q.4. Enumerate the difference between a human and a frog's heart.

S. No.	Characteristics of frog's heart	Characteristics of the human heart
	Pacemaker–sinus venosus	Pacemaker–sinoatrial node (SA)
	Two atria, one ventricle (3 chambers)	Two atria, two ventricles (4 chambers)
	No special conduction system in the heart	Special conduction system in the heart
	No coronary circulation	Coronary circulation
	Can withstand change in pH, O_2 content of blood	Cannot withstand changes in pH and O_2 content of blood

Q.5. Why frog's heart is preferred in experimental studies?

- Frog is cold-blooded and thus can withstand changes in temperature, pH and O_2 content of the blood.
- At the cellular level as physiology is the same, results obtained in frogs can be extrapolated.

■ COMMON STATIONS – SPOTS IN PRACTICAL EXAMINATION (2/3 MARKS)

Q.1. Identify the graph: Answer any one or two questions.

Q.2. Enumerate the differences between the frog and human heart.

Q.3. Graph: Identify atrial systole, diastole, and ventricular systole.

■ KEY POINTS TO REMEMBER

- In contrast to the human heart, a frog's heart is a three-chambered structure.
- Sinus venosus is the pacemaker of a frog's heart.
- After impulse generation at the sinus venosus, the impulse goes to the atria followed by the ventricle.

Effect of Heat and Cold on Frog's Heart

Competency:

PY 3.18: With computer-assisted learning observe amphibian cardiac experiments.

Learning Objectives

After completion of this practical, students shall be able to:

- Identify the graph of the normal cardiogram of the frog
- Identify the effects of heat and cold temperature on a frog's heart
- Enlist reasons for the change in activity of the heart with respect to changes in temperature

Apparatus

Dissection apparatus, Starling's heart lever, Lucas chamber, amphibian Ringer solution (warm and cold), kymograph and drum.

■ INTRODUCTION

A normal cardiogram is recorded of a frog's heart. The effect on cardiac activity of a frog's heart is studied with exposure to different temperatures.

Principle

We try to understand how temperature affects various chemical reactions in the heart and affects its beating ability.

Procedure

- Expose the frog's heart and remove the pericardium.
- Pass the bent pin (attached to Starling's heart lever) via the apex of the heart. Care is taken not to puncture the ventricle.
- Record normal cardiogram on moving drum.
- Pour a few drops of 0.65% saline with a temperature of less than 50°C on the frog's heart and record the cardiogram.
- As the effect of warm saline is over again normal cardiogram is recorded.
- Now, pour a few drops of cold saline on the frog's heart and record the cardiogram.

Observations

- Normal cardiogram shows impulse generated from sinus venosus and then impulse going to atria and ventricle of frog's heart.
- *Effect of hot saline:* When hot saline is poured on the frog's heart, heart rate and force of contraction of the heart increase. Due to warm saline, the rate of all chemical processes increases which is responsible for increasing heart rate and force of contraction **(Fig. 73.1)**.
- *Effect of cold saline:* When cold saline is poured on the frog's heart, heart rate and force of contraction of the heart decrease. Due to cold saline, the rate of all chemical reactions slows down which is responsible for reducing heart rate and force of contraction.

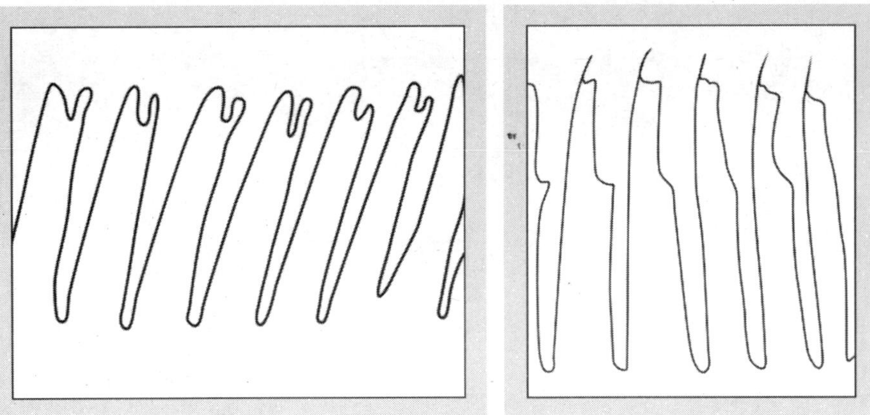

Fig. 73.1: Effect of cold and warm saline on frog's heart

Precautions

- A normal cardiogram has to be recorded before observing the effect of hot and cold saline on a frog's heart.
- Too hot and too cold saline has to be avoided.
- Frequently heart needs to be moistened with the help of Ringer's solution.

■ IMPORTANT QUESTIONS AND ANSWERS

Q.1. Why heart rate and force of contraction increase when hot saline is put in? Why heart rate and force of contraction decrease when cold saline is put in?

Warm saline effects:
- Increase in enzymatic activity
- Decrease in the viscosity
- Both effects combined cause an increase in heart rate and force of contraction on the use of hot (warm) saline.

Cold saline effects:
- Decrease in enzymatic activity
- Increase in enzymatic activity
- Both effects combinedly cause a decrease in heart rate and force of contraction on the use of cold saline.

■ COMMON STATIONS – SPOTS IN PRACTICAL EXAMINATION (2/3 MARKS)

Q.1. Identify the graph and answer any one or two questions from above.

Q.2. Write the difference between stimulation of the heart with warm saline and cold saline and the causes for the same.

■ KEY POINTS TO REMEMBER

- With the use of warm saline, heart rate and force of contraction increases
- With cold saline, heart rate and force of contraction decreases.

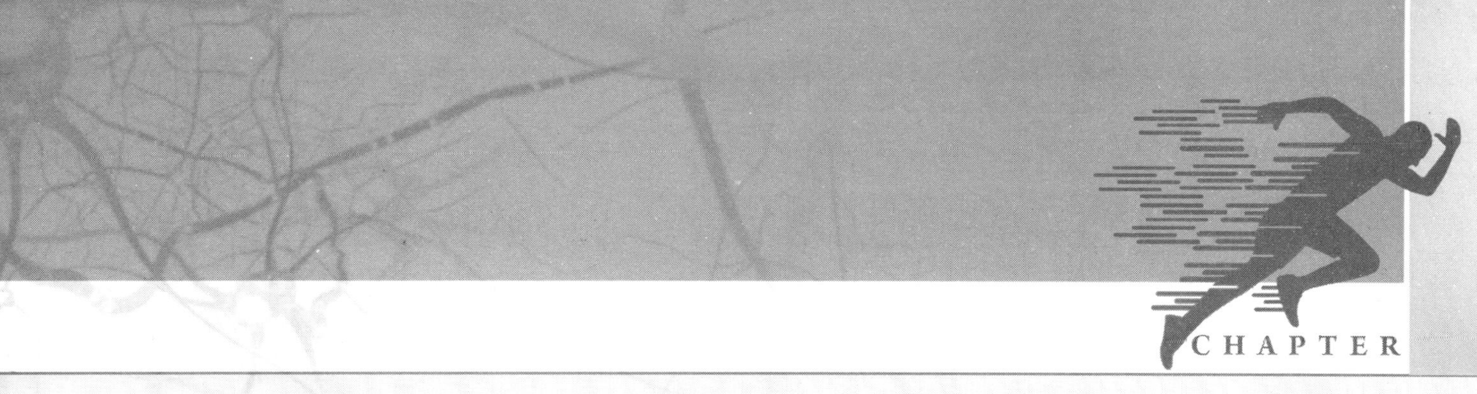

To Study Properties of Cardiac Muscle of Frog's Heart

Competency:

PY 3.18: With computer-assisted learning, observe amphibian cardiac experiments.

Learning Objectives

At the end of this practical student shall be able to:
- Enlist properties of cardiac muscle
- Differentiate absolute and relative refractory period
- Explain the cause of the staircase phenomenon
- Explain the physiological basis of compensatory pause

■ INTRODUCTION

In this experiment, different cardiac muscle properties are studied like auto rhythmicity, long refractory period, compensatory pause, staircase phenomenon, and all or none law.

Principle

- With the help of electrodes, the heart is stimulated in systole and diastole. When an extrastimulus is given, the cardiac muscle responds as extrasystole followed by a compensatory pause due to stimulus.
- Stannius ligature helps to understand conductivity as a property of cardiac muscle.
- For studying other properties, the heart is made quiescent and then various properties are studied.

Apparatus

Kymograph with drum, starling's heart lever, Ringer solution, pins, electrical circuit for cardiac stimulation.

Procedure

- Prepare to make and break the circuit with a time marker in the primary circuit.
- Record graph on slow-moving drum.
- Expose the frog's heart and remove the pericardium. Pass bent pin attached to Starling's heart lever through the apex of the heart and record normal cardiogram (excitability, contractility, auto rhythmicity and conductivity properties are studied).
- With the help of electrodes stimulate the heart during systole and we observe that the heart does not respond at all during systole.
- Now stimulate the heart during diastole with the help of an electrode and extra-contraction of the heart is recorded. The extra-contraction recorded due to additional stimulus is called as extrasystole. After that follows a compensatory pause and again record normal cardiogram. This shows the property of the long refractory period as the absolute refractory period extends throughout the systole of the heart, no response is obtained during systole **(Fig. 74.1)**.
- After making the heart quiescent, by giving increasing strength of stimuli all or none law property is studied. When the strength of the stimulus is below threshold no response is obtained and the response obtained with threshold stimuli and above threshold stimuli are the same.
- **Staircase phenomenon:** When more than a couple of threshold stimuli are applied to the heart, successive contractions are observed to be of higher magnitude.

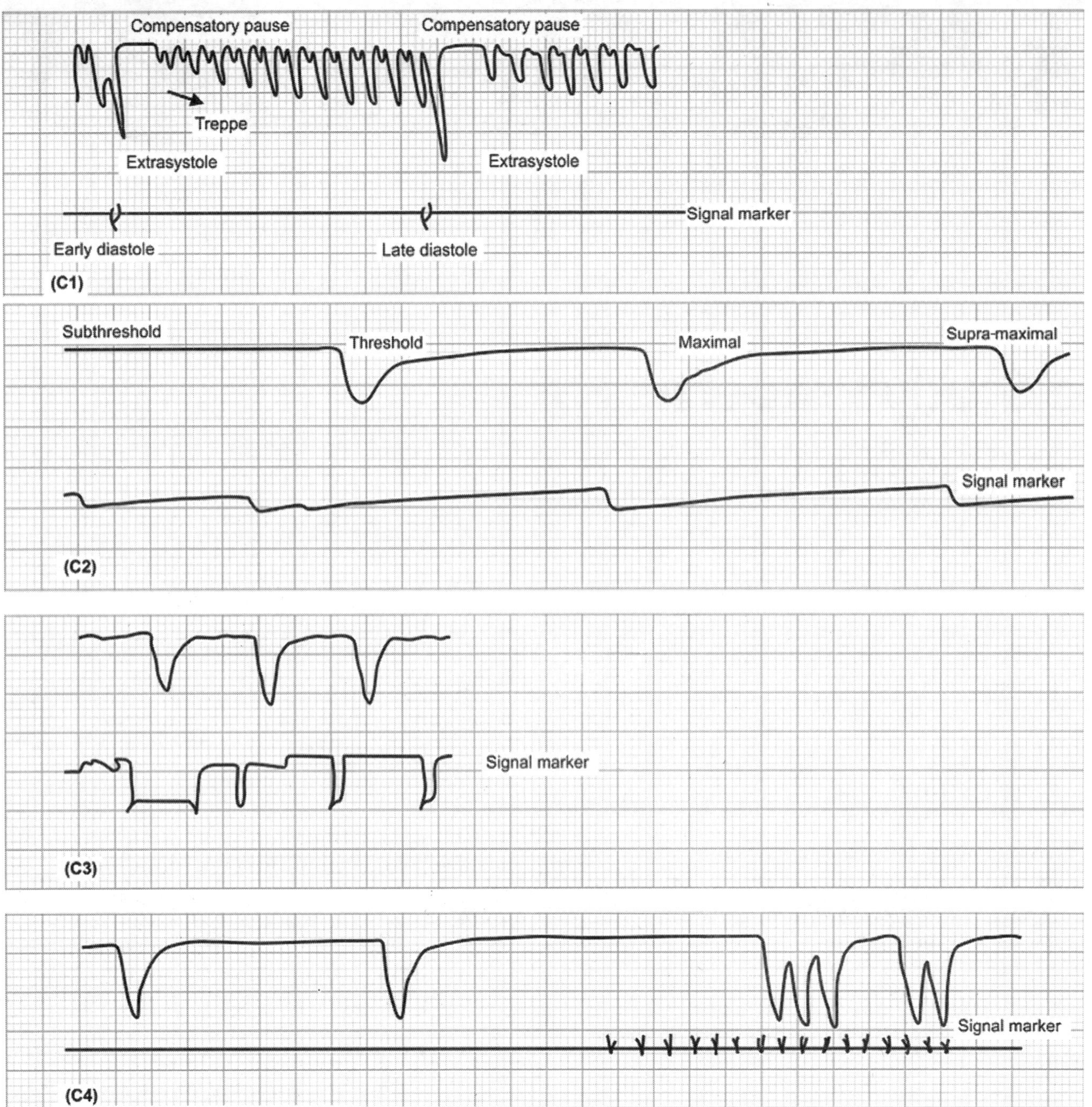

Fig. 74.1: (C1) Extrasystole and compensatory pause; (C2) All or none law; (C3) Staircase phenomenon (Beneficial effect); (C4) Summation of subliminal stimuli

This is called the beneficial effect and is observed due to increased temperature and accumulation of metabolites due to previous contractions.

- Taking Kneef's hammer in a circuit and stimulating the heart with more than 30 stimuli/second, the heart does not maintain a continuous state of contraction. This shows the property of non-tetanizability.

Precautions

- Take care not to puncture the ventricle while passing the pin through the apex of the heart.
- Use only scissors not knives during the experiment.

■ IMPORTANT QUESTIONS AND ANSWERS

Q.1. State all or none law.

- **All or none law:** Within physiological limits, any excitable tissue when stimulated with threshold stimulus either responds to its maximum or does not respond at all.
- Each individual motor unit in skeletal muscle obeys all or none law. In the case of the heart, the whole of the heart obeys all or none law.

Q.2. What is absolute and relative refractory period?

- **Refractory period:** It is the loss of excitability of excitable tissue due to a previous stimulus.

- **Absolute refractory period**: In this period there is complete loss of excitability. This is the first part of the refractory period.
- **Relative refractory period**: This period is followed by an absolute refractory period where there is a partial loss of excitability. When one stimulates tissue in this period with a higher strength of stimulus, excitable tissue might respond.

Q.3. What is the advantage of a long refractory period of cardiac muscle?
- Heart muscle has got long refractory period as compared to smooth and skeletal muscle.
- Due to a long refractory period, the heart muscle does not get fatigued and cannot get tetanized. Thus, we have the myocardial pump, pumping effectively without getting fatigued throughout the person's life.
- Normal refractory period of the heart is about 250 to 350 ms.

Q.4. What is the beneficial effect?
- **Beneficial effect**: An increase in the strength of contraction due to repeated stimulation is known as a beneficial effect.
- This is due to an increase in the temperature of muscle (due to previous stimulus), release of more Ca^{+} for sarcoplasmic reticulum, and decrease in viscosity of muscle. This is seen as a staircase phenomenon as seen in **Fig. 74.1.**

Q.5. What is a compensatory pause?
- When a stimulus is given to cardiac muscle, extrasystole is recorded due to that stimulus, which is followed by a compensatory pause.
- When there is extrasystole, it appears before the next sinus beat therefore when the next impulse comes from the sinus the muscle is in a refractory period due to that extra-stimulus. Therefore, extrasystole is followed by a compensatory pause.

Q.6. Why extrasystole is called as premature beat?
As this beat comes earlier than the normal beat of the heart, it is called as extrasystole/premature beat.

Q.7. What is a threshold, sub-threshold and supra-threshold stimulus?
- **Threshold stimulus**: It is the minimum strength of stimulus that can elicit a response from excitable tissues.
- **Sub-threshold stimulus**: A stimulus with a strength less than the threshold stimulus is called subthreshold stimulus.
- **Suprathreshold stimulus**: A stimulus with a strength more than the threshold stimulus is called as suprathreshold stimulus.

Q.8. Which tissues obey all or none law?
- **Nerve and skeletal muscle**: Every single unit in the case of the nerve (single nerve fibre) and skeletal muscle (each motor unit) obeys all or none law.
- **Cardiac muscle:** The whole of the cardiac muscle obeys all or none law.
- **Smooth muscle:** Single-unit smooth muscle as a whole and single unit of multiunit smooth muscle obeys all or none law.

Q.9. What do you mean by intercalated extrasystole?
When the heart rate is very low, extrasystole is not followed by a compensatory pause, this is known as intercalated extrasystole.

Q.10. What are experiments (graphs) that demonstrate that the heart has a long refractory period?
Graphs that demonstrate a long refractory period of the heart are:
- Extrasystole with compensatory pause
- Two successive stimuli
- Incomplete tetanus

Q.11. Heart obeys all or none law. Give its physiological significance.
- In the case of the heart, the whole heart obeys the all or none law (in contrast to each motor unit in the case of skeletal muscle).
- As the whole heart contracts as one powerful unit, an adequate amount of cardiac output can be obtained.

Q.12. What is partial or incomplete tetanus?
On repeated stimulation, cardiac muscle cannot be thrown into a sustained state of contraction (tetanus). It shows intermittent relaxation (incomplete tetanus).

Q.13. Why contraction that follows the compensatory pause is of greater amplitude?
- During the compensatory pause, there is an increased filling of the heart which causes increased stretch on cardiac muscle fibre (initial length).
- According to Frank Satrling's law, the magnitude of the contraction is directly proportional to the initial length of muscle fibre. Hence, contraction that follows compensatory pause is of greater magnitude.

■ COMMON STATIONS– SPOTS IN PRACTICAL EXAMINATION (2/3 MARKS)

Q.1. Any of the graphs: Identify the property of cardiac muscle. Answer any one or two questions from the above.

■ KEY POINTS TO REMEMBER

- Properties of cardiac muscle are excitability, contractility, conductivity, all or none law, long refractory period, non-fatigability, non-tetanizability and auto-rhythmicity.
- Due to a long refractory period, cardiac muscle cannot get fatigued or tetanized.
- Compensatory pause followed by extrasystole indicates a long refractory period property of the heart.

Effect of Stannius Ligature on Frog's Heart

Competency:

PY 3.18: With computer-assisted learning, observe amphibian cardiac experiments.

Learning Objectives

At the end of this practical, the students shall be able to:
- Understand that each chamber of the heart has the property of autorhythmicity
- Sinus venosus is a pacemaker in a frog's heart
- Describe the first and second stannius ligature and its effects

■ INTRODUCTION

In this experiment stannius ligatures are tied to specific regions in the heart of a frog and the effect of each is seen. This helps to understand different autorhythmic structures in the heart. It also helps to understand the conductivity property of the heart.

Apparatus

Kymograph, drum, Starling's heart lever, pins, thread.

Procedure

- The heart of the frog is exposed and the pericardium is exposed.
- Bent pin which is attached to Starling's lever, is passed through the apex of the heart.
- Normal cardiogram is obtained on a moving drum.
- First stannius ligature is tied with the help of thread at the junction of sinus venosus and atria. As impulse generated from the sinus venosus stop reaching to atria and ventricle, they stop beating.
- After some time, atria start their own rhythm. This is called atrial or auricular rhythm **(Fig. 75.1)**.
- Due to this now atria and ventricle contractions are recorded but the rate is much less than when sinus venosus rhythm.

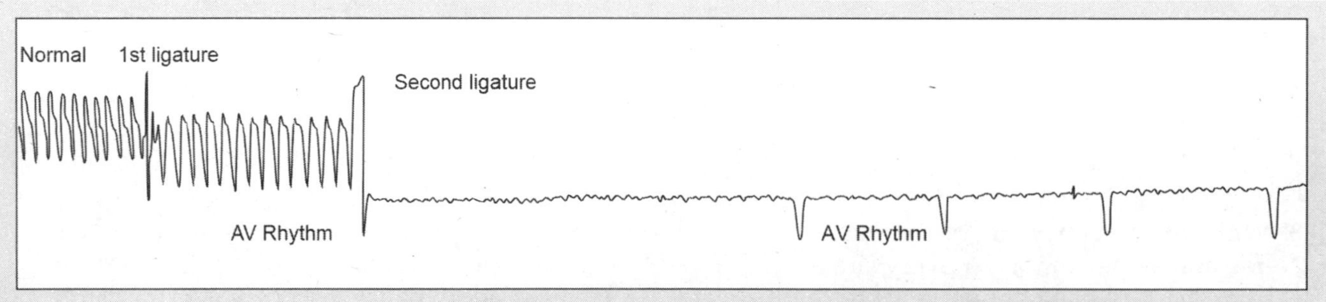

Fig. 75.1: Effect of stannius ligature on frog's heart

- The second stannius ligature is tied between the atria and ventricle. Now ventricle stops contracting as impulse generated from the atria cannot pass to ventricle.
- After some time, the ventricle starts beating at its own rhythm, called idioventricular rhythm, which is still slower than auricular.

■ IMPORTANT QUESTIONS AND ANSWERS

Q.1. What does the stannius ligature experiment proves?

This experiment proves that:

- In frog's heart, the sinus venosus acts as a pacemaker and has the highest rate of impulse generation as compared to atria and ventricle rhythm.
- Each chamber of the heart can generate its own rhythm, thus demonstrating the property of autorhythmicity.
- As far as the rate of impulse generation capacity is concerned, sinus venosus has the highest capacity followed by atria and then the ventricle.

Q.2. Can one try to put the first stannius ligature in the mammalian heart?

In the mammalian heart there is a sinoatrial node which is the pacemaker of the heart, thus the first stannius ligature can not be tied in the mammalian heart.

Q.3. Can one try to put a second stannius ligature in a mammalian heart?

- No, one cannot tie a second stannius ligature in the mammalian heart. The mammalian heart is thick-walled as compared to the amphibian heart, so cannot obtain the required amount of nutrients and O_2 from the blood present in it. That is the reason the mammalian heart is supplied by coronary arteries, which are present in an atrioventricular grove.

- As the second stannius ligature is tied at the junction of atria and ventricle in mammalian, it will obliterate coronaries and then the heart will not be able to continue beating due to lack of O_2 and nutrients.
- Thus, the second stannius ligature cannot be tied to the mammalian heart.

Q.4. Explain the graph obtained when the first and second stannius ligature is tied.

- **Effect of first stannius ligature:** After tying the first stannius ligature (between sinus venosus and atria), atria and ventricles stop beating as impulse from sinus venosus do not reach them.
- After some time, atria takes its own rhythm (atrial or auricular rhythm) and atrial and ventricular contractions are recorded but the rate is much slower than that of sinus venosus rhythm.
- **Effect of second stannius ligature:** After tying the second stannius ligature at the junction of the atria and ventricle, the ventricle stops contracting as an impulse from the atria cannot reach to the ventricle.
- After some time, the ventricle starts its own rhythm which is called as idioventricular rhythm but is much slower than the auricular rhythm.

■ COMMON STATIONS – SPOTS IN PRACTICAL EXAMINATION (2/3 MARKS)

Q.1. Identify the graph and answer any one or two questions from the above.

■ KEY POINTS TO REMEMBER

- The pacemaker of the heart generates impulses (sinus venosus in amphibians and sinoatrial node in mammalians).
- The pacemaker of the heart has the highest rate of impulse generation followed by atria and ventricle.

Effect of Heart Block on Frog's Heart

Competency:

PY 3.18: With computer-assisted learning, observe amphibian cardiac experiments.

Learning Objectives

After this practical, students shall be able to:
- Understand the concept of heart block
- Describe the effects of heart block and its effects on ECG waves and intervals

■ INTRODUCTION

By blocking impulse conduction through the heart at different places heart blocks can be created. In this experiment specific areas in the heart are tied to block impulse conduction at various places and effects are seen.

Procedure

- Expose the frog's heart and remove the pericardium.
- Cardiogram is recorded by passing a bent pin which is attached to the starling's lever.
- Make a loop of thread by passing thread through the glass tube.
- Loop is passed around the heart at the atrioventricular junction.
- Pull the thread to partially compress the atrioventricular junction. This helps produce partial heart block.
- After every 3 to 4 atrial contractions, ventricular contraction is obtained.

- This helps in producing different degrees of heart blocks like 3:1, 4:1 and so on where these numbers indicate atrial and ventricular contractions respectively.
- After some time idioventricular rhythm is initiated which is slower than sinus venosus rhythm.

■ IMPORTANT QUESTION AND ANSWERS

Q.1. How one can diagnose heart block in human beings?
- Heart blocks can be diagnosed with the help of electrocardiogram (ECG).
- Incomplete heart block is characterized by a prolongation of the P-R interval. The normal P-R interval ranges from 0.12 to 0.16 seconds. If the P-R interval exceeds 0.2 seconds, it indicates a partial heart block.
- Complete heart block occurs when no impulses can travel from the atria to the ventricles. As a result, the ventricles generate their own rhythm, known as an idioventricular rhythm, which is about 40 beats/minute and much slower than the sinus rhythm. In complete heart block, there is no impulse conduction from the pacemaker to the atria and then to the ventricles, leading to a complete dissociation of P waves and QRS complexes.

Q.2. Is complete heart block compatible with life?
Yes, complete heart block is compatible with life.

Q.3. What is the clinical application of this experiment?
- This experiment makes us understand that there are different types of heart blocks.
- It also shows that ventricles have got capacity to generate and beat at their own rhythm (auto-rhythmicity) when there is complete blockage of impulse transmission from the SA node to the ventricles.

■ KEY POINTS TO REMEMBER
- Normal rate of sinus rhythm– 40 to 60 beats/min
- Atrioventricular rhythm– 25 to 40 beats/min
- Idioventricular rhythm– less than 15 beats/min

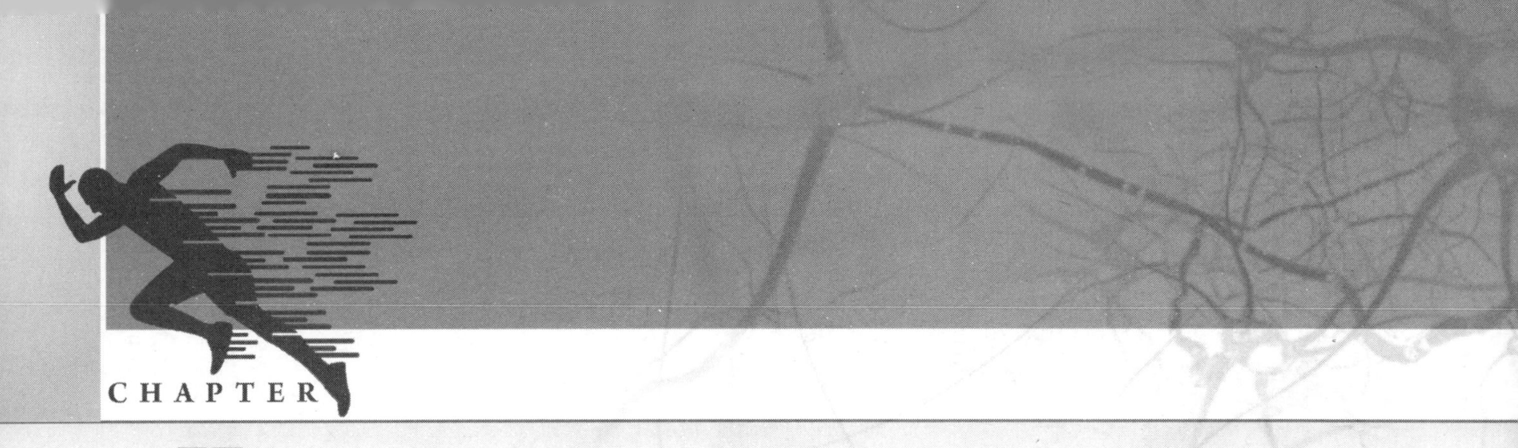

Effect of Vagus and Crescent Stimulation on Frog's Heart

Competency:

PY 3.18: With computer-assisted learning, observe amphibian cardiac experiments.

> ### *Learning Objectives*
> After completion of this practical, the students shall be able to understand:
> - What is crescent and understand the effects of crescent stimulation
> - Mechanism that causes vagus and crescent stimulation
> - Enumerate causes of vagal escape

■ INTRODUCTION

- The nerve supply of the frog's heart is via the vagosympathetic trunk which contains 75% of parasympathetic preganglionic fibres and 25% of sympathetic postganglionic fibres.
- Stimulation of the vagus and crescent causes the heart to stop in diastole. The staircase effect is observed when one stops vagus and crescent stimulation.

Apparatus

Same as that for recording a normal cardiogram of the frog.

Procedure

- Remove the pericardium and expose the frog's heart.
- Record the cardiogram as one passes the bent pin through the apex of the heart.
- Dissect the vagus on one side and stimulate it. The heart does stop in diastole. As one stops stimulating the vagus, a gradually normal cardiogram is recorded (staircase observed).
- As normal tracings are recorded, now stimulate crescent. The crescent lies at the junction between the sinus venosus and atrium **(Fig. 77.1)**.

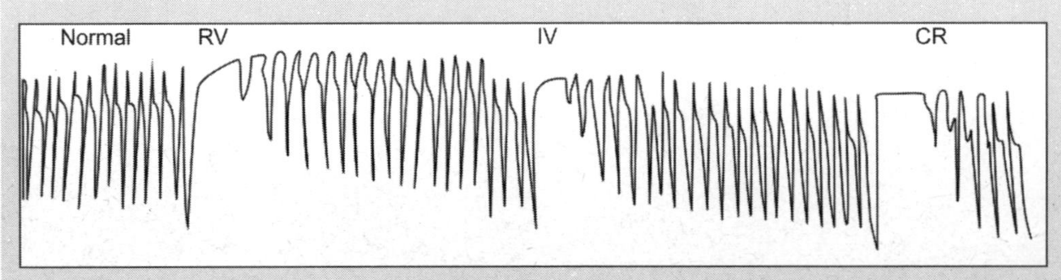

Fig. 77.1: Effect of the vagus and crescent stimulation

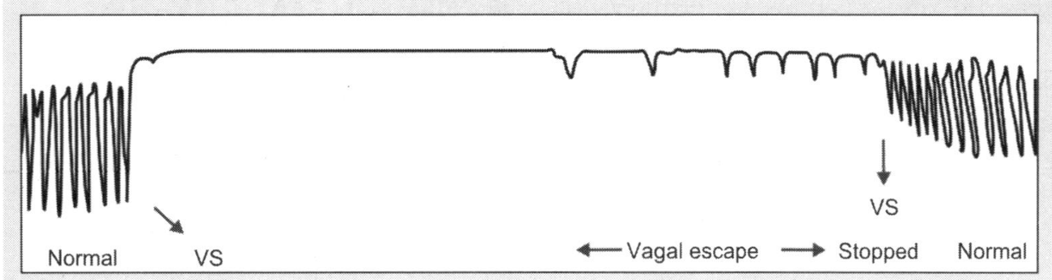

Fig. 77.2: Vagal escape

- Stimulation of the crescent also causes inhibition of the heart and as one stops crescent stimulation normal cardiogram is recorded.
- As normal tracings are recorded, the vagus is stimulated. With initial stimulation of the vagus, inhibition is obtained followed by solitary ventricular contractions, indicating that the heart has escaped the effect of vagus stimulation **(Fig. 77.2)**.
- Normal cardiogram is recorded despite of continuous vagal stimulation.

■ IMPORTANT QUESTIONS AND ANSWERS

Q.1. What is the nerve supply of a frog's heart?
Nerve supply is via ANS through the vagosympathetic trunk (explained above).

Q.2. Enumerate the parasympathetic ganglia of a frog's heart.
Parasympathetic ganglia lie near the organ. In frogs, there are three ganglia.
1. **Remark's ganglia** (present at the junction of sinus venosus and atria)
2. **Bidder's ganglia** (present at the atrioventricular junction
3. **Ludwig's ganglia** (lies in interatrial septum)
   When one stimulates the crescent, postganglionic parasympathetic fibres are stimulated.

Q.3. What does the vagus contain?
- In frogs it is the vagosympathetic trunk that contains 75% parasympathetic and 25% sympathetic fibres.
- In mammals, vagus is purely parasympathetic and thus contains only preganglionic parasympathetic fibres.

Q.4. Describe the mechanism by which vagus and crescent stimulation cause inhibition.
- Parasympathetic nerve endings release acetylcholine therefore both vagus and crescent stimulation cause the release of acetylcholine at their endings.
- Acetylcholine acts on the myocardium, it increases the permeability of the cardiac muscle membrane for potassium K^+ ions. This causes K^+ ions to diffuse outward from the inside of the membrane.

- This leads to hyperpolarization (potential becomes even more negative than RMP). This is responsible for the inhibition of the heart.

Q.5. What is vagal escape? Describe the causes of the same.
When the vagus nerve is continuously stimulated at first heart is inhibited. After some time even if vagus stimulation is continued, the heart escapes its action and continues beating. This is called a vagal escape.
Causes of vagal escape:
- In frog vagus is the vagosympathetic trunk, thus along with parasympathetic fibres even sympathetic fibres are also stimulated which releases adrenaline at their nerve endings. Adrenaline stimulates the heart.
- Another cause of vagal escape is, there is an exhaustion of acetylcholine released from parasympathetic nerve endings.
- Idioventricular rhythm—prolonged inhibition due to vagus stimulation, initiates idioventricular rhythm (ventricles start beating on their own) as there is no vagus supply to ventricles.
- In the case of intact animals, as heart stops beating with vagus stimulation, which leads to the accumulation of blood on the venous side which in turn initiates the Bainbridge reflex.
- In intact animals, with vagus stimulation, as the heart stops beating, there is a lowering of BP which initiates Mary's reflex.

Q.6. What is the importance of vagal escape?
Due to vagal escape, the heart does not remain inhibited for long, so it is life-saving, e.g. in human beings with strong emotional disturbance, the vagus nerve can get stimulated (vagal syncope) and this causes inhibition of the heart but due to immediate vagal escape, the heart starts beating again.

Q.7. After stopping vagus and crescent stimulation why staircase phenomenon is observed?
- When vagal stimulation is stopped, there happens gradual hydrolysis of accumulated acetylcholine by cholinesterase.

- This helps to restore cardiac activity to normal with a gradual increase in the force of contraction, exhibiting the staircase phenomenon.

Q.8. Name neurotransmitters released at sympathetic and parasympathetic nerve endings.

Sympathetic preganglionic nerve endings	Acetylcholine
Sympathetic postganglionic nerve endings	Noradrenaline
Parasympathetic preganglionic nerve endings	Acetylcholine
Parasympathetic postganglionic nerve endings	Acetylcholine

■ COMMON STATIONS – SPOTS IN PRACTICAL EXAMINATION (2/3 MARKS)

Q.1. Identify the graph and answer any one or two questions from the above.

Q.2. After vagus and crescent stimulation, the staircase phenomenon is observed justify.

■ KEY POINTS TO REMEMBER

- Nerve supply to frog's heart has vagosympathetic trunk.
- Acetylcholine released with vagus and crescent stimulation, causes inhibition of the heart.
- The heart can escape the effect of vagal stimulation.

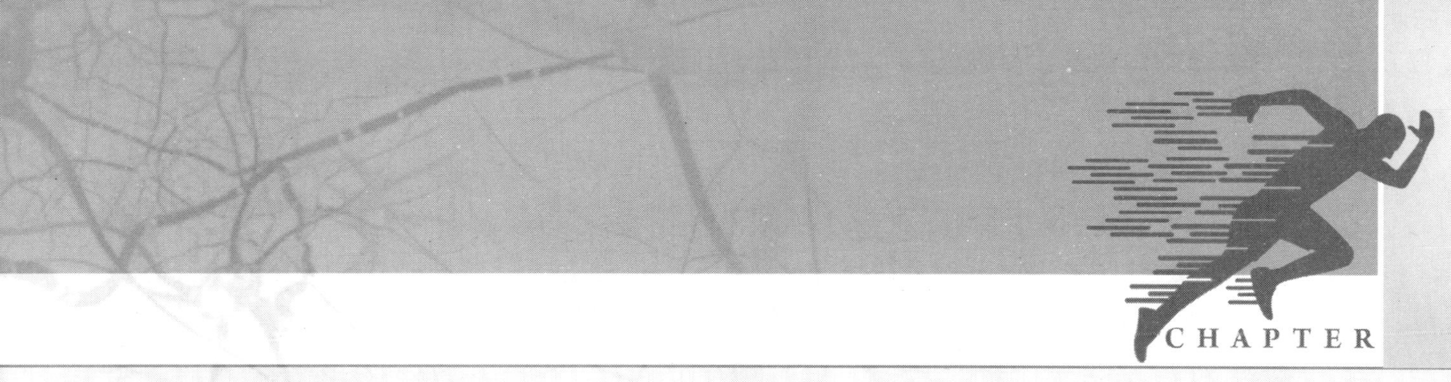

Effect of Acetylcholine on Frog's Heart

Competency:
PY 3.18: With computer-assisted learning, observe amphibian cardiac experiments.

Learning Objectives

After completion of this practical, the students shall be able to:

- Describe the mechanism of action of acetylcholine on a frog's heart
- Identify the graph of the effect of acetylcholine on the heart

■ INTRODUCTION

- Acetylcholine is a neurotransmitter released at the parasympathetic nerve endings. Its action on the heart is inhibitory in nature. Acetylcholine is known to increase the permeability of membranes for K^+ ions.
- With increased permeability of the membrane for K^+ ions, there is rapid repolarization that shortens action potential. When a large number of K^+ ions diffuse out, it leads to hyperpolarization, i.e. potential of the membrane becomes more negative than RMP.
- This decreases the excitability of excitable tissue and it takes much more time for potential to return back to the threshold voltage (threshold voltage for opening of Na^+ Ca^{++} channels) in the pacemaker to fire an action potential.

Principle

To study the effect of acetylcholine on a frog's heart.

Apparatus

Same as for recording a normal cardiogram in a frog, Syme's cannula, 1 in 1000000 acetylcholine.

Procedure

- Kneef's hammer is taken in circuit with the slow speed of the drum (pulley 4:1 slow gear)
- Normal cardiogram is recorded
- The vagus is stimulated causes inhibition of the heart
- After stopping vagus stimulation, a normal cardiogram is recorded again. Then crescent is stimulated which again records inhibition of the heart.
- After stopping crescent stimulation, again normal cardiogram is recorded.
- Now few drops of acetylcholine are directly applied to the heart **(Fig. 78.1)**. This causes a decrease in heart rate and force of contraction of the heart.
- Vagus and crescent are again stimulated to obtain inhibition.

■ IMPORTANT QUESTIONS AND ANSWERS

Q.1. Why is vagus and crescent stimulation done before and after the application of acetylcholine?

- To demonstrate if the action of acetylcholine is direct or through nerves, the vagus and crescent are stimulated before and after the application of acetylcholine to the frog's heart.
- They show the same effect before and after the application of acetylcholine, thus we can conclude

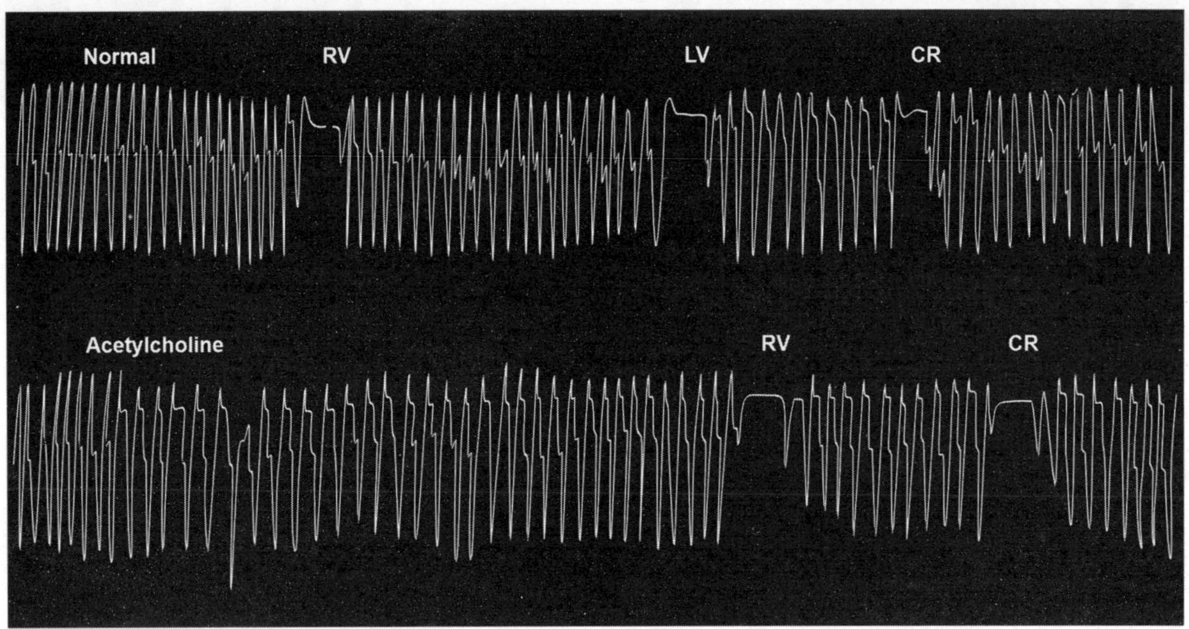

Fig. 78.1: Effect of acetylcholine on frog's heart

that the action of acetylcholine is direct on the heart (muscarinic receptors).

Q.2. What are the different types of actions of acetylcholine?

Actions of acetylcholine: It normally acts on two types of receptors.

A. Muscarinic action: These receptors are present on gland cells, smooth muscles and myocardium.

B. Nicotinic action: These receptors are present on motor end plates of skeletal muscle, adrenal medulla and autonomic ganglia.

Q.3. What is the effect of acetylcholine on a frog's heart?

Acetylcholine is inhibitory to the myocardium. It acts by combining with cholinergic receptors in the postsynaptic membrane. It increases the permeability of the membrane for K^+ ions (as explained above) and inhibits the heart.

Inhibitory effects of acetylcholine on the heart are:
- Decrease in heart rate-negative chronotropic effect
- Decrease in force of contraction-negative ionotropic effect
- Decrease excitability of myocardium-negative bathmotropic effect
- Decrease rate of impulse conduction-negative dromotropic effect.

Q.4. Enumerate different sites where acetylcholine is liberated.
- Acetylcholine is synthesized in terminal nerve endings of cholinergic nerve fibres.
- Acetyl– CoA + Choline → Acetylcholine (in the presence of acetylcholine transferase)

Acetylcholine is liberated at the following sites:
- Pre- and postganglionic parasympathetic nerve endings
- Preganglionic sympathetic nerve endings
- Neuromuscular junction in skeletal muscle
- Postganglionic sympathetic nerves supplying sweat glands
- Various synapses in the brain.

Q.5. What is the fate of acetylcholine?
- Acetylcholine is removed from the site by the action of cholinesterase present in the synaptic cleft. It splits acetylcholine into choline and acetic acid, where choline is reused for the synthesis of acetylcholine.
- Diffused acetylcholine is destroyed by pseudo-cholinesterase present in plasma or RBCs.
- Some acetylcholine reuptake happens by presynaptic membrane.

Q.6. What is anticholinesterase? What is their clinical importance?

Anticholinesterases are drugs that inhibit the action of cholinesterase enzymes. It means they prevent acetylcholine degradation. They are physostigmine, neostigmine, di- isopropyl fluorophosphate and tetra-ethyl pyrophosphate.

Clinical significance:
- In treatment of myasthenia gravis.
- To reduce intraocular tension in glaucoma (normal intraocular pressure is about 15–20 mm Hg).

Q.7. What are anticholinergic drugs? What is their clinical use?

Anticholinergic drugs – Atropine, homatropine

Clinical uses:

- Used as an antispasmodic to relieve abdominal pain
- Used as pre-anaesthetic medicine
- In treatment of organophosphorus poisoning.

■ COMMON STATIONS – SPOTS IN PRACTICAL EXAMINATION (2/3 MARKS)

Q.1. **Effect of acetylcholine on frog's heart:** Identify the graph and answer any one or two questions from the above.

Q.2. Acetylcholine inhibits myocardium. Justify.

■ KEY POINTS TO REMEMBER

- Acetylcholine is inhibitory to the myocardium.
- It decreases heart rate and force of contraction, excitability of myocardium and rate of impulse conduction of the heart.
- Acetylcholine does this by increasing the permeability of the membrane of cardiac muscle fibres to K^+ ions.

79

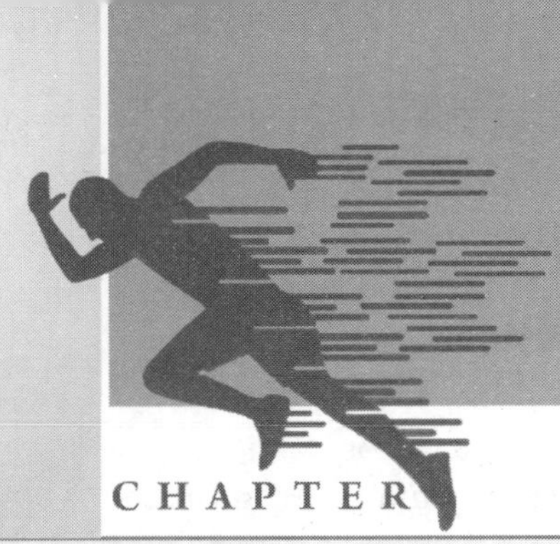

Effect of Adrenaline on Frog's Heart

Competency:

PY 3.18: With computer-assisted learning, observe amphibian cardiac experiments.

Learning Objectives

After completion of this practical, the students shall be able to:

- Describe the mechanism of action of adrenaline on the frog's heart
- Identify the graph of the effect of adrenaline on the heart.

■ INTRODUCTION

- Adrenaline is a neurotransmitter which is released by the adrenal medulla. It acts on the myocardium.
- It is known to increase the permeability of the myocardium for sodium and calcium ions. This makes the myocardium more excitable. It helps to increase the force of contraction of the heart.
- Due to its effect on the sinus venosus (which is the pacemaker of the frog's heart) it increases heart rate.

Aim

To study the effect of adrenaline on a frog's heart.

Apparatus

Same as for recording a normal cardiogram in a frog, Syme's cannula, 1 in 1000000 adrenaline.

Procedure

- Take Keef's hammer in the circuit.
- Record the graph at slow speed (pulley connection 4:1, slow gear).
- Record normal cardiogram.
- Record the effect of the vagus and crescent stimulation.
- Put a few drops of adrenaline in the frog's heart. An increase in heart rate and force of contraction are recorded **(Fig. 79.1)**.
- Again stimulate the vagus and crescent and record the effect.

■ IMPORTANT QUESTIONS AND ANSWERS

Q.1. What are the sites of adrenaline release in the body?

Sites of adrenaline release in the body are:

- Adrenal medulla
- Synapses at various places in the CNS

Q.2. Why vagus and crescent are stimulated before and after the adrenaline application?

To prove that adrenaline acts directly on the heart and the effect is not via nerves, the vagus, as well as the crescent, are stimulated before and after adrenaline application.

Q.3. What are adrenergic and cholinergic fibres?

- **Adrenergic fibres**: They release adrenaline at their nerve endings
- **Cholinergic fibres**: They release acetylcholine at their nerve endings

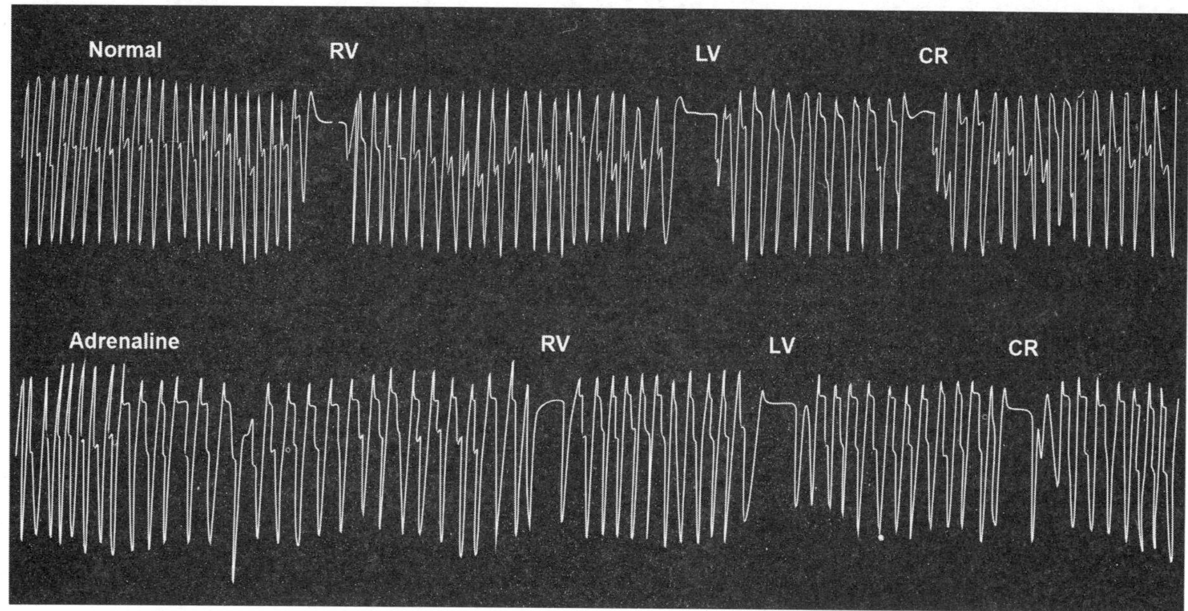

Fig. 79.1: Effect of adrenaline on frog's heart

Q.4. Write the fate of adrenaline in the body.

Adrenaline is converted to vanillylmandelic acid (VMA) in the body by action of the enzyme COMT (Catechol-O-methyltransferase) and MAO (Monoamine oxidase) as follows:

- Epinephrine (in the presence of MAO) forms dihydroxymandelic acid which in the presence of COMT forms VMA.
- Epinephrine (in the presence of COMT) forms metanephrine (which is in the presence of MAO) forms VMA.
- VMA is a 3-methoxy-4-hydroxymandelic acid which is excreted in urine.

Q.5. What are the different receptors on which adrenaline acts?

Adrenaline acts on alpha- and beta-receptors.

Sites of alpha-receptors	Sites of beta-receptors
- Sweat glands	
- Blood vessels of skin and mucosa	- Heart
- Piloerector muscle	- Bronchial muscles

Q.6. Name adrenergic drugs and adrenergic blocking drugs.

Adrenergic drugs: As the name suggests these classes of drugs mimic the action of adrenaline, e.g. isoprenaline, ephedrine.

Clinical use of adrenergic drugs:
- Anaphylactic shock
- Bronchial asthma
- **Adrenergic blocking drugs:** As the name suggests these classes of drugs block the receptors on which adrenaline acts thus preventing the effect of adrenaline.

- Alpha blockers like dibenzamine, and beta-blockers like propranolol. They are important members of antihypertensive drugs.

Q.7. Explain the effect of adrenaline on a frog's heart.

Adrenaline is stimulatory to the myocardium. It acts by combining with adrenergic receptors in the postsynaptic membrane. It increases the permeability of the membrane for Na^+ ions (as explained above) and stimulates the heart.

Stimulatory effects of adrenaline on the heart are:
- **Increase in heart rate:** Positive chronotropic effect
- **Increase in force of contraction:** Positive ionotropic effect
- **Increase excitability of myocardium:** Positive bathmotropic effect
- **Increase rate of impulse conduction:** Positive dromotropic effect.

COMMON STATIONS– SPOTS IN PRACTICAL EXAMINATION (2/3 MARKS)

Q.1. Effect of adrenaline on frog's heart: Identify the graph and answer any one or two questions from the above.

Q.2. Adrenaline stimulates the myocardium. Justify.

KEY POINTS TO REMEMBER

- Adrenaline is stimulatory to the myocardium.
- It increases heart rate and force of contraction, excitability of myocardium and rate of impulse conduction of the heart.
- Adrenaline does this by increasing the permeability of the membrane of cardiac muscle fibres to Na^+ and Ca^+ ions.

Effect of Nicotine on Frog's Heart

Competency:

PY 3.18: With computer-assisted learning, observe amphibian cardiac experiments.

Learning Objectives

After completion of this practical, the students shall be able to:

- Describe the mechanism of action of nicotine on a frog's heart
- Identify the graph of the effect of nicotine on the heart

■ INTRODUCTION

- Nicotine is an alkaloid. It is found in tobacco. It does act on autonomic ganglia (sympathetic as well as parasympathetic)
- Nicotine is known to stimulate the ganglion and later on paralyse the ganglion. When there is functional paralysis of the ganglion, there is failure of transmission of impulse across it.

Principle

To study the effect of nicotine on a frog's heart.

Procedure

- Take Keef's hammer in the circuit.
- Record the graph at a slow speed (pulley connection 4:1, slow gear).
- Record normal cardiogram.
- Record the effect of the vagus and crescent stimulation.

- Put a few drops of dilute nicotine (2 to 3%) on the frog's heart.
- Initially there is a reduction in heart rate as nicotine stimulates parasympathetic ganglion. Afterwards, the heart rate increases as nicotine paralyses the ganglion which will prevent the effect of the parasympathetic nerve, i.e. vagus.
- Initial reduced heart rate (with stimulation of ganglion) is recorded as stage I, later on, heart rate increases (with functional paralysis of ganglion) is recorded as stage II.
- After recording stages I and II, stimulate the vagus, but no inhibition is obtained.
- However, with crescent stimulation, inhibition is recorded **(Fig. 80.1)**.

■ IMPORTANT QUESTIONS AND ANSWERS

Q.1. What is the site of action of nicotine?

The site of action of nicotine is the parasympathetic ganglion of the heart.

Q.2. What is the action of nicotine on sympathetic ganglia?

Nicotine blocks or paralyses the sympathetic ganglia.

Q.3. Why vagus and crescent are stimulated before and after seeing the nicotine effect?

- The vagus and crescent are stimulated before and after nicotine to demonstrate the site of action of nicotine.

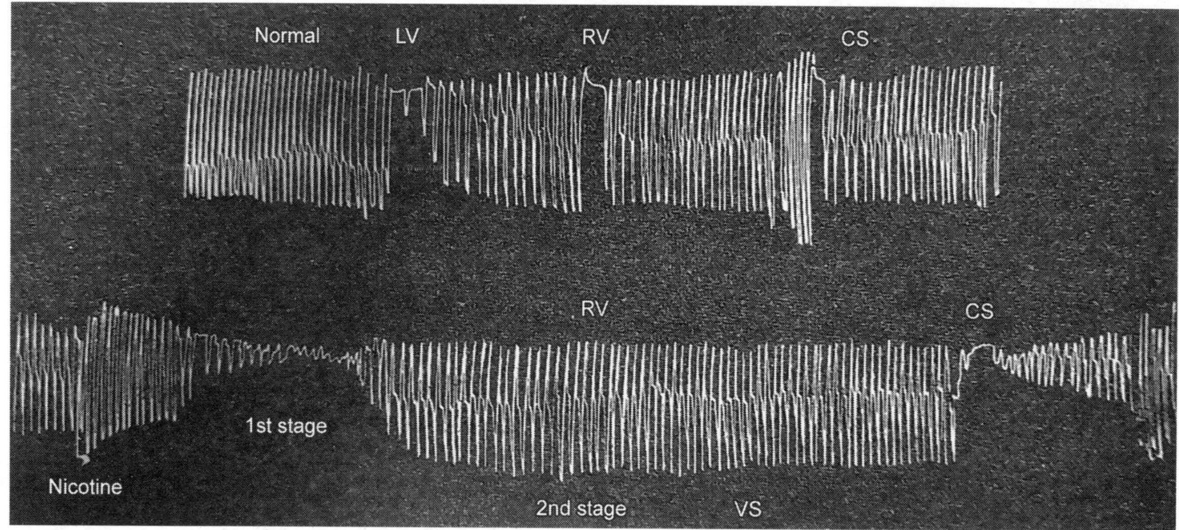

Fig. 80.1: Effect of nicotine on frog's heart

- Vagus contains preganglionic parasympathetic fibres. The parasympathetic ganglion lies at the crescent. Thus, when we stimulate the crescent, post-ganglionic parasympathetic fibres are stimulated. When nicotine is applied to a frog's heart, transmission of impulses through the frog's heart is blocked as nicotine causes functional paralysis of the ganglion.
- After nicotine action when we again stimulate the vagus, crescent stimulation does show inhibition.

Q.4. Explain how this experiment helps trace the autonomic pathway in a frog's heart.

- The parasympathetic ganglion lies near the organ. In this experiment, we stimulate the vagus and crescent before as well as after observing the action of nicotine.
- Nicotine is a ganglion-blocking agent. After the application of nicotine, stimulation of the vagus becomes ineffective in causing inhibition of the heart.

- However crescent stimulation does inhibit the heart even after nicotine action. This proves that the parasympathetic ganglion lies at the crescent.

Q.5. Name ganglion-blocking agents.
Ganglion-blocking agents are guanethidine and hexamethonium. Both drugs are used to treat hypertension (anti-hypertensive drugs).

COMMON STATIONS – SPOTS IN PRACTICAL EXAMINATION (2/3 MARKS)

Q.1. Action of nicotine on frog's heart: Identify the graph and answer any one or two questions from the above.

KEY POINTS TO REMEMBER

- Nicotine is a ganglion-blocking agent. First, it stimulates the ganglion and later on paralyses the ganglion.
- Ganglion-blocking agents are one of the important classes of antihypertensive drugs.

Effect of Perfusion on Frog's Heart

Competency:
PY 3.18: With computer-assisted learning, observe amphibian cardiac experiments.

Learning Objectives

After completion of this practical, the students shall be able to:
- Describe the effect of perfusion of different ions on a frog's heart
- Identify the graph of the effect of perfusion of different ions on a frog's heart.

■ INTRODUCTION

- Cardiac muscle has the property of auto rhythmicity. It can initiate its own rhythm without any external stimulus. Even if the heart is isolated from the body, it can do its function of beating if adequate amounts of nutrients are supplied to it.
- In this experiment frog's heart is isolated and perfused with Ringer Lock's solution.

Principle

To study the effect of perfusion on a frog's heart.

Procedure

- Record the graph on a slow-moving drum (pulley connection 3:1 and slow gear).
- Expose the frog's heart and pass a thread behind the sinus venosus.
- Take a small cut in the sinus venosus and introduce Syme's cannula to it. Tie a thread around the neck of the cannula.
- Isolate the heart from the body by cutting the aorta and pulmonary vessels.
- Through a side tube of Syme's cannula, connect to a reservoir containing Ringer Locke's solution.
- Keep the reservoir at a height of 1 to 1.5 feet above the level of the heart for adequate perfusion.
- Fluid flows from reservoir to heart via Syme's cannula, first in sinus venosus, then in atria and then in ventricle. From the ventricle, fluid flows out through the cut aorta.
- Pass bent pin attached to lever through the apex of the heart and normal contractions are recorded. Systole is recorded as upstroke and diastole as downstroke.
- Clamp the tubing of the reservoir after recording normal contractions. Put some drops of NaCl (0.65%) from the vertical limb of the cannula.
- After observing the effect, wash the heart with Ringer Locke's solution and again record normal contractions **(Fig. 81.1)**.
- Repeat the procedure for studying the effects of KCl (1%) and $CaCl_2$ (1%).

■ IMPORTANT QUESTIONS AND ANSWERS

Q.1. Define perfusion.
The passage of fluid or blood through any tissue or organ is termed as perfusion.

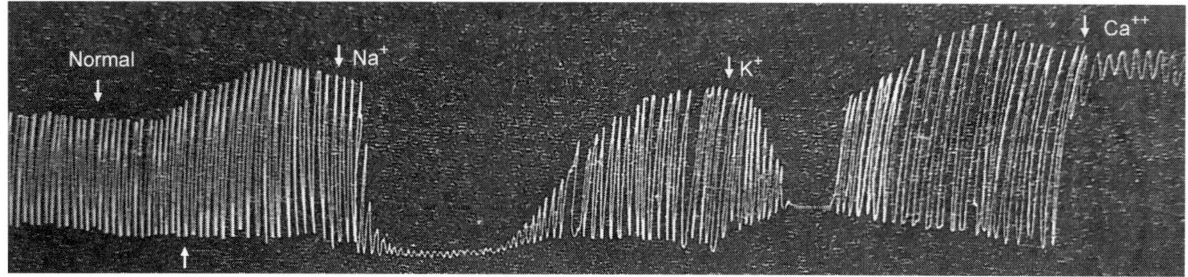

Fig. 81.1: Effect of perfusion of frog's heart with effect of ions

Q.2. What is the mechanism of action of sodium on a frog's heart?

- **Action of sodium**: The addition of NaCl causes the heart to contract less and less and ultimately heart stops in diastole.
- **Mechanism of action**: Increased concentration of Na^+, interferes with Ca^{++} which couples excitation with contraction.

Q.3. What is the mechanism of action of potassium on a frog's heart?

- **Action of potassium**: The addition of KCl causes a decrease in heart rate, and a decrease in height of contraction, making ultimately the heart stop in diastole.
- **Mechanism of action**: High K^+ concentration in ECF causes a change in resting membrane potential in cardiac muscle fibres due to a reduction in concentration gradient for potassium ions across the membrane (if resting membrane potential is –90 mV then due to entry of positively charged K^+ ions, it will become less negative say –80 mV, –70 mV etc.). This causes a decrease in the intensity of action potential which makes weaker contractions of the frog's heart (this causes an increase in the diastolic period of the heart).
- When KCl is added in excess, ECF concentration of K^+ ions increases further and resting membrane potential falls still further (becomes still more positive) and at some point, it remains in a depolarized state. Height of contraction gradually reduces and at one point heart stops as propagated action potential cannot develop. The heart becomes unexcitable and stops in diastole.

Q.4. What is the mechanism of action of calcium on a frog's heart?

- **Action of calcium**: The addition of calcium chloride increases the height of contraction of the heart and the addition of excess calcium ions causes the heart to stop in systole (calcium rigour).
- **Mechanism of action:** The effect of calcium ions is due to the direct effect in the exciting cardiac muscle process. Calcium ions are responsible for excitation-contraction coupling in cardiac muscle.
- With more addition of calcium ions, there is a decrease in the diastolic period of the heart causing the heart to go into a contracted state which is calcium rigour.

- Due to excess perfusion with calcium ions, besides calcium ions released from sarcoplasmic reticulum to sarcoplasm during contraction, more calcium ions do flow from ECF through T tubules.
- This additional availability of calcium increases the strength of the contraction of cardiac muscle as the contraction of the cardiac muscle depends to a great extent on the concentration of calcium ions in ECF.

Q.5. Enumerate differences between amphibian and mammalian heart perfusion.

S. No.	Amphibian heart perfusion	Mammalian heart perfusion
1.	For passing perfusion fluid cannula is put in sinus venosus	For passing perfusion fluid cannula is put in aorta
2.	Fluid flows from the sinus venosus to the ventricle and then comes out from the aorta	Fluid flows via coronary arteries
3.	O_2 in perfusion fluid is sufficient for heart nutrition	O_2 supplied in perfusing fluid is not sufficient and thus additional O_2 has to be added to the fluid
4.	The temperature of perfusion fluid need not be maintained (amphibians are cold-blooded animals)	The temperature of perfusion fluid must be maintained at 37°C (mammals are hot-blooded animals)
5.	pH of perfusion fluid need not be maintained	pH of perfusion fluid has to be maintained at 7.4 to 7.6
6.	The height of the reservoir via which perfusion fluid is passed is about 1 to 1and half feet from the heart	The height of the reservoir via which perfusion fluid is passed is about 3 to 4 feet from the heart
7.	The heart is thin-walled and thus can take nutrition from perfusion fluid	The heart is thick-walled and thus cannot get sufficient nutrition from perfusion fluid

Q.6. Define the following terms.

- **Hypokalemia**: Decrease in the concentration of potassium ions in ECF
- **Hyperkalemia**: Increase in the concentration of potassium ions in ECF
- **Hypocalcemia**: Decrease in the concentration of calcium ions in ECF
- **Hypercalcemia**: Increase in the concentration of calcium ions in ECF

Q.7. Write normal values of sodium and potassium ions in ECF and ICF.

Name of the ions	ECF (mEq/L)	ICF (mEq/L)
Na^+ (Sodium)	140	14
K^+ (Potassium)	4	140
Ca^{++} (Calcium)	2.4	0.0001

Q.8. What is the composition of Ringer Locke's solution for frogs?

NaCl	0.65 g%
$CaCl_2$	0.012 g%
KCl	0.014 g%
$NaHCO_3$	0.010 g%
Na_2HPO_4	0.001 g%
Glucose	0.1g % (just added prior to use)
O_2	Atmospheric O_2 dissolved in fluid is sufficient

COMMON STATIONS – SPOTS IN PRACTICAL EXAMINATION (2/3 MARKS)

Q.1. **Effect of perfusion of different ions on the frog's heart:** Identify and answer any one or two questions from the above.

KEY POINTS TO REMEMBER

- Different ions will have different effects on cardiac activity in the frog.
- Alterations in the levels of ions, do alter function of myocardium.

Index